OPERATIVE OBSTETRICS

An Illustrated Manual

OPERATIVE OBSTETRICS

An Illustrated Manual

Arup Kumar Majhi
MD DNB FICOG
Professor, Department of Obstetrics and Gynecology
Santiniketan Medical College, Bolpur, Birbhum, West Bengal, India
Formerly Professor and Head, Department of Obstetrics and Gynecology
RG Kar Medical College, Kolkata and Bankura Sammilani Medical College, Bankura
Associate Professor, Department of Obstetrics and Gynecology
Nil Ratan Sircar Medical College, Kolkata
Assistant Professor, Department of Obstetrics and Gynecology
Burdwan Medical College, Burdwan, West Bengal, India

JAYPEE BROTHERS MEDICAL PUBLISHERS
The Health Sciences Publisher
New Delhi | London

Jaypee Brothers Medical Publishers (P) Ltd.

Headquarters
Jaypee Brothers Medical Publishers (P) Ltd
EMCA House, 23/23-B
Ansari Road, Daryaganj
New Delhi 110 002, India
Landline: +91-11-23272143, +91-11-23272703
+91-11-23282021, +91-11-23245672
Email: jaypee@jaypeebrothers.com

Corporate Office
Jaypee Brothers Medical Publishers (P) Ltd
4838/24, Ansari Road, Daryaganj
New Delhi 110 002, India
Phone: +91-11-43574357
Fax: +91-11-43574314
Email: jaypee@jaypeebrothers.com

Overseas Office
JP Medical Ltd.
83, Victoria Street, London
SW1H 0HW (UK)
Phone: +44 20 3170 8910
Fax: +44 (0)20 3008 6180
Email: info@jpmedpub.com

Website: www.jaypeebrothers.com
Website: www.jaypeedigital.com

Operative Obstetrics: An Illustrated Manual

First Edition: **2023**

ISBN: 978-93-5465-988-1

Printed at: Samrat Offset Pvt. Ltd.

Dedicated
to

All Mothers

Foreword

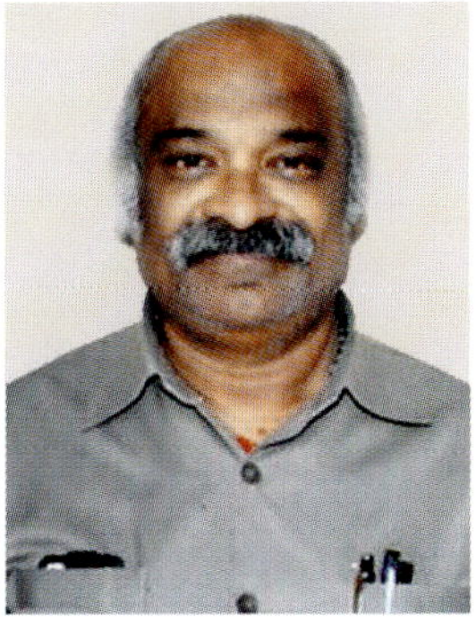

The evolution of Obstetric Practice over the last few decades has witnessed a sea change in the context of the Obstetricians as well as the beneficiaries. The changing concepts with the advancing technologies have added a new dimension in the obstetric practice. Keeping pace with this, there is a need for updating the knowledge and skill of Practitioners in Obstetrics.

Viewed in these contexts, Dr Arup Kumar Majhi, a teacher of teachers is bringing out this *Operative Obstetrics: An Illustrated Manual*. The contents of this manual are absolutely precise and extending from early pregnancy procedures to intrapartum and postpartum problems with special emphasis on operative interventions. The changing trends in practice at present have been vividly coined for the benefit of practitioners as well as postgraduate students across the globe.

I am sure the great effort of the author for years which culminated in this illustration will certainly enrich and update the knowledge and skill of the Practitioners in Obstetrics and proved to be a *Bible for Obstetricians* so as to fulfil the concept of *Tricks of Obstetrics*.

7th December 2022

Dr PC Mahapatra MD FICMCH
Ex-Professor and Head
Department of Obstetrics and Gynecology
SCB Medical College
Cuttack, Odisha, India

Preface

Surgical skills are developed from the very inception of medical careers. Surgery is learnt through observation, assistance, practicing on model or mannequin and by consulting books, literature, illustration and videos. Obstetrics involves not only operative surgery but it also consists of various maneuvers and procedures, unique to the specialty. Obstetrics differs from the other streams of medicine as in most of the situations, operation is done on emergency basis in order to save life of baby, mother or for both.

Learners learn how to do surgery in most of the cases. More important is, what to do, and when to do, to learn what is the future effect of surgery, and what is to be done to prevent the complications and adverse sequelae as a result of surgery. With increase in rate of cesarean delivery this has become very relevant. Injury of birth canal and anal sphincters during vaginal birth is quite common, however, the magnitude of the problem is often underestimated.

During last few decades, there has been a sea change in obstetric practice due to evolution of various new technologies and availability of guideline-based and evidence-based medicine.

There is no dearth of learning materials today, however dearth is in the availability of a good compendium to get everything under a single umbrella in very precise manner including the titbits of surgical methods and the tricks of obstetric procedures.

Keeping this in mind, a great challenge has been taken by me to make such a manual which is led by my vast teaching and clinical experience and extensive dealing with the numerous obstetrics patients of versatile nature for over three and half decades. During my early days of my professional career and thereafter, I have been associated with several stalwarts and many colleagues who are great obstetricians in true sense, which has helped me to take up this herculean task.

Starting from the basic surgical principle and development of skill, tackling of the obstetric patients extending from early pregnancy to intrapartum and postpartum periods, every aspect has been described with huge number of illustrations, both original and diagrams with special emphasis on procedures and operative steps.

Hope this unique book of operative obstetrics will be thoroughly useful, which will help to update the knowledge and skill of the postgraduates and practitioners in obstetrics and be a companion in day-to-day practice.

Arup Kumar Majhi
drarupkmajhi@yahoo.com

Acknowledgments

Without the help, support, encouragement and blessings from many it was not possible to publish this amazing book.

This book would never come into light without the active support and direct involvement of my wife Swapna who always cared in every step in spite of several constrains. I also got a lot of support from my son Debanjan on various aspects.

I got aspiration from the approach and surgical techniques of my teachers Professor BB Sarkar and late Professor BN Chakravarty for which I should always remember them.

I am very grateful to Professor Kusagradhi Ghosh, Director, Institute of Fetal Medicine, Kolkata not only for the contribution a chapter 'Invasive Prenatal Testing and Fetal Therapy', but for his constant encouragement and support. I am obliged to Dr Abhinibesh Chatterjee, an advanced Laparoscopic Surgeon for writing the chapter of 'Laparoscopic procedure in obstetrics'.

I am deeply indebted to Professor Kamal Oswal (Department of Radiodiagnosis, Vivekananda Institute of Medical Sciences, Kolkata) and Professor M Karmakar (Department of Radiodiagnosis, Institute of Postgraduate Medical Education and Research, Kolkata), for their contribution in imaging.

I like to express my thanks to Professor PC Mahapatra, a man of very high gesture for writing the foreword of this book.

Mr Dipankar Dhar, Academic Publishers, Kolkata, publisher of my book, *Bedside Clinics in Obstetrics*, from which I have used many figures and materials for this new book of *Operative Obstetrics: An Illustrated Manual* deserves special mention for the support from the beginning of writing of this operative obstetrics.

My special acknowledgment and thanks to Professor Abhijit Rakshit, Department of Obstetrics and Gynecology, RG Kar Medical College, Kolkata, who has actively supported me continuously for this work. My special thanks to Dr Anirban Mondal, Associate Professor, Bankura Sammilani Medical College for uninterrupted input of various materials of the book.

My special acknowledgement to Dr Tulika Jha, Associate Professor, Rampurhat Government Medical College, West Bengal and Dr Pradipto Sanyal, Senior Obstetrician and Gynecologist for the contribution in various ways.

The support and encouragement of my friends Professor Pratip Kumar Kundu, Dean, Santiniketan Medical College and Professor Sobhan Kumar Das, Head, Department of Forensic and Toxicology, Santiniketan Medical College, Bolpur, Birbhum, West Bengal have encouraged me a lot to complete this mega task.

I must show my gratitude to many of my friends, senior and junior colleagues, the names of whom could not be mentioned individually.

This book could not be completed without the active involvement of many of my postgraduate students. I am really indebted to them.

Finally, I find myself extremely fortunate to have Shri Jitendar P Vij (Group Chairman), Mr Ankit Vij (Managing Director), Mr MS Mani (Group President), Ms Chetna Malhotra (Senior Director–Professional Publishing, Marketing and Business Development), Ms Pooja Bhandari (Production Head), Ms Sunita Katla (Executive Assistant to Group Chairman and Publishing Manager) and the team of M/s Jaypee Brothers Medical Publishers (P) Ltd, New Delhi, India, who have given tremendous efforts to release this book within stipulated time. I especially mention the staff of Kolkata branch, Mr Sabyasachi Hazra, who has given relentless effort and constant encouragement for this project.

Arup Kumar Majhi
drarupkmajhi@yahoo.com

Contents

CHAPTER 1

Instruments, Basic Surgical Techniques, Incision and Closure in Obstetrics

Learning Objectives

- Scissors
- Scalpel Blades and Handles
- Artery Forceps, Tissue Forceps, and Clamps
- Tissue Dissecting Forceps or Dissecting Forceps
- Needle Holders
- Retractors
- Suction During Surgery
- Surgical Drains
- Electrosurgical Systems
- Surgical Needle
- Suture Materials
- Suture Tie and Knots
- Suture Techniques
- Staplers
- Abdominal Incisions and Closure
- Anatomy of Anterior Abdominal Wall
- Types of Incision
- Incision in Obese Woman

INTRODUCTION

Surgical instrument is one of the important components for success and perfectness of surgery. As the tissue characteristics vary in pregnant mother than those of normal individual proper selection of instruments are important to make the procedures easy, rapid, and secured. The instruments commonly required for the obstetric surgery and procedures and their handlings are discussed in this chapter. Surgical skill develops by observing more and more good surgery and by regular practice. Knowledge of right selection of instruments and of its perfect use make an operator a good and finer surgeon. The perfect practice and correct technique should start from the very beginning of the career.

SCISSORS (FIGS. 1A TO F)

Various types of scissors are available, each type is used for various tissue textures and different purposes. The common types are Mayo scissors both curved and straight, Metzenbaum fine blade scissors, and Monaghan's scissors.

Mayo's scissors **(Fig. 1A)**, also called Bonney's dissecting scissors are heavy, ends are relatively blunt, but suitable for accurate gentle dissection "separate and cut type". Curved Mayo scissors are used for dissection of anterior abdominal fascia and dense tissue. These are also used for separating uterus from the vagina at terminal part of hysterectomy. Straight variety of Mayo's scissors **(Fig. 1B)** consists of blunt and flat blades and reserved for suture cutting purpose. Fine tissue dissecting scissors should not be used for suture cutting to avoid the dullness of blades.

Metzenbaum scissors **(Fig. 1C)** are used to dissect and define the natural tissue planes. It is useful for adhesiolysis in thin adhesion of peritoneum or vaginal epithelium. Dissection is done in the same plane not to injure deeper or unintended tissue. In closed condition, a small nick is given to enter into tissue plane, tissue dissection done, opened, and removed in slightly close condition.

Monaghan's scissors **(Fig. 1D)** are dissecting scissors with lighter pair with the tips relatively blunt to prevent trauma to the unintended tissues. In fact, these scissors are ideal for lymph node dissection around blood vessels.

Episiotomy scissors **(Fig. 1E)** are typically curved scissors with one blunt end and the other sharp end and blunt end is placed inside to prevent injury of fetal head.

Stitch removal scissors **(Fig. 1F)** are used for stitch removal.

Correct handling is important for correct dissection. To hold the scissors, usually thumb and fourth finger are introduced into rings of scissors **(Fig. 2)**, and index finger is placed over the crosspiece thus, a good grip called "tripod grip" is obtained for good functioning of the scissors.

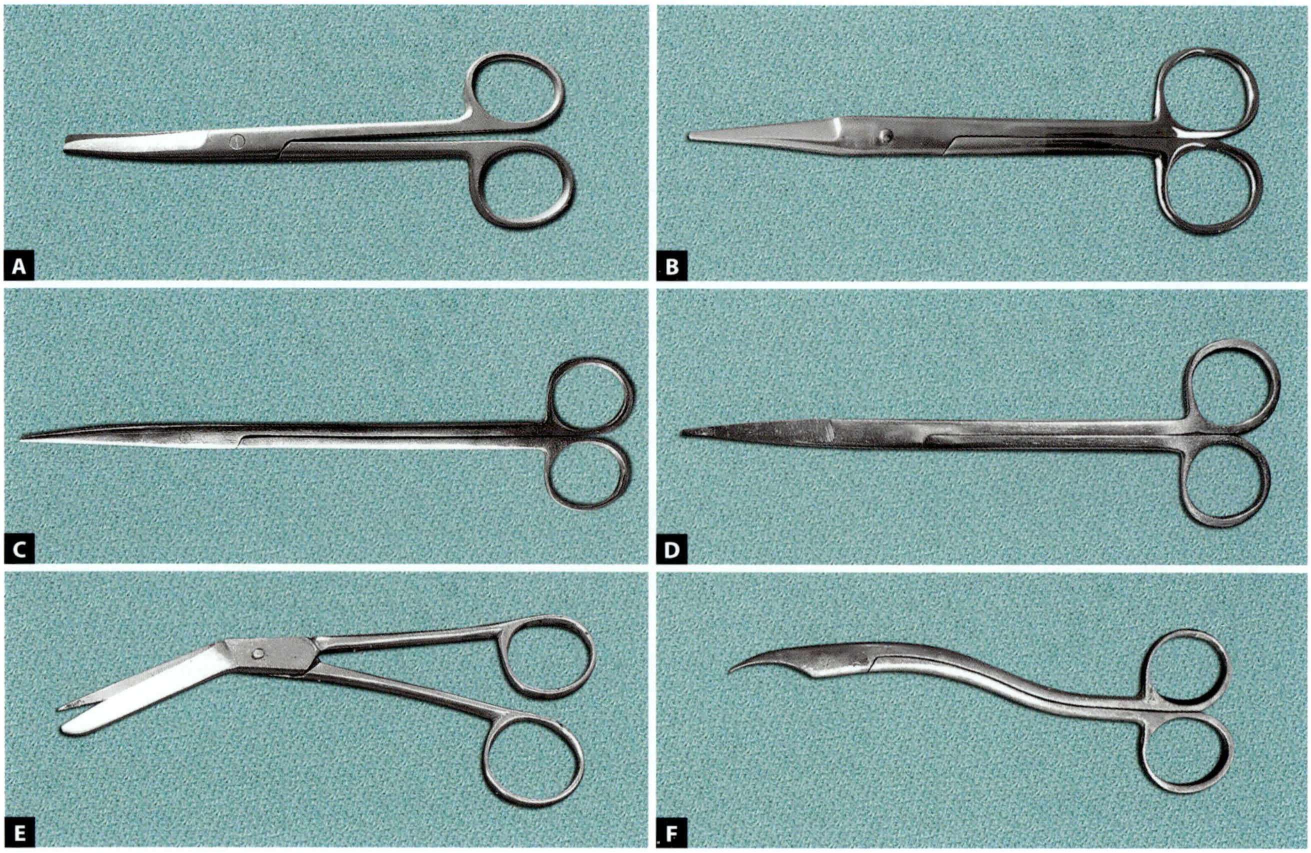

Figs. 1A to F: (A) Mayo scissors (Bonney's dissecting scissors)—bent on flat type; (B) Mayo scissors straight; (C) Metzenbaum scissors; (D) Monaghan's gynecological dissecting scissors; (E) Episiotomy scissors; (F) Stitch removal scissors.

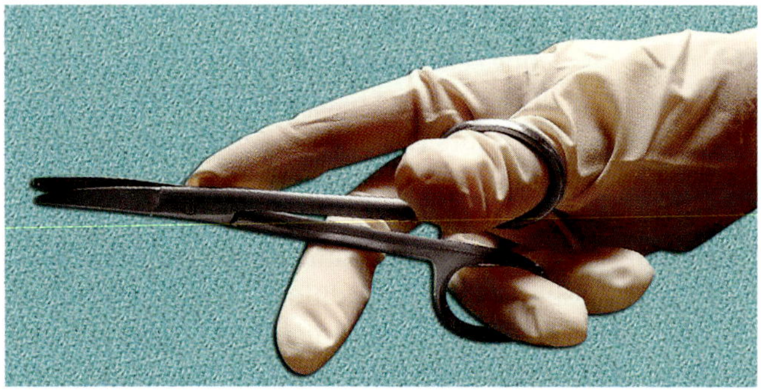

Fig. 2: Holding of scissors showing thumb and fourth finger inside the rings.

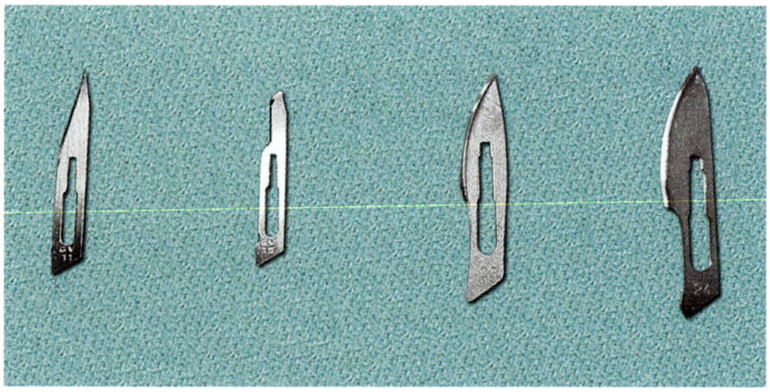

Fig. 3: Varieties of blade No. 11, 15, 23, and 24.

SCALPEL BLADES AND HANDLES

Surgical blade has basic components of sharp edge, unsharpened edge, and a slot where the handle is fitted. Surgical blades are basically of two types. Those which are used in obstetric practice are No. 11, 15, 23, and 24 and are shown in **Figure 3**. There may be other numbers also. Each type has different purpose to use and technique of use is also different.

For each type blade knife, there is a specific handle **(Fig. 4)**. To get the maximum benefits, correct holding

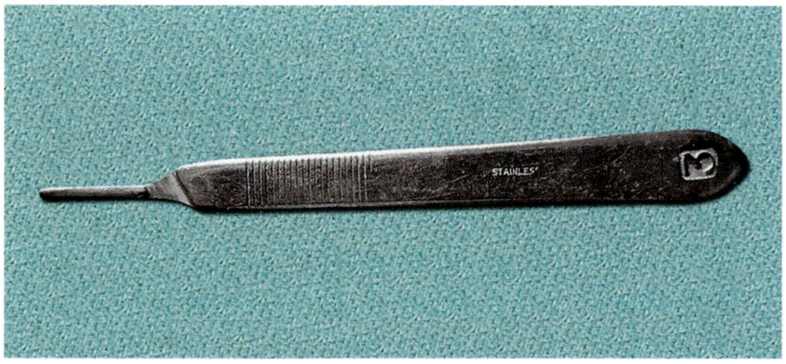

Fig. 4: Scalpel handle.

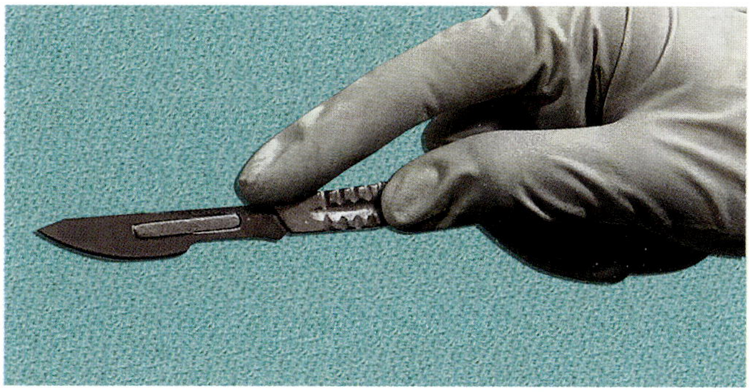

Fig. 5: Pencil grip of holding scalpel.

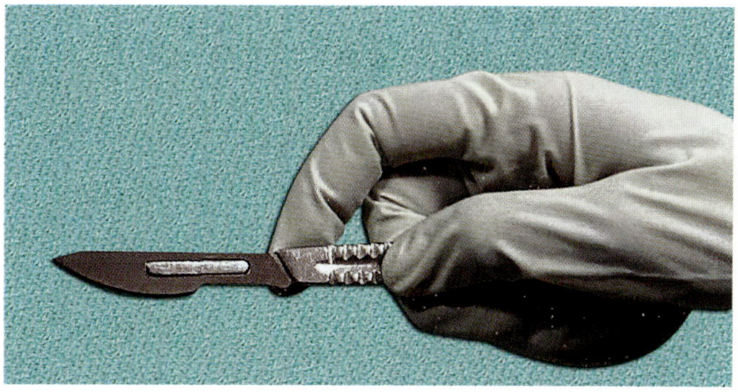

Fig. 6: Power grip of holding scalpel.
Courtesy: Professor Abhijit Rakshit, Department of Gynecology and Obstetrics, RG Kar Medical College, Kolkata, West Bengal, India.

of the scalpel is very important. Basically, there are two types of grip "pencil grip" **(Fig. 5)** and another is "power grip" **(Fig. 6)**. Pencil grip is also called precision grip and power grip is regarded as violin grip or bow grip. In pencil grip, index finger lies directly on blunt edge and in power grip, index finger is placed over the flat surface of blade.

During incision, skin surface is stretched. It will take little force and make controlled depth of incision.

No. 11 blade is sharp pointed and used to incise tough wall structure like tough wall of Bartholin abscess. No. 15 blade is used for more finer incision. Both 11 and 15 numbers are held in pencil grip to make precise and pointed incision and the tip is used for incision. No. 11 scalpel is placed at almost 90° over the surface and also called stab knife whereas no. 15 scalpel is held at about 45° to the surface of the skin.

No. 23 and 24 are similar type of surgical blades and sharp margin is used for incision. No. 23 is smaller than No. 24. Both these blades are placed 25–30° with the surface during incision and full length of the sharp margin comes in contact with surface for incision and tip is not used. Blade is used to incise skin first keeping the flat of blade perpendicular to skin to avoid beveling. Good pressure is given to apply traction on lateral aspects of incision which helps for straight and single incision line.

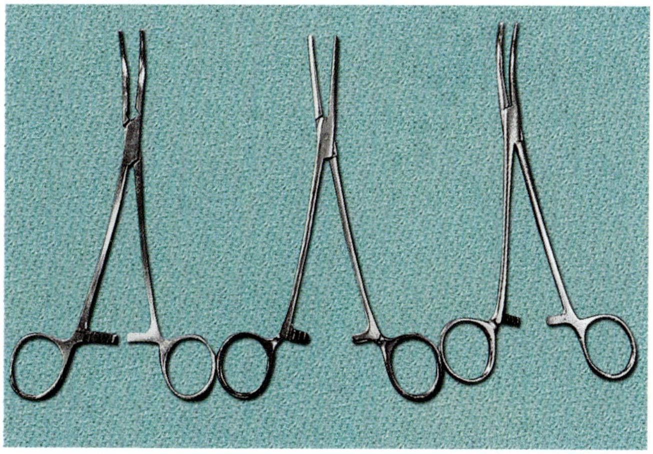

Fig. 7: Varieties of artery forceps (hemostatic forceps).

ARTERY FORCEPS, TISSUE FORCEPS, AND CLAMPS

Artery forceps may be of different types **(Fig. 7)**. Both straight and curve artery forceps are used as vascular clamp. Mixter right-angle clamps, tonsil clamp are suitable for grasping delicate tissue like vessels. Long hemostatic forceps are used in hysterectomy **(Figs. 8A and B)**. **Figure 9** shows Spencer Wells straight type. Heavier clamps are Kelly clamps, Kocher clamp or Ochsner clamps. They are used to grasp and manipulate stiffer tissues and used to grasp hysterectomy pedicles. Kocher clamps (forceps) may also be used in hysterectomy **(Fig. 10)**. Kocher's artery forceps are used for cord clamping and artificial rupture of membranes in obstetrics.

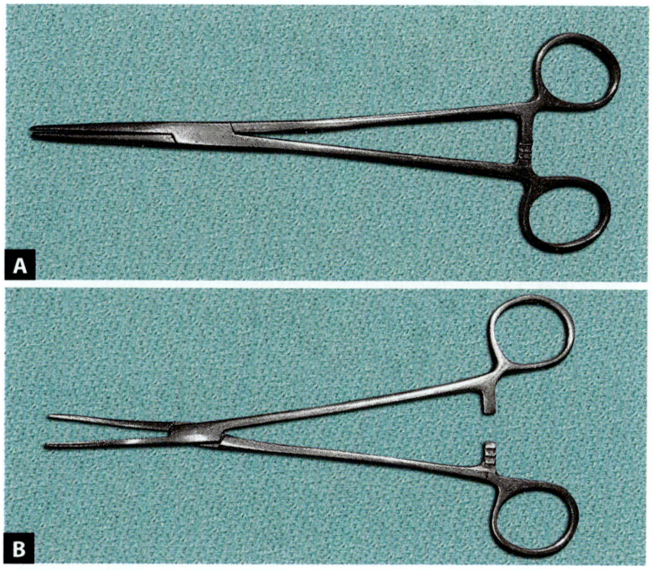

Figs. 8A and B: Long hemostatic forceps used as hysterectomy clamp.

Example of other heavy clamps are Heaney clamp and Zeppelin clamp. The jaws of the clamp are made with deep

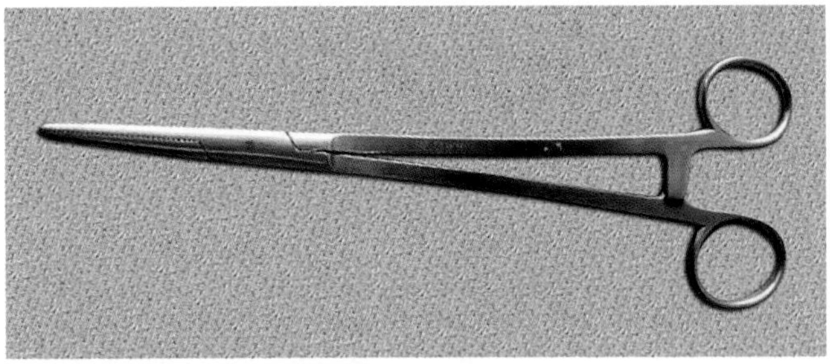

Fig. 9: Spencer Wells straight.

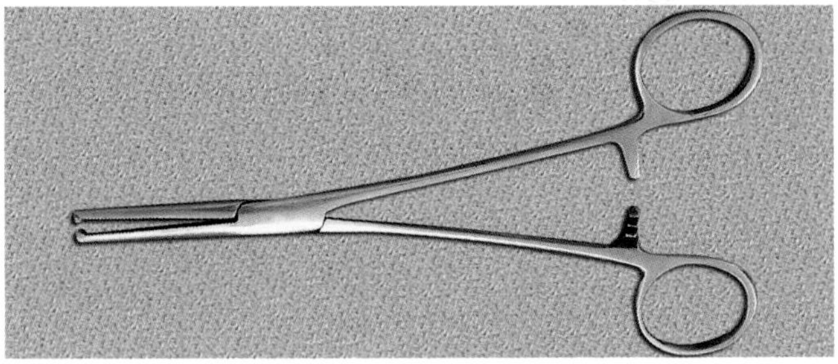

Fig. 10: Kocher clamps.

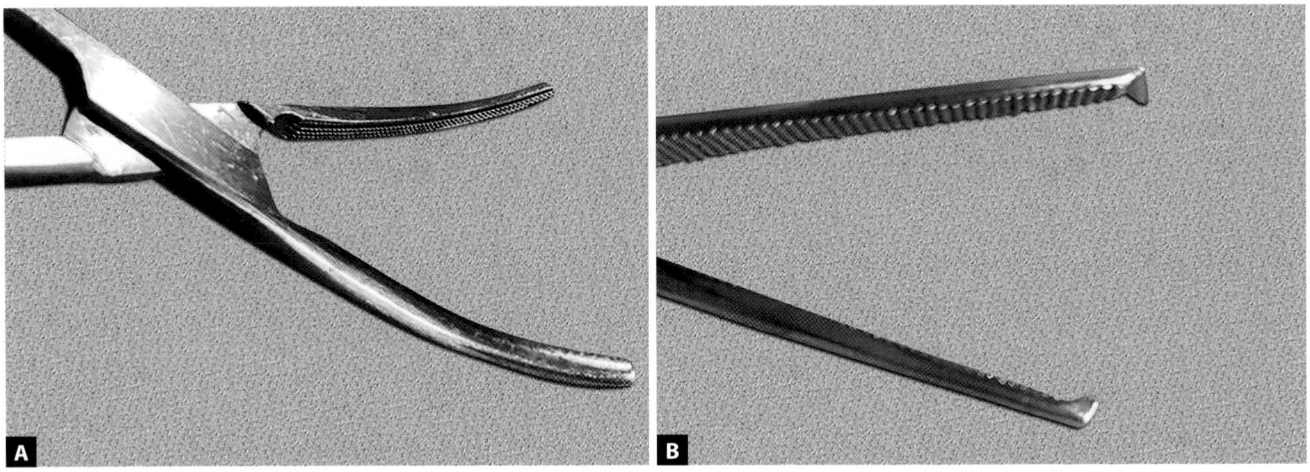

Figs. 11A and B: (A) The jaws of the clamp are made with deep groove or longitudinal serrations; (B) The jaws of the clamp with transverse serrations with teeth.

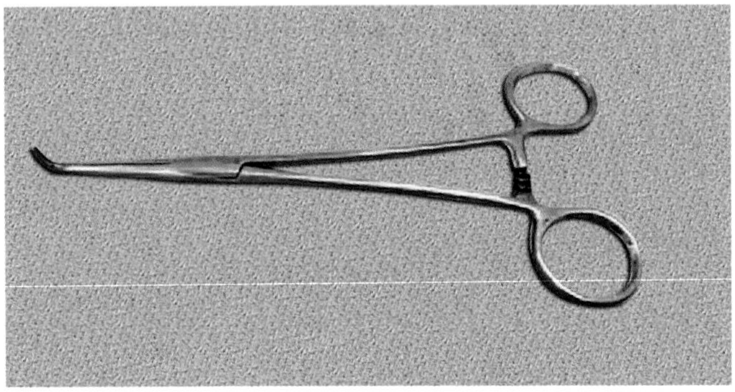

Fig. 12: Meigs-Navratil forceps which is also called right-angled forceps.

groove or longitudinal serrations **(Fig. 11A)** or transverse serrations with teeth **(Fig. 11B)** for firm tissue gripping.

Large Meigs-Navratil forceps which is also called right-angled forceps **(Fig. 12)** is used to clamp vessels in deep in the pelvis and also for internal iliac ligation. Kelly placental forceps **(Fig. 13)** is used for postpartum intrauterine contraceptive device (IUCD) insertion.

Tissue forceps are of several varieties, e.g., Allis tissue forceps **(Fig. 14)**, Babcock tissue forceps **(Fig. 15)**, and Lane's tissue forceps **(Fig. 16)**.

Allis tissue forceps **(Fig. 14)** is used in various purposes. In dilation and evacuation (D&E) operations, it is used to

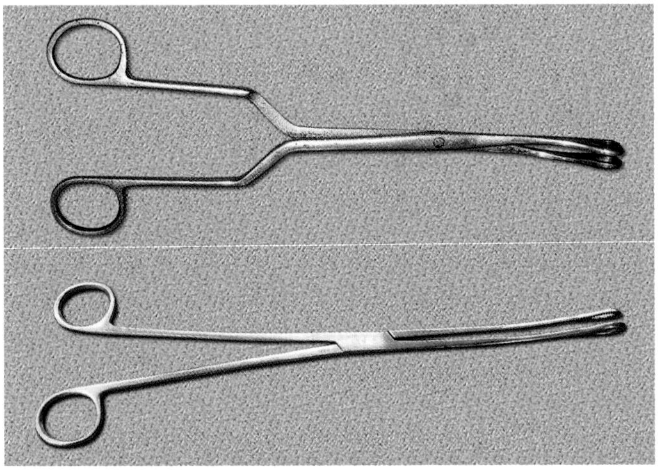

Fig. 13: Kelly placental forceps (long size—lower). Ovum forceps (upper) is shown to compare the size.

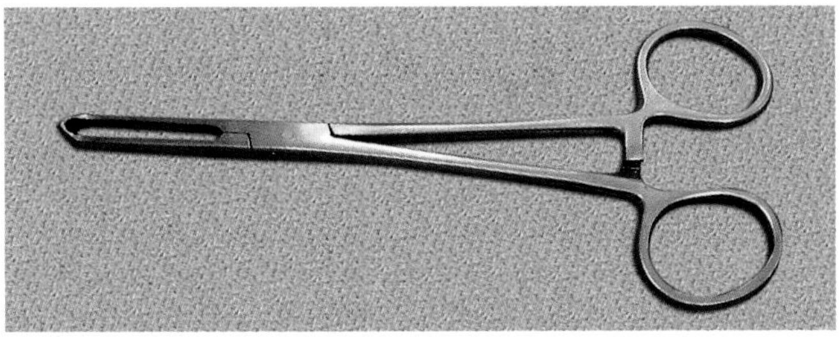

Fig. 14: Allis tissue forceps.

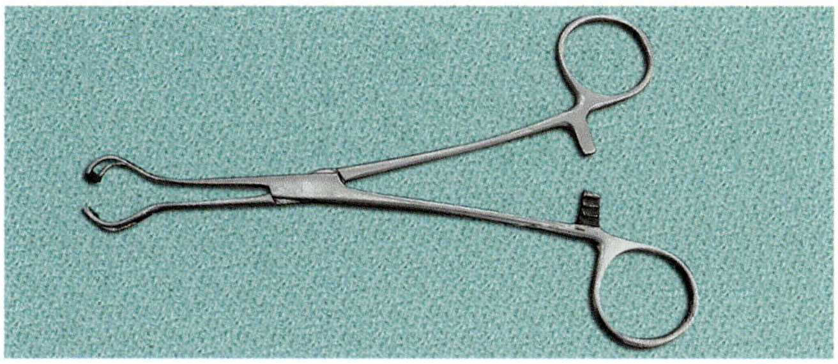

Fig.15: Babcock tissue forceps.

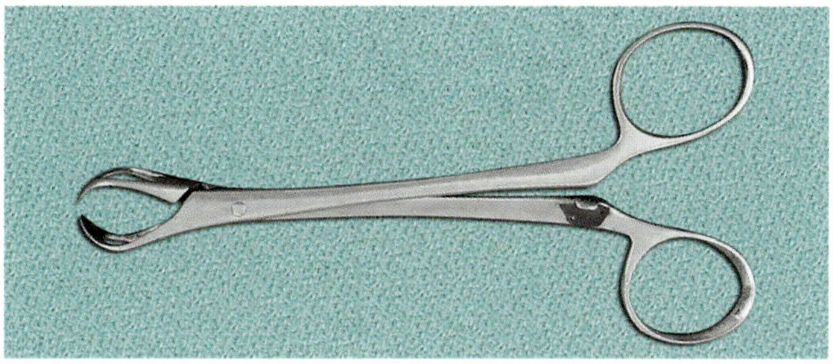

Fig. 16: Lane's tissue forceps.

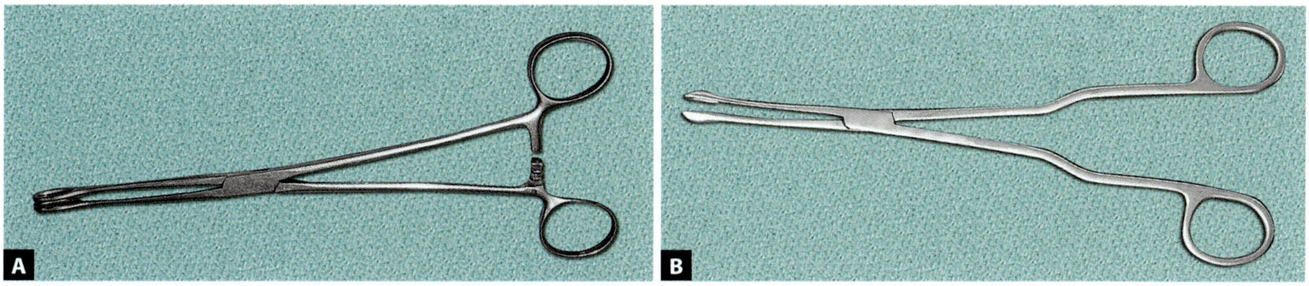

Figs. 17A and B: (A) Sponge forceps or ring forceps; (B) Ovum forceps.

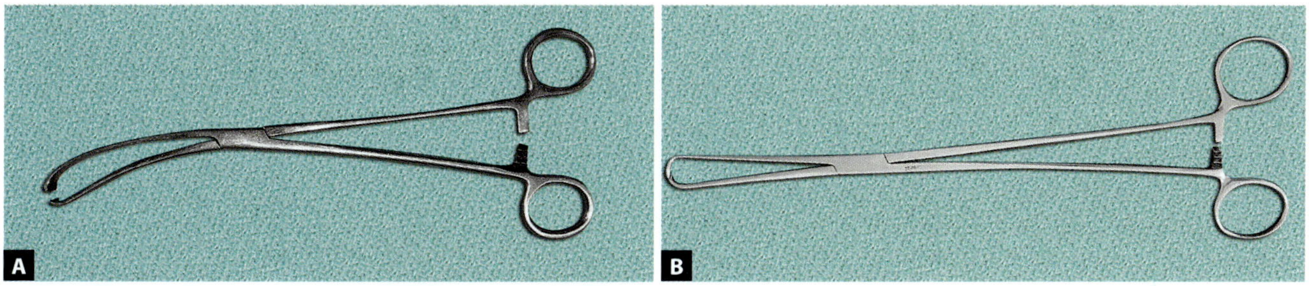

Figs.18A and B: (A) Multiple toothed vulsellem; (B) Single tooth tenaculum.

grasp the anterior lip of the cervix and to hold the lips of the cervix in cerclage operations. In cesarean section, it is used in various steps—during skin incision, it is used to hold the skin margins, to hold the peritoneal and rectus fascial margins. Four Allis forceps are used to hold the cut margins and two angles of uterine wound during hysterotomy. Allis tissue forceps are used to hold the rectal fascia margins during laparotomy and also to hold the cuff of the vagina during peripartum hysterectomy.

Sponge forceps or ring forceps **(Fig. 17A)** are used in various situations in obstetrics. It is used to hold soft tissue like cervix due to its wide area, but less traumatic. Its other uses in obstetrics are antiseptic dressing of abdominal operations like cesarean delivery or for vaginal operations like D&E, suction and evacuation (S&E), normal delivery, instrumental delivery, and cerclage operations. It is used to grasp the lip of the cervix for diagnosis and repair of cervical tear, to remove the membranes in normal delivery or following cesarean delivery. In case of extension of uterine wound and tear of blood vessels during cesarean delivery, it can be used to hold the margins and torn blood vessels for hemostasis. It is also used instead of ovum forceps **(Fig. 17B)** for D&E operations or removal of placental bits in postpartum hemorrhage (PPH) or septic abortion.

Babcock tissue forceps **(Fig. 16)** are specially used to hold the fallopian tubal in tubal ligation.

Multiple toothed vulsellum **(Fig. 18A)** can be used to hold the lip of the cervix, but largely replaced by Allis tissue forceps. Single tooth tenaculum **(Fig. 18B)** can be used for its firm grip, but less traumatic to cervix. It is also used for gynecological purpose to hold nulliparous cervix or amputated cervical stump. Lane's tissue **(Fig. 16)** forceps is used to hold tough structures in gynecology.

TISSUE DISSECTING FORCEPS OR DISSECTING FORCEPS (FIGS. 19A AND B)

These are of simple and toothed varieties and of different sizes.

Nontooth or smooth forceps **(Fig. 19A)**, due to presence of serrations at tip can grip the tissue well. They are used to

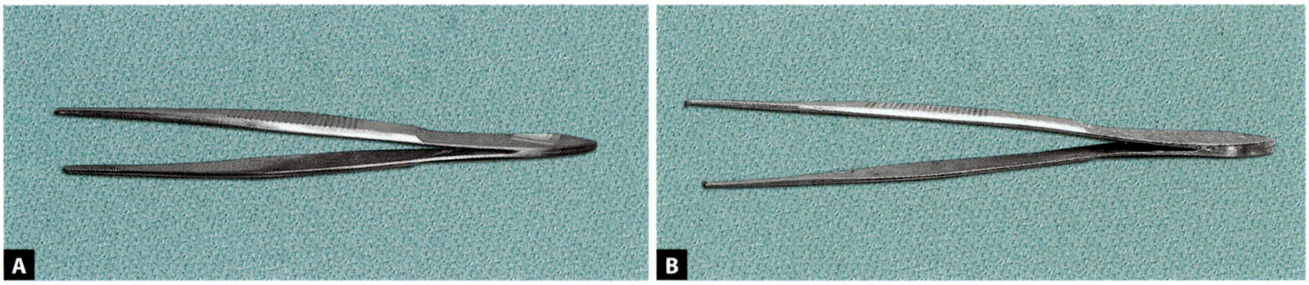

Figs. 19A and B: (A) Nontoothed or smooth forceps; (B) Tooth forceps.

hold tissue to stabilize for suturing, to pass ligature around hematoma, to fix tissue for cutting, to extract needle, to grasp vessels for diathermy coagulation, and to pack sponges. Small simple dissecting forceps are used to handle the delicate structure like peritoneum with minimal injury.

Shallow-grooved tips forceps are used for hysterotomy closure during cesarean delivery. Heavy tooth forceps **(Fig. 19B)** are used to catch fascia for abdominal wound closure.

NEEDLE HOLDERS (FIGS. 20A AND B)

Needle holders, also called needle drivers, may have curved or straight jaws. Straight jaws are commonly used. Needle holders with curved jaws are used in needle placement in angled or confined areas. Transverse serrations or cross hatching of the needle holder in the inner surface of jaw help to grip the needle securely. Needle is grasped by needle holder at right angle at point two-thirds from the needle tip that site is called swage which is usually flattened in contrast to cylindrical body of needle **(Fig. 20C)**.

Needle holder is commonly held by the thumb and fourth finger introducing into the rings and this method helps to grip with precision **(Fig. 20C)**. Other method is by "palmar grip" when the holder is held by the ball of the thumb and base of the fingers, no finger is introduced into the ring. Palmar grip is used for time saving during continuous suturing. Needle holders are used in episiotomy repair, in perineal laceration, in cesarean delivery, and also for obstetric hysterectomy.

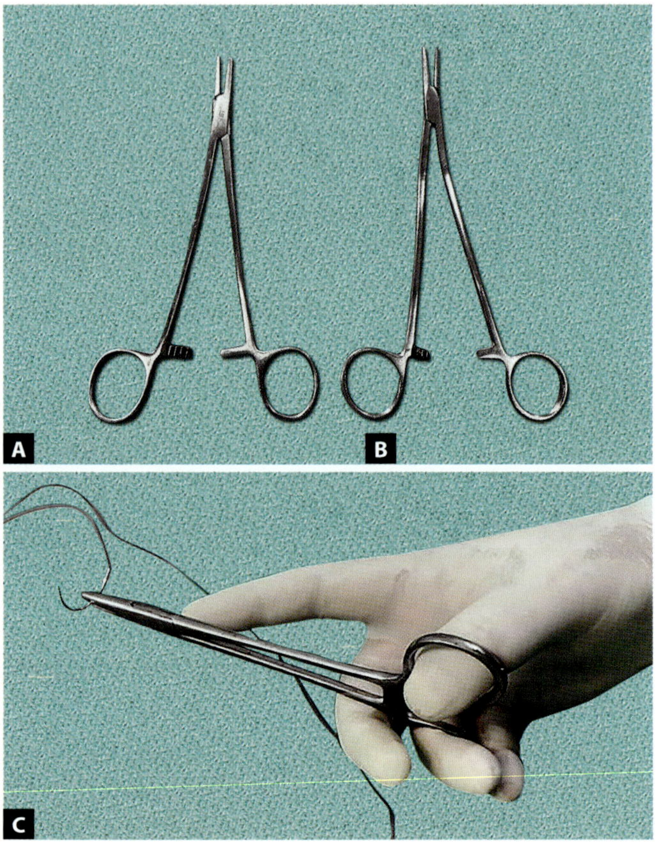

Figs. 20A to C: Needle holder (A) curve (upper); (B) straight (lower); (C) Needle is grasped by needle holder at right angle at point two-thirds from the needle tip. Needle holder is commonly held by the thumb and fourth finger introducing into the rings and this method helps to grip with precision.

Courtesy: Professor Abhijit Rakshit, Department of Gynecology and Obstetrics, RG Kar Medical College, Kolkata, West Bengal, India.

RETRACTORS

Retractors are used to retract the surrounding tissue to visualize properly the area of working field. They may be abdominal or for vaginal use. They may be self-retaining or handheld.

Self-retaining retractors are reusable, metallic, or may be disposable.

Self-retaining reusable retractors are Balfour retractor and Bookwalter retractor. Commonly used retractor is Balfour retractor **(Fig. 21)**. It can retract three sides; blades retract bladder caudally and abdominal muscles on two sides. Upper abdomen structures are packed. An additional attachment may retract cephalad or other handheld retractor is used by an assistant to retract the cephalad structures. Retraction by self-retaining retractor may injure the femoral nerves for which precaution to be taken so that retractors retract the anterior abdominal muscles, not the psoas. Disposable self-retaining retractors contain equal sized two plastic rings.

There are several varieties of *handheld retractors* shown in **Figure 22**. For example Deaver retractor, Richardson retractor, and Doyen's retractor. Doyen's retractor **(Fig. 23A)**

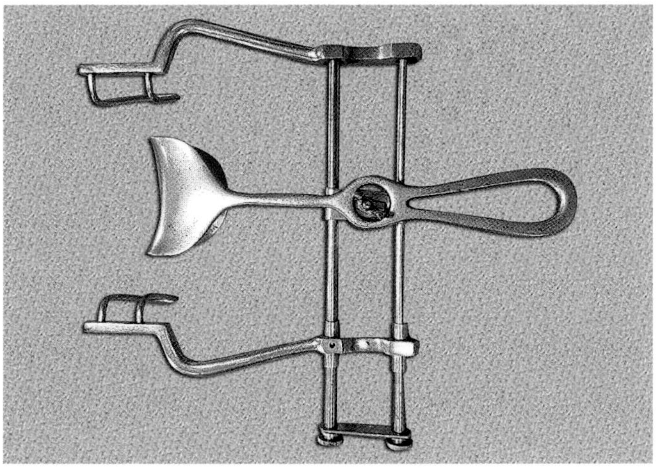

Fig. 21: Balfour retractor.

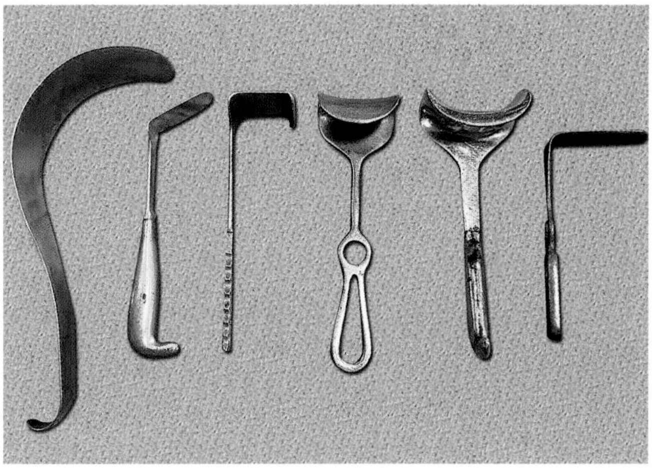

Fig. 22: Varieties of handheld retractors.

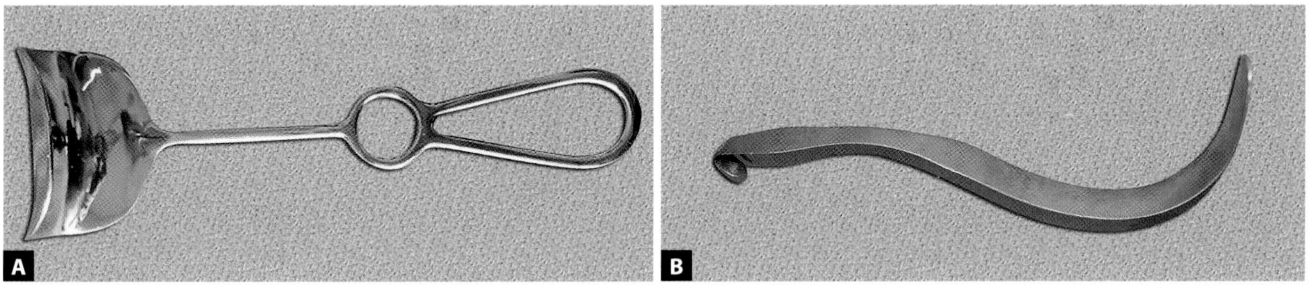

Figs. 23A and B: (A) Doyen's retractor; (B) Deaver retractor.

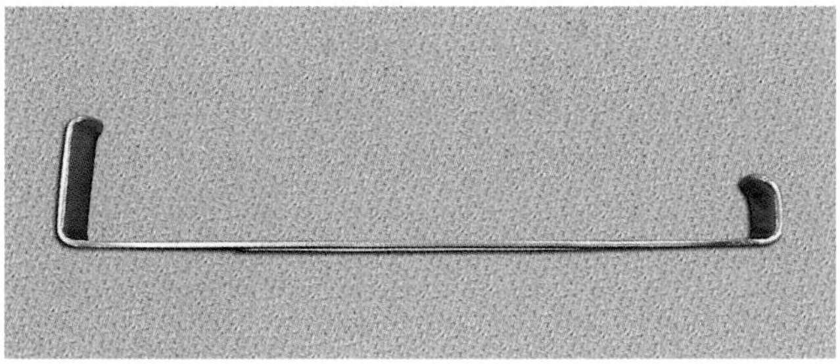

Fig. 24: Short retractor. Army–Navy retractor.

is routinely used for cesarean delivery. Deaver retractor **(Fig. 23B)** is better than Richardson as better depth can be achieved and commonly used for retracting bowel, bladder, and anterior abdominal wall muscles. Some short blade retractors are also available for minilaparotomy wounds and laparoscopy wound. These are Army–Navy retractor **(Fig. 24)** and S retractors.

Among vaginal wall retractors, Sims posterior vaginal wall speculum, single or double blade **(Figs. 25A and B)**, is commonly used to retract the posterior vaginal wall. Landon retractor or right angle retractor **(Fig. 26)** is used to retract bladder, commonly in vaginal hystetrectomy. They can also be used to retract lateral wall to repair vaginal wall laceration. Auvard self-retaining **(Fig. 27)** posterior wall retractor is not

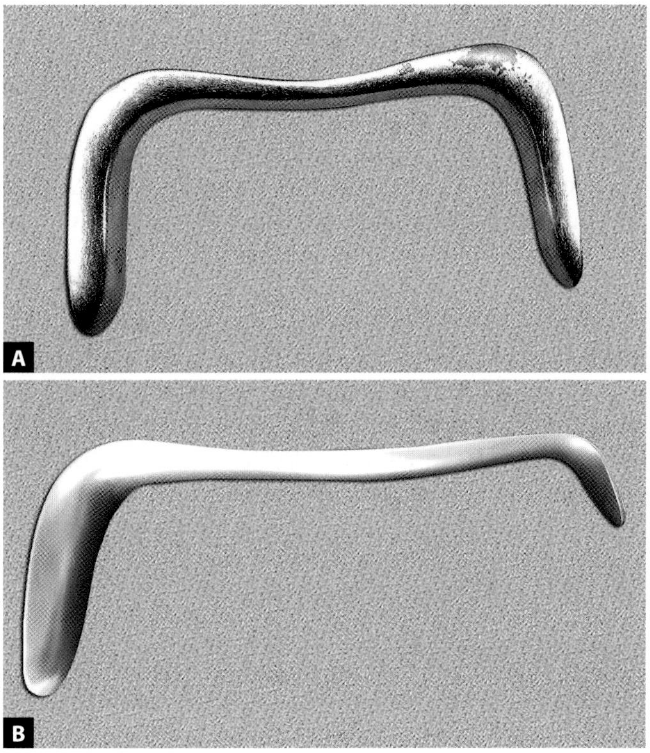

Figs. 25A and B: (A) Sims posterior vaginal wall speculum, double bladed; (B) Sims posterior vaginal wall speculum, single bladed.

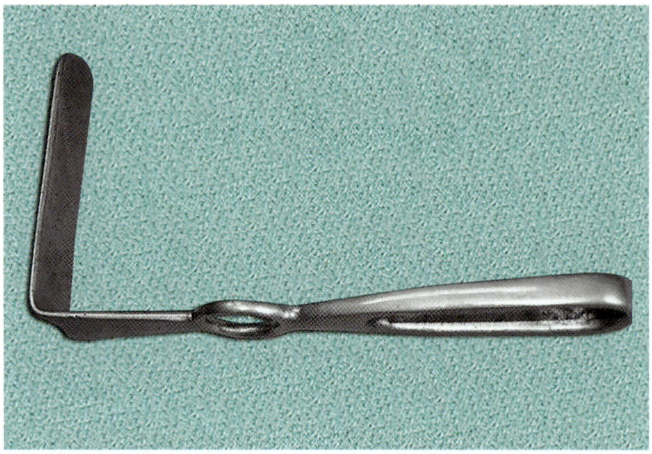

Fig. 26: Landon retractor or right angle retractor.

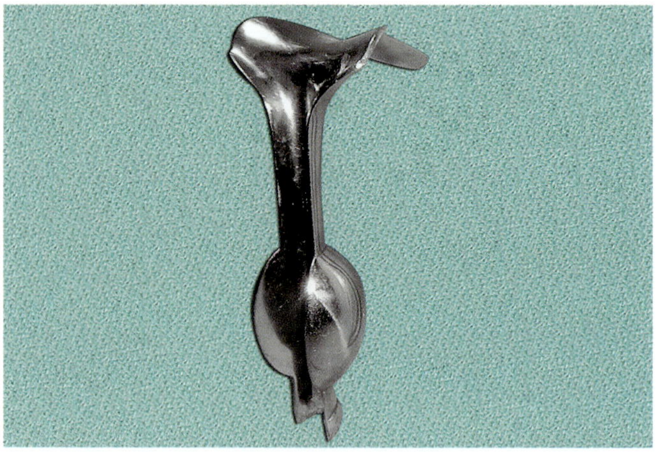

Fig. 27: Auvard self-retaining.

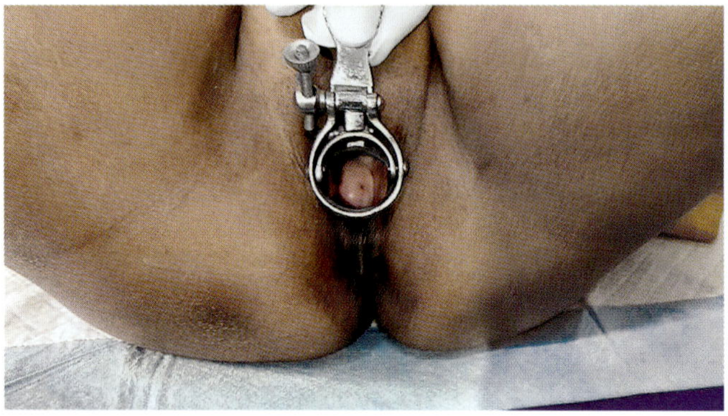

Fig. 28: Cusco's self-retaining speculum is used for inspection of cervix and cervical os.

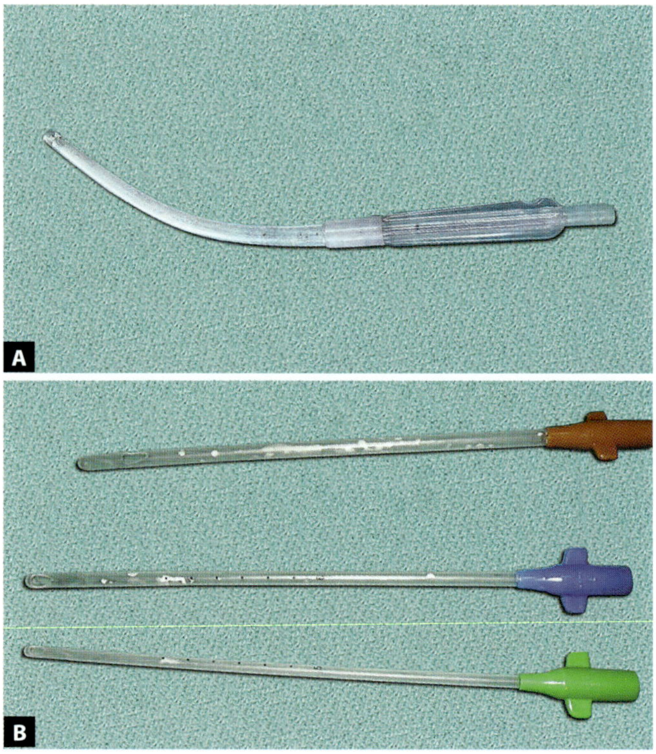

Figs. 29A and B: (A) Plastic suction tip for use during laparotomy; (B) Suction cannula used for manual vacuum aspiration.

used commonly for its weight. Gelpi retractor with small blades or Rigby retractor with longer blades are useful for use in perineal and lateral vaginal wall, respectively. Cusco's self-retaining speculum is used for inspection of cervix and cervical os **(Fig. 28)** for any pathology or leakage of liquor in prelabor rupture of membranes (PROM).

SUCTION DURING SURGERY

Varieties of suction system and cannula are used. Those may be metallic or plastic blade. **Figure 29A** shows a common plastic suction tip for use during laparotomy. Suction cannula, which is used in evacuation of product of conception, is described in chapter of Early Pregnancy Procedure and (Chapter 3) and Molar Pregnancy (Chapter 5). Suction cannula **(Fig. 29B)** used for manual vacuum aspiration (MVA) is made-up of plastics.

SURGICAL DRAINS

Indications of drainage is reduced today due to liberal use of antibiotics and proper hemostatic technique.

Suction drain in postoperative period may be therapeutic or prophylactic. Role of prophylactic drain is controversial. Following a major abdominal surgery or drainage of an abscess keeping a drain is an established procedure.

The indications of surgical drain are: (1) where complete perfect hemostasis could not be achieved and significant postoperative oozing is expected, (2) where there is danger of urine leakage, and (3) in case of huge contamination by abscess formation or fecal peritonitis following gut injury.

Drain is needed sometimes following drainage and repair of vulvar hematoma. Drain may be active or passive. Active drain may be close or open. Example of passive drain is keeping a Malecot catheter. One example of closed drainage following laparotomy is using ROMO ADK (Abdominal drainage kit) collection bag **(Fig. 30A)**. Corrugated rubber drain is also used for passive drainage **(Fig. 30B)**.

Vacuum-assisted wound closure (negative pressure wound therapy) is one therapeutic method of suction drain which is described in Chapter 30 with figures of postoperative complications.

ELECTROSURGICAL SYSTEMS (FIGS. 31 AND 32)

All obstetrician should have knowledge of electrosurgical system. Electrosurgery differs from electrocautery. In electrosurgery, electric current passes through the tissue to get the effective result. In electrocautery, current passes through a metal-like loop which is heated and destroys the tissue and current does not pass directly through the body of the patient. In monopolar system, current passes from the generator, passes through the tip of the electrosurgical instrument, and then into the grounding pad and current returns to the generator, thus circuit is completed. In bipolar device **(Fig. 32)**, both active electrode and return electrode are there and there is no need of grounding return pad.

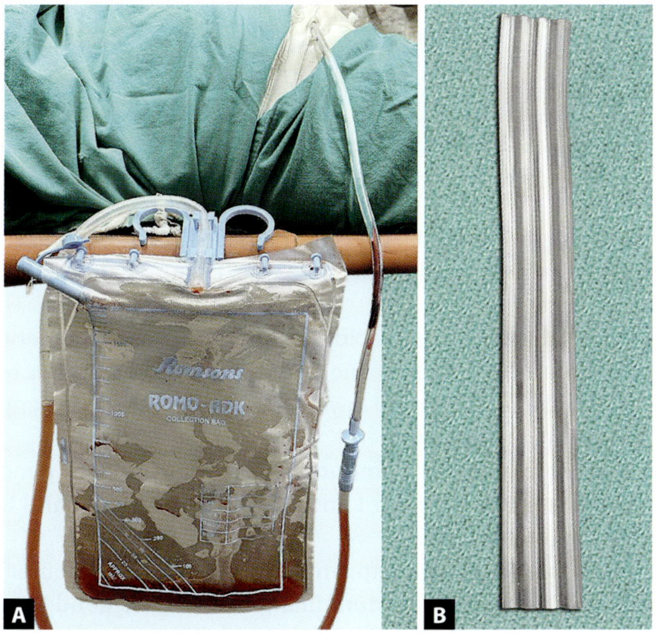

Figs. 30A and B: (A) Closed drainage following laparotomy using ROMO ADK collection bag; (B) Corrugated rubber drain is also used for passive drainage.

SURGICAL NEEDLE (FIG. 33)

Surgical needle has three parts, namely tip (point), body, and swage or eye. They differ in length, shape, curvature, and attachment of the suture. The needle may be straight or curved.

The types of surgical needle are swagged, control release or "pop off", and open variety. Powerful bondage occurs between the needle and suture material due to modern swaging technique; there is no change of diameter or little change requiring smallest necessary hole in the tissues. In swaged needle, the suture is fixed with the hollowed end of the needle. Suture needs to cut to free the needle. Swaged needle is ideal for application in obstetrics specially for running suture line. The control release needle is ideal for interrupted or ligation of vascular pedicle. Open-eyed needle has an advantage of using different suture types, but disadvantage of consumption time for threading and chance of frequent displacement of suture material. In modern obstetrics and gynecological practice, virtually there is no place of eyed needle.

Body may be round or ovoid. The ovoid type is flattened on top and bottom. Needle shape may be 1/4, 3/8, 1/2, and 5/8 circle. Most of the needles used are 1/2 or 3/8 circle. In obstetrics, 3/8 circle is used commonly. Needle is usually grasped by needle holder at right angle at point two-thirds from the needle tip. This site may be changed in specific places. Curve needles should never be grasped by hand, straight needles are sometimes used manually.

Needle tip or point may be taper point, blunt point, conventional cutting, and reverse cutting. Conventional cutting needles are useful for very fine skin stitches. Needle stick

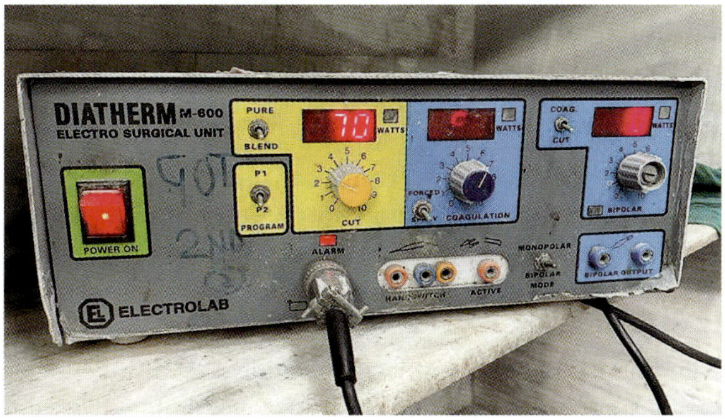

Fig. 31: Electrosurgical system.

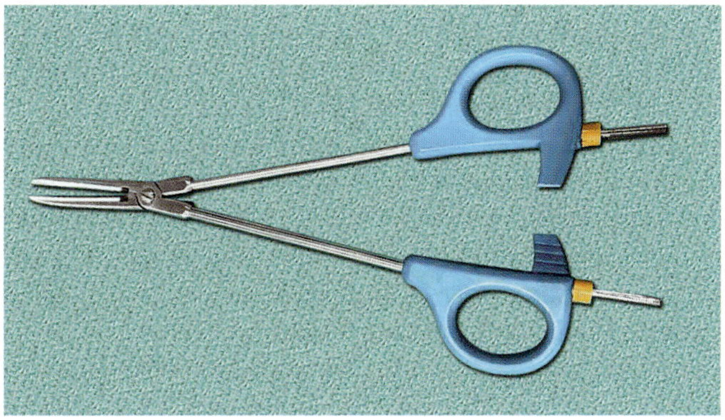

Fig. 32: Bipolar device.

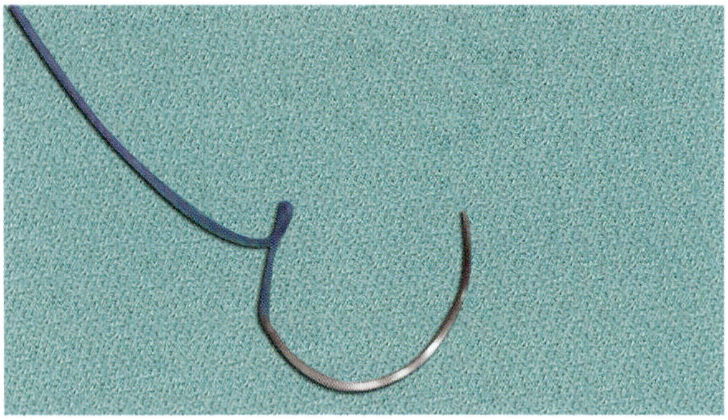

Fig. 33: Surgical needle attached with vicryl.

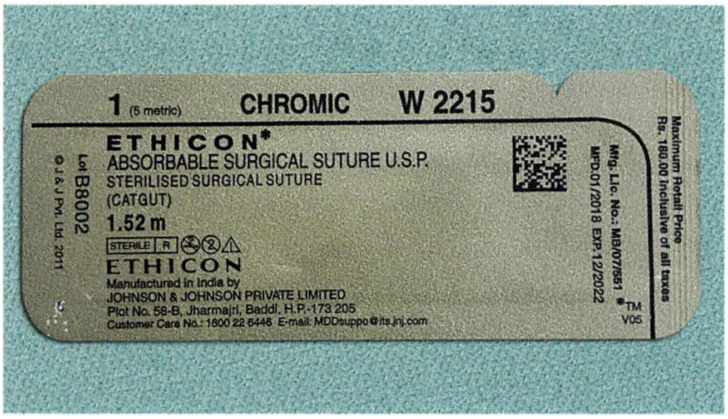

Fig. 34: Catgut.

injury is less in blunt needles and in episiotomy suturing blunt eye is suitable to prevent needle stick injury.

Cutting needle is not so used for obstetric surgeries for fear of tear of soft tissues. Reverse cutting needle is good for subcuticular skin repair.

SUTURE MATERIALS

There is no ideal suture material in true sense. It should be economic, can be tied easily and securely with good knot strength, superb tensile strength, not cutting through the tissue, capability of recoiling to initial length, and should have no adverse effect on wound healing.

The term catgut came from the term "kit gut". "Kit" means violin. The source of violin strings were intestines of sheep or ox.

Various suture materials used are silk, nylon, catgut, Vicryl, Dexon, polydioxanone (PDS), Prolene, Mersilene, Monocryl, Biosyn, etc.

Silk and catgut are traditional suture materials.

Silk is natural protein produced during cocoon development by the silkworm larva. It is easy to handle, less knot slippage, and less tear during suturing. One disadvantage is absorption of fluid and harboring bacteria for which it is not used in infected tissue. Cotton suture is rarely used in obstetrics.

Nylon is polyamide polymer synthetic suture, either monofilament or multifilament. It has excellent tensile strength, but cut through the thin tissue and is stiff and needs several knotting for good tying. Nylon is degraded with time and tensile strength remains little after 6 months.

Catgut **(Fig. 34)** is made from submucosa of sheep intestines or serosa of cattle intestine. It is chromicised by treating with chromium salts to increase strength and to delay in absorption. Tensile strength of catgut is poor, becomes minimal after 10 days, knot security is poor and is absorbed completely within 2–3 weeks.

Vicryl (polyglactin 910) **(Fig. 35)** is delayed synthetic suture. It is braided, good tensile strength, knot security fair, and absorbed in 80 days. Vicryl is associated with less

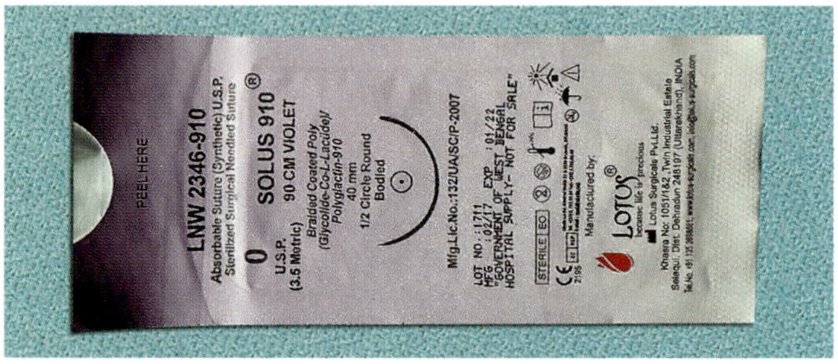

Fig. 35: Polyglactin 910 (Vicryl).

pain, less dyspareunia, and less risk of dehiscence in perineal suturing. Cutting through the tissue is important disadvantage.

Dexon (polyglycolic acid) is another delayed synthetic suture, braided, good tensile strength, knot security fair to good, and absorbed in 90 days. It has similar advantage and disadvantage like Vicryl.

Polydioxanone II is monofilament, not braided, good tensile strength, but poor knot security, fair to good, and is absorbed in 180 days.

Monocryl (Poliglecaprone) and Biosyn (Glycomer) both are configured as monofilament and have good knot security. Biotin is better than Monocryl in respect to tensile strength.

Prolene is prepared by propylene polymerization, it is similar to polythene suture dermalene. It has very little tendency of friction for which it is ideal for cervical cerclage and intradermal closure.

Mersilene is uncoated polyester synthetic suture and is commonly used for cervical cerclage. They are unabsorbable and tensile strength is very strong and remains indefinitely.

Stainless still suture is rarely used nowadays.

Vicryl is superior to catgut for use in vaginal lacerations and episiotomies.

SUTURE TIE AND KNOTS

Tying knots is important part of surgical technique, every young surgeon should learn from very beginning. Everyone should practice a wide variety of knots, not depending on a single type, and should learn which one to be applied when. Being an assistant, a young surgeon will learn to cut the tails of sutures quickly and accurately leaving a short but adequate length. Scissors are used to cut the suture with the tip of blades after making it stationery. Surgeon should also present the suture such a way that it will be well approachable for assistant to cut. It is very wrong to take short length suture to use in difficult places. For knot tying at least half lengths of sutures to be provided to the surgeon.

There are three components of a suture tie. These are loop, knot, and tears. Loop approximates the wound or make hemostasis, knot makes the tie secured, and the tears ensure that suture will not become untied due to knot slippage.

The different knots are Granny knot, common square knot, Square surgeon's knot, and simple slipknot.

Knot can be given doublehanded, single-handed, and by using forceps (forceps knot).

Granny knot is the simplest and can be applied quickly with two identical hitches by two-handed techniques. The reef knot consists of two hitches and this is also two-handed techniques and make a firm knot.

A square knot is more secure than a granny (cross) knot. Both these knots are superior to slipknot.

The single-handed knot is fast and of simple technique without using special instruments **(Figs. 36A to E)**.

Forceps knot is useful in case of short length of suture material **(Figs. 37A to D)**. Suture strength is reduced by stray knots and suturing with use of any instrument.

Knot in depth: It is best dealt with Meigs-Navratil right-angled forceps **(Fig. 38)**.

Ligature Tying of a Pedicle (Fig. 39)

Small vascular pedicle is tied with a single tie beneath the ti. If the tissue becomes edematous as seen in pregnancy or seems not secured along with a free tie, a transfixing suture is given distal to the first tie for proper hemostatic control and also prevents ligature slip.

SUTURE TECHNIQUES

Sutures may be interrupted suture and continuous suture.

Continuous suture: Simple, locked or blanket sutures **(Fig. 40)**, and continuous locked figure-of eight sutures **(Fig. 41)**.

Interrupted suture: Simple **(Fig. 42)**, vertical mattress **(Fig. 43)**, and horizontal mattress **(Fig. 44)** and Lembert sutures **(Fig. 45)**.

Mass closure of parieties: Smead-Jones or mass closure incorporating peritoneum, rectus abdominis muscle,

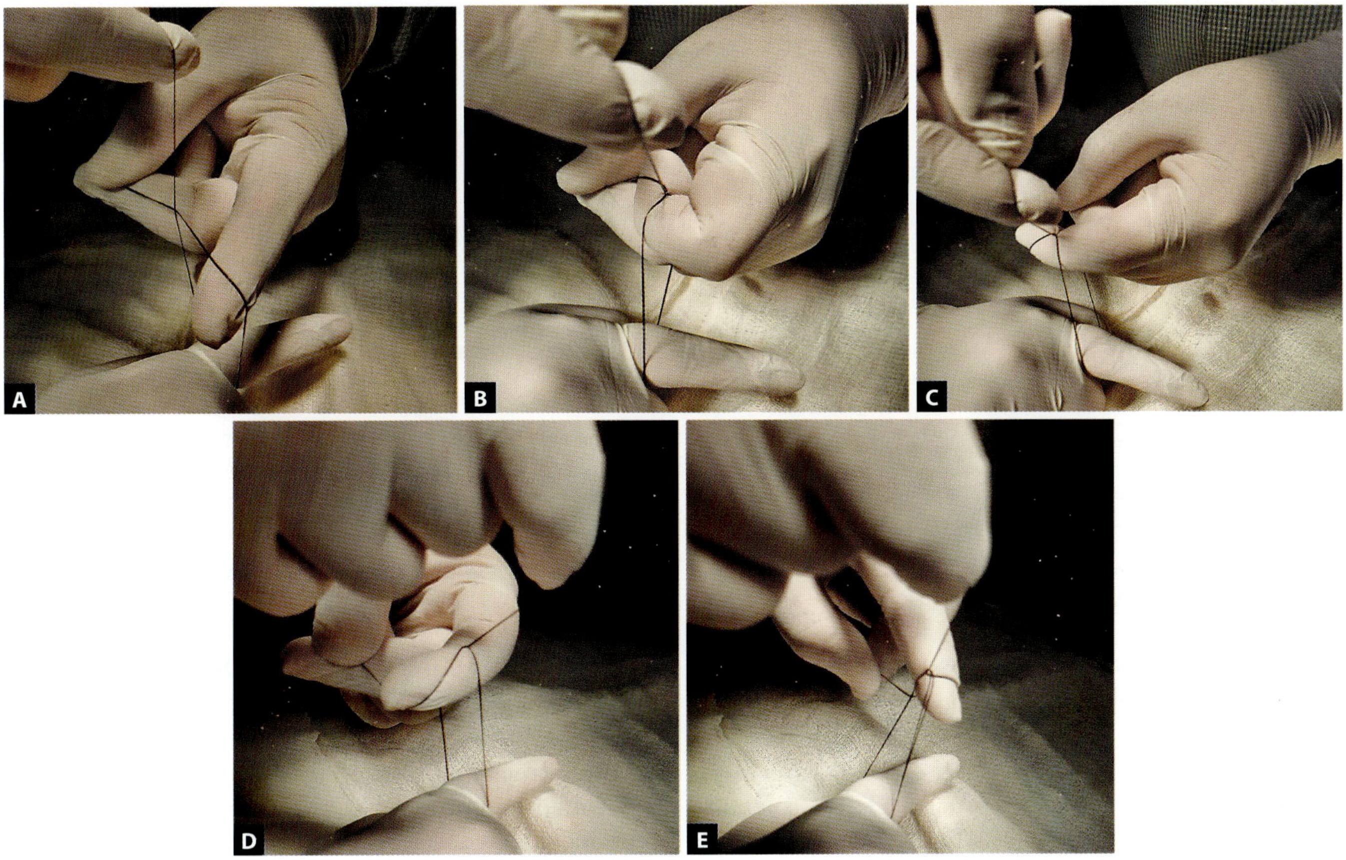

Figs. 36A to E: Single-handed knot—steps.
Courtesy: Dr Pradipto Sanyal, Senior Consultant Gynecologist.

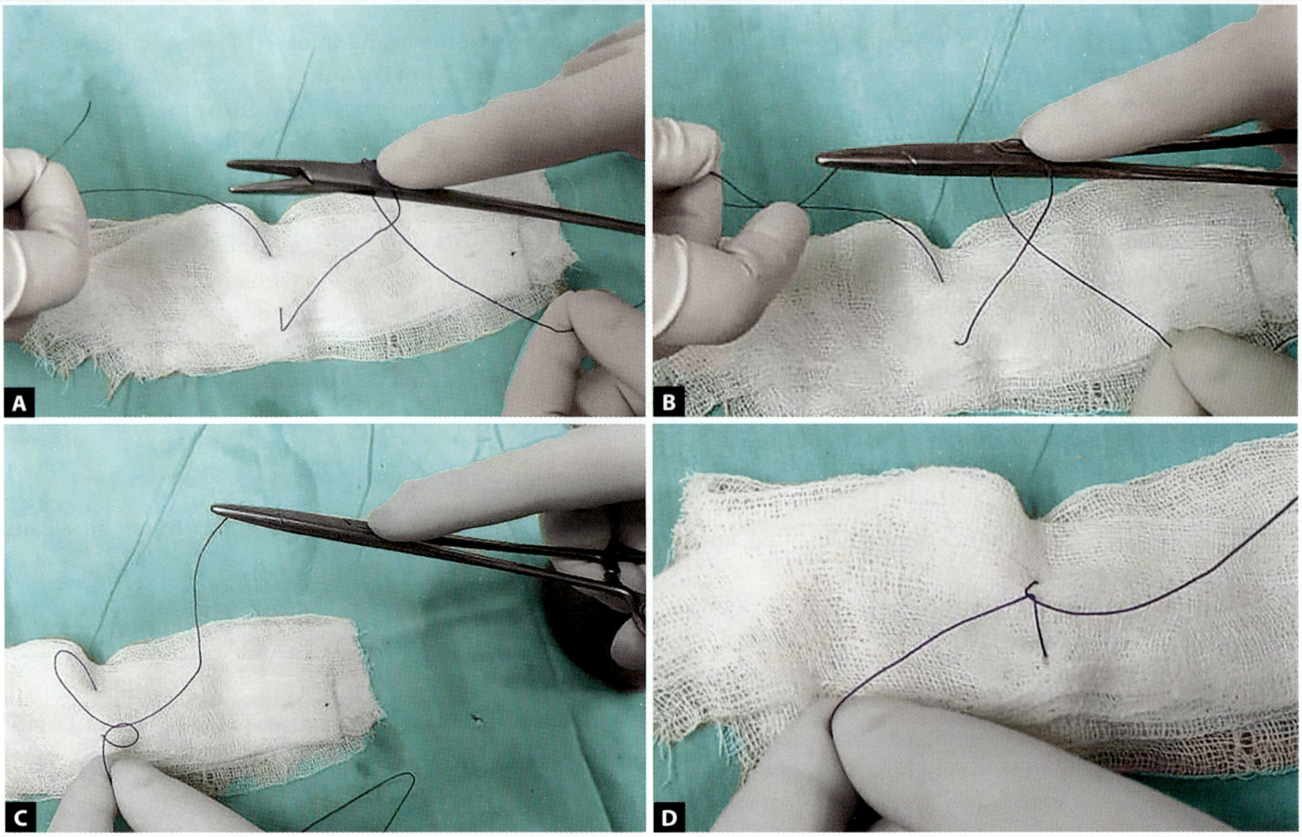

Figs. 37A to D: Forceps knot.
Courtesy: Professor Abhijit Rakshit, Department of Gynecology and Obstetrics, RG Kar Medical College, Kolkata, West Bengal, India.

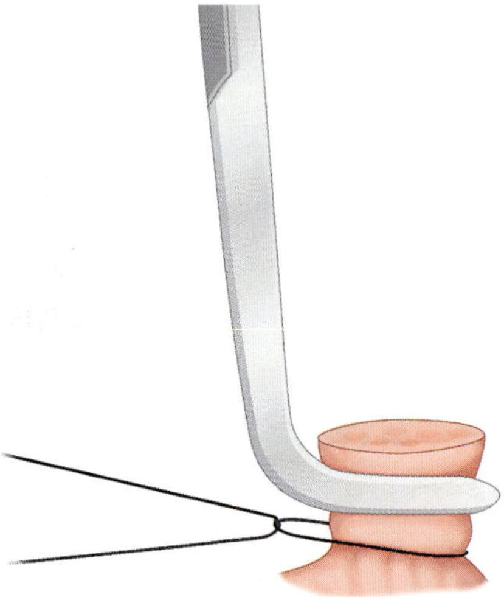

Fig. 38: Knot in depth is dealt with best by Meigs-Navaratil right-angled forceps.

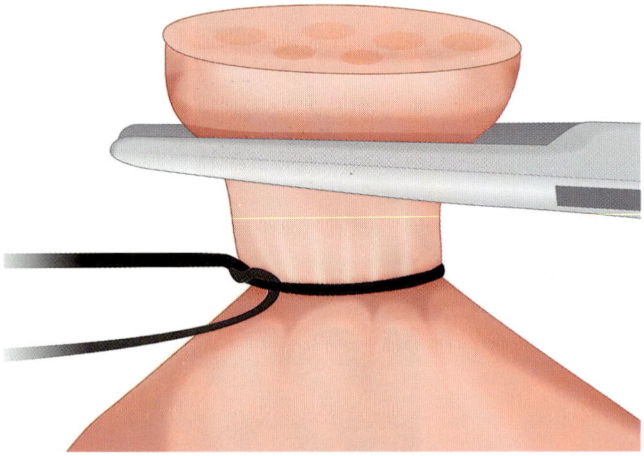

Fig. 39: Ligature tying of a pedicle.

and rectus sheath together are described in Chapter 30 Postoperative Complications.

STAPLERS

In obstetrics and gynecology, use of stapler is not so popular. In this stream, use of stapler is limited to skin closure. Recently, use of staplers has become popular in minimal access surgery.

ABDOMINAL INCISIONS AND CLOSURE

Abdominal incision in obstetric patient varies and depends on various factors. These are surgeon's choice, indication of surgery, whether it is elective or emergency, patients-associated comorbidity specially obesity, presence of previous scar, and its type. In cesarean delivery, quick entry and ease of baby delivery are important factors for choosing a type of incision.

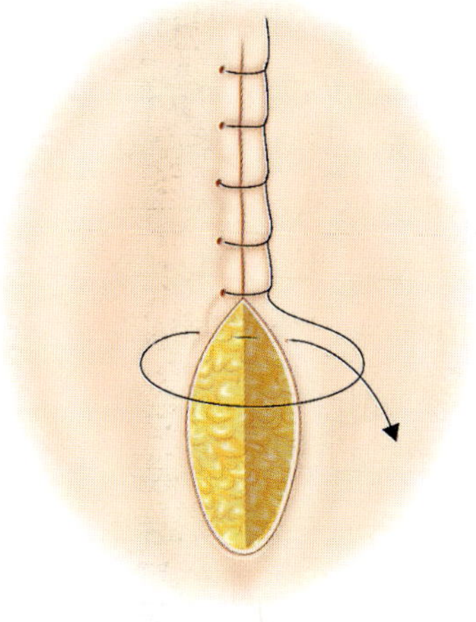

Fig. 40: Continuous suture—locked or blanket sutures.

ANATOMY OF ANTERIOR ABDOMINAL WALL (FIGS. 46 TO 48)

Thorough knowledge of anterior abdominal wall is imperative for any incision and choosing an incision type. These include disposition of abdominal muscles, fascia, aponeurosis, vessels on anterior abdomen, and nerve distribution.

Anterior abdominal wall consists of skin, superficial fascia, deep fascia then laterally external oblique, internal oblique, and transversus abdominis muscle. Their aponeurosis fuse medially to form rectus sheath, anterior rectus sheath, and posterior rectus sheath in between which lies rectus abdominis muscle and below pyramidalis. In lower abdomen below the arcuate line, there is no rectus sheath posteriorly and weak transversalis fascia and peritoneum support the rectus.

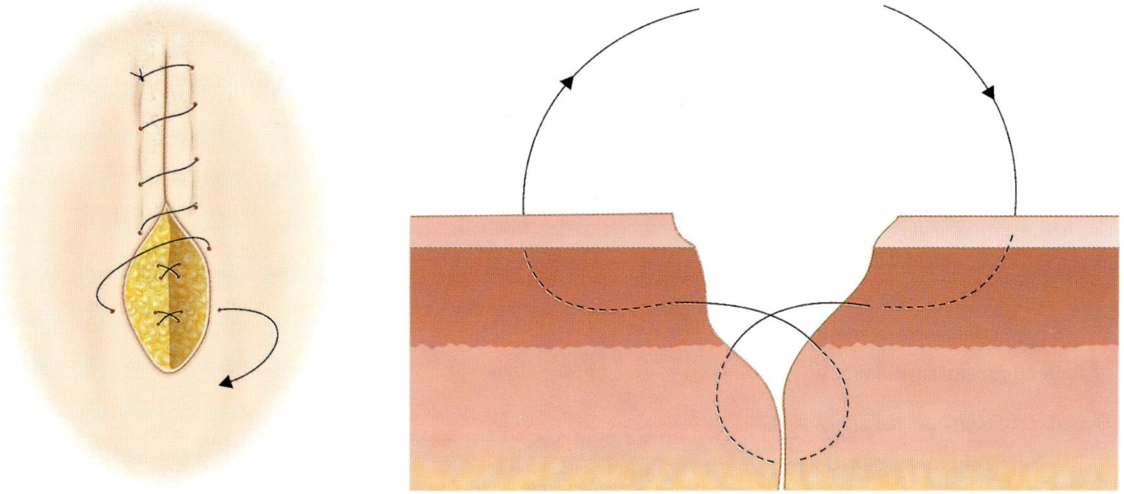

Fig. 41: Continuous suture—continuous locked figure-of-eight sutures.

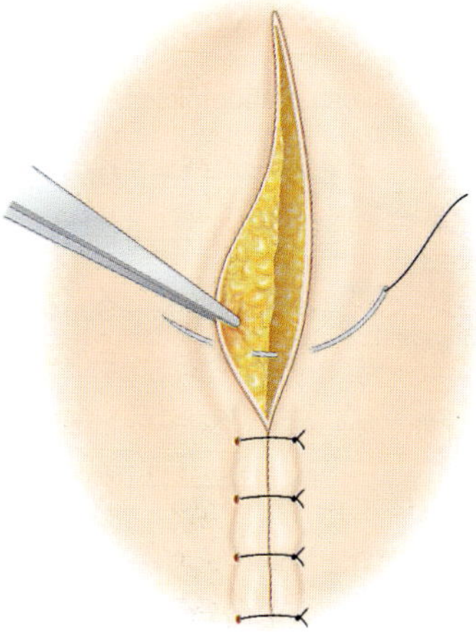

Fig. 42: Interrupted suture—simple.

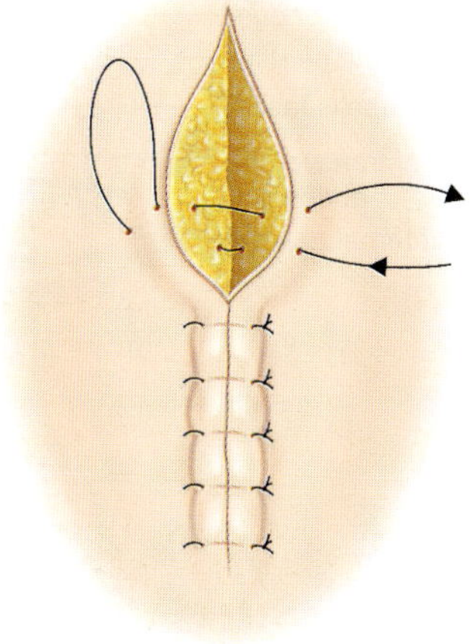

Fig. 43: Vertical mattress.

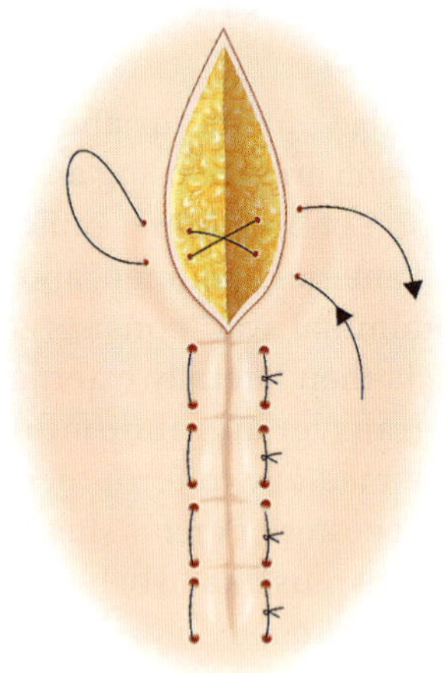

Fig. 44: Horizontal mattress.

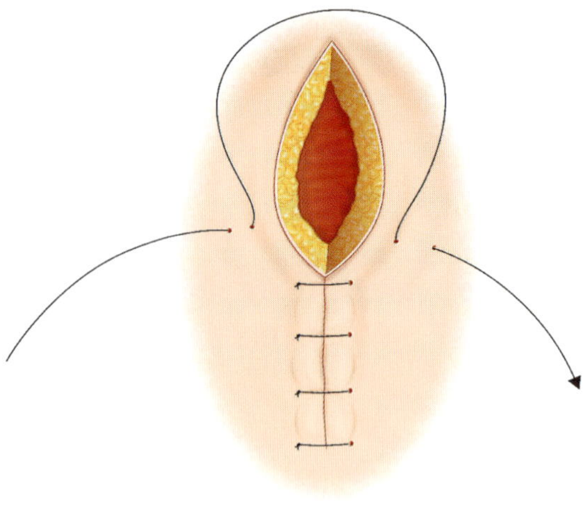

Fig. 45: Lembert stitches.

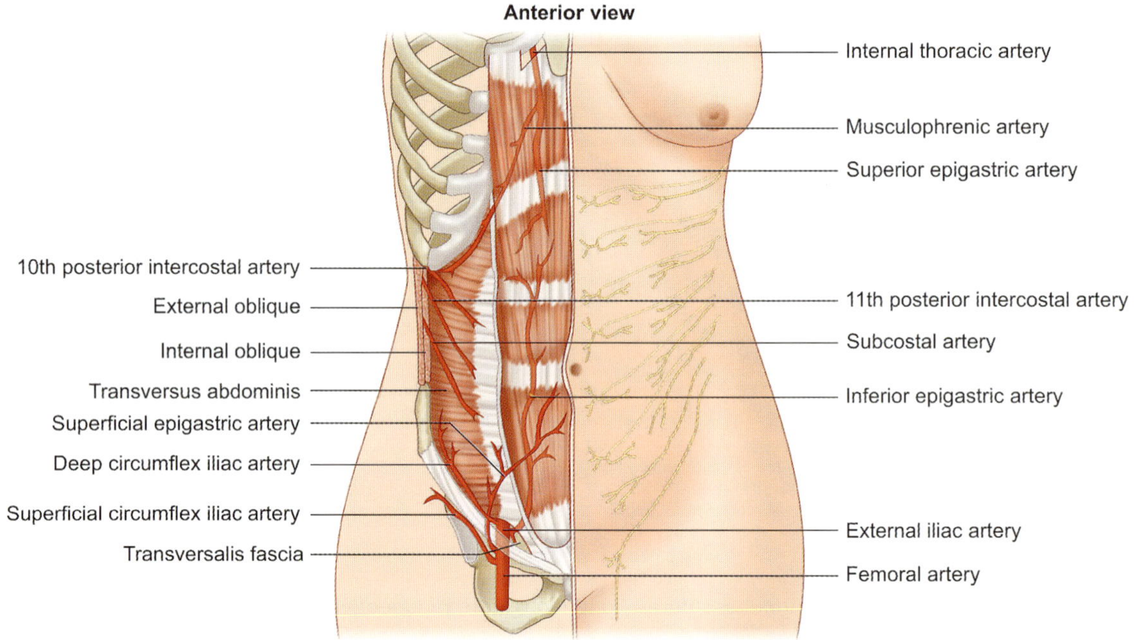

Fig. 46: Anatomy of anterior abdominal wall including disposition of vessels.

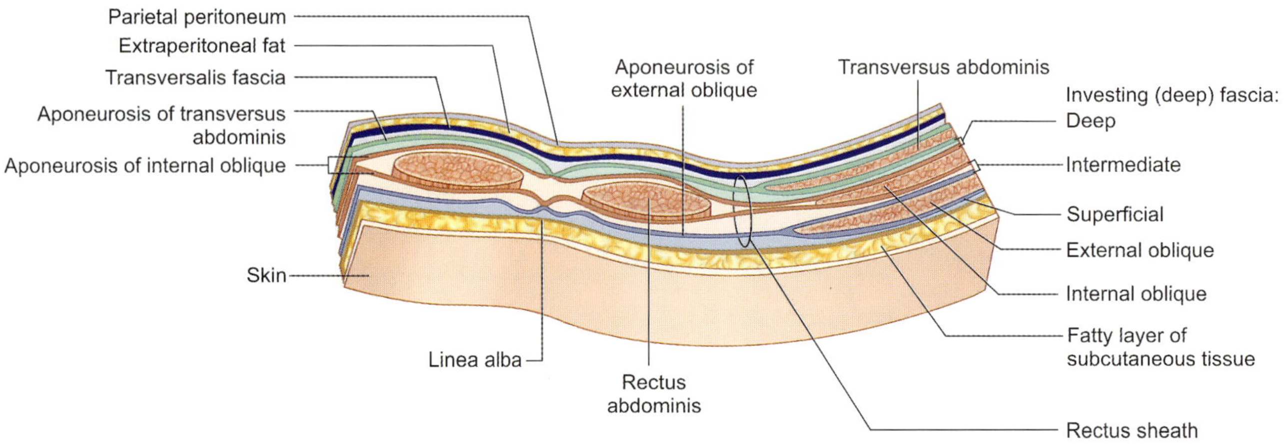

Fig. 47: Anatomy of anterior abdominal wall—transverse section.

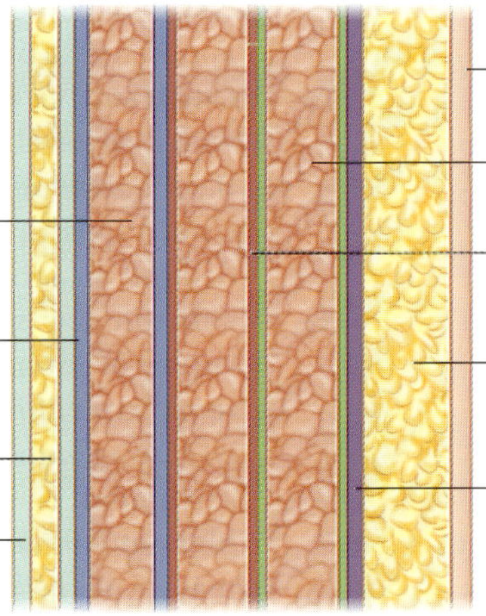

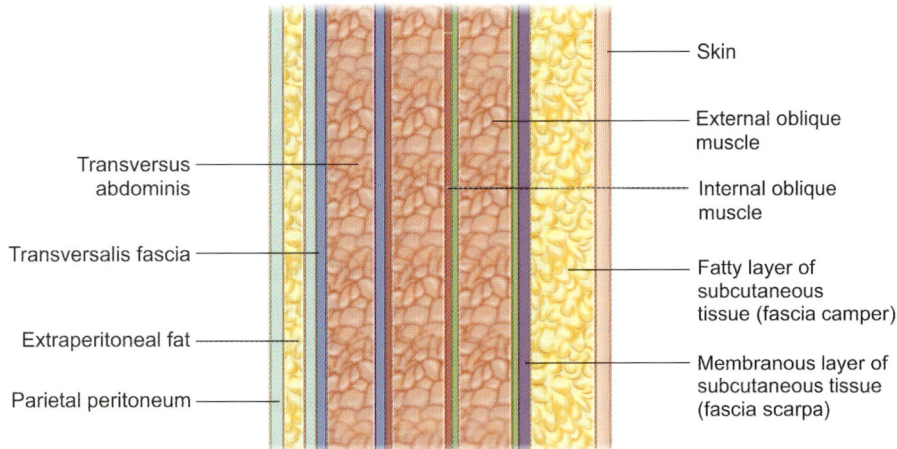

Fig. 48: Anatomy of anterior abdominal wall—longitudinal section.

Important vessels of anterior abdominal wall are superior epigastric artery, inferior epigastric artery (IEA), and perforator arteries.

Superior epigastric artery (thoracic artery) and musculophrenic artery are terminal branches of internal thoracic artery which is a branch of subclavian artery and which lies beneath the rectus muscle and in front of posterior rectus sheath. These are not of obstetric concern.

Inferior epigastric artery, branch of the external iliac artery, which runs upward behind the rectus muscle is loosely supported by weak transversalis fascia and peritoneum as rectus sheath is deficient below arcuate line, is more prone to be injured, and there is chance of formation of large hematoma on injury which is the main obstetrical concern.

Deep circumflex iliac artery is another branch of external iliac artery. Perforator arteries which have origin in bifurcations of the IEAs perforate the rectus abdominis muscle, traversing to the superficial tissues of the abdomen, and are most commonly injured while lifting the anterior rectus sheath from the rectus abdominis muscle. Care must be taken during incision and proper hemostasis, if injured. Superficial circumflex iliac and superficial epigastric vessels are branches of femoral artery.

TYPES OF INCISION

Most common incisions for obstetric surgery are midline (vertical) incision and Pfannestiel incisions. Other abdominal incisions are Maylard, Cherney, and supraumbilical (transverse) incisions.

Advantage and Disadvantage of Transverse Incision

A transverse incision is preferred where it is feasible, due its various advantages. The advantages of transverse incision of skin are cosmetic, chance of wound dehiscence is less, and probability of incisional hernia is also less.

The disadvantage of transverse incision is less exposure, especially in obese women and also in situations where wide operating space is required, and access to upper abdomen is needed. Incision cannot be extended. Anatomically, more chance of blood loss and hematoma formation due to involvement of superficial and inferior epigastric vessels and higher rate of neural injury of ilioinguinal and iliohypogastric nerves are encountered in transverse incision. Dead spaces are formed more due to the division of multiple layers of muscle layers and fascia. More time is also needed. There is difficulty in delivery of nonengaged head. Repeat cesarean delivery is more time consuming and difficult due to scarring in Pfannenstiel incision.

Advantage and Disadvantage of Midline Vertical Skin Incision

Emergency entry is quicker in vertical incision during primary and repeat cesarean delivery. With high-infection-risk patients, midline incision is favored as in transverse incision, chance of collection of purulent fluid is more in layers of parieties. Important neurovascular structures are not damaged by this incision, and it becomes almost bloodless procedure. There is often no need to separate recti due to naturally occurring diastasis in pregnancy.

Pfannenstiel Incision

Skin incision: Pfannenstiel incision is a suprapubic low transverse "smile" like incision **(Figs. 49A to D)** 2–3 cm above the symphysis pubis at the level of pubic hairline, slightly curved, 12–15 cm in length (see below). Actual length depends on need of exposure. It starts 2–3 cm below the anterior iliac crest and ends at the same point on opposite side.

Subcutaneous tissue layer is sharply dissected to reach rectus sheath. Superior epigastric vessels may be encountered much lateral to midline which is either diathermy coagulated or ligated with plain catgut (3-0).

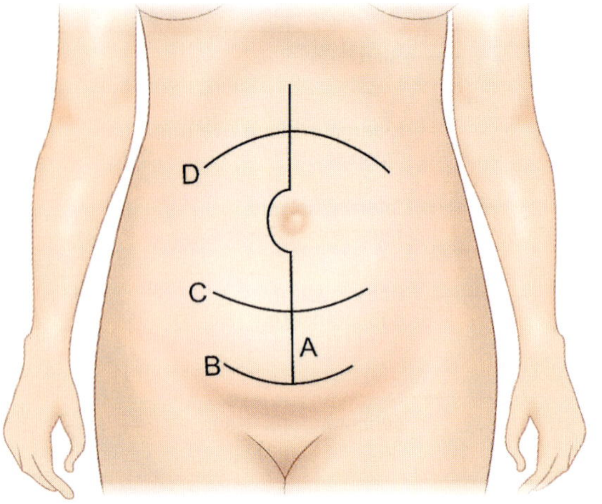

Figs. 49A to D: Types of abdominal incision in obstetrics. (A) Vertical incision including supraumbilical extension; (B) Pfannenstiel; (C) Maylard incision; (D) transverse supraumbilical incision.

Recuts sheath is cut transversely with sharp incision. Anterior rectus sheath is composed of two layers, external oblique aponeurosis and fused aponeurosis of internal oblique and transverse abdominis muscles. Inferior epigastric vessels which lie lateral to rectus abdominis is not usually injured and if injured, needs ligation or coagulation. By holding the cut margins of rectus sheath at midline both below and above flaps are separated from rectus abdominis below up to symphysis pubis and above to the extent as needed. The vessels coursing between muscle and sheath are secured by coagulation or stitches and complete hemostasis done. Careful hemostasis is very crucial to prevent hematoma and infection prevention.

Rectus muscles and pyramidalis are retracted laterally starting from above (there is no posterior layer of rectus sheath in lower abdomen).

Opening of peritoneal cavity: Transversalis fascia with Preperitoneal fat are dissected to reach peritoneum which is opened very carefully by lifting with two artery forceps and not to do any inadvertent injury of omentum, bowel, and bladder. Holding the peritoneum in upper part prevents injury of bladder. Before opening it, the peritoneum is palpated to exclude the inclusion of omentum, bowel, and bladder. The incision is then extended below up to the bladder reflection and superiorly above the arcuate line where transverse fibers of posterior layer of rectus sheath may need to be cut. It is to be remembered that bladder is elevated and edematous in obstructed labor. One must also be careful regarding the presence of any intra-abdominal adhesion in case of previous abdominal surgery.

Closure of Abdomen

The layers are peritoneum, rectus muscle, rectus sheath, and skin. Peritoneum closure is not recommended, due to lack of benefit by the recent studies. Rectus muscles may be apposed with one or two figure-of-eight sutures with 0 or no. 1 catgut stitches but not mandatory. Rectus sheath is repaired with delayed absorbable continuous and nonlocking suture. If subcutaneous tissue is >2 cm, it is closed separately with continuous or interrupted stitches with plain catgut or delayed absorbable suture. Skin is sutured with continuous subcuticular stitch using 3-0 or 4-0 delayed absorbable suture or interrupted nonabsorbable suture which needs removal on fifth or sixth day. Alternatively, skin can be closed by glue, or with staples. Staples are associated with more skin separation. There is no evidence of good result with negative pressure wound dressing in obese women. Secondary closure may be needed sometimes and is described in Chapter 30 of Postoperative Complications.

Cherney Incision

In Cherney incision, caudal tendons of both rectus abdominis muscle are divided at their insertion to get adequate operative exposure. In this incision, 25% more space is available than infraumbilical midline vertical incision. Caution is taken not to injure the bladder during cutting of tendon and a finger is kept behind the tendon. With blunt dissection space of Retzius is made, the muscles are reflected above, and the incision over exposed peritoneum is extended laterally.

Peritoneum is closed by catgut or Vicryl. Drain is usually not needed. Rectus tendon is approximated by six to eight interrupted or horizontal mattress stitches, with distal cut edge of rectus sheath, not directly with symphysis bone to prevent osteomyelitis.

Maylard Incision (Figs. 49C)

In Maylard incision, a transverse muscle cutting skin incision is given. A transverse skin incision is given 3–8 cm above the symphysis pubis depending on the patient's size. Skin, subcutaneous tissue, and rectus fascia are cut up to the lateral border of rectus muscles. One must be cautious about the injury of IEA or it can be ligated beforehand. During closure, margins of rectus muscle is stitched with fascia. Only fascia is approximated with sutures, thus there is no need of further muscle suture. A subfascial drain may be given. In Pfannenstiel incision, as the rectus muscle is separated from the fascia (not done in Meylard type), converting Pfannenstiel incision to Maylard incision there will be a problem for muscle approximation, for which Maylard incision should be also planned prior. Maylard incision is not preferred in cesarean delivery. It is mostly done in cancer radical surgery. In obstetrics, it is reserved for laparotomy for peripartum hysterectomy, management of PPH, and internal iliac ligation.

Supraumbilical transverse incision **(Fig. 49D)** which is given 6 cm above the umbilicus is indicated in pregnant woman with a large uterus and large adnexal mass.

Vertical Incision

Vertical incision may be midline vertical and paramedian.

Midline Vertical (Fig. 49A)

Infraumbilical midline vertical skin incision is about 12–15 cm length extended below up to 2–3 cm above the superior border of symphysis pubis. Subcutaneous layer is cut by scalpel or diathermy to expose the rectus sheath. Linea alba is opened starting first in upper part very gently by lifting to avoid injury to intra-abdominal structures. Rectus muscle and pyramidalis are separated in midline. Peritoneum is opened carefully similar to transverse incision extension of vertical incision is needed sometimes in laparotomy or cesarean delivery in obese woman.

Paramedian Incision

The disadvantages of paramedian incision are more bleeding during surgery, more time consuming, more infection, and more postoperative pain though healing is said to be good in paramedian incision. It is not preferred incision in obstetrics.

INCISION IN OBESE WOMAN

It varies from surgeon to surgeon. For morbid obese woman, periumbilical midline incision is preferred. In midline vertical incision, the lower end should begin above the thick panniculus crease. So, the incision extends upward above the umbilicus. Supraumbilical transverse incision is another alternative for obese woman. A subcutaneous drain is also suggested. Negative pressure wound therapy has been tried, but its cost effectiveness is not well established.

CHAPTER 2

Obstetric Emergencies: Dealing with Critically Ill Mothers

Learning Objectives

- Obstetric Emergency
- Maternal Emergencies
- Maternal Mortality—Reflection of Country's Health Status
- Preeclampsia/Eclampsia
- HELLP Syndrome
- Amniotic Fluid Embolism
- Obstetric Shock
- Hemorrhagic Shock
- Septic Shock (Endotoxic Shock)
  Syn: Endotoxic Shock/Bacteremic Shock/Septicemic Shock
- Acute Kidney Injury in Obstetrics
- Disseminated Intravascular Coagulation
- Blood and Blood Products

INTRODUCTION

Obstetric care refers to the care of the mother and her fetus during pregnancy, care during intrapartum period and management of puerperal mother and her neonate. It includes prevention, detection and treatment of complications through this spectrum of antenatal period, during delivery and puerperium. Obstetric emergencies may appear in two groups; one group, the known high-risk pregnant women which can be predicted, and another group, so called low-risk women facing sudden obstetric emergency. While the percentage of deaths may be higher among high-risk women, the greatest total number of deaths takes place among women considered to be of low-risk which constitutes more than 80% pregnancies. The implementation of emergency obstetrics care (EmOC) was stressed by UNFPA in the millennium development goals (MDG) in 2000. Care and management of critically ill mother during obstetric emergencies can save majority of the lives.

OBSTETRIC EMERGENCY

Obstetric emergency is defined as a critical situation that occurs suddenly and unexpectedly and needs immediate action. Emergency may be of mother and fetus.

MATERNAL EMERGENCIES

Maternal emergencies are given below.

- *Hypertensive diseases:* Preeclampsia, eclampsia, and HELLP (hemolysis, elevated liver enzymes, and low platelets) syndrome
- *Hemorrhages*: Antepartum hemorrhage (APH) and postpartum hemorrhage (PPH), disseminated intravascular coagulation (DIC), retained placenta, excessive bleeding in abortion, uterine inversion, uterine rupture
- Shoulder dystocia
- Sudden maternal collapse

Sudden Maternal Collapse

Sudden maternal collapse may be due to various reasons. These are obstetric shock for any reason, septic shock, hemorrhagic shock, anaphylactic shock, pulmonary embolism, amniotic fluid embolism (AFE), and cardiac cause (myocardial infarction, cardiomyopathy, aneurysm rupture, arrhythmia, and aortic dissection). Cerebral hemorrhage, cerebral thrombosis, deep vein thrombosis, illegal drugs (benzodiazepines, amphetamines, heroin, and cocaine), common medications (overdoses of magnesium sulfate, opioids, and local anesthetics), hypoglycemia, and anesthetic hazards.

Hypovolemia due to hemorrhage is the most common cause of maternal collapse.

Management of Obstetric Emergencies

Best way to tackle the situation is the *ABC approach* [Royal College of Obstetricians and Gynaecologists (RCOG), 2011].

A—maintenance of *Airway*
B—*Breathing* and ventilation
C—*Circulatory* support

Components of steps of management are:

- Ask for assistance
- Speak with the patient
- Tilt the patient to left
- Breathing, O_2, bag mask, intubation, if positive pressure ventilation is needed.
- Intravenous (IV) channel with large bore cannula
- Defibrillator and if cardiac arrest → management on that line
- Treatment of the cause

MATERNAL MORTALITY—REFLECTION OF COUNTRY'S HEALTH STATUS

Maternal mortality ratio (MMR) reflects the country's status of healthcare system. There has been remarkable improvement of healthcare system globally; still in many of the states in developing world, maternal mortality is high. Risks lie in every pregnancy, in every childbirth, in every society, and in every setting. In developed countries, risks have been largely overcome by providing access to special care during pregnancy and childbirth to every pregnant woman. The picture is reverse in many developing countries where pregnancy represents a journey into an unknown from where many women never return. The tragedy is that majority of these deaths are preventable.

Maternal death is defined as the death of a woman while pregnant or within 42 days of delivery, irrespective of the duration and site of pregnancy, from any cause related to or aggravated by the pregnancy or its management but not from accidental or incidental causes.

Maternal mortality ratio is calculated as the number of maternal deaths during a given year per 100,000 live births during the same period. MMR represents the risk associated with each pregnancy, i.e., the obstetric risk.

The global annual number of maternal deaths is estimated to be 295,000 in 2017. Global maternal death is reduced by 38% from 2000 to 2017. Global number of daily maternal deaths is 810. 94% deaths occur in low and lower-middle class countries. India contributes one-fifth of world's maternal deaths.

More than 80% of maternal death is due to three causes, namely hypertensive disorder of pregnancy (HDP), PPH, and sepsis. In India, anemia is a major contributory factor. During last three decades, the number of maternal deaths has been remarkably reduced. Death from preeclampsia/eclampsia has been prevented by regular antenatal care, antihypertensives, and $MgSO_4$ as anticonvulsant that of PPH-by-PPH drill with timely use of oxytocics, blood transfusion, and other management, and death from sepsis has been reduced by delivery in clean environment, antibiotics, and immunization. In India, institutional delivery rate is increased to 89% (in urban 94%) according to National Family Health Survey 5 (NFHS 5) (2019–2021) data. The "Anemia Mukt Bharat 2018" program launched by India shows that iron supplementation of 6 months during antenatal period and another 6 months after delivery has an impact on improvement of anemia. Overall care of the mother with easy access to high dependency unit (HDU) and critical care facility has played important role to minimize number of maternal deaths. There are many to be achieved as many of the maternal deaths are preventable.

In fact, main drive was taken from the 1990s following first international safe motherhood program in Nairobi in 1987 with an aim to reduce the maternal mortality by 50% in 2000 as compared to in 1990. First global maternal audit report was published in 1996 on the basis of 1990 data. Various global organizations like World Health Organization (WHO), United Nations International Children's Emergency Fund (UNICEF), [United Nations Population Fund (UNFPA)], the World Bank, and United Nations Fund for Population Activities (UNFPO) are highly active to be associated with the issue of maternal mortality in most countries. Thereafter, Child Survival and Safe Motherhood (CSSM) program (1989) and International Conference on Population and Development (ICPD) (Cairo, 1994) agenda were initiated. Government of India launched a Reproductive and Child Health (RCH) program in 1997 and expanded later.

In 2000 at the Millennium summit, safe motherhood was viewed as a top priority in Millennium Development Goal 5 (MDG 5) among eight MDGs. The aim was to reduce 75% maternal mortality rate within 2015 in comparison to the level of 1990. Emergency obstetric care (EmOC) was started in India in 2003.

India's care on maternal and child health was dramatically improved following implementation of National Rural Health Mission (NRHM) program in 2005 which later changed to National Health Mission (NHM).

In 2016, Sustainable Development Goals (SDGs) are initiated. SDG3 includes the health of all ages. Target 1 of SDG3 is to reduce MMR <70/100,000 live birth by 2030. Laqshya (labor room quality improvement initiative) has been launched by Government of India in December, 2017.

Present global MMR has come down to 211 maternal deaths per 100,000 live births (2017 estimate), from MMR of 385 per 100,000 live births in 1990.

In countries like South Sudan, Chad, and Sierra Leone MMR is >1,000/100,000 live births. Lowest MMR is 2/100,000 live births in Belarus, Poland, Italy, and Norway. MMR of United Kingdom is 7, United States 19, Russia 17, China 29, Sri Lanka 36, Bangladesh 173, Pakistan 140, and Nepal 186/100,000 live births (all 2017 estimates).

According to the Sample Registration System (SRS) used by Registrar General of India, the MMR of India has declined to 103/100,000 live birth in 2017–2019 from estimate of 398/100,000 live birth of 1997–98. Five states of India already achieved SDG target of 70/100,000 live birth. Undoubtedly, India has to achieve more.

PREECLAMPSIA/ECLAMPSIA

Among all the HDPs, severe preeclampsia/eclampsia is an obstetric emergency and poses a great challenge for high maternal and perinatal morbidity and mortality.

Classification and Incidence of Hypertensive Disorder of Pregnancy

In basic classification of HDP complicating pregnancy [(Modified from NHBPEP—(2000)] four types are categorized.

1. *Gestational hypertension:* There is no evidence of development of preeclampsia syndrome and hypertension resolves by 12 weeks postpartum. Prevalence is 6–7% of pregnancy.
2. Preeclampsia and eclampsia which are found in 5–7% of pregnancy.
3. Preeclampsia superimposed on chronic hypertension complicating 1–5% of pregnancy.
4. Chronic hypertension (of any etiology—primary or secondary) constitutes 20–25% of chronic hypertension.

Definition and Diagnostic Criteria of Preeclampsia/Severe Eclampsia (American College of Obstetricians and Gynecologists 2020)

According to American College of Obstetricians and Gynecologists (ACOG) 2020, preeclampsia/severe eclampsia is associated with ≥140 mm Hg systolic or ≥90 mm Hg diastolic after 20 weeks of gestation in a woman with a previously normal blood pressure (BP) (on two occasions at least 4 hours apart) and proteinuria or, in the absence of proteinuria, new onset hypertension with the new onset any of the five features, namely thrombocytopenia, renal insufficiency, impaired liver function, pulmonary edema, cerebral symptoms or visual symptoms.

For severe hypertension, BP ≥160 mm Hg systolic or ≥110 mm Hg diastolic, severe hypertension can be confirmed within a short interval (minutes) to administer timely antihypertensive therapy.

Severe preeclampsia is a variety of preeclampsia which is associated with any of the following findings—severe hypertension, thrombocytopenia, renal insufficiency, impaired liver function, pulmonary edema, and new onset cerebral symptoms or visual symptoms.

Eclampsia is defined by the occurrence of generalized tonic-clonic convulsion (seizures) in a woman with preeclampsia, not attributed to other causes.

Complications of Preeclampsia/Severe Eclampsia and Eclampsia

Maternal complications are eclampsia, abruptio placentae, cerebral hemorrhage/posterior reversible encephalopathy syndrome (PRES), cardiac failure, oliguria and anuria, HELLP syndrome, eye complications (scotoma, blurring of vision and diplopia, and few incidences of blindness), coagulation failure, preterm labor, and PPH.

Fetal complications are intrauterine growth restriction (IUGR), intrauterine death, asphyxia, and prematurity.

Outline of Management of Preeclampsia, Severe Preeclampsia, and HELLP Syndrome

Nonsevere variety of preeclampsia is managed with frequent antenatal visit with rest, oral iron, folic acid, calcium, aspirin, and close maternal and fetal surveillance. Recent guideline [National Institute for Health and Care Excellence (NICE) 2019] suggests antihypertensive, if BP remains above 140/90 mm Hg. Target BP is 135/85 mm Hg or less on antihypertensive treatment. First line is oral labetalol, nifedipine when labetalol is not suitable, and methyldopa if labetalol or nifedipine is not suitable. Injection $MgSO_4$ is given in severe preeclampsia as prophylactic anticonvulsant. Patient should be warned regarding the ominous features of fulminating preeclampsia and should attend the hospital immediately, if any feature develops.

Severe preeclampsia is an obstetric emergency and management of severe preeclampsia is in the line of eclampsia—admission in HDU, antihypertensive, prophylactic $MgSO_4$, intense monitoring, and decision of termination of pregnancy. The management outline of severe preeclampsia is given in **Flowchart 1**.

Time of Delivery in Pregnancy-induced Hypertension

In pure gestational hypertension advice is to wait till term, no indication for induction earlier.

In nonsevere preeclampsia with no other complications, termination is done at or beyond 37 weeks. There is no benefit to continue the pregnancy beyond that (ACOG).

In severe preeclampsia <24 weeks and >34 weeks period of gestation, pregnancy is terminated. In severe preeclampsia, before 24 weeks severe morbidity of mother develops and survival chance of fetus is less, hence conservative approach is not advisable. In severe preeclampsia at or beyond 34°/7 weeks of gestation, delivery is recommended. When pregnancy is <34 weeks of gestation but with unstable maternal or fetal conditions delivery is planned soon after maternal stabilization. In severe preeclampsia at <34°/7 weeks of gestation with stable maternal and fetal conditions, continuation of pregnancy is undertaken only at facilities with adequate maternal and neonatal intensive care facilities. Injection betamethasone—12 mg intramuscular (IM) two doses 12 hour apart is given for fetal lung maturation. Hypertension is not worsened by corticosteroid. Vaginal delivery with induction of labor is tried when possible.

Flowchart 1: Management of severe preeclampsia.

Approach of management of severe preeclampsia (how would you manage severe preeclampsia)?

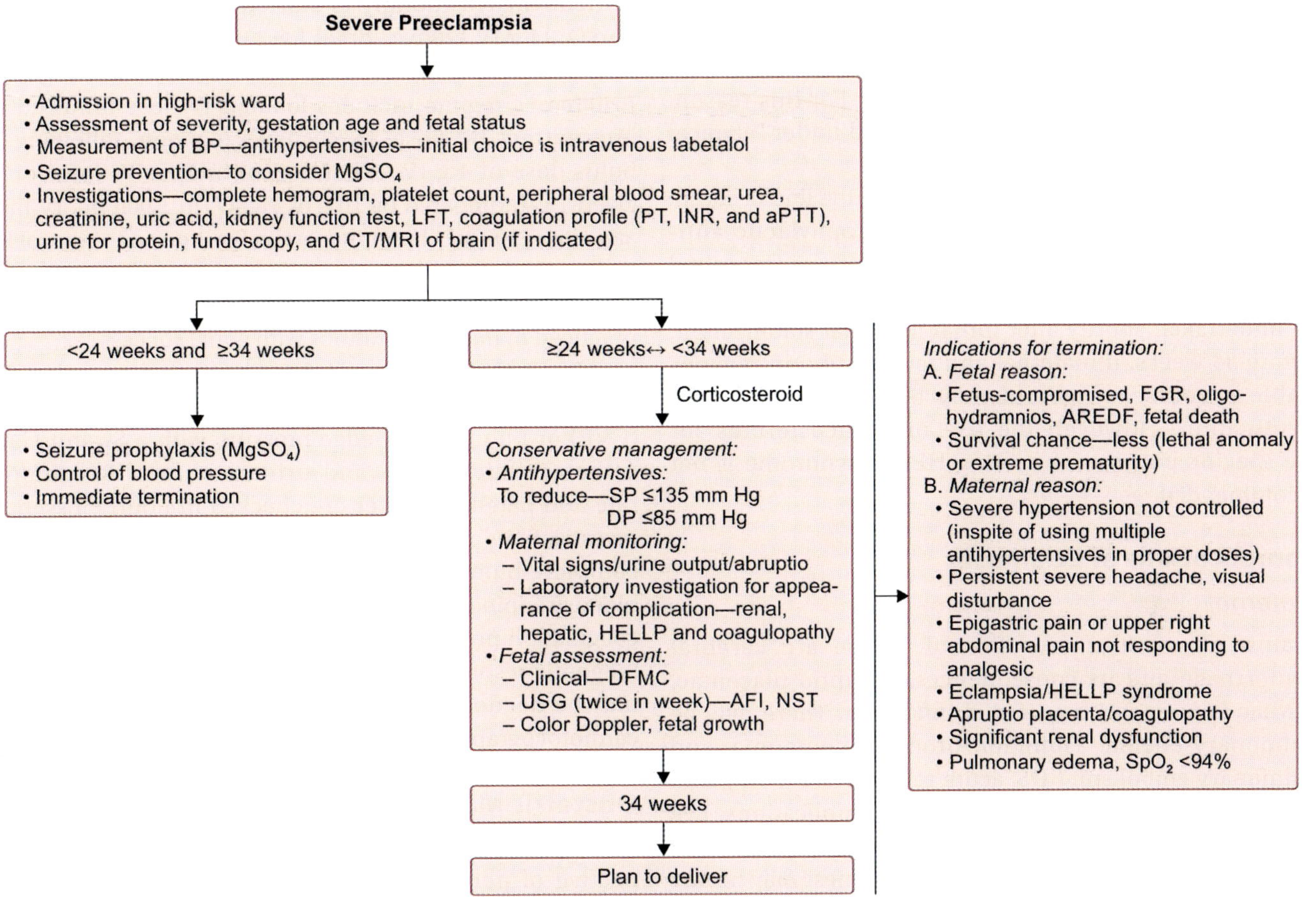

(AREDF: absent or reversed end-diastolic flow; aPTT: activated partial thromboplastin time; AFI: amniotic fluid index; BP: blood pressure; CT: computed tomography; DP: diastolic blood pressure; DFMC: daily fetal movement count; FGR: fetal growth restriction; HELLP: hemolysis, elevated liver enzymes, and low platelets; INR: international normalized ratio; LFT: liver function test; MRI: magnetic resonance imaging; NST: nonstress test; PT: prothombin time; SP: systolic blood pressure; USG: ultrasound)

Indications of cesarean section are when cervix is unfavorable for surgical induction but immediate termination is needed, imminent eclampsia not responding to induction, severe preeclampsia with IUGR. Other indications of cesarean delivery are for obstetric reasons like contracted pelvis, placenta previa, malpresentation, elderly primi, bad obstetric history (BOH), etc.

HELLP SYNDROME

HELLP syndrome is an acronym of *hemolysis, elevated liver enzyme, and low platelet* counts and a subsyndrome of severe form of preeclampsia (Weinstein-1982). It is rare, but may occur up to 10–15% cases of preeclampsia. HELLP syndrome mostly occurs in third trimester, but in 30% cases it is first expressed or progresses postpartum. In 15% cases of HELLP syndrome, there may be insidious and atypical onset without hypertension or proteinuria (ACOG 2020). *Hemolysis* is due to the passage of red cells through partially obliterated vessels (microangiopathic hemolysis), as evidenced by schistocytes in blood smear, hyperbilirubinemia, and absent plasma haptoglobin. *Elevated liver enzymes* are due to liver dysfunction. Serum glutamic-oxaloacetic transaminase (SGOT) or aspartate aminotransferase (AST) and lactate dehydrogenase (LDH) are mostly elevated. LDH increases to 600 IU/L or more. AST and alanine aminotransferase (ALT) increased more than twice the upper limit of normal. *Low platelet count* (100×10^9/L) is a late feature and is probably due to platelet aggregation and platelet deposition at the sites of endothelial damage. In 90% cases presenting symptom is right upper abdominal pain and malaise and in 50% cases there is nausea and vomiting.

It is classified as partial when one or two abnormalities are present and complete when all three abnormalities are present.

Complications of HELLP syndrome: Serious complications are risk of hepatic hematoma and rupture of liver. The other complications are eclampsia, placental abruption, acute kidney injury (AKI), pulmonary edema, stroke, coagulation disorder, acute respiratory distress syndrome (RDS), and sepsis. HELLP syndrome is associated with high perinatal and maternal mortality and once diagnosed, needs aggressive treatment usually by termination of pregnancy. The complication rates of HELLP syndrome are much higher than those of the isolated preeclampsia. For this reason, HELLP syndrome is sometimes described under "atypical preeclampsia—eclampsia" (Sibai 2009).

Management of HELLP syndrome is in the line of severe preeclampsia, *i.e.*, antihypertensive, prophylactic anticonvulsive, close monitoring, and delivery as described above. For women with HELLP syndrome, delivery should be undertaken shortly after initial maternal stabilization. Before 34 weeks, if maternal and fetal condition remains stable a course of steroid may be completed before termination. However, the use of corticosteroids for the specific purpose of treating HELLP syndrome is not recommended.

Complications of Eclampsia

Maternal

Almost all systems are affected. These are cerebral hemorrhage and its consequences, abruptio placentae, cardiac failure, and myocardial infarction. There may be pulmonary edema, aspiration bronchopneumonia, and pulmonary embolism. RDS, acute renal failure (ARF), and hepatic necrosis and DIC are serious complications. Eye complications are blurring of vision scotoma, diplopia, and blindness which is usually reversible. Blindness may be due to retinal detachment or sometimes, as a result of cortical necrosis. Effects of convulsion are injuries to tongue and other parts of body due to fall and aspiration.

In puerperium, patient may develop postpartum shock, sepsis, and psychosis. Residual neurological damage is rare, but may have short- and long-term effects like impaired memory, cognitive functions, cytotoxic edema, infarction, and impaired limb movement.

Case fatality rate in eclampsia varies from 1 to 10%. Causes of maternal death are cerebral hemorrhage and pyrexia (most common cause), cardiac failure, lung complications, e.g., asphyxia due to aspiration, pulmonary edema and bronchopneumonia, renal failure, and postpartum shock and sepsis.

Fetal complications are asphyxia, prematurity—spontaneous or iatrogenic, hypoxia, and fetal death.

Management of Eclampsia

Three basic principles of management of eclampsia are: (1) to control the convulsions and support during convulsions, (2) to reduce BP, and (3) obstetric management.

Tongue spatula is introduced in mouth to prevent tongue bite, suction is given to clear airway passage. Moist oxygen inhalation is given. The patient is kept on a railed cot in dedicated eclampsia room. IV drip 60 to <125 mL/h (80 mL/h) is started with crystalloid (Ringer lactate). Anticonvulsive therapy is started with loading dose of $MgSO_4$ [4 g IV (20 c.c. 20%)] for 3–5 minutes immediately followed by 5 g IM in each buttock (Pritchard regime). Pritchard's regime includes loading IV dose followed by intermittent IM dose. In Zuspan's regimen, following IV bolus dose of 4 g IV as before, continuous IV infusion is given 1 g/h prepared by 10 g of $MgSO_4$ in 1,000 mL IV fluid at a rate of 100 mL/h. Antihypertensive is given to control BP. IV labetalol, hydralazine or nifedipine are the antihypertensives commonly used. Low-dose therapy of $MgSO_4$ is also practiced in many institutions with equal success.

Maternal monitoring is done by recording pulse, BP, respiratory rate, and measuring central venous pressure (CVP) or pulmonary wedge pressure with a Swann-Ganz catheter, fluid intake, and urinary output. Respiratory rate and patellar reflexes are checked in hourly. Essential investigations are arterial blood gas (ABG), urine for albumin, complete blood count, platelet count, peripheral smear, blood grouping, liver function test (LFT), renal function test, coagulation profile, and computed tomography (CT) scan/ magnetic resonance imaging (MRI) of brain and others as may be needed. Fetal monitoring is done by continuous cardiotocography.

Obstetric Management in Eclampsia

Once eclampsia develops pregnancy is terminated irrespective of period of gestation because continuation of pregnancy is dangerous for mother as well as for baby. In many of the cases, patient goes into spontaneous labor. In rest of the cases, termination is done either by induction or by lower segment cesarean section (LUCS). Delivery is planned as soon as possible after stabilization of mother. If there is no spontaneous onset, termination is done by induction or by cesarean section according to the situation.

If patient is in labor, vaginal delivery not contraindicated augmentation with artificial rupture of membranes (ARM) and oxytocin drip is done to hasten the delivery. In case of patient not in labor, route of delivery is determined by: (1) period of gestation, (2) status of cervix (Bishop score), (3) fetal condition, and (4) maternal condition.

When period of gestation is >34 weeks, cervix is favorable, no fetal compromise and no other obstetric complication vaginal delivery is planned by induction with intracervical prostaglandin E2 (PGE2) gel, ARM, and oxytocin.

If period of gestation is <34 weeks, corticosteroid is administered for fetal lung maturity followed by termination. In prematurity, it is unlikely to respond successful rapid induction and cesarean section is indicated.

Cesarean section is indicated in very unfavorable cervix where induction is unlikely to be successful, prematurity, fetal compromise, fetal growth restriction, and obstetric reasons like abruptio placentae and malpresentation, induction failure, and slow progress of labor.

The details have been described in author's *Bedside Clinics in Obstetrics*, fifth edition revised reprint 2022 published by Academic publishers, Kolkata.

AMNIOTIC FLUID EMBOLISM

When amniotic fluid enters into the maternal circulation, AFE may occur.

It is a catastrophic event in obstetrics and often fatal, and characterized by the *classic triads*, namely acute onset of respiratory distress, sudden hemodynamic compromise, and coagulopathy (DIC).

Amniotic fluid embolism usually occurs (1) following ARM, (2) in late labor or immediate postpartum period, and (3) during cesarean delivery or immediately after it and rarely during external version.

Risk factors of AFE are induction of labor, multiple pregnancy, cervical and vaginal laceration, and cesarean section.

Etiopathology is exactly not known. Multiple small emboli enter inside the lungs and pulmonary pressure is increased. Fibrin clots and amniotic emboli are formed inside the vessels. In some cases, the reaction of anaphylaxis is evident.

Causes of DIC in AFE—thromboplastin like material is liberated in AFE which leads to activation of factor X, which in turn activates factor X, which activates thrombin. C1 esterase inhibitor (C1INH) is another marker to identify AFE which becomes low.

Incidence is 1 in 30,000 pregnancies.

Diagnosis of Amniotic Fluid Embolism

Diagnosis is very difficult and sudden peripartum collapse followed by death is the usual scenario.

Diagnostic criteria (Clark et al., 2016) are (1) sudden onset of cardiorespiratory arrest, or both hypotension and respiratory compromise, (2) DIC (coagulopathy) must be detected prior to sufficient blood loss, (3) clinically detected during labor or within 30 minutes of delivery of placenta, and (4) no fever. There is no specific diagnostic investigation marker to confirm AFE, it is solely clinical diagnosis.

Clinical Presentations

Symptoms are respiratory distress and acute severe chest pain. Physical findings are tachycardia, tachypnea, hypotension, cyanosis, pulmonary edema/bronchospasm, peripheral collapse, hemorrhage from multiple sites due to coagulation failure, and consumptive coagulopathy (DIC). There may be convulsion due to cerebral anoxia or cardiac arrest and sudden death.

Investigations suggested are coagulation screening, electrocardiography (ECG)—right ventricular strain, ABG analysis—reduced O_2 tension.

Diagnosis is only confirmed at postmortem. Emboli of vernix and abundant squamous cells are found in pulmonary vessels.

Management

Intubation and mechanical ventilation with 100% oxygen are immediately done. Resuscitation and circulatory support (advance cardiac support) are given. Extracorporeal membrane oxygenation (ECMO) is suggested (2020) for management of AFE. Hydrocortisone and dopamine are administered. Treatment of coagulation failure is done by whole blood, platelets, and fresh frozen plasma (FFP). Patient is shifted to intensive care unit (ICU).

Prognosis is very poor. Overall survival rate is 10%. Maternal death is more common after cesarean delivery than vaginal delivery. In an average, 30% mothers die within an hour.

OBSTETRIC SHOCK

Definition

Shock is a clinical condition characterized by inadequate tissue perfusion and resulting from inability of the circulatory system to meet the tissue demands of oxygen and nutrients and to remove metabolites.

Types and Causes

Hemorrhagic shock (excessive blood loss) may be due to: (1) bleeding in early pregnancy, (2) antepartum hemorrhage, and (3) PPH.

Septic shock (endotoxic shock): Generalized vascular disturbance due to release of toxins due to various causes.

Neurogenic shock (painful conditions) may be due to disturbed ectopic pregnancy, concealed accidental hemorrhage, forceps, or breech extraction before full cervical dilatation. Rupture uterus, acute inversion of uterus, and intrauterine manipulation including internal podalic version and Crédé's method of placental removal are other causes.

Cardiogenic shock: Myocardial infarction and heart failure

Anaphylactic shock: Caused by sensitivity to drugs.

Other causes are (1) embolism—amniotic fluid, air, or thrombus and (2) anesthetic complications as Mendelson's syndrome.

Classic Clinical Picture of Shock

Pallor, rapid, weak and thready pulse, low BP, oliguria or anuria, cold clammy extremities, cyanosis, air hunger, and restlessness.

HEMORRHAGIC SHOCK

Classification of Hemorrhage

Depending on the amount of blood loss hemorrhage can be classified in four classes, namely class I (15% blood loss), II (20–25%), III (30–35%), and IV (40–45%). In class I, vitals are normal with normal pulse and BP. In stage IV there is profound hypotension, carotid pulse palpable only, and reversible shock.

Phases of Hemorrhagic Shock

There are three phases: (1) phase of compensation, (2) phase of decompensation, and (3) phase of cellular damage and danger of death.

Management of Hemorrhagic Shock

Urgent interference is indicated, preferably in HDU. Arrest of hemorrhage by detecting the cause is the priority. Airway establishment and oxygen administration by mask or endotracheal tube are done. Legs are elevated to encourage return of blood from the lower limbs to the central circulation.

Two or more IV access with large bore needle are started for administration of blood, fluids (crystalloids and colloids), and drugs.

Analgesics is given if there is pain, tissue damage, or irritability. Role of corticosteroids and its mode of action are controversial; it may decrease peripheral resistance and potentiate cardiac response so it improves tissue perfusion. Sodium bicarbonate is administered, if metabolic acidosis is demonstrated.

Vasopressors are given to increase the BP, so as to maintain renal perfusion.

Monitoring is done by measurement of CVP, pulse rate, BP, urine output, and pulmonary and capillary wedge pressure (PCWP). Clinical improvement is assessed by improvement of pallor, cyanosis, air hunger, sweating, and consciousness.

Complications of hemorrhagic shock are ARF, pituitary necrosis (Sheehan's syndrome), and DIC.

SEPTIC SHOCK (ENDOTOXIC SHOCK) SYN: ENDOTOXIC SHOCK/BACTEREMIC SHOCK/ SEPTICEMIC SHOCK

Septic shock has been defined as systemic inflammatory response due to infection causing hypotension which persists after adequate fluid resuscitation with or without lactic acidosis, oliguria or an acute alteration in mental state (The American College of Chest Physicians and the Society of Critical Care Medicine).

Sepsis is defined as infection plus systemic manifestation of infection. Severe sepsis is caused when sepsis is associated with organ dysfunction or tissue hypoperfusion. Septic shock is the persistence of hypoperfusion in spite of adequate fluid replacement therapy.

Causes of Septic Shock

The causes are septic abortion, prolonged rupture of membranes, manipulations and instrumentations, trauma, retained placental tissues, puerperal sepsis, severe acute pyelonephritis, etc.

Pathogenesis of Septic Shock

Septic shock begins when organisms (commonly gram-negative organisms, *Escherichia coli, Klebsiella, Proteus mirabilis, Pseudomonas aeruginosa*) proliferate locally and invade the maternal circulation, where various exotoxins (lipoprotein-carbohydrate complex) are released. Exotoxins interact with leukocytes and endothelial cells, causing release of different mediators such as cytokines, platelet activating factor, nitric oxide, prostaglandins, leukotrienes, and tissue necrosis factor which are thought to be responsible for various clinical manifestations.

Organisms involved are gram-positive (30–50%), gram-negative (25–30%), fungus (1–3%), and virus (2.4%) are parasite (1–3%).

Most of the genital tract infections are polymicrobial.

Aerobes-gram positive: Group A *Streptococcus*, Group B *Streptococcus*, *Staphylococcus*. *Gram negative*: *E. coli*, *Klebsiella*, and *Pseudomonas*.

Anaerobes—anaerobic *Streptococcus, Bacteroides*, and *Clostridia*.

Phases of Endotoxic Shock

Reversible stage: It has two phases: (1) Early (warm) phase: Hypotension, tachycardia, pyrexia, rigors, flushed skin, patient is alert, and leukocytosis develops within hours and (2) *Late (cold) phase:* Cold and clammy skin, mottled cyanosis, purpura, jaundice, progressive mental confusion, and coma.

Irreversible stage: Prolonged cellular hypoxia leads to—metabolic acidosis, ARF, cardiac failure, pulmonary edema, adrenal failure, multiorgan failure, and ultimately death.

Management of Endotoxic Shock

Restoration of Circulatory Function and Oxygenation

Replacement of blood loss is done by whole blood; if not available, then colloids or crystalloids should be started. CVP measurement is essential to guard against circulatory overload. Corticosteroids—(hydrocortisone or dexamethasone) is given. β-adrenergic stimulants—isoprenaline—cause arteriolar dilatation, increase in heart rate and stroke volume, thus improving tissue perfusion. Blood volume must be normal prior to its administration. Oxygen is administered, if respiratory function is impaired. Administration of aminophylline improves respiratory function by alleviating bronchospasm.

Eradication of infection is done by antibiotics and surgery, if needed.

Endotoxin is released by lysis of cell envelope of gram-negative bacilli like *E. coli*, *Proteus*, *Pseudomonas*, bacteroides and exotoxin by β-hemolytic streptococci, anaerobic streptococci, and clostridia.

Antibiotic therapy: Swabs and blood for culture and sensitivity are taken first. Antibiotic is started immediately and should be given by intravenous route before waiting for the result of culture and sensitivity report. The therapy should cover the wide range of organisms. Regimen 1—ampicillin or cephalosporines (500–1,000 mg 6 hourly), gentamycin and metronidazole (500 mg 8 hourly) and regimen 2—clindamycin (600 mg 6 hourly) and gentamycin (80 mg 8 hourly).

Surgical treatment: Surgery is indicated when there is retained infected tissues as in septic abortion. It should be removed as soon as antibiotic therapy and resuscitative measures have been started. Suction evacuation, digital evacuation or hysterectomy in advanced infection with a gangrenous (*Clostridium Welchii*) or traumatized uterus are the usual options.

Correction of Fluid and Electrolyte Deficits

Extensive monitoring in HDU is required. General nursing care and frequent change of position are of utmost importance. Establishment of IV access and Foley catheterization with maintenance of intake-output chart is done. Regular measurements of ABG and electrolytes and correction, if needed, are of vital importance for the management.

Prevention of DIC: Prophylactic heparin therapy is started as and when indicated in high-risk conditions.

ACUTE KIDNEY INJURY IN OBSTETRICS

Acute kidney injury, previously known as acute renal failure (ARF), is defined as the sudden impairment of kidney function, resulting in reduction of urine volume, thus leading to an increase in the plasma or serum creatinine, other nitrogenous and waste products. Incidence of ARF in pregnancy is less and prognosis is relatively better due to current management.

Acute renal failure may be: (1) prerenal, (2) renal, and (3) postrenal due to obstruction.

Causes of Acute Kidney Injury in Obstetrics

Early pregnancy causes are hemorrhage due to abortion, ruptured ectopic pregnancy, hydatidiform mole, severe volume depletion due to hyperemesis gravidarum, ovarian hyperstimulation syndrome, and septicemia in septic abortion.

Causes in late pregnancy and peripartum are hemorrhage in abruptio placentae, placenta previa, PPH; hypertension for preeclampsia/HELLP syndrome, eclampsia; infection—chorioamnionitis, puerperal sepsis, obstruction in the renal tract due to renal calculi, ureteric damage in cesarean hysterectomy, and ruptured uterus. Other causes are AFE, acute fatty liver of pregnancy (AFLP), hemolytic uremic syndrome, thrombotic thrombocytopenic purpura, and drugs like nonsteroidal anti-inflammatory drug (NSAID) and aminoglycosides.

The common causes of ARF in pregnancy are severe preeclampsia/eclampsia, obstetric hemorrhage—abruptio placentae, PPH, septicemia, and hyperemesis gravidarum.

Pathophysiology

Acute prerenal insult like dehydration, hemorrhage, or septic shock may develop into renal cortical necrosis with permanent renal impairment, if inadequately treated. Risk increases in presence of consumptive coagulopathy or preeclampsia/HELLP syndrome. Prerenal failure is caused by moderate degrees of renal ischemia and if renal perfusion is restored adequately, it is reversible. Renal cortical necrosis is now uncommon.

Acute tubular necrosis is caused by more prolonged renal ischemia and changes limited to the tubular cells and it occurs commonly. It is also reversible. Acute cortical necrosis results from more severe renal ischemia that causes diffuse renal cortical necrosis with permanent renal impairment. It is difficult to diagnose in early phase between acute tubular necrosis and acute cortical necrosis.

Obstructive renal failure may rarely develop due to bilateral ureteral compression by a very large pregnant uterus or ureteric injury.

Diagnosis

Diagnosis is based on diminished urinary output, revealing the etiology, clinical symptoms, and signs and blood values.

A careful history may reveal poor fluid intake or fluid loss (hemorrhage, diarrhea, and vomiting), intake of nephrotoxic drugs, heart failure, recent blood transfusion, history of severe preeclampsia/eclampsia.

Urine output becomes less initially. ARF passes in three phases: (1) Phase of oliguria or anuria, (2) phase of diuresis or polyuria, and (3) phase of recovery.

1. *Phase of oliguria/anuria*: Oliguria means urine output usually <400–500 mL in 24 hours. In cases of anuria (absence of excretion of urine to <100 mL in 24 hours) urinary tract obstruction must be excluded first.
2. *Polyuria or phase of diuresis*: Following oliguric or anuric phase, there is markedly increase in urine output lasting for several days. During this phase, renal tubular cells start recovering, but not able to concentrate urine.

   Plasma urea and creatinine levels usually continue to raise.

3. *Recovery phase:* Urine output tends toward normal. The concentrating power gradually returns to normal.

Initially, patient may not experience any symptom, but gradually develops anorexia, nausea, vomiting, mental changes, abdominal distension, and shortness of breath. Physical examination may reveal features of shock, peripheral edema, pericardial or pleural rub, and pulmonary rales. Concentration of plasma urea, creatinine, potassium, and phosphate rise gradually. The plasma concentration of bicarbonate and calcium decrease with simultaneous increase in magnesium concentration.

Management of Acute Kidney Injury in Pregnancy

Principles of Management

Identification and correction of the precipitating insult and optimal fluid balance should be done. Monitoring is best done by measurement of the CVP and ideally by pulmonary artery wedge pressure. Dose of drugs, e.g., magnesium sulfate, aminoglycosides, NSAIDs, and iodine-containing contrast agents, are adjusted. Dialysis is started after evaluation of indication (see below).

As in majority of the cases AKI develops in postpartum period, there is no issue on fetal problems in such cases.

Correction of the Precipitating Insult and Prevention of Acute Renal Failure

Termination of pregnancies is done in severe preeclampsia/eclampsia. Correction of hypovolemia by blood product and whole blood transfusion in massive hemorrhage, such as in abruptio placentae, placental previa, uterine rupture, and PPH. Septic syndrome is detected early and to start antibiotics to control sepsis, e.g., septic abortion, pyelonephritis, chorioamnionitis, urinary tract infection (UTI), and other pelvic infections. Diuretic is not started before correction of hypervolemia so that cardiac output is sufficient for renal perfusion. Vasoconstrictor should not be given until and unless it is evident that vasodilation is the cause of the hypotension.

Fluid Balance and Monitoring

Fluid balance is the most crucial in the management of ARF. Monitoring is done by clinical examination and thorough biochemical markers. Volume overload is prevented by restriction of fluid and sodium and with the use of diuretics. Dialysis may be avoided in some cases, if diuretic is used timely. *Furosemide* may be given as a bolus (200 mg) followed by an IV drip at a rate of 10–40 mg/h in cases of severe volume overload.

Dopamine may be used in low doses to increase salt and water excretion.

Calculation of fluid—insensible water loss (the amount of fluid lost from the lungs, skin, respiratory tract, and in the feces) is estimated to be in an adult is about 800 mL/day under normal circumstances (from skin 400 mL and respiratory tract about 400 mL). Metabolic water production by endogenous oxidation is considered to be 400 mL/day. Thus, to maintain adequate fluid balance approximately 500 mL of fluid plus the amount lost by vomitus, gastric aspirate or due to diarrhea should be replaced daily. A further fluid supplementation is needed, if there is any urine output, hot climate, or raised body temperature.

Monitoring—in anuric phase, it is very much important to assess intravascular volume. An indwelling bladder catheter and a CVP line should be established. A separate IV line should also be established for IV therapy and intake output should be carefully monitored. Blood parameters (complete blood count, urea, creatinine, electrolytes, and acid–base status) are monitored routinely and urine sample examination one as needed. In diuresis phase, fluid supplementation is done on the basis of total urine output in previous 24 hours plus 500 mL. Salt supplementation is usually needed in this stage to compensate increase urinary loss. In recovery phase, fluid replacement is totally guided by patients need. Nutrition is maintained by avoiding negative nitrogen balance and supplementation of adequate calorie.

Obstetric management: Timing and route of delivery must be considered according to the clinical condition of the patient. Pregnancy termination should be considered in patients who need dialysis for renal failure.

Evaluation for need of dialysis: Persistent oliguria, deteriorating renal function, or fluid overload are the indications for renal replacement therapy.

Hemodialysis

When oliguria continues and there is persistent high level of creatinine, dialysis is the treatment of choice. Early dialysis improves the prognosis dramatically and renal function usually returns to normal.

Prognosis

Acute renal failure following postabortal sepsis, severe preeclampsia/HELLP syndrome or abruptio placentae has poor maternal outcome as they are often associated with bilateral renal cortical necrosis which causes irreversible renal damage. As ARF in pregnancy is mostly due to obstetric-related problems and not due to chronic renal disease, prognosis is relatively better if diagnosed early and quick management is done.

In spite of significant improvement, maternal mortality still now is in the range of 15–20% and perinatal mortality ranges from 30 to 70% according to the severity of the illness.

DISSEMINATED INTRAVASCULAR COAGULATION

Disseminated intravascular coagulation is a serious acquired disorder in obstetrics. DIC is associated with 25% of maternal deaths globally and associated with severe maternal morbidity like AKI. Incidence of DIC in obstetrics is not very high and it is 0.03–0.35%.

De Lee in 1901 described this entity in a woman in abruptio placentae and in another woman with prolong retained dead fetus.

Disseminated intravascular coagulation or consumptive coagulopathy or defibrination syndrome occurs when there is consumption of procoagulants within the intravascular system. Due to *intravascular activation of coagulation* natural hemostasis mechanism is disrupted with imbalance of natural anticoagulant mechanism which results fibrin (microthrombi) deposition leading to multiorgan failure.

When there is a huge loss of procoagulants due to bleeding, it is called *dilutional coagulopathy*. Treatment with crystalloids and packed red blood cells (PRBC) in massive hemorrhage depletion of platelets and coagulation factors occur leading to dilutional coagulopathy which is indistinguishable from DIC (consumptive coagulopathy), however, treatment for both is same.

Causes of Disseminated Intravascular Coagulation in Obstetrics

Abruptio placentae is the most common cause of severe consumptive coagulopathy (DIC) and most probably in entire spectrum of medicine. Consumptive coagulopathy is more in concealed type as due to pressure by retroplacental clot, more thromboplastin is drained into large veins. DIC is seen in 37% cases of severe abruptio. Other clinical obstetric conditions which may be complicated with DIC are AFE, AFLP, severe preeclampsia, eclampsia, HELLP syndrome, intrauterine fetal death (IUFD), massive PPH, placenta accreta spectrum, sepsis syndrome, cesarean section, massive blood transfusion (old blood), molar pregnancy, ruptured uterus, and intra-amniotic hypertonic saline. DIC is found in 15% cases of HELLP syndrome and uncommon in preeclampsia without HELLP syndrome.

Pathophysiology of Disseminated Intravascular Coagulation

The process of DIC starts with activation of tissue factor (TF) which is found in subendothelial cells, amniotic fluid, and placenta. Proinflammatory cytokines [interleukin-6 (IL-6), IL-1, and tumor necrosis factor-α] which are released causes increased expression of TF which in turn results activation of factors VII and X, which results fibrin formation. Normally, this coagulation process is checked by natural anticoagulant proteins—protein C, protein S, and antithrombin (AT). Due to increased consumption and degradation and decreased synthesis, these proteins are markedly decreased in DIC. Newly synthesized fibrinogen is converted to fibrin and fibrin degradation products (FDPs). This fibrinolysis is facilitated by plasminogen converted into plasmin by thrombin. Plasminogen activator inhibitor 1 (PAI1) inhibits fibrinolytic activity. Elevated PAI1 is found in DIC. Platelets and leukocytes are also activated enhancing fibrin formation by the activation of TF. Hemorrhage and coagulation defect both occurs in DIC though attention is given to hemorrhage primarily by the obstetrician.

Tissue damage causes (1) release of *thromboplastin* which results in fibrin clot formation with depletion of fibrin and (2) release of plasminogen activator which causes lysis of clot formation. Both these factors (1) cause coagulation defect due to depletion of fibrinogen and (2) increase fibrinolysis and formation of FDP including D-dimer resulting in increase in hemorrhage.

Diagnosis of Disseminated Intravascular Coagulation

There is presence of underlying etiology, blood loss, bleeding from venepuncture sites, nose bleeding, gum bleeding, hematuria, and bleeding from any operative site and PPH following delivery in hard-contracted uterus in absence of any trauma. There may be features of shock and hypotension. Bleeding time, clotting time, clot observation test, and peripheral smear are done.

Other conventional laboratory investigations are plasma fibrinogen estimations, plasma FDP (evidence of fibrinolysis), D-dimer, platelet count, activated partial thromboplastin time (aPTT)—intrinsic coagulation, prothrombin time (PT)—extrinsic coagulation and thrombin time. Low-platelet count is an important diagnostic feature of DIC. Other causes of low-platelet count in pregnancy are gestational thrombocytopenia, preeclampsia, HELLP syndrome, or idiopathic thrombocytopenic purpura.

D-dimer is one of the end products of fibrin degradation. In both acute and chronic DIC, it is increased.

Thrombin time assay measures the clotting pathway from conversion of fibrinogen to fibrin. Due to formation of thrombin–AT complexes, AT levels are decreased. The tests are repeated at a minimum interval of 6–12 hours.

Serum markers, values, and their changes in DIC are given in the **Table 1**.

Scoring for Diagnosis of Disseminated Intravascular Coagulation

Various scoring systems have been developed to define uniform definition of DIC. Currently three scoring systems

TABLE 1: Serum markers, values, and their changes in disseminated intravascular coagulation (DIC).

Tests	*Normal values in pregnancy*	*Values in DIC*
Plasma fibrinogen	• 300–600 mg/dL (physiological increase) • Normal average prepregnancy level 250 mg increases by 50% in pregnancy average level 450 mg	<150 mg/dL. May as low as 100 mg/mL
PT	9.5–13.5 seconds	Prolonged >1.5 × mean control
aPTT	22.6–38.9 seconds	Prolonged >1.5 × mean control
INR	0.80–1.09	Increased
Thrombin time	16.5 ± 2.4 seconds	Prolonged
D-dimer	0.05–1.7 µg/mL	Increased
FDP	<40 µg/mL	Increased
Antithrombin III	76–128%	Decreased
Platelet count	140–400 × 10^9/L	Decreased. Also decreased in gestational thrombocytopenia, preeclampsia, HELLP syndrome, or ITP

(aPTT: activated partial thromboplastin time; FDP: fibrin degradation product; HELLP: hemolysis, elevated liver enzymes, and low platelets; ITP: idiopathic thrombocytopenic purpura; INR: international normalized ratio; PT: prothombin time)

are in use: (1) International Society of Thrombosis and Hemostasis (ISTH 2001), (2) Japan Association of Acute Medicine (JAAM 2005), and (3) Pregnancy-modified scoring system by Erez (2014).

Scoring system is based on the common tests, e.g., PT, aPTT, plasma fibrinogen, D-dimer, and FDPs. Other workers used only fibrinogen, platelet count, and PT difference.

Management of Obstetrical Disseminated Intravascular Coagulation

Disseminated intravascular coagulation should always be based on multidisciplinary approach. Hematologist and critical care specialist are consulted for management.

Fluid balance is restored. Choice of fluid is crystalloids and Hartman's solution before blood and blood products are available. Principle is to transfuse volume two to three times more than the estimated blood loss.

Blood and blood products are transfused to replace coagulation factors in consumptive coagulopathy and transfusion is also needed in acute bleeding. The guideline is in the ratio of 1:1:1 of FFP, PRBC transfusion, and platelets. FFP is started immediately to correct coagulation in bleeding patient irrespective of Rh type. Cryoprecipitate in a dose of 10–15 mL/kg is given to correct hypofibrinogenemia, commonly found in DIC. At least 10 units of cryoprecipitate is needed when fibrinogen level is <100 mg/dL to raise >200 mg/dL. There is risk of transmission of viral infections with cryoprecipitate. To avoid risk of bleeding platelet count is maintained ≥50,000. Target value of Hb is 7 g/dL. For the treatment of hypovolemia, due to catastrophic hemorrhage compatible whole blood is the ideal but may not be readily available. Shelf life of whole blood is 24 days. 70% remain functioning for 24 hours after transfusion. Three to four volume percent of hematocrit increases (equivalent to 1 g% Hb) for one unit of whole blood **(Table 2)**. After five units or more transfusion of RBC platelet count, clotting tests, and fibrinogen should be evaluated.

Massive transfusion means 8–10 units or more transfusion within 24 hours.

Tranexamic acid is an antifibrinolytic agent that reduces blood loss by inhibiting enzyme breakdown of fibrinogen and fibrin by plasmin. It is not used in renal impairment patient as it is cleared by kidney. It is used early in hemorrhages, no clinical data for use in obstetric-related DIC is available (WOMAN trial).

Other hemostatic agents under consideration are fibrinogen concentrate, human recombinant thrombomodulin (rhTM), activated recombinant factor VII, AT III, and prothombin complexes.

Treatment of underlying cause: Immediate delivery is indicated in abruptio placentae, IUFD, and HELLP syndrome. Any surgical cause of hemorrhage is ruled out. Antibiotic is given in sepsis.

Supportive care: To avoid tissue hypoxia adequate tissue perfusion is done.

Massive transfusion protocol and blood product replacement are the essential tool in management in obstetric hemorrhage with DIC.

BLOOD AND BLOOD PRODUCTS

Packed red blood cell has very little amount of soluble coagulation factors and in stored whole blood, there is deficiency of platelets and factors V, VIII, and XI. Massive transfusion with RBCs only without the factor replacement, hypofibrinogenemia and prolongation of PT and PTT occur.

TABLE 2: Blood products—characteristics, indications, effects, and complications.

Blood product	***Contents in each unit***	***Volume/unit***	***Indications***	***Effects***	***Complications***
Whole blood	RBCs, plasma, and fibrinogen (500–700 mg), no platelet	500 mL	Hypovolemia from catastrophic hemorrhage	• Blood volume and fibrinogen are restored • Hematocrit increased 3–4% by volume in each unit	• Hemolytic reaction, infection, and TRALI • Human error
pRBCs	Mainly RBCs, no platelet, minimum fibrinogen	300 mL	Hematocrit <18 Hematocrit <30 in unstable patient or active bleeding	Hematocrit* increased 3% in each unit	• Hemolytic reaction, infection, and TRALI • Human error
FFP	600–700 mg fibrinogen, colloid, no platelets	250 mL	• INR >2 × normal • aPTT >1.5 × normal • Massive: 1:1 with RBC	Fibrinogen raised by 10–15 mg/dL/unit	• Hemolytic reaction, infection, and TRALI • Human error
Platelets	One unit raises platelet count 5,000/µL	50 mL	• Platelets count < 50,000 • Massive transfusion: 1:1 with RBC • Microvascular bleeding	To raise 30,000/µL at least 6 units required	• Hemolytic reaction, infection, and TRALI • Human error
Cryoprecipitate	200 mg fibrinogen, other clotting factors per unit, no platelet	40 mL	Fibrinogen <100 mg/dL	Fibrinogen increases by 10–15 mg/dL/unit	• Hemolytic reaction, infection, and TRALI • Human error

(aPTT: activated partial thromboplastin time; FFP: fresh frozen plasma; INR: international normalized ratio; pRBCs: packed red blood cells; TRALI: transfusion related acute lung injury)

*The ratio of hematocrit to Hb is 3:1. Increase of 3% hematocrit is considered as 1 g% Hb increase.

Thrombocytopenia is also most common coagulation defect in blood loss and in multiple transfusions. This "dilutional coagulopathy" is indistinguishable from DIC (consumptive coagulopathy) as later may also occur in obstetric hemorrhage, however, treatment for both is same.

Table 2 shows the contents, indications, effects, and complications of transfusion of one unit of blood or blood products.

Obstetric hemorrhages of different etiologies are discussed in respective chapters. (Chapter 3 Early Pregnancy Procedure, Chapter10 Antepartum Hemorrhage, Chapter 11 PAS, Chapter 17 Rectus Sheath Hematoma, Chapter 20 Inversion of Uterus, and Chapter 21 Genital Tract Injuries). Other details are available in author's *Bedside Clinics in Obstetrics*, fifth edition revised reprint 2022 published by Academic Publishers, Kolkata.

CHAPTER 3

Early Pregnancy Procedures: Abortion—Spontaneous and Induced

Learning Objectives

- Definition and Terminology
- Classification of Abortion
- Spontaneous Abortion
- Different Methods of Evacuation of Uterus
- Induced Abortion—Medical Termination of Pregnancy
- Medical Abortion
- Septic Abortion
- Medical Termination of Pregnancy Act of India Following its Amendments 2021

INTRODUCTION

Surgical method for abortion is a well-known procedure for a long time with little changes, but many medications have been added and introduced both for induced or spontaneous abortions. The incidence of spontaneous abortion varies from 10 to 15% which occurs more in earlier gestations. After legalization of abortion in most of the countries the incidence of safe abortion has been increased and the subsequent complications both morbidity and morbidity from unsafe abortion have been significantly decreased. Very recently (2021), India has widened the scope of medical termination of pregnancy (MTP) in some special situations. In country like United States following recent Supreme Court verdict on restriction on induced abortion a lot of hue and cry is going on. According to the present National Family Health Survey-5 (NFHS-5) (2019–2021) report overall contraceptive prevalence rate (CPR) of India has increased substantially from 54 to 67%. Total unmet Need for Family Planning (currently married women age 15–49 years) is 9.4% and unmet need for spacing is 4.0%. Therefore, unintended pregnancy occurs in a significant number of Indian women who either seek for MTP or the pregnancy may end in unwanted childbirth, where many younger women are involved. According to NFHS-5 (2019–21), 23.3% women surveyed got married before attaining the legal age of 18 years and teenage pregnancies are 6.8%. A significant number of women with unwanted pregnancies opt for induced abortion. Procedures involved in induced abortion and also for spontaneous should be safe and service providers should have thorough knowledge.

DEFINITION AND TERMINOLOGY

"Abortion is the termination of pregnancy, either spontaneously or intentionally, before the fetus develops sufficiently to survive." In order to survive, the fetus must weigh 500 g. The fetus of 500 g corresponds to 22 weeks of pregnancy in developing country and 20 weeks in developed country. Previously, the age of viability was considered as 28 weeks of pregnancy. With improvement of neonatal care, the age of viability is decreased. According to Royal College of Obstetricians and Gynaecologists (RCOG), the limit of viability is considered at 24 weeks of pregnancy. Hence, the definition of abortion varies according to state laws for reporting abortions, fetal death, and neonatal death.

World Health Organization (WHO) defines abortion as pregnancy termination or loss before 20 weeks' gestation or with a fetus delivered weighing <500 g. The terms "miscarriage" and "abortion" are very often used interchangeably. However, for layperson, abortion is popularly used as intended pregnancy termination but miscarriage always implies spontaneous loss. The age old definition of abortion—"*it is the expulsion or extraction of a fetus or embryo weighing <500 g*". One important point needs to be clarified in the definition of abortion. In all types of abortion cases, expulsion of product of conception does not occur. Like, in threatened abortion there is no expulsion of product, instead there is a chance of continuation of pregnancy.

CLASSIFICATION OF ABORTION

Abortion is broadly classified into: (1) spontaneous abortion and (2) induced abortion.

Spontaneous abortion can be subdivided into: (1) threatened abortion, (2) inevitable abortion, (3) incomplete abortion, and (4) complete abortion.

Missed abortion and recurrent abortion are special varieties of spontaneous abortion.

Induced abortion can be subdivided into (1) MTP where all legal procedures are maintained and (2) criminal abortion, also called illegal abortion. Most of the criminal abortions are unsafe abortion.

Septic abortion: Any type of abortion which becomes complicated with infection, as clinically evident is called septic abortion.

SPONTANEOUS ABORTION

Abortion occurring without medical or mechanical means to empty the uterus is referred as spontaneous abortion. Spontaneous abortion is also called miscarriage. Majority (80%) of spontaneous miscarriage occurs within first 12 weeks of pregnancy. It has been found that in some conceptions in about one-fifth of cases conception is diagnosed by elevated by serum human chorionic gonadotropin (hCG) levels and there is no clinical manifestation of pregnancy loss, but diagnosed by decrease of serum β-hCG levels, these are called biochemical pregnancy loss. Many factors are responsible for abortion. The most important factors in early pregnancy are fetal factors of which genetic factors due to chromosomal abnormality either numeral (aneuploidy) or structural are most common (50–60%). Important maternal factors are uncontrolled diabetes mellitus, thyroid disease, systemic lupus erythematosus (SLE), infections, mullerian defects, cervical incompetence, immunological, complicated laparotomy, and environmental factors. In significant number of cases of spontaneous abortion no cause could be detected.

Threatened Abortion (Figs. 1 and 2)

Threatened abortion is the type of spontaneous abortion where there is a possibility of continuation of pregnancy.

Inevitable Abortion (Figs. 3 and 4)

Inevitable abortion is the type of abortion where the expulsion of product of conception is inevitable as evidenced by dilatation of cervical os but still there is no expulsion, but may have severe hemorrhage necessitating urgent evacuation.

Incomplete Abortion (Fig. 5)

Incomplete abortion is the kind of abortion where part of the product of conception has been expelled but some parts are retained within the uterus. It may be spontaneous or sequelae of induced abortion. Bleeding and potentiality of sepsis warrant immediate intervention.

Complete Abortion

Complete abortion is the type of abortion where the product of conception has been expelled completely.

Missed Abortion

In *missed abortion* **(Fig. 6)** the fetus is dead and retained inside the uterus for a variable period of time. *Carneous mole* is one type of missed abortion before 12 weeks where repeated small hemorrhage in the choriodecidual space separates the fetus from the uterine wall and the fetus usually dies and becomes a mole-like structure. It is also called blood mole or fleshy mole. The treatment is same as that of missed abortion. *Blighted ovum* (anembryonic miscarriage) **(Fig. 7)** is the ultrasonographic diagnosis of abortion where there is absence of fetal pole in the gestation sac (anembryonic sac). The diameter of gestation sac should be 3 cm or more.

Recurrent Abortion

Recurrent abortion or recurrent miscarriage (habitual abortion) refers to three or more consecutive spontaneous abortions. Induced abortion is not included in recurrent abortion or recurrent miscarriage. The pregnancy is <20 weeks or with a fetal weight <500 g. The American Society for Reproductive Medicine (2020) defines recurrent pregnancy loss as two or more failed clinical pregnancies confirmed by either sonographic or histopathological reports. *Recurrent pregnancy loss* is a broader term which includes recurrent abortion and also the pregnancy wastages in later months of pregnancy.

In majority of the cases (two-thirds) of threatened abortion there is continuation of pregnancy however, there is increased chance of placenta previa, abruptio placentae, prematurity, premature rupture of membrane (PROM), fetal growth restriction (FGR) or fetal anomaly, and increase fetal and neonatal death. In rest of the cases (one-third) of

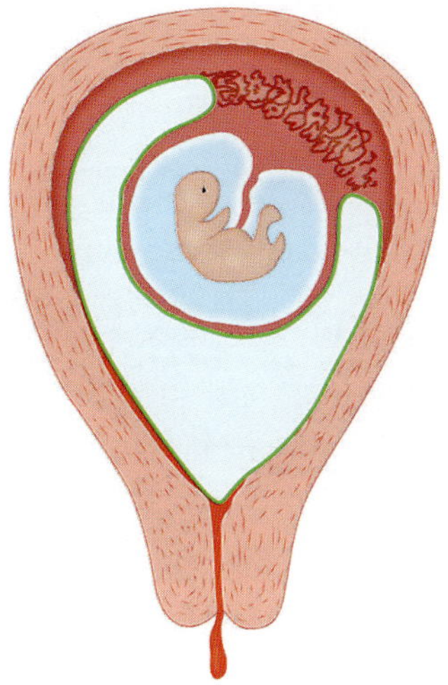

Fig. 1: Threatened abortion.

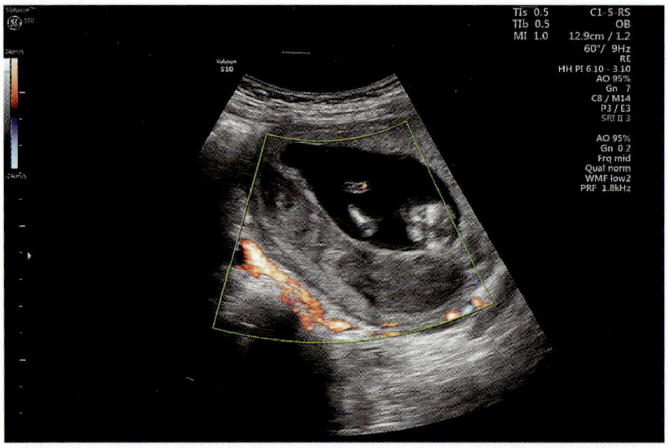

Fig. 2: Ultrasound showing subchorionic hemorrhage.
Courtesy: Professor Kamal Oswal, Head, Department of Radiodiagnosis, Vivekananda Institute of Medical Sciences, Kolkata, West Bengal, India.

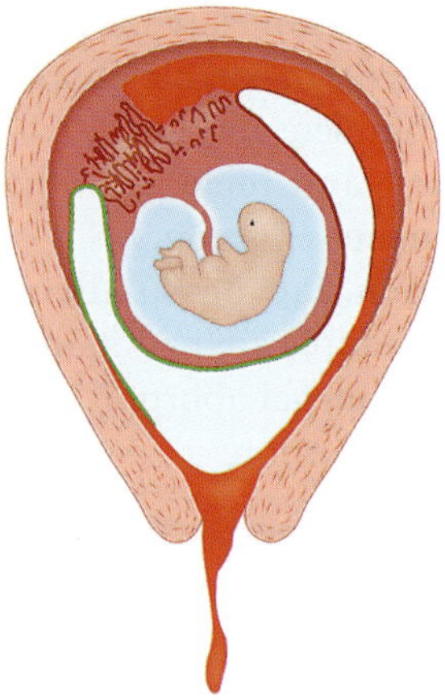

Fig. 3: Inevitable abortion. (OS is open and retroplacental hemorrhage)

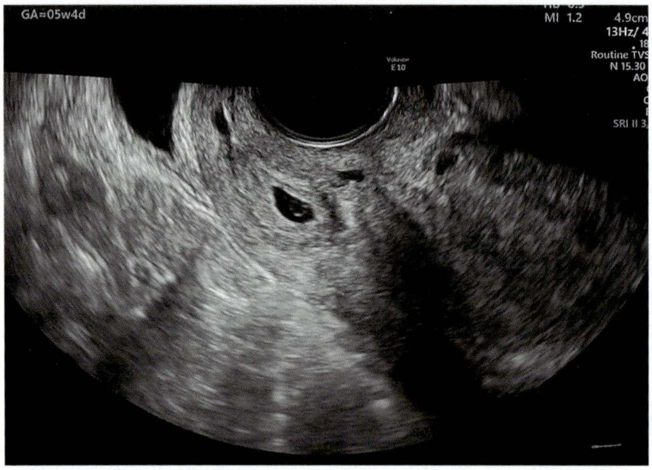

Fig. 4: Ultrasound showing products in the process of expulsion (inevitable abortion).
Courtesy: Professor Kamal Oswal, Head, Department of Radiodiagnosis, Vivekananda Institute of Medical Sciences, Kolkata, West Bengal, India.

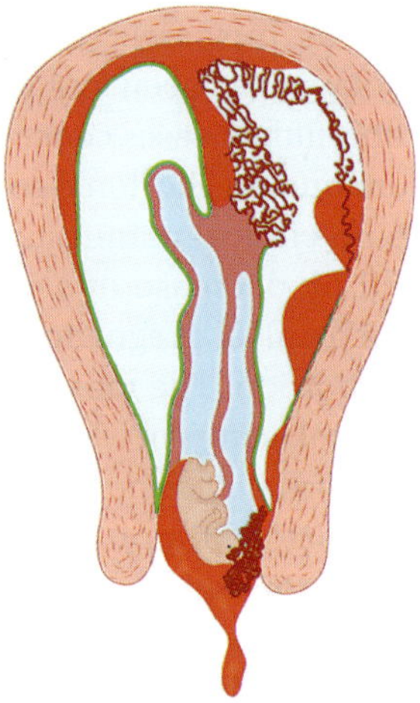

Fig. 5: Incomplete abortion (product partly expelled, OS is open and profuse bleeding).

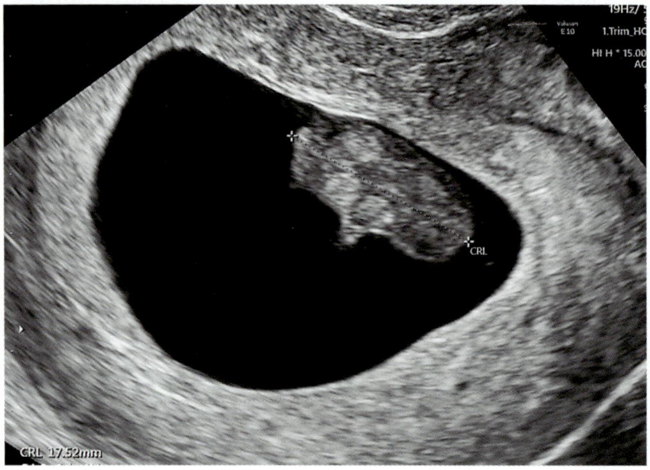

Fig. 6: Missed abortion with absent fetal cardiac activity at 8 weeks.

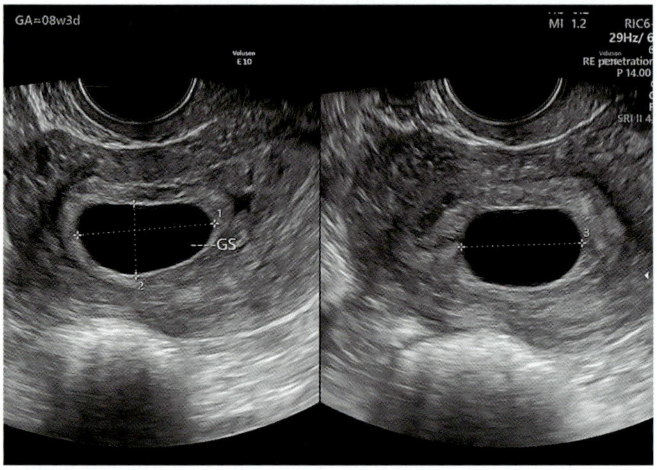

Fig. 7: Anembryonic pregnancy of 6 weeks 3 days.
Courtesy: Professor Kamal Oswal, Head, Department of Radiodiagnosis, Vivekananda Institute of Medical Sciences, Kolkata, West Bengal, India.

threatened abortion pregnancy is wasted either in the form of missed, inevitable, incomplete, or complete abortion.

Diagnosis of individual spontaneous abortion is done by history, clinical symptoms, physical findings, sonography, and serum β-hCG measurement.

Management of threatened abortion is conservative that of inevitable and incomplete abortion is surgical evacuation and missed abortion needs evacuation by medical and/or surgical methods. Confirmed complete abortion needs no treatment.

Preoperative evaluation—every woman should be assessed by proper history taking, physical examination, investigations with hematocrit, blood grouping, Rh status, routine urine analysis, serology [including human immunodeficiency virus (HIV)], sonography, and other investigations as indicated.

Depending upon the degree of bleeding, vitals, and hematocrit value resuscitative measure is taken. Prophylactic antibiotic is given in all surgical abortions.

Rh anti-D immunoglobulin should be administered to Rh negative woman undergoing abortion—spontaneous or induced in the dose of 50–120 μg intramuscular (IM) in pregnancies ≤12 weeks gestation, 300 μg in ≥13 weeks of gestation. American College of Obstetricians and Gynecologists (ACOG) (2019) recommends 300 μg IM irrespective of gestation age. In medical abortion or in expectant management it is given within 72 hours. In threatened abortion, though controversial it is better to administer.

DIFFERENT METHODS OF EVACUATION OF UTERUS

The various methods are:

- Dilatation and curettage (D&C) and dilatation and evacuation (D&E)—rapid method and slow method
- Vacuum aspiration
- Suction evacuation by electric sucker or electric vacuum aspiration (EVA).

The term dilatation and curettage is usually confined to early pregnancy, not beyond first trimester abortion and D&E is applied thereafter, usually for second-trimester evacuation. The term dilatation and evacuation is used also in first trimester in many places. The term dilatation and curettage is popularly used for endometrial curettage for gynecological indications like abnormal uterine bleeding, etc.

Dilatation and Evacuation

Indications of Dilatation and Evacuation Operations

The indications of D&E operations are: (1) inevitable and incomplete abortions, (2) missed abortions, (3) hydatidiform mole (H. mole), and (4) induced abortion (MTP).

Instruments Needed for Dilatation and Evacuation Operation (Fig. 8)

- Sponge holding forceps
- Simple rubber catheter
- Sims vaginal speculum
- Allis tissue forceps/multiple teeth vulsellum
- Uterine sound
- Cervical dilators
- Ovum forceps or ovum holding forceps
- Uterine curette—sharp, blunt, and flushing curette
- Uterine dressing forceps.

Steps of Rapid Method of Dilatation and Evacuation Operations (Figs. 9 to 20)

Patient is made to lie in lithotomy position. Anesthesia is given by sedation with paracervical block or general anesthesia

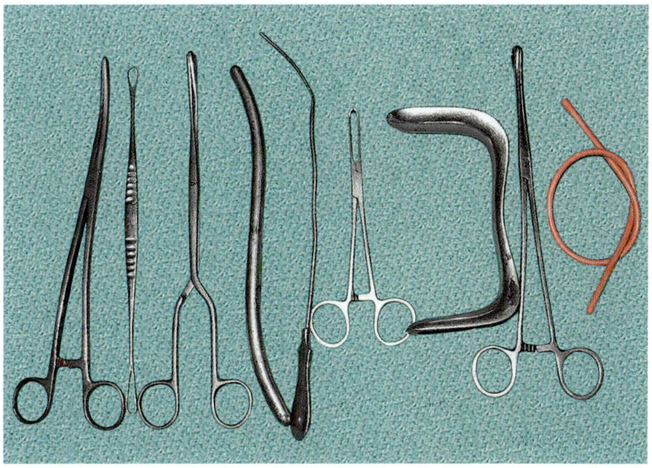

Fig. 8: Instruments used in dilatation evacuation operation. (Individual instrument is to be labeled as from right to left: (1) Simple rubber catheter, (2) Sponge holding forceps, (3) Sims posterior vaginal speculum, (4) Allis tissue forceps, (5) Uterine sound, (6) Cervical dilators, (7) Ovum forceps or ovum holding forceps, (8) Uterine curette—sharp and blunt curette, and (9) Uterine dressing forceps).

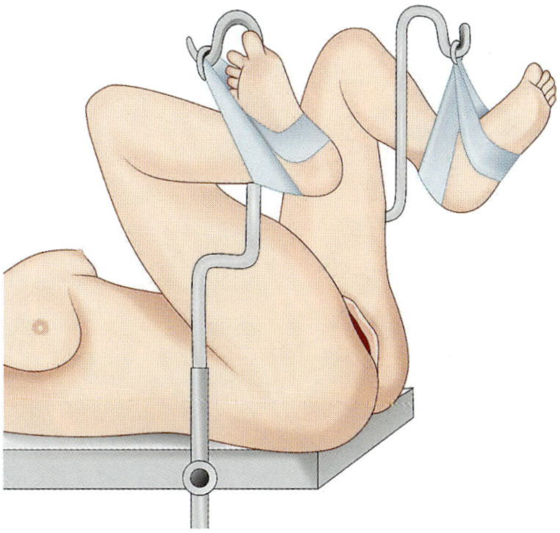

Fig. 9: Lithotomy position.

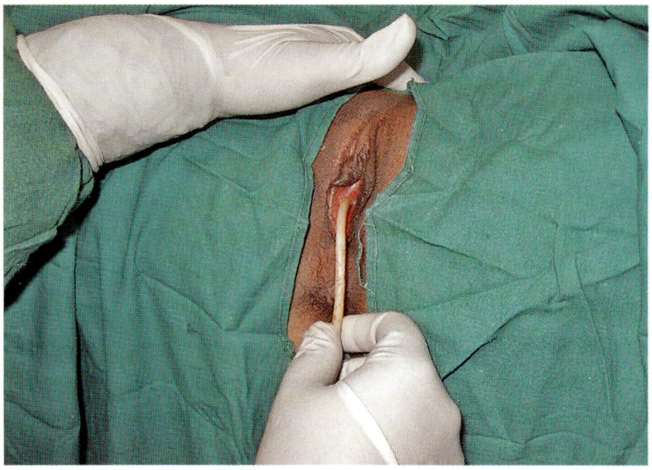

Fig. 10: Catheterization.

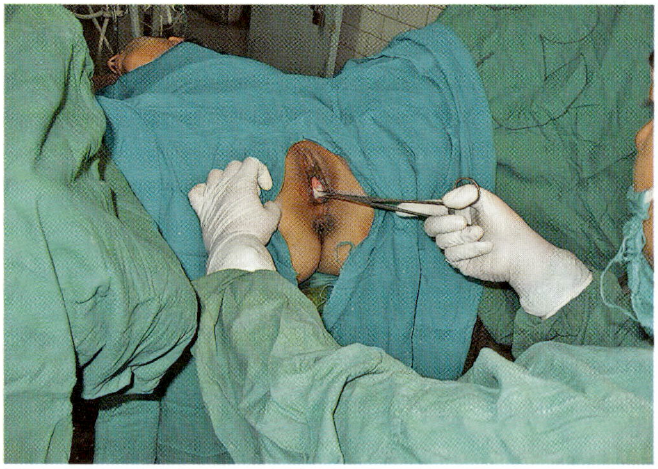

Fig. 11: Vaginal swab with the help of sponge-holding forceps.

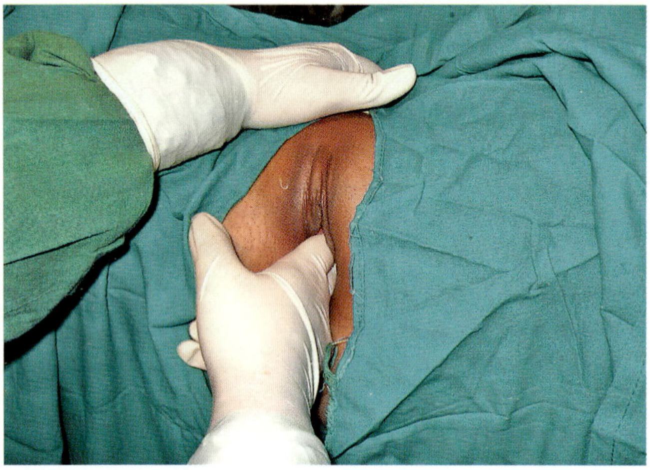

Fig. 12: Pervaginal examination to note the size, and position of the uterus and any other pathology.

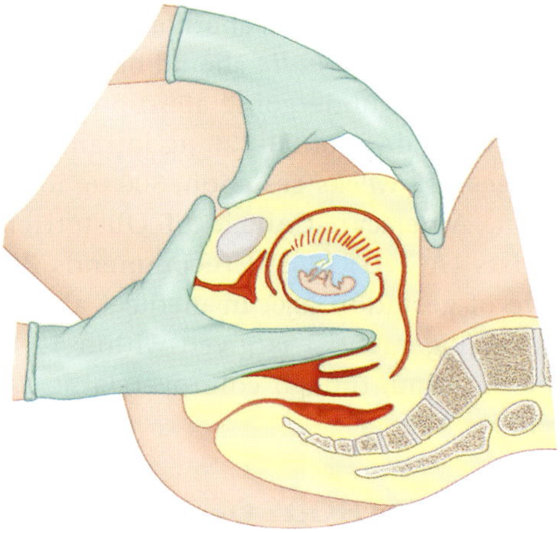

Fig. 13: Pervaginal examination to note the size, and position of the uterus and any other pathology (diagrammatic).

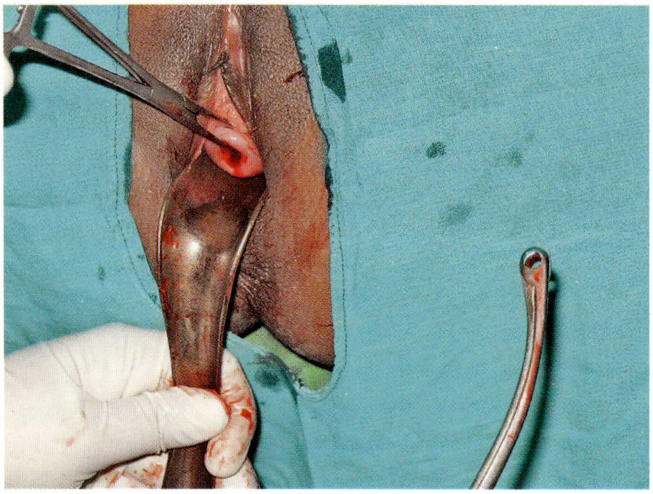

Fig. 14: Posterior vaginal wall is retracted by Sims speculum and anterior lip of cervix is held by Allis' tissue forceps.

in few cases. Following antiseptic dressing and draping catheterization is done. Bimanual vaginal examination is done to note the uterine size, position, cervical dilatations, and also to exclude any other pathology. Sims speculum is introduced through the vagina, and posterior wall of vagina is depressed and held by an assistant. Anterior lip of the cervix is grasped by Allis tissue forceps or multiple teeth vulsellum. Uterine sound is introduced through the cervical canal inside the uterine cavity by which the length of the uterine cavity is assessed and position of uterus determined. Dilatation of the cervical canal is done first, passing the smallest dilator through the cervical canal. Then cervical dilators of gradually increased diameter are introduced. The maximum size of the cervical dilator is chosen so that ovum forceps can be introduced depending on the size of the uterus (see below). In incomplete or inevitable abortions, where the cervix is already dilated, larger dilator can be introduced

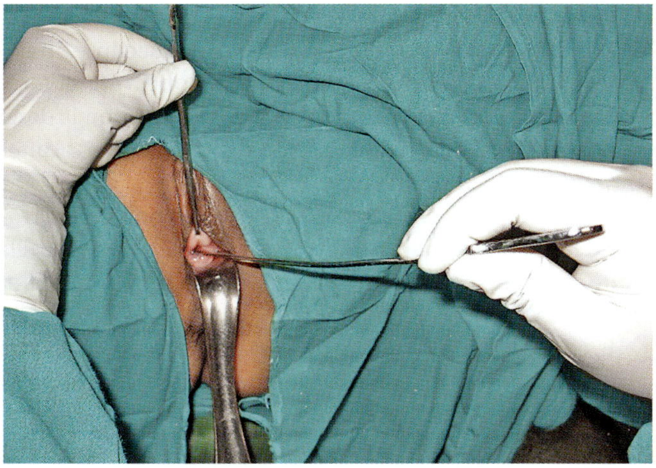

Fig. 15: Introduction of sound to determine the length and position of uterus.

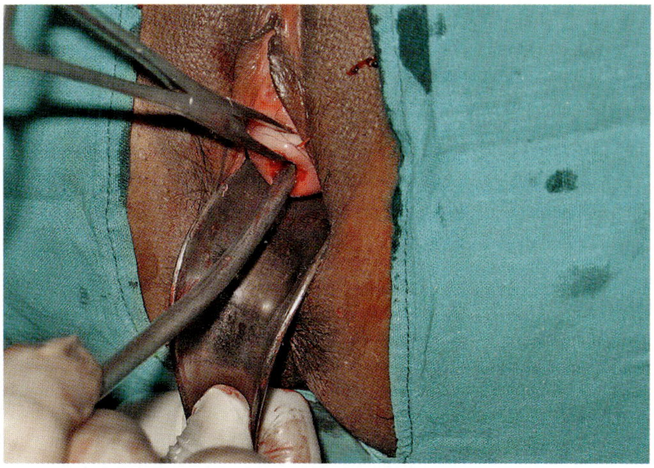

Fig. 16: Dilatation of cervical canal with cervical dilators.

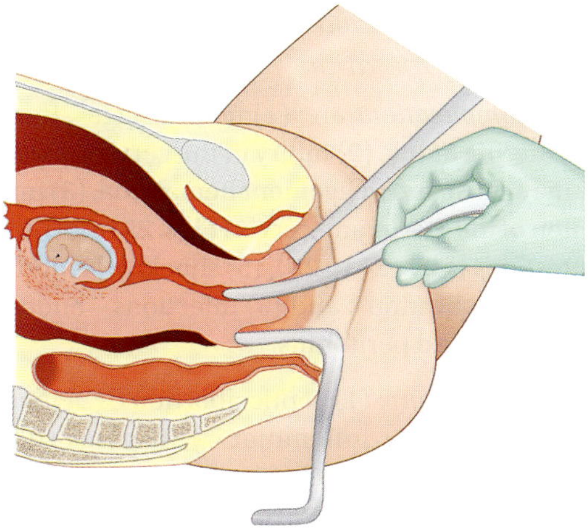

Fig. 17: Dilatation of cervical canal with cervical dilators (diagrammatic).

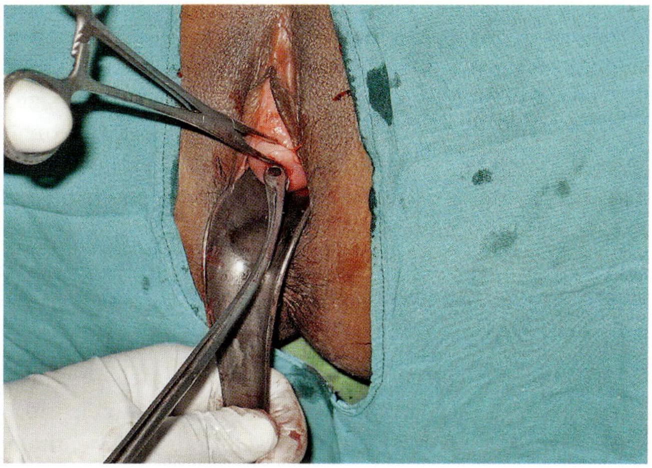

Fig. 18: Ovum forceps is used for evacuation of product of conception.

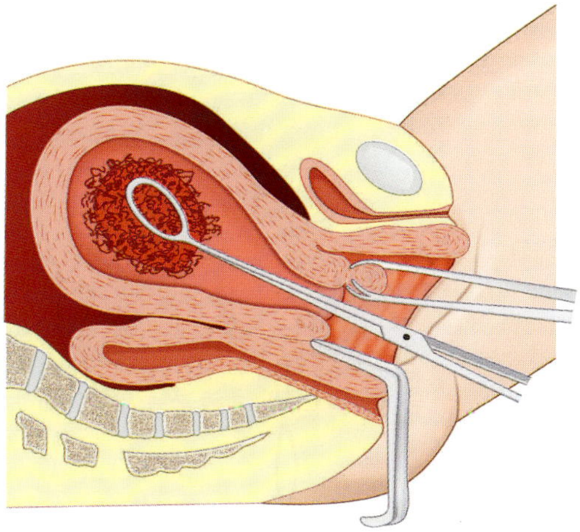

Fig. 19: Ovum forceps is used for evacuation of product of conception (diagrammatic).

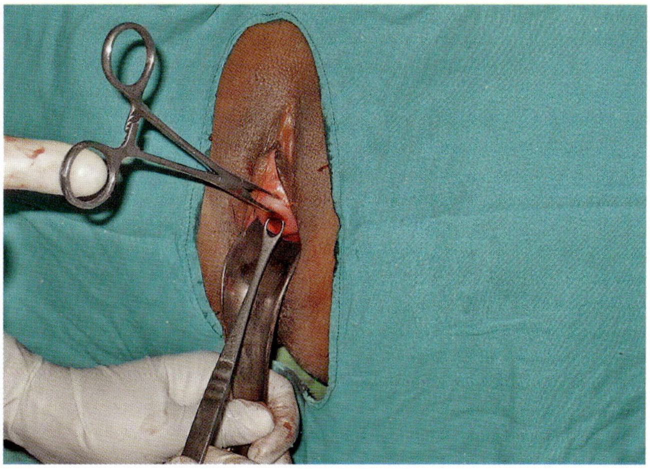

Fig. 20: Uterine curette is being introduced to curette uterine wall.

first or no dilatation is needed at all. Ovum forceps are introduced and the product of conception is grasped and removed gradually till no products are found to come out. Blunt uterine curette is introduced to curette all the walls of the uterine cavity. Emptiness of uterine cavity is identified by the feeling of gritting sensation, less bleeding, gripping, and appearance of bubbles/frothing. Uterine cavity is dressed with uterine dressing forceps covered with a betadine gauge (not mandatory). Injection Methergine 0.2 mg intravenous (IV) is administered. It can also be given earlier. Sims speculum and Allis tissue forceps are removed. Uterine massaging is done bimanually (by keeping two fingers inside the vagina and left hand over the fundus). Uterus is felt well contracted and no bleeding per vagina is seen. At the end of the procedure, patient is observed for pulse, blood pressure (BP), and vaginal bleeding. Uterine emptiness is understood by hardness of uterus and absence of bleeding per vagina.

Maximum sizes of dilators to be introduced in different situations: In MTP and missed abortion—dilatation is made up to the sizes that will allow the introduction of ovum forceps, and the size of which depends on the size of the uterus (up to 12 weeks—9/12 Hawkin's Ambler size). In incomplete and inevitable abortion no dilatation is needed in most of the cases as cervical os becomes already dilated. If there is no sufficient dilatation it should be dilated so that an index finger (16/19 mm) can be introduced. For suction evacuation one size smaller than suction cannula is used for proper airtightness.

Various mechanical and pharmacological methods for preabortion cervical ripening: Mechanical—osmotic dilators—laminaria tent, Dilapan-S, and Lamicel; intrauterine balloon inflated with sterile solution—Foley catheter

Pharmacological: Prostaglandins (misoprostol, dinoprostone, carboprost), antiprogestin (mifepristone), nitric oxide donor (nitroglycerine), and letrozol

Cervical dilatation may be done by slow method or by rapid method. Slow method is a two-stage procedure. In the first stage, slow dilatation of the cervix is done by *laminaria tent* or *isaptent*. In the second stage, rapid dilatation is done by metal cervical dilators following a significant interval after laminaria tent is introduced.

Laminaria tent is Chinese seaweeds. When it is introduced in cervical canal and kept in situ for 12 hours, it swells up by its hygroscopic nature about four times its diameter and makes the cervix soft and dilatable.

It should be inserted properly so that the tip of the laminaria tent is just placed at the level of internal os **(Figs. 21 and 22)**. These tents are sterilized in absolute alcohol, which are kept for 24 hours at least.

Drug used preoperatively for softening of cervix is misoprostol which is a prostaglandins PGE1—200–400 µg inserted 3–4 hours before D&E makes the cervix soft and the procedure becomes easier.

Complications of the Dilatation and Evacuation Operation

Immediate complications are: (1) hemorrhage—from injury or due to uterine atony, (2) injury of the cervix—extension of the tear may cause broad ligament hematoma, (3) injury and perforation of the uterus and cervix **(Figs. 23 to 26)**, (4) injury of the intestines **(Figs. 27 to 29)**, (5) shock, (6) embolism, (7) anesthetic complications, and (8) infections—endometritis, pelvic infection, and peritonitis.

Late complications are: (1) septic abortions, (2) incomplete evacuation, (3) pelvic inflammatory diseases (PIDs), (4) infertility—due to tubal block, (5) uterine synechia—due to vigorous uterine curette, and (6) cervical incompetence—due to forceful dilatation of the cervix. The most common complication of D&E operation is incomplete evacuation of product of conception and its sequels.

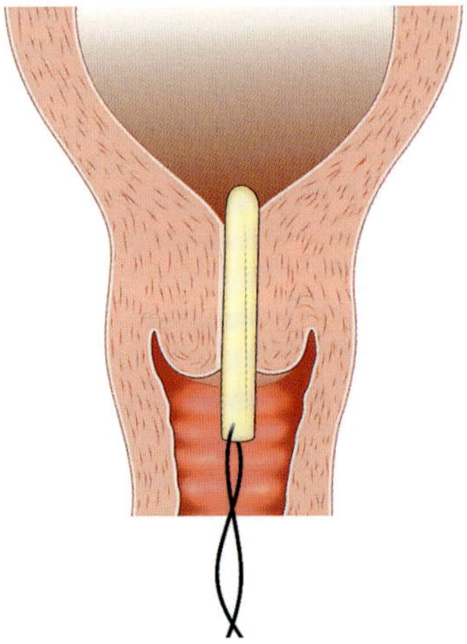

Fig. 21: Correct application of laminaria tent. Upper end laminaria tent is placed up to the internal os.

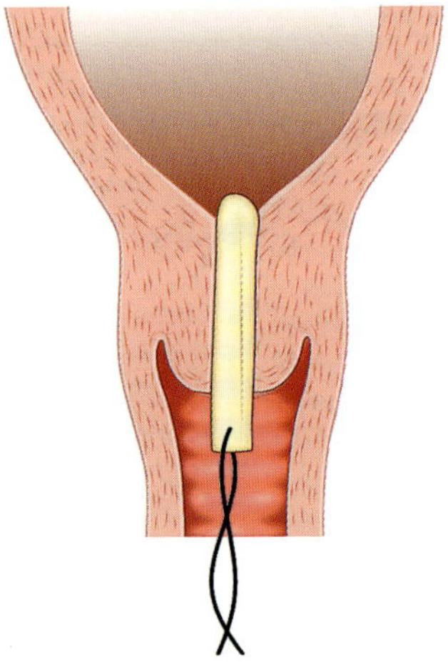

Fig. 22: Laminaria tent is swollen after several hours.

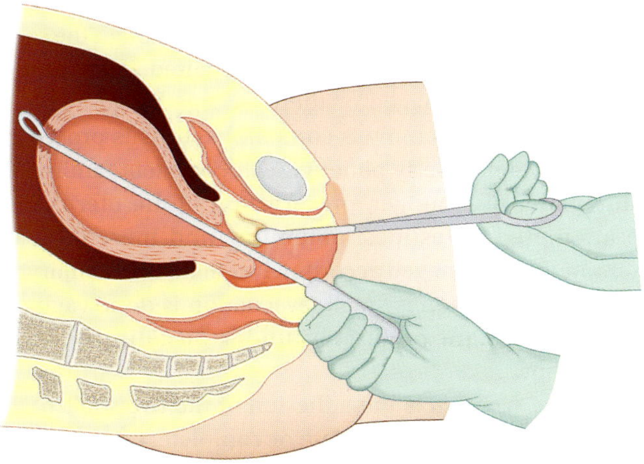

Fig. 23: Perforation of the uterine fundus by the uterine curette.

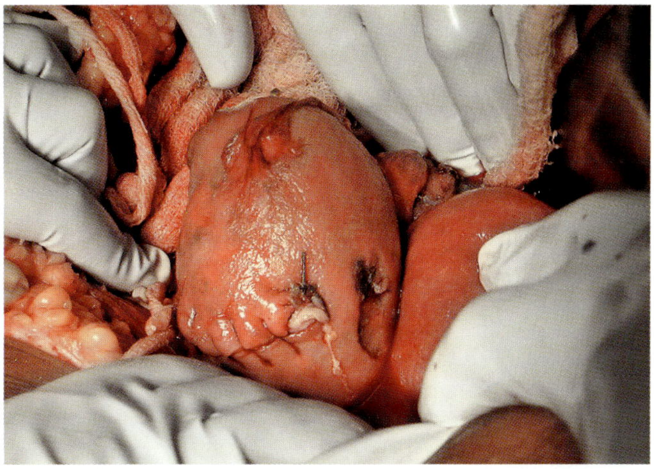

Fig. 24: Multiple perforation sites of the uterus following dilatation and evacuation operation. Wounds have been repaired with catgut stitches.

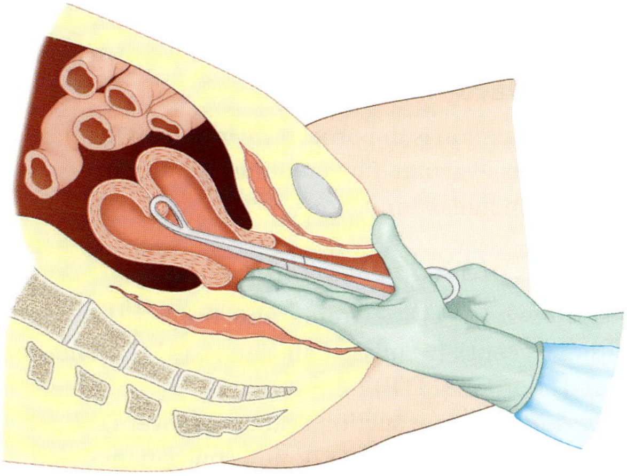

Fig. 25: Ovum forceps grasping the wall of the fundus injuring the fundus.

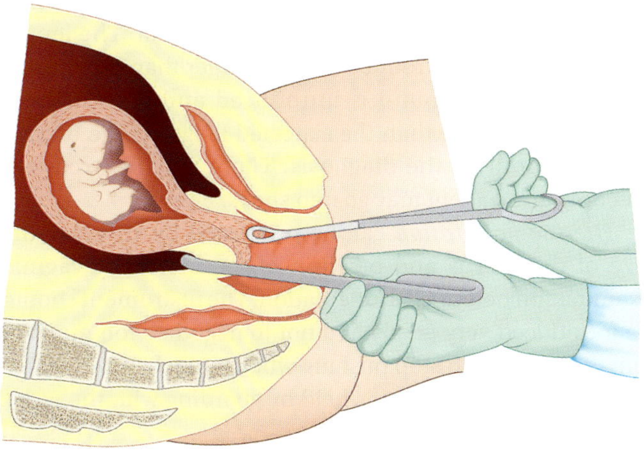

Fig. 26: Perforation through the posterior wall of the cervix by the dilator to reach POD (more common when uterus is acutely anteflexed).

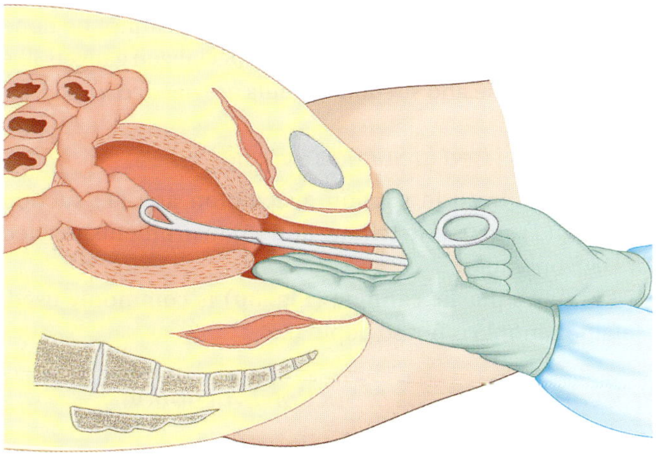

Fig. 27: Ovum forceps grasping the loop of the bowel through the perforation wound and the loop may come outside vagina.

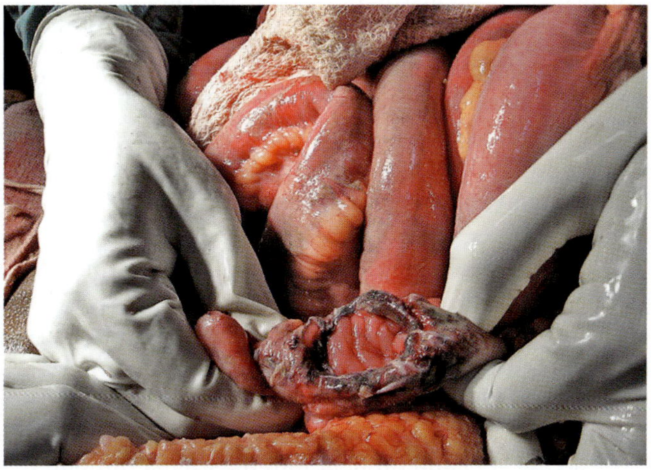

Fig. 28: Injury of sigmoid colon during dilatation and evacuation operation (Same case as in Figure 24).

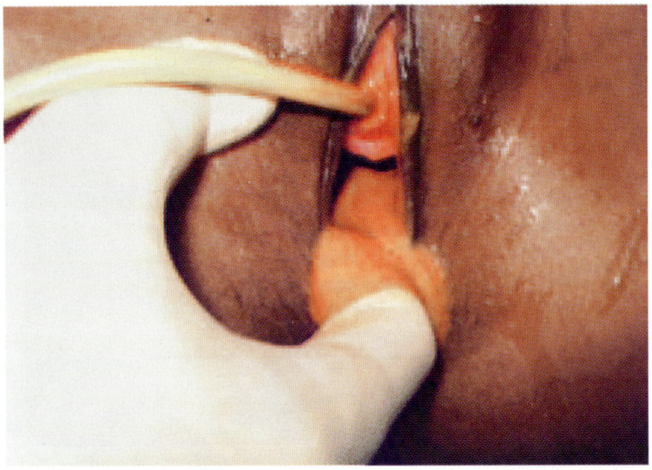

Fig. 29: Stool coming out through cervical canal due to formation of sigmoidouterine fistula after 25 days of dilatation and evacuation operation due to intestinal injury.

Diagnosis of uterine perforation is done by sudden loss of resistance and feeling give-way to uterine wall. The length of the instrument introduced will be larger than the uterine size. If a uterine sound is introduced and goes without resistance for more than the expected length of the uterine cavity it confirms the diagnosis. There may be excessive bleeding and patient may go into shock.

Uterine perforation can be prevented by knowing the size of the uterus and position of the uterus by vaginal examination before instrumentation. The instrument should be introduced very gently and not to negotiate too much of length initially and stop pushing when it touches the fundus felt by resistance. Dilator is held by guarding with the index finger.

If perforation does occur or suspected the procedure is stopped immediately. The extent of perforated wound is assessed and its effects which depend on the type of instruments used for perforation. If perforation is done with a small instrument like uterine sound or dilator of small size, then the patient is observed by noting the pulse and BP and pallor. Conservative management is given with antibiotics if patient's condition remains stable. If the condition of the patient deteriorates (evidenced by tachycardia, hypotension) laparotomy is done following IV fluid and blood requisition. In uncertainty, diagnostic laparoscopy may be performed. If perforation is caused by a large-sized dilator or ovum forceps or suction cannula, immediate laparotomy is planned for. Before that, diagnostic laparoscopy is helpful to see the site, size, and extent of the perforation. During laparotomy the intestines, omentum, and mesentery are examined to look for any injury or hemorrhage. It is not unlikely that sometimes intestines are grasped by ovum forceps **(Fig. 27)** and brought into the vagina through the perforated uterine wound.

Following laparotomy if the products of conception seem to remain inside the uterus, it is evacuated through the same rent or by hysterotomy and the rent is repaired. If the wounds are irreparably damaged or there is large broad ligament hematoma, hysterectomy is contemplated. This procedure is applicable in elderly patients with complete family. But if the patient is younger, preservation of the uterus is to be attempted. Intestines, omentum, and mesentery are examined and managed accordingly if there is any injury.

If the perforation is small, evacuation is done vaginally with utmost care preferably under visualization with laparoscopy.

Uterine synechia is the adhesion of the two walls of the uterus. This may be incomplete or complete, depending on which amenorrhea or scanty period may occur. The woman may suffer from infertility and the treatment is D&C and introduction of Cu-T or hysteroscopic synechiolysis followed by cyclical estrogen and progesterone therapy. There is a possibility of morbid adhesion of the placenta in future pregnancy.

Suction Evacuation

Suction evacuation is the procedure by which the product of conception is evacuated by creating negative pressure with the help of suction cannula.

Indications of Suction Evacuation

Indications are: (1) inevitable abortions, (2) incomplete abortion (recent), (3) missed abortions, (4) H. mole, and (5) induced abortion (MTP).

The advantages of suction evacuation over D&E are—it is more simple and safe, can be done as outpatient department (OPD) procedure and time required is less, blood loss is less (20–25 cc), chances of injury are less, chance of perforation is less, milder form of anesthesia is sufficient, and overall complications are less than D&E.

Disadvantages are—this procedure becomes difficult when the fetal parts are well formed, i.e., it cannot be done after 10 weeks of pregnancy and also specialized gadgets like suction machine and suction cannula are needed.

Instruments Used in Suction Evacuation

Instruments used in suction evacuation are: (1) suction cannula, (2) suction machine, and (3) instruments needed for D&E operation.

Karman's plastic cannula **(Fig. 30)** is commonly used. Metallic cannula is not so popular.

Procedures and Steps of Suction Evacuation (Figs. 31 to 33)

Patient is placed in lithotomy position. For anesthesia—deep sedation with IV diazepam or pethidine with atropine

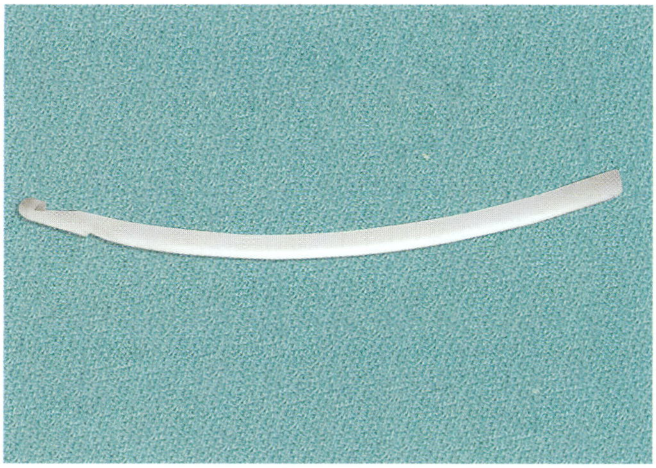

Fig. 30: Karman suction cannula.

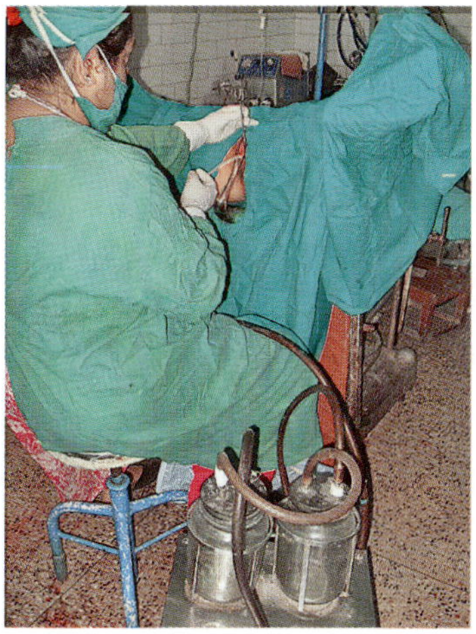

Fig. 31: Procedure of suction evacuation.

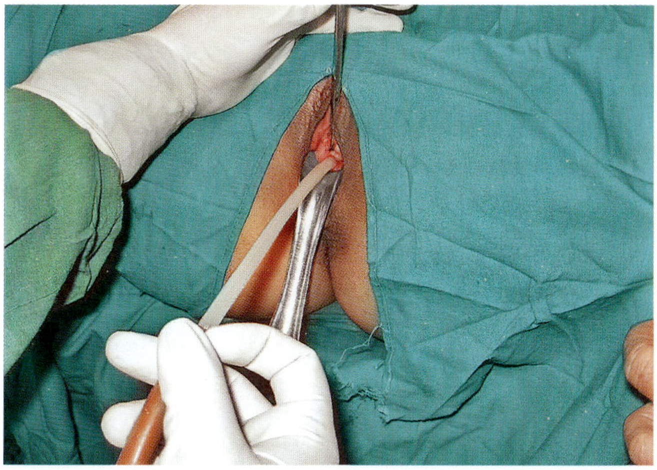

Fig. 32: Using suction cannula fitted with electric sucker machine for suction evacuation.

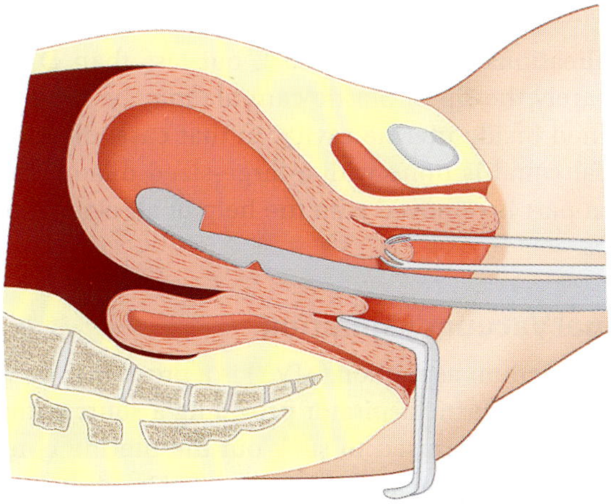

Fig. 33: Evacuation with plastic suction cannula.

and paracervical block are sufficient. Following antiseptic dressing and draping evacuation of the bladder is done. Usually, patient passes urine herself before shifting to the operation theater (OT) table. Bimanual examination is done, then posterior vaginal speculum is introduced and is held by an assistant. Anterior lip of the cervix is grasped by Allis tissue forceps. Uterine sound is introduced to note the length and position of the uterus. Dilatation of the cervix is done with a dilator smaller than the size of suction cannula. If misoprostol (400 mg) is administered per vaginally 3–4 hours before the procedure further dilatation is usually not needed. Suction cannula of appropriate size fitted with suction machine by rubber tubing is introduced in the cervical canal. Injection Methergine 0.2 mg is given IV. The cannula is pushed inside the uterine cavity up to the midway inside the cavity. Negative pressure is created up to 400–600 mm Hg (0.6 kg/sq cm) in the suction machine. The cannula is moved up and down and rotated, and the products of conception are sucked out to be collected in the suction bottle and the procedure is continued till the uterus becomes empty. The negative pressure is released before removal of the cannula. Uterine cavity is finally curetted with blunt curette. All the instruments are removed and vaginal examination is done to look for any bleeding. The completion of evacuation is determined by no material is seen to come out more, cannula is gripped tightly as uterus contracts and becomes small, there will be formation of bubble at the end, during curetting, there will be gritting sensation and no materials come out and bleeding becomes less.

The size of the cannula used depends on the size of the uterus. 8 mm cannula is used for 8-week-sized uterus, 6 mm size is used for 6-week-sized uterus, and so on. Five sizes are available. These are 4, 6, 8, 10, and 12 mm. Karman's cannula is sterilized by keeping it in Savlon solution for 12 hours.

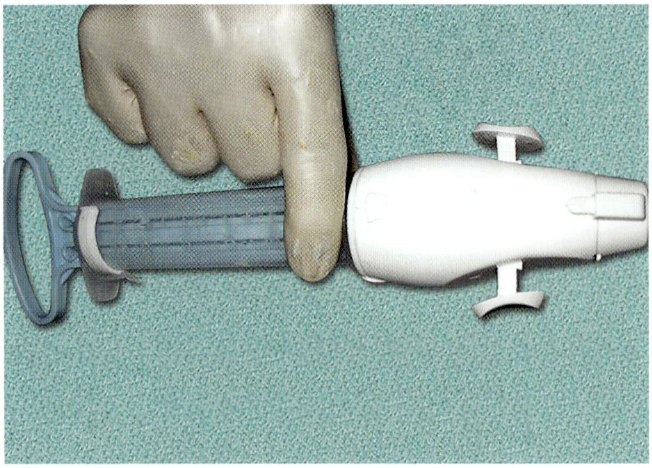

Fig. 34: Manual vacuum aspiration plus aspirator.

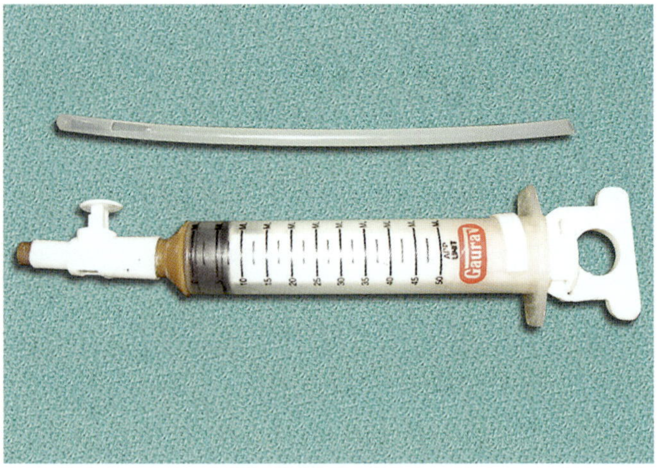

Fig. 35: Menstrual regulation syringe.

Complications of Suction Evacuation

Complications are like D and E but less than D and E. Very rarely the tip of plastic cannula may be broken and remained inside uterine cavity. In that case, dilatation of cervical canal is done with a large-sized dilator and the broken part is removed with the help of an ovum-holding forceps.

Manual Vacuum Aspiration

Manual vacuum aspiration (MVA) is a procedure by which a hand-held plastic aspirator providing a source attached with a cannula is used to suck out the uterine contents. The negative pressure is manually created inside it.

Manual vacuum aspiration plus aspirator (Ipas), a double valve aspirator is used to terminate the pregnancy up to 12 weeks using the larger cannula as needed up to 12 mm size **(Fig. 34)**.

Menstrual regulation (MR) syringe (single valve aspirator) **(Fig. 35)** can terminate the pregnancy ≤7 weeks using small cannula up to 6 mm size. This method was classically called *the MR or menstrual extraction method*. No dilatation is needed and no premedication is given except preoperative nonsteroidal anti-inflammatory drug (NSAID).

Manual vacuum aspiration plus aspirator (Ipas) is made up of silicone and autoclavable whereas MR syringe is made up of latex and nonautoclavable, and cold sterilization is needed.

Advantages of Manual Vacuum Aspiration in Comparison to Electric Vacuum Aspiration

The most important advantage is that it can be used in rural settings with intermittent electrical supply since no electricity is needed. It is also convenient for mobile services. MVA creates little noise. Products of conception can be examined very well for completeness of evacuation.

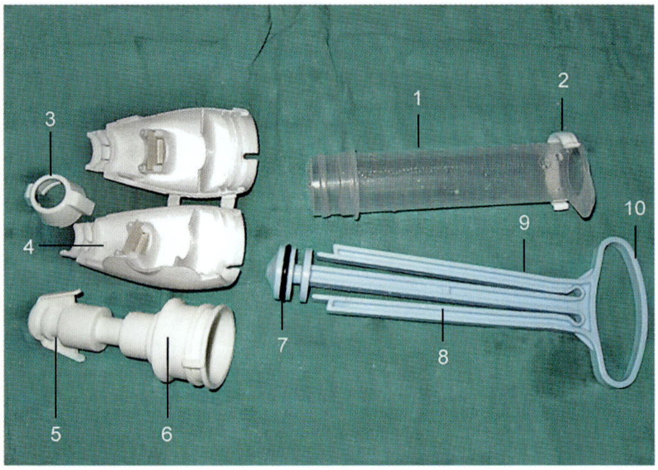

Fig. 36: Different parts of manual vacuum aspiration. (1) Cylinder, (2) Collar stop, (3) Cap, (4) Valve, (5) Valve buttons, (6) Valve liver, (7) Plunger O-ring, (8) Plunger arm, (9) Plunger, and (10) Plunger handle]

Similarities of the two are both have high level of safety and effectiveness, both have low complication rates, same amount of negative pressure is created in both the methods (24–26 inches or 609.6–660.4 mm of mercury).

Different Parts of Manual Vacuum Aspiration (Figs. 36 and 37)

- 60 cc cylinder for holding the product of conception.
- Plunger with handle which is pulled out to create vacuum.
- Valve buttons to control formation and release of vacuum.
- Hinged valve with cap and removal liner
- Collar stop with retaining clip which prevents to come out.

Cannula used in Ipas MVA are same dimension and apertures as Karman's cannula. 4, 5, 6, 7, 8, 9, 10, and 12 mm sizes are available, slightly rigid, bases are permanently affixed with wings, cannula are used as per uterine size:

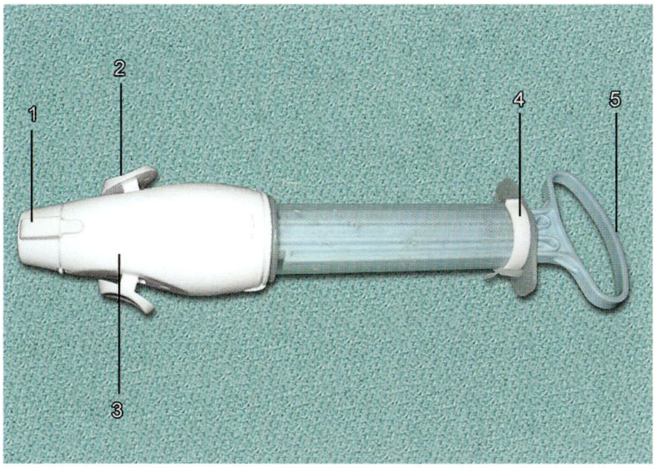

Fig. 37: After assembling the different parts: (1) Cap, (2) Valve button, (3) Hinged valve, (4) Collar stop, and (5) Plunger handle.

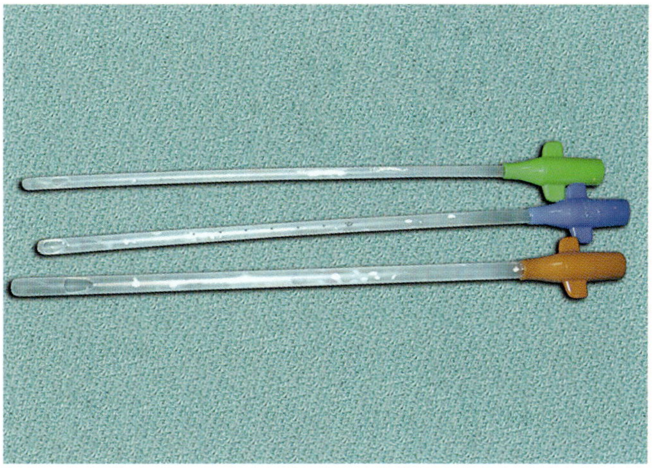

Fig. 38: Different sizes of cannula. Each cannula is available in sterile pack.

4–7 mm for 4–6 weeks, 6–10 mm for 7–9 weeks, and 8–12 mm for 9–12 weeks duration MTP **(Fig. 38)**.

Indications of Manual Vacuum Aspiration

Indications are: (1) MTP up to 12 weeks, (2) incomplete abortion, (3) missed abortion, (4) blighted ovum, (5) H. mole up to 12 weeks uterine size, and (6) endometrial biopsy/aspiration.

Contraindications of Manual Vacuum Aspiration

It is contraindicated, rather it is difficult for MTP in >12 weeks pregnancy and incomplete abortion >12 weeks uterine size. Other contraindications are multiple fibroids, acute cervicitis/PID, bleeding disorder, and uterine perforation.

Instrumental Setup for Manual Vacuum Aspiration (Fig. 39)

- Swab holding forceps
- Rubber catheter
- Allis tissue forceps
- Sims speculum
- Syringe with lignocaine
- MVA
- Cannula
- Container for collection of tissue

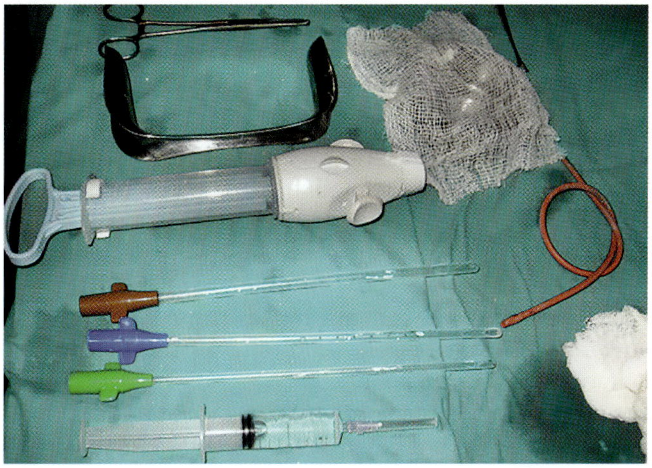

Fig. 39: Instrument setup for manual vacuum aspiration. (To be labeled individually (1) Rubber catheter, (2) Allis tissue forceps, (3) Sims speculum, (4) Syringe with lignocaine, (5) MVA, (6) Cannula, and (7) Container for collection of tissue).

Disassembling the Instrument

- Cylinder is removed from valve by pulling it.
- Cap is removed by pressing cap-release.
- By pulling open latch, hinged valve is opened and valve liner is removed.
- Collar stop is disengaged by sliding under retaining clip or is removed completely.
- O-ring is displaced by squeezing its sides and is rolled down into the groove below.

Procedure of Assembling

- Valve liner is placed in valve by aligning ridges.
- Valve is closed and it is ensured that it snaps in place.
- Cap is snapped onto the end of valve.
- O-ring is placed into groove near the tip of plunger and one drop of lubricant around O-ring is spread.
- Plunger arms after squeezing is pushed.
- Collar stop tabs is inserted into holes in cylinder.

"Charging" or "Preparing" the Instrument (Creation of Negative Pressure)

- To start with—valve buttons are open, plunger is kept all the way in, and collar stop is locked in place.
- Valve is closed by pushing the buttons down and forward until they are locked.

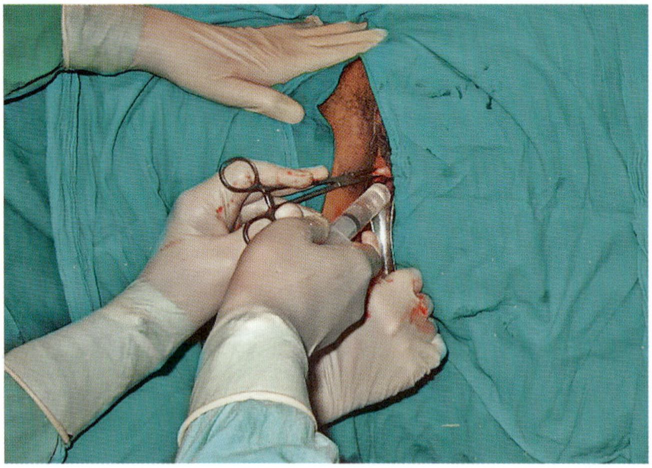

Fig. 40: Paracervical block.

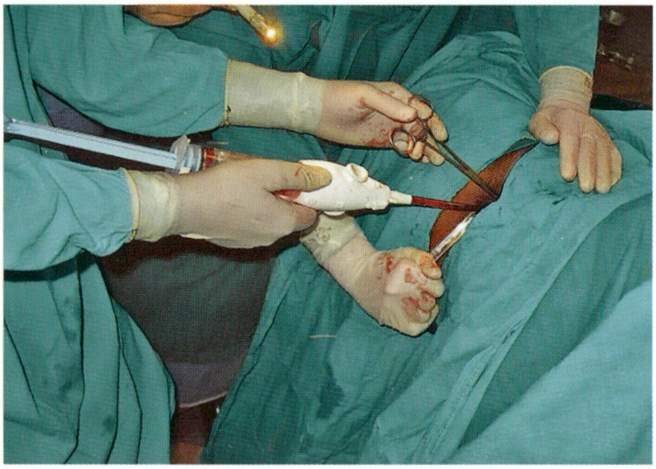

Fig. 41: Aspiration of product of conception by manual vacuum aspiration following release of buttons.

- Plunger is pulled back until plunger arms catch on the wide sides of cylinder and it is ensured that both plunger arms are extended and secured over the edge of cylinder.
- Now the "charged" instrument is ready for use.

Steps of Manual Vacuum Aspiration (Figs. 40 and 41)

Manual vacuum aspiration is done as an office procedure in the following 10 steps:

1. Prepare the instruments—following assembling, instrument is charged (negative pressure is created).
2. Preparation of woman—passes urine, sedation and analgesics are given, lithotomy position, bimanual examination are done.
3. Antiseptic swabbing of cervix and vagina. Speculum is inserted and anterior lip is held by Allis tissue forceps.
4. Paracervical block **(Fig. 40)**—10–20 mL of 1–2% xylocaine is infiltrated at 4 and 8 o' clock position following aspiration to check whether blood is coming.
5. Cervical canal is dilated with dilators. Cannula can be used in place of dilator. Misoprostol 400 µg given vaginally 3–4 hours before makes the procedure easy, especially when the pregnancy is >9 weeks.
6. Cannula is inserted gently by rotating until the tip touches the fundus.
7. Suction of products of conception—the charged aspirator is attached to cannula first and the buttons are released to start the suction **(Fig. 41)**. Cannula is rotated in all directions, moving up and down till the uterine cavity is completely aspirated. Red or pink foam without tissue passing through the cannula indicates emptiness of uterus. After closing valve, cannula is disconnected.
8. Evacuated tissue is examined after pouring from the aspirator into a container **(Fig. 42)**.
9. Concurrent procedure like intrauterine contraceptive device (IUCD) application or female sterilization may be performed.

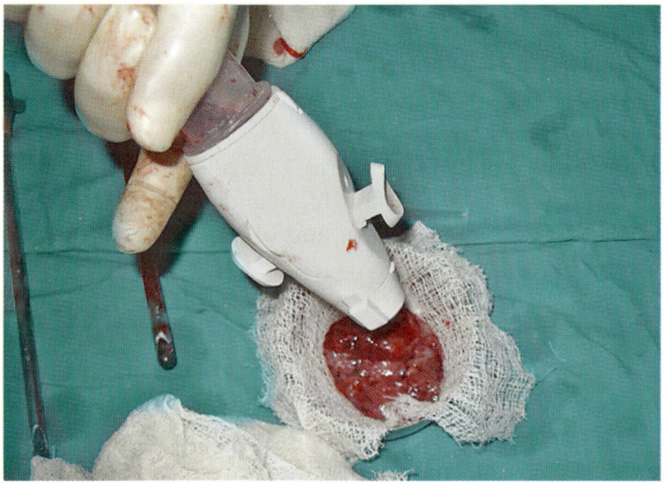

Fig. 42: Evacuated tissue is examined after pouring from the aspirator.

10. Instrument is disassembled and processing is done for cleaning and disinfection for next procedure.

Prophylactic antibiotic is given in all surgical abortions.

Examination of the Extracted Product

It is crucial to confirm the tissue consistent with products of conception in all surgical abortions specially in early pregnancy. If tissue is not obtained and not identified ectopic pregnancy, molar gestation, or failed abortion are suspected and evaluated. For identification of tissue it is taken in a container and allowed to float in normal saline for examination. Below 9 weeks pregnancy part of gestational sac (transparent) and trophoblastic tissue (frond-like projections) are identified beyond which fetal parts are visible. Continuation of pregnancy may occur in <0.5% cases. It is possible lesser period of gestation and also in multiple pregnancy. Ectopic pregnancy is excluded by transvaginal sonography (TVS) and serum β-hCG level. Tissue is sent for histopathology (H/P) examination.

Instrument Disinfection

Disinfection is done either by sterilization or high-level disinfection. Sterilization is done by steam autoclaving or by 2% Cidex for 10 hours. High-level disinfection is carried out either with boiling in water for 20 minutes, immersing in 2% Cidex for 20 minutes, or in 0.5% chlorine solution **(Fig. 43)** for 20 minutes.

Complications of Manual Vacuum Aspiration

Complications are perforation, infection, cervical injury, incomplete evacuation, vagal reaction, and acute hematometra.

Cervical Dilators

The use of cervical dilators is to dilate the cervical canal, external os, and internal os gradually. They are usually made of metal.

Different varieties of cervical dilators are Hegar's dilator, Das's dilator **(Fig. 44)** and Hawkin-Ambler's dilator **(Fig. 45)**. Dilator may be single-ended or double-ended. Hawkin-Ambler's dilator is always single-ended.

Any dilator can be used for dilatation and evacuation procedures. In D&C (gynecological) operations where cervix is hard, Das's or Hegar's dilators are preferred as these are more gradual dilators.

Measurements of Different Cervical Dilators

Hawkin-Ambler's dilators: The lowest size is 3/6 mm and maximum size is 18/21 mm. One set consists of 16 dilators. In 3/6, 3 and 6 denote diameters at the tip and at the widest part behind the tip, respectively.

Das's dilator or Hegar's dilator: In double-ended dilators the lowest size is 1/2 mm and the largest size is 23/24 mm. So one set consists of 12 dilators **(Fig. 46)**. However, as the larger dilators are not used now-a-days, the dilators from 1/2 to 15/16 mm sizes (a set of eight dilators) are sufficient. Single-ended dilator is also available. Double-ended dilators are commonly used.

Hegar's dilators and Das's dilators are of similar types, but Das's dilator is more gradual (longer) than Hegar's

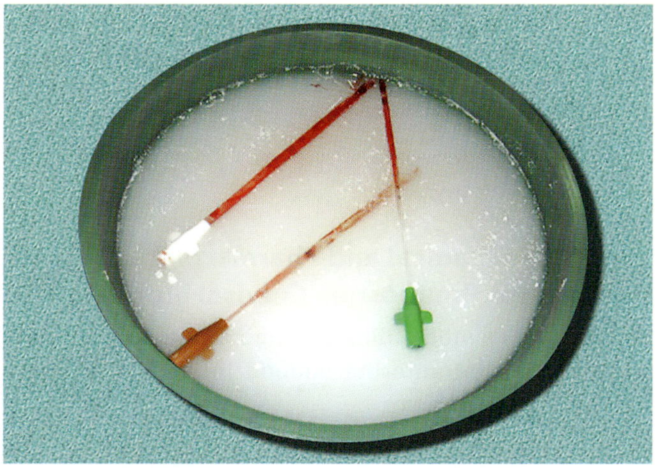

Fig. 43: Disinfection is done in chlorine water.

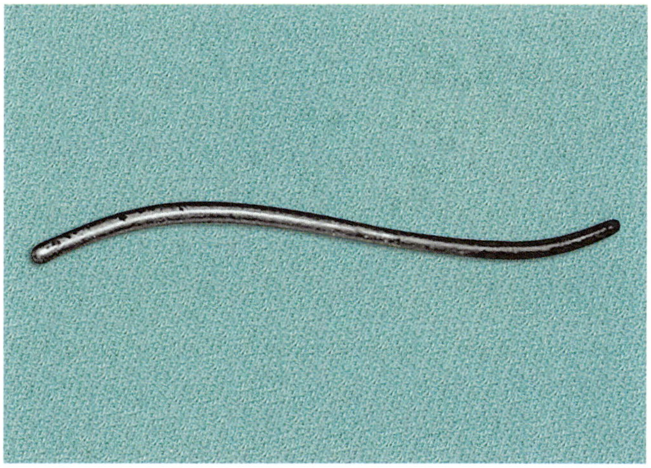

Fig. 44: Das's dilator.

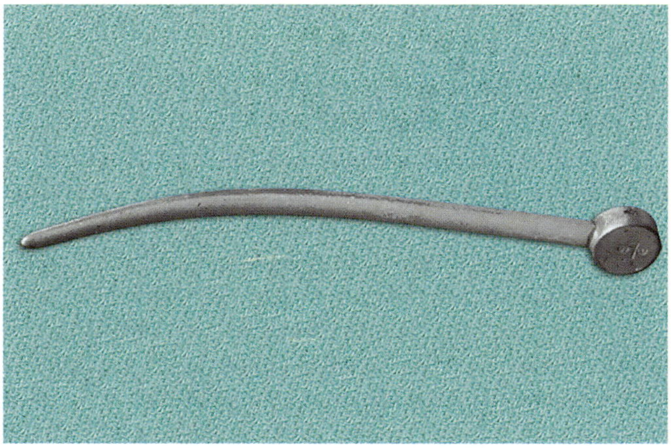

Fig. 45: Hawkin-Ambler's dilator.

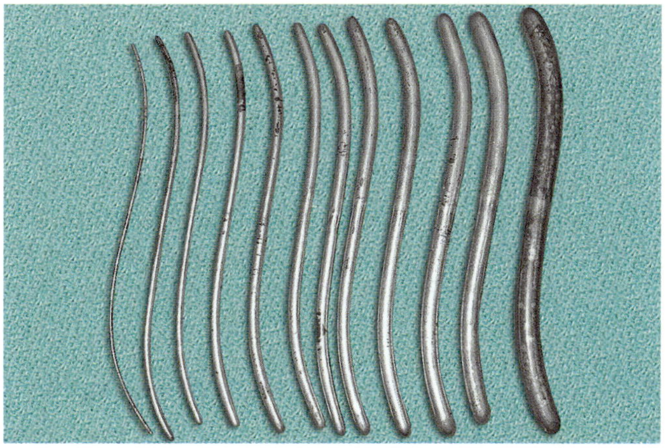

Fig. 46: One set of Das's dilators.

dilator. The name of Das's dilator is after the name of its inventor, Sir Kedar Nath Das, a famous obstetrician. The length of the uterus is measured by introducing uterine sound before introduction of dilators, otherwise there is a chance of perforation. The purpose of use of dilator is fulfilled when its maximum diameter crosses the internal os.

Passage of maximum diameter of cervical dilator through the internal os is understood by feeling of loss of resistance following resistance at a point during introduction. There will be also gripping of dilator by internal os and it will not fall down if left without any support.

INDUCED ABORTION—MEDICAL TERMINATION OF PREGNANCY

Induction of Abortion

Induction of abortion is the deliberate termination of pregnancy before the viability of fetus. It may be *legal* or *criminal (illegal)*. *Unsafe abortion* is a popular term used which means induction of abortion where all necessary precautions are not taken to make the procedure safe.

Prerequisites of Termination of Pregnancy

- Approach by the woman for termination with genuine indication.
- Counseling—regarding procedures and potential complications.
- Evaluation of the patient-history—accurate gestation age, previous obstetric history, prior cesarean delivery, medical and surgical history, any drug allergy
- Physical examination—general and gynecological examination, vital parameter including cardio-pulmonary status. Speculum examination and bimanual examination to detect any cervical infection and to determine the size of uterus and any other pelvic pathology.
- Investigations—hematocrit, urine for albumin, and sugar and blood group. Sonography in discrepancy of gestational age and also in suspected scar ectopic should be done.
- *Rh anti-D immunoglobulin* should be administered to Rh negative woman—50–120 μg IM in pregnancies ≤12 weeks gestation, 300 μg in ≥13 weeks of gestation. ACOG (2019) recommends 300 μg IM irrespective of gestation age. In medical abortion or in expectant management, it is given within 72 hours. In threatened abortion though controversy it is better to administer.

Methods of Medical Termination of Pregnancy

Medical termination of pregnancy methods are categorized according to first and second trimester.

Methods of Medical Termination of Pregnancy in the First Trimester (Up to 12 Weeks)

- Medical methods (medication abortion)
- MVA
- EVA or commonly called suction evacuation
- D&C and D&E.

Methods of Medical Termination of Pregnancy in the Second Trimester (13 Weeks Onward)

- *Medical methods of induction of abortion (medication abortion):*
  - Intra-amniotic hyperosmotic solution (IAHS)—saline (20%)
  - Hyperosmolar urea (40%) and prostaglandins (PGF2α)
  - Extra-amniotic installation of ethacridine lactate
  - PGE1 (misoprostol) alone or combined with mifepristone—commonly used now.
  - Other prostaglandins—PGE2, PGF2α (see later)
  - Oxytocin—it can be used either:
    - In adjunct to other drugs which is used in intra or extra-amniotic route through IV drip, or
    - Concentrated oxytocin in escalating sequentially in five to six cycles which is more effective (see below).
- *Surgical methods:*
  - D&E (13–15 weeks)
  - Hysterotomy.

Various Mechanical and Pharmacological Methods for Preabortion Cervical Ripening

Mechanical: Osmotic dilators-Laminaria tent, Dilapen-S, and Lamicel, intrauterine balloon inflated with sterile solution—Foley catheter

Pharmacological: Prostaglandins (misoprostol, dinoprostone, carboprost, antiprogestin (mifepristone), nitric oxide donor (nitroglycerine), and Letrozol.

MEDICAL ABORTION

Medical abortion is special subcategory of medical method of abortion or medication abortion.

Termination of pregnancy using mifepristone followed by misoprostol up to 9 weeks of pregnancy is an established and safe method for inducing abortion and is called *medical abortion*. Initially in India, it was recommended up to 7 weeks (49 days) of amenorrhea from the first day of last menstrual period. In April 2002, Drug Controller of India approved mifepristone along with misoprostol for termination of early pregnancy and it was included under the purview of MTP Act, 1971 as MTP rules 2003. From December 2008, Government of India has approved medical abortion up to

63 days gestation using Combipack (mifepristone 200 mg one tablet and misoprostol 200 µg four tablets). US Food and Drug Administration (FDA) approved mifepristone in September 2000.

Regime of Medical Abortion

Mifepristone is given orally as a single dose of 200 mg followed by 400 µg of misoprostol orally or vaginally on day 3. In many countries, mifepristone is licensed while using as a single dose of 600 mg. Vaginal misoprostol is superior to oral with higher efficacy and lower side effects.

Mifepristone is a derivative of norethindrone with anti-progestin action. It is also called RU-486. RU is derived from the pharmaceutical company "Roussel-Uclaf", which made it available and 486 is the laboratory serial number of the compound.

Mifepristone binds to progesterone receptors at endometrium and decidua resulting necrosis and detachment of placenta. It also softens the cervix and causes mild uterine contractions. It sensitizes the uterus to the effect of prostaglandin. Mifepristone alone is not used as it is less effective and success rate is 50–60% only.

Contraindications of mifepristone are history of smoking, heart disease, hypertension, anemia (Hb <8 g%), renal disease, and seizure disorder.

Misoprostol is a synthetic PGE1 analogue. It is well absorbed through gastrointestinal (GI) tract and vaginal mucosa. It has no significant effects on bronchi and blood vessels. It is stable at room temperature. Other than medical abortion, it has many uses in obstetrics.

It binds to myometrial cells resulting in strong myometrial contraction and causes cervical softening and dilatation, and ultimately leads to expulsion of product of contraction.

Misoprostol has little contraindication. Unlike other prostagladin it may be used in bronchial asthma as it is selective for PGE1 receptors and no effect on bronchus and blood vessels.

Efficacy of medical abortion: Medical abortion has a success rate of 95–99% in cases where it is done within 7 weeks of pregnancy. 1% of the women may require surgical evacuation for heavy bleeding, 1% may fail to abort, and 2–3% may be incomplete.

Three visits are needed for medical abortion. Day 1—for intake of mifepristone 200 mg orally, day 3—two tablets (400 mg) of misoprostol orally or vaginally, day 15—to ensure that abortion is complete.

Side effects of combination of mifepristone and misoprostol used in medical abortions are pain, nausea, vomiting, feeling of warmth, bleeding, diarrhea, chills, headache, dizziness, and fatigue. Yes, as there is risk of teratogenesis, it is advisable to terminate pregnancy surgically if there is failure of abortion following administration of mifepristone and misoprostol. Use of misoprostol in first trimester may cause *Mobius syndrome*, a multifacial anomaly of fetus.

Use of Methotrexate in Medical Abortion

Methotrexate 50 mg/m^2 is administered orally or commonly IM alternative to mifepristone followed by 800 µg misoprostol vaginally after 3–7 days. This gives >90% success rate.

Intra-amniotic Hypertonic Saline

Intra-amniotic hypertonic saline (IAHS) is used to terminate the pregnancy in midtrimester by instillation of hypertonic saline in amniotic cavity by amniocentesis method. It is suitable from *16 weeks onward.* Though it was a very popular method previously, this procedure is not commonly practiced nowadays due to its *serious complications* and availability of better alternative method.

Most accepted mechanism of action of IAHS is the liberation of prostaglandins due to necrosis of placenta and decidua which in turn excites uterine contraction and leads to expulsion of fetus. Overdistention of uterus by drawing fluid is another contributory factor.

Procedure of Administration of Intra-amniotic Hypertonic Saline (Fig. 47)

The woman lies in supine position after emptying her bladder. Under aseptic condition, skin in the midline below the fundus is infiltrated with 1% lignocaine. An 18-gauge lumbar puncture needle is passed through the abdominal wall into the uterine cavity. When clear amniotic fluid is found to flow freely through the needle after withdrawal of stylet, a drip set is attached to the needle and 20% normal saline is slowly infused. If there is bloody tap instead of clear amniotic fluid, the needle is pushed further or position is changed to get clear fluid. If no free fluid comes out, the procedure is abandoned. Woman's pulse and BP is monitored and she is observed for appearance of flushing, thirst, abdominal

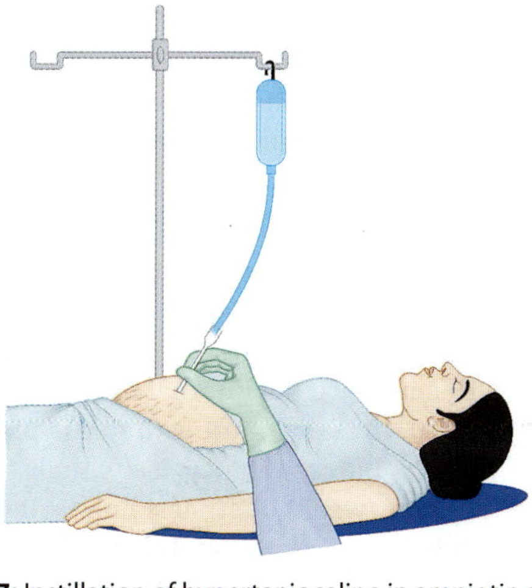

Fig. 47: Instillation of hypertonic saline in amniotic cavity.

pain, and headache during and in immediate postoperative period. Postoperatively, an antibiotic is given for 5 days.

Very rarely unusual symptoms and signs appear during and in immediate postoperative period and is usually due to accidental IV administration of hypertonic saline. 5% dextrose solution—1,000 mL infusion and diuretics in IV route is given rapidly.

Amount of hypertonic saline needed is calculated by the number of weeks multiplied by 10, hence maximum is 200 mL.

Contraindications of IAHS are heart disease, renal disease, and hypertension.

Success rate: Intra-amniotic hypertonic saline method becomes successful in 95% cases with a mean induction-abortion interval of 30–36 hours. Use of oxytocin drip lowers the induction-delivery interval. When abortion does not occur within 48 hours, it is declared as method failure.

If IAHS fails alternative method is applied. Ethacridine lactate or prostaglandins are used. IAHS can also be repeated. In case of repeated failure, possibility of extrauterine pregnancy is doubted.

Advantages of IAHS are high success rate and fetus is delivered dead (fetus dies within an hour of instillation.

Complications of intra-amniotic hypertonic saline: Minor complications are nausea, vomiting, headache, flushing, thirst, abdominal pain, and fever. Major complications are incomplete abortion, bleeding, cervical tear, infection. More serious complications are hypotension and shock due to hypernatremia following intravascular injection of hypertonic saline, renal failure, pulmonary and cerebral edema, and disseminated intravascular coagulation (DIC).

Mortality rate is 0–0.5%. Due to some of its life-threatening complications, this procedure has become almost *abandoned* in spite of high success rate.

Extra-amniotic Ethacridine Lactate

Ethacridine lactate **(Fig. 48)** is a dye which is used extra-amniotically through transcervical route to induce abortion in midtrimester (13 weeks onward).

Mechanism of action: Separation of membranes with release of prostaglandins and dilatation of cervix are the probable causes of abortion.

*Procedure of administration **(Fig. 49)**:* Patient is placed in lithotomy position. After antiseptic dressing and draping following pulling of cervix with Allis tissue forceps, a 14 or 16 no. Foley catheter is introduced through cervical canal for about 10–15 cm above the internal os. Catheter balloon is inflated with 10 mL saline and catheter is pulled down so that the balloon blocks the cervical canal. Now about 0.1% 150 mL (10 mL/week) of ethacridine lactate solution **(Fig. 48)** is instilled extra-amniotic. The catheter is removed after 4 hours.

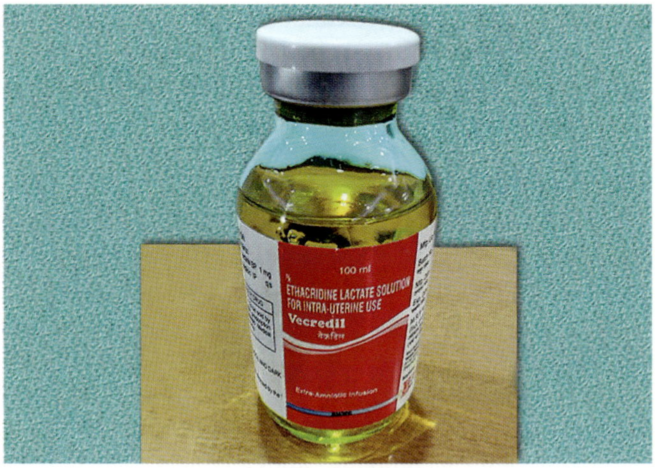

Fig. 48: Ethacridine lactate solution.

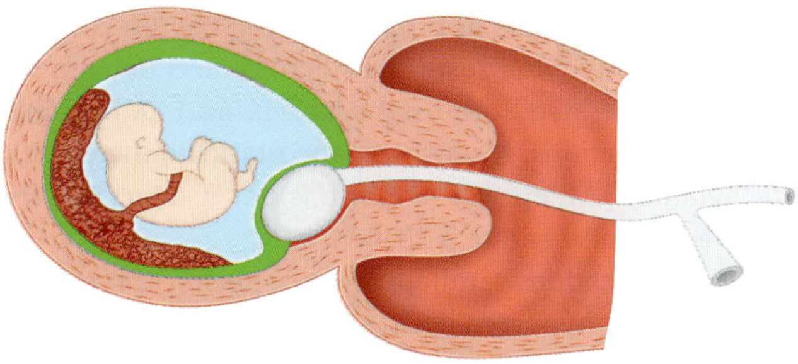

Fig. 49: Transcervical administration of extra-amniotic ethacridine lactate by Foley catheter.

Success rate is 95% with similar induction-abortion interval like IAHS. Adding of oxytocin drip increases the success rate and decreases induction-abortion interval.

Complications: There is no major complication like IAHS. High rise of temperature and incomplete abortion are the important complications.

It is a good option and a popular method for second-trimester abortion.

Prostaglandins in Induction of Abortions

With the availability of different prostaglandins and their analogues, MTP in midtrimester has become easier and safer. Prostaglandins are 20 carbon carboxylic acid containing a cyclopentene ring. It has various uses in obstetrics including MTP. The different preparations used are PGE2, PGF2α, and PGE1 which can be administered in various routes orally, vaginally, rectally, and parenterally. PGE2 is five times more potent than PGF2α. These act on the myometrium or on the cervix or both.

Different Preparations of Prostaglandins, their Doses, and Various Routes

PGE1 (misoprostol): In second-trimester abortion, dosage and route of misoprostol vary. One recommended regime is to give 400 μg of vaginal misoprostol, repeated every

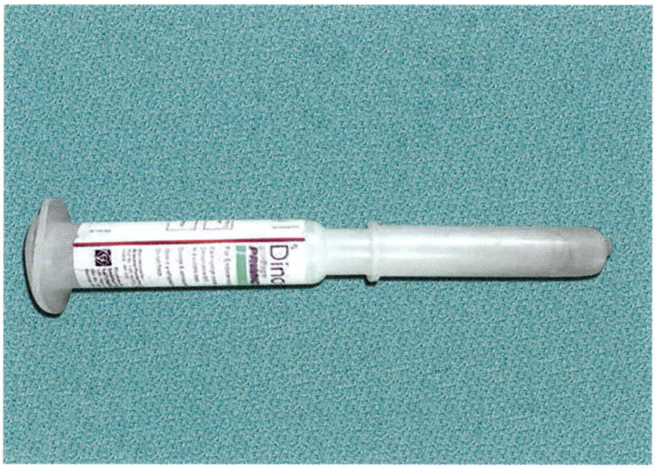

Fig. 50: Dinoprostone gel.

3–6 hours (average 4 hours) up to five total doses. Initially, it can also be started with 600 μg vaginally or sublingually. It can also be used along with oral mifepristone to increase efficacy. When, mefipristone is used, following 200 mg of mifepristone, misoprostol 400 or 600 μg is administered after 36–48 hours sublingually or vaginally followed by repeated dose of 400 μg misoprostol every 3–6 hours in vaginal, sublingual, or oral route up to five doses. If not successful following five doses it is repeated after 24-hour gap. Misoprostol is equally effective in buccal, sublingual, and vaginal route but less in oral route. Recently, misoprostol has become the most popular agent for midtrimester termination of pregnancy.

PGE2: PGE2 (*dinoprostone*) is used vaginally as suppository, and 20 mg every 3 hours or gel form in the dose of 500 μg intracervically or vaginally.

Cervical gel (**Fig. 50**) is very popular and relatively safe. Another PGE2 analogue (sulprostone) 500 μg is used intramuscularly every 8 hours. PGE2 200 μg in repeated doses can be used extra-amniotically through cervix with the help of Foley catheter.

Dinoprostone vaginal insert (tape) (Cervidil/Propess 10 mg) is also available (see pages 455 & 461).

PGF2α: 15 methyl PGF2α (carboprost tromethamin) 250 μg every 3 hours are administered in *IM route* for maximum of 10 doses. 15 methyl PGF2α (carboprost tromethamin) is also used as intra-amniotic instillation in the dose of 2 mg like IAHS. Combining with hyperosmotic urea the induction-abortion interval can be reduced. PGF2α can also be used in a dose of 200–500 μg extra-amniotically through transcervical route with repeated doses maximum up to 10 such with the help of Foley catheter (14 no.) like ethacridine lactate.

Advantages and Success Rate of Prostaglandin for Using in Midtrimester Abortion

Success rate is as high as 90% with lesser induction-abortion of 15–20 hours. Accidental IV injection has minimal

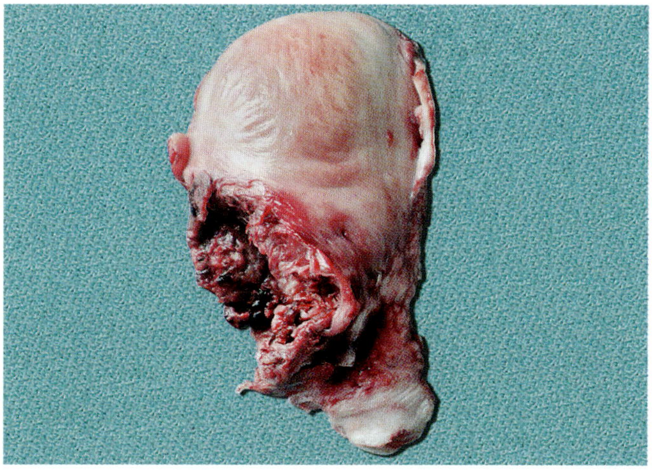

Fig. 51: Specimen of total hysterectomy for rupture uterus following attempt of induced midtrimester abortion with misoprostol in a post-cesarean delivery pregnancy.
Courtesy: Dr Subrata Samanta, RG Kar Medical College, Kolkata, West Bengal, India.

side effects. PGE1 (misoprostol) is not contraindicated in bronchial asthma where the other prostaglandins are contraindicated. Prostaglandins are used safely.

Complications of Prostaglandin

- Nausea, vomiting, diarrhea, and pain abdomen. Prior use of antiemetic reduces the side effects.
- Cervical tear and rarely rupture of uterus (**Fig. 51**).
- Incomplete abortion
- Fetus may be delivered alive in contrast to IAHS.

Concentrated High-dose Oxytocin

Oxytocin solution which is used in labor induction is not effective for midtrimester abortion and concentrated oxytocin solution becomes effective with or without vaginal PGE2 50 units of oxytocin in 500 mL normal saline infused IV in 3 hours (278 mU/min) following which 1 hour diuresis done without oxytocin. It is followed by escalating sequence of 150 units, 200 units, 250 units, and 300 units each in 500 mL normal saline in similar manner with 1 hour diuresis after each bottle. High-dose oxytocin become successful in 80–90% cases of second trimester. In comparison misoprostol is more effective with quicker expulsion for which misoprostol is preferred to oxytocin.

Hysterotomy

Hysterotomy is an operative method by which the product of conception is removed by incising the anterior wall of the uterus before 28 weeks of pregnancy. However, in broader perspective hysterotomy term is used irrespective of period of gestation, as such, cesarean delivery (CD) is also included in hysterotomy.

Abdominal or vaginal, both are possible, but it is mostly done through abdominal route.

Indications of hysterotomy:

- MTP in second trimester (13 weeks onward) when other methods fail or contraindicated.
- Second-trimester MTP with tubal ligation
- Midtrimester uncontrolled vaginal bleeding due to low-lying placenta
- In H. mole, when there is failure of vaginal method.
- Hysterotomy is not encouraged as a method of MTP due to its complications.

Procedure of abdominal hysterotomy ***(Figs. 52 to 55)****:* Woman is placed in supine position, general or epidural anesthesia is administered, antiseptic dressing, and draping done.

Low transverse or infra umbilical longitudinal incision is given to open the peritoneal cavity. Uterus is brought out through the incision and abdominal wound is fully covered with pack to prevent spillage of product of conception over the cut margins of the parieties.

The bladder peritoneum (uterovesical pouch) is incised transversely and the bladder is pushed down. Uterine cavity is opened by a longitudinal or transverse incision on its lower part in the mid-line. The products **(Figs. 56 to 58)** are gently delivered. Precautions are taken not to contaminate abdominal wound with products by surrounding the abdominal gauze. This precaution may prevent deposition of placental tissue to the wound and prevent scar endometriosis. The uterine cavity is cleaned with gauze piece. Uterine incision is closed by two layers (deep muscles and superficial muscles) with 1-0 continuous catgut stitches using round needle. Visceral peritoneum is closed transversely with continuous 1-0 catgut stitches. Injection Methergine 0.2 mg is given IM. Injection Methergine 0.2 mg IV before uterine incision is preferred by many as it makes the uterus hard and operative procedure becomes easier.

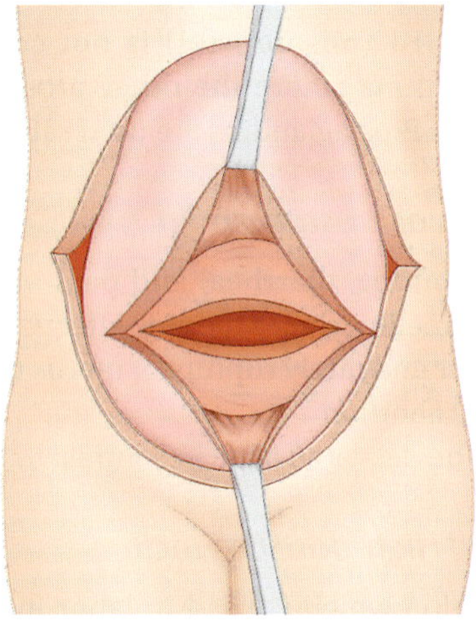

Fig. 52: Procedure of hysterotomy. Uterine cavity is opened by transverse incision at its lower part.

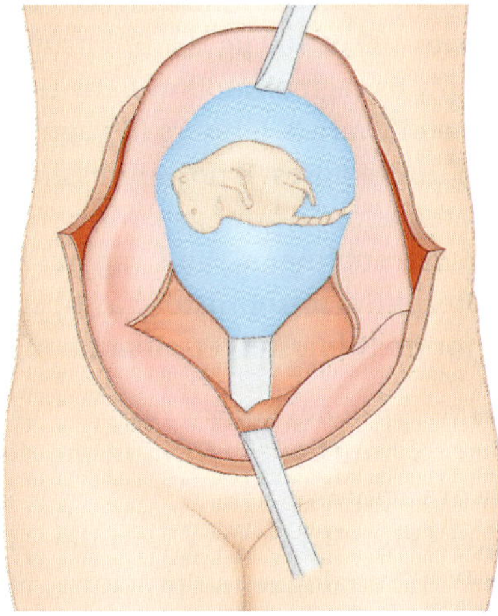

Fig. 53: Procedure of hysterotomy. The product of conception is delivered.

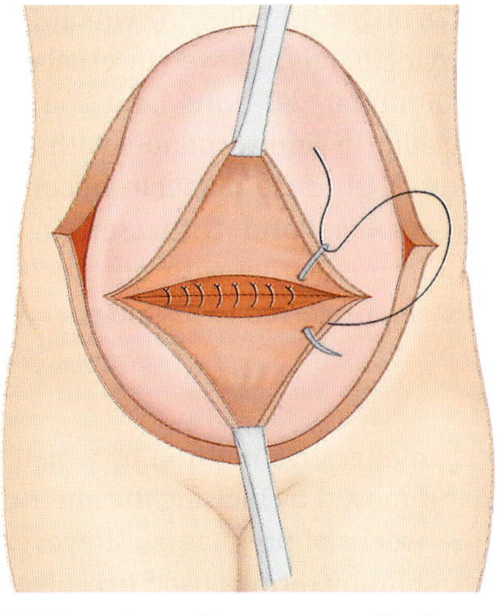

Fig. 54: Procedure of hysterotomy. Uterine wound is closed in two layers, first layer.

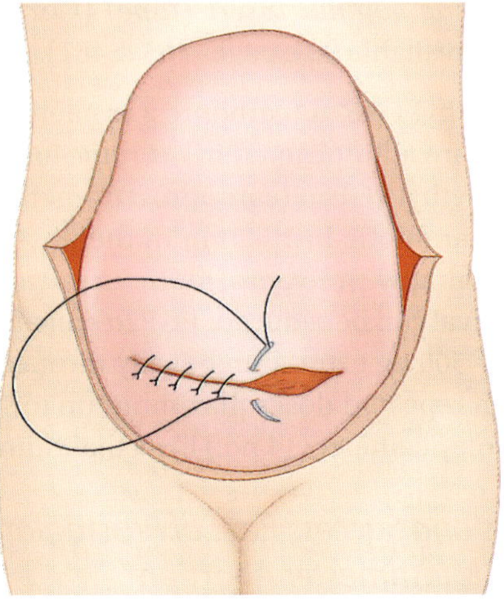

Fig. 55: Procedure of hysterotomy, closure of second layer.

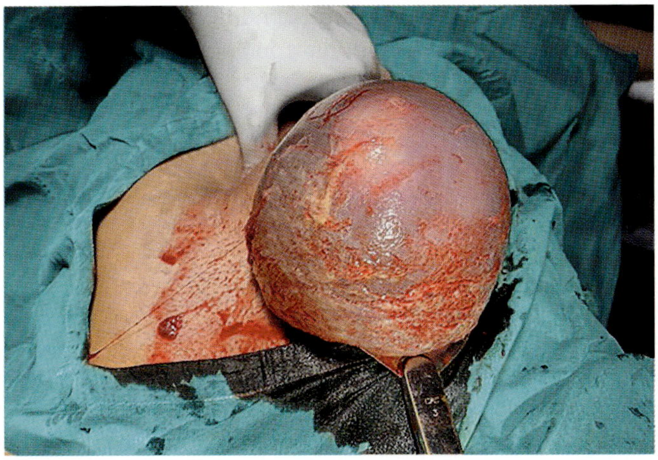

Fig. 56: Hysterotomy in previous two LSCS mother with Down syndrome positive on amniocentesis at 19 weeks + GA.
Courtesy: Professor Abhijit Rakshit, Department of Gynecology and Obstetrics, RG Kar Medical College, Kolkata, West Bengal, India.

Packings are removed and peritoneal cavity is cleaned. Abdominal wound is repaired in layers.

Complications of hysterotomy: Immediate complications are bleeding, infections, intestinal obstruction, and anesthetic hazards.

Remote complications are scar endometriosis (0.5–1%), rupture in future pregnancy, scar ectopic, adherent placenta, and menstrual abnormalities.

Indications of hysterectomy: Abortion and hysterectomy are done concurrently in cancer cervix, uncontrolled bleeding, and septic abortion.

Complications of Medical Termination of Pregnancy

The complications depend on the gestational age when abortion is being done and the methods applied.

Overall complication rate is 5% following MTP. Midtrimester abortion is always more hazardous than first trimester. Complication rate is five times more in midtrimester abortion. Termination within 8 weeks is much safer.

Immediate Complications

- Complications due to abortion process are hemorrhage, shock, incomplete abortion (most common complication), injury to cervix, uterus, and intestines, thrombosis and embolism, infection, anesthetic complications, lower abdominal pain, and fever.
- Complications which are method specific:
  - *IAHS*—hypernatremia, renal failure, DIC
  - *Ethacridine lactate*—hyperpyrexia
  - *Prostaglandins*—vomiting, diarrhea, and injury of cervix. There is slight risk of uterine rupture in repeat doses of misoprostol **(Fig. 51)** especially in scarred uterus [post-CS, postmyomectomy) for which one should be cautious.

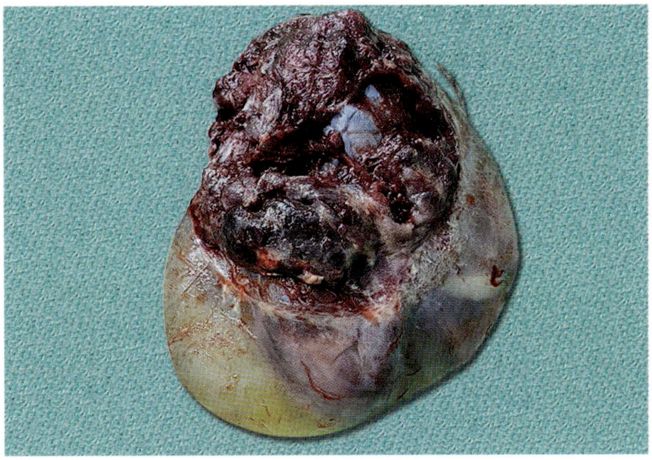

Fig. 57: Delivered intact sac to prevent spillage in the patient as in Figure 56.

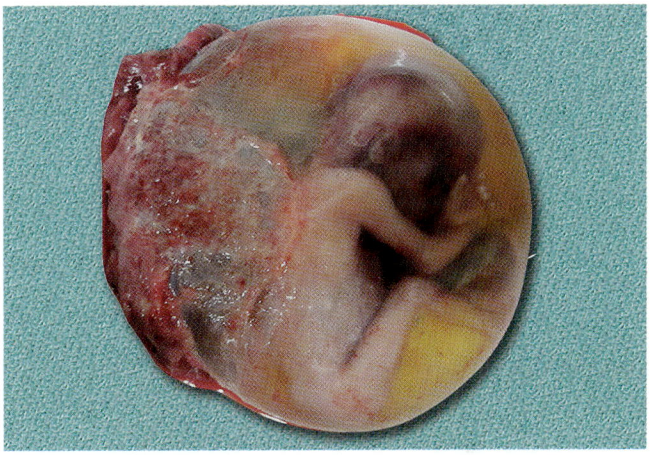

Fig. 58: Delivered intact sac in hysterotomy to prevent spillage in another patient.

  - *Oxytocin*—water intoxications
  - *Hysterotomy*—peritonitis, intestinal obstruction

Delayed Complications

- *Effect on future pregnancy:* Cervical incompetence—recurrent abortion, preterm labor, ectopic pregnancy (2–3 fold rise), chance of uterine rupture and retained placenta increases and increases perinatal death.
- *Gynecological problems:* Chronic pelvic infection, infertility (2–5%)—tubal block, uterine synechiae—amenorrhea, scanty
  - Period and menstrual abnormality. Scar endometriosis (0.5–1%) is a remote complication of hysterotomy.

Mortality Following Medical Termination of Pregnancy

0.6/1 lac abortions in first trimester and it increases 5–6 folds in midtrimester abortion. In the United States, the rate is 0.4/1 lac (2020).

SEPTIC ABORTION

Any abortion complicated with infection of the uterus and its contents as clinically evident (pyrexia, metritis, and Parametritis) is called septic abortion.

Most common cause of septic abortion is induced abortion performed without maintaining the criteria of MTP Act. Sometimes, spontaneous abortion may be complicated with infection if not cared properly.

Unsafe abortion is one kind of induced abortion which is done by an unskilled person and/or done in an environment lacking standard quality. Unsafe abortion contributes to 13% of all maternal deaths in the world and mostly (90%) are from the developing countries.

Reasons of Infection in Induced Abortion

- Proper antiseptic and aseptic precautions are not taken during evacuation.
- Preoperative presence of infection, particularly cervicitis which are not eradicated and need prior antibiotic therapy.
- Product of conception is retained where colonization of *N gonorrhea*, *Chlamydia trachomatis*, and other clostridial organism occur.
- Injury to the uterus (perforation) and adjacent structures like intestine.

Diagnostic Criteria of Septic Abortion

- Fever with a temperature of at least 100.4°F or more for 24 hours or more
- Offensive vaginal discharge
- Pain and tenderness in lower abdomen and uterus

There may be still serum/urinary β-hCG positive.

Causative Organisms of Septic Abortion

The organisms are *polymicrobial,* mainly from the normal flora of the genital tract.

Microorganisms are:

- Aerobic—*Escherichia coli, Klebsiella, Staphylococcus,* hemolytic *Streptococcus, Pseudomonas*
- Anaerobic—anaerobic streptococci, bacteroids, and *Clostridium welchii*

In 80% cases of septic abortion, infection is localized within the conceptus. In 15% cases infection extends to the other pelvic structures and only in 5% cases there may be septic peritonitis and/or generalized septicemia.

Different Grades of Septic Abortion

Grade I—localized within the uterus.

Grade II—involvement of the parametrium, Adnexae, and other pelvic structures.

Grade III—general peritonitis, endotoxic shock, or acute renal failure. Grade III septic abortion is usually sequelae of induced abortion.

Clinical Features of Septic Abortion

History of induced abortion, fever, pain abdomen, offensive purulent discharge.

On examination: Tachycardia, raised temperature, and there may be hypotension in severe cases.

Per abdominal examination: Tenderness present, distention of the abdomen, and there may be presence of muscle guard in presence of peritonitis.

Per vaginal examination: Offensive discharge may be mixed with blood. Cervix may be soft with open cervical os and tenderness over the fornices and on movement of uterus. In case of pelvic abscess, a boggy mass may be felt through posterior fornix.

Investigations for septic abortions are blood for complete blood count, ABO grouping and Rh typing, blood for urea, creatinine, and serum electrolytes and cervical or high vaginal swab for culture and sensitivity, blood culture in case of systemic spread, and urine for routine examination.

Ultrasound (USG) of pelvis and whole abdomen is done for any pelvic mass, retained products, presence of any foreign body, fluid level in intestines, and free fluid in the POD; X-ray of chest and straight X-ray abdomen to detect gas under the diaphragm in suspected bowel injury.

Complications of Septic Abortion

Complications of septic abortion are bleeding per vagina, septic shock, injury of the uterus and intestines, pelvic thrombophlebitis, generalized peritonitis, DIC, and acute renal failure.

Delayed complications of septic abortion are chronic pelvic pain, secondary infertility, ectopic pregnancy, and chronic debilitative disorder.

The mortality rate in septic abortion is about 20–25%, the most important factor is delay in seeking treatment—mostly following illegal or criminal abortion.

Septic abortion can be prevented by taking proper family planning measures to prevent unwanted pregnancy, performing abortion while maintaining the criteria of MTP act, *i.e.,* it should be done in proper place by qualified persons and in properly indicated cases and maintaining antiseptic and aseptic precautions during vaginal examinations or during any surgical procedure.

Prophylactic antibiotic during or before procedures reduce the postabortal infection. A regime like doxycycline 100 mg orally prior to procedure and 200 mg after surgery is suggested by ACOG (2015). A course of metronidazole (500 mg orally twice daily) for 5 days is a good choice.

Management of Septic Abortion

The aim of management is to control the infection, evacuate the uterine cavity, give supportive measures, and to interfere surgically according to the severity of the cases.

General care includes hospitalization, broad spectrum antibiotics and IV fluid, blood transfusion, high vaginal swab, and other investigations as mentioned above. Antibiotic is chosen properly depending on culture sensitivity report.

Specific management depends on the grade of the disease:

- *Grade I*—antibiotics and evacuation of the uterus. Antigas gangrene serum of 8,000 units and antitetanus serum of 3,000 units are given in case of criminal abortion.
- *Grade II*—antibiotics, IV fluid with crystalloids, central venous pressure monitoring, and blood arrangement for blood transfusion. Continuous bladder catheterization is done to maintain input and output chart. A specific antibiotic is given after getting culture sensitivity report. Evacuation of the uterus is done after 4–6 hours of starting the antibiotics. Posterior colpotomy may be needed where there is formation of pelvic abscess.
- *Grade III*—patient is managed in intensive therapeutic unit. Gastric suction, intravenous fluid, and sedation are given. Broad-spectrum antibiotic is continued. Routine investigations and investigations for the vital organ functions are performed. Intense monitoring is done. Surgery is indicated in specific indications.

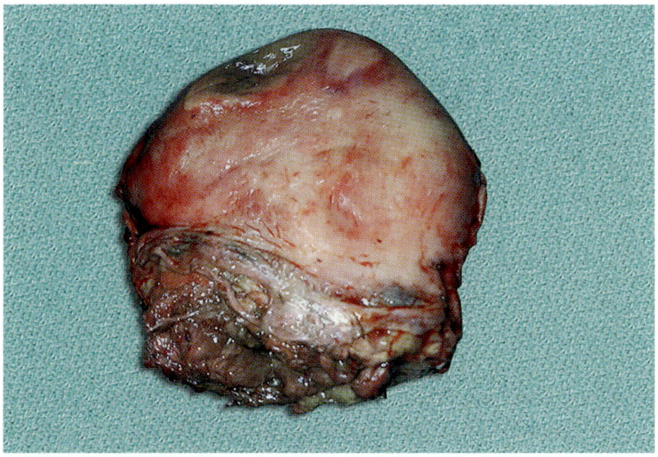

Fig. 59: Hysterectomy specimen in a 22 year P2+0 women with two living issue, referred from a remote place with history of attempt of midtrimester abortion (the method not clear) by quack about 4 weeks back. She was admitted in emaciated condition, low GC and lump abdomen with features of septic peritonitis. Following course of antibiotic and resuscitation laparotomy decision was taken. Uterus was found unhealthy and adhered with the surrounding structures and anterior wall was found opened containing placenta, with a dead macerated fetus outside. Peritoneal cavity was full of thick pus. No obvious gut injury was detected. Life of the patient was saved.

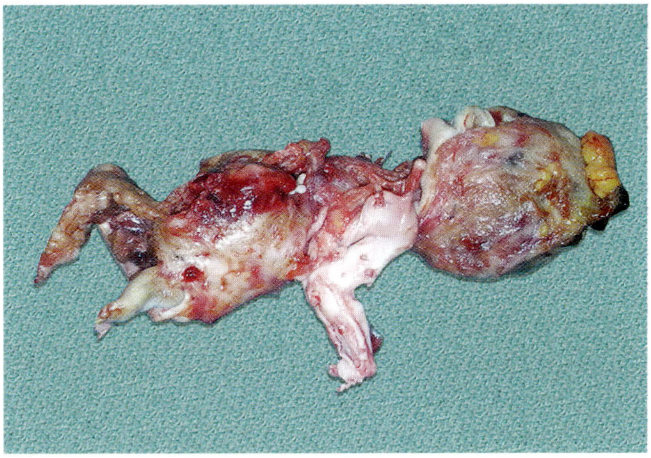

Fig. 60: Dead macerated fetus found in the abdominal cavity in the patient as described in Figure 59.

Indications of Exploratory Laparotomy in Septic Abortion

Exploratory laparotomy is done in suspected cases of bowel injury, uterine perforation, presence of foreign body inside the uterus, and collection of loculated pus (abscess) and/or peritonitis not responding to conservative management.

Computed tomography (CT)-guided pus aspiration can be attempted for pelvic abscess.

Hysterectomy may be needed in longstanding neglected cases **(Figs. 59 and 60)**. With improved care the incidence of such cases has declined.

MEDICAL TERMINATION OF PREGNANCY ACT OF INDIA FOLLOWING ITS AMENDMENTS 2021

The MTP Act was passed in 1971 and came into force from April 1, 1972 (except in Jammu and Kashmir where it became effective from November 1, 1976). The MTP Act was revised in 1975. The act has been amended in 2002 as "MTP (amendment) Act, 2002". This has been further amended in 2003 under the title "Medical Termination of Pregnancy Rules and Regulations" where the medical method of abortion has been included in the purview of MTP Act. Medical Termination of Pregnancy (Amendment) Bill, 2021 had been passed by Rajya Sabha to amend the MTP Act, 1971 ("MTP Act") on March 17, 2021 and Parliament received the assent of the President on March 25, 2021. Central Government has made the Medical Termination of Pregnancy (amendment) rules, 2021 by amending MTP rules, 2003. They came into force on the date of their publication in the official gazette by Ministry of Health and Family Welfare notification on October 12, 2021.

The Act lays down the *conditions* (indications) for which termination of pregnancy can be done, *who* (all person or persons) can perform such termination and *where* (place) can it be performed. This act also specifies the *higher limit* of period of gestation for induction of abortion.

Indications of Medical Termination of Pregnancy

Therapeutic: Heart disease (grades III and IV), severe hypertension, renal disease (chronic glomerulonephritis), diabetic retinopathy, epilepsy, severe psychiatric illness, and uncontrolled hyperemesis gravidarum. These conditions may involve a risk to the life or a grave injury to the physical health of the pregnant woman.

Eugenic: Anencephaly, Down syndrome, uncorrecv multiple anomalies, malformation due to teratogenesis, and rubella in the first trimester. These conditions involve the substantial risks to the child.

Humanitarian: Caused by rape.

Social: (1) Pregnancy due to contraceptive failure and (2) Unplanned pregnancy in a parous woman. The option (2) is the most common (80%) indication for MTP. These causes may result in a grave injury to the mental health of the pregnant woman.

Period of Gestation Up to When Medical Termination of Pregnancy is Allowed

- Up to 20 weeks MTP is allowed in all indications.
- Beyond 20 weeks till 24 weeks it is allowed in some special situations (see below).
- Beyond 24 weeks onward, *no upper limit of gestation* is specified only in *fetal malformation* decided by the medical board.

Indications of Medical Termination of Pregnancy According to Length of Pregnancy

Up to 20 Weeks

- Therapeutic
- Eugenic
- Humanitarian
- Social grounds.

In *the amendment 2021, any woman irrespective of marital status* is eligible for MTP on ground of contraceptive failure.

Beyond 20 Weeks till 24 Weeks [MTP (Amendment) Bill, 2021]

Following categories of women shall be considered:

- Survivors of sexual assault or rape or incest
- Minors
- Change of marital status during the ongoing pregnancy (widowhood and divorce)
- Women with physical disabilities [major disability as per criteria laid down under the Rights of Persons with Disabilities Act, 2016 (49 of 2016)]
- Mentally ill women including mental retardation
- The fetal malformation that has substantial risk of being incompatible with life or if the child is born, may suffer from such physical or mental abnormalities to be seriously handicapped.
- Women with pregnancy in humanitarian settings or disaster or emergency situations as declared by government.

Beyond 24 Weeks Onward [MTP (Amendment) Bill, 2021]

The fetal malformation has substantial risk of it being incompatible with life or if the child is born it may suffer from such physical or mental abnormalities to be seriously handicapped as decided by the *medical board* only after due consideration and ensuring that the procedure would be safe for the woman at that gestation age.

Eligibility Criteria of Service Providers

The practitioners are categorized in five groups, e.g., (a), (b), (c), (ca), (d).

a. In case of a medical practitioner who was registered in a state medical register immediately before the date of commencement of the Acts—he or she had experience in the practice of gynecology and obstetrics for a period of not <3 years.

b. In the case of a medical practitioner who was registered in a state medical register on or after the date of commencement of the Act, either:
   i. He or she has completed 6 months of house surgency in gynecology and obstetrics.
   ii. He or she had experience at any hospital for a period of not <1 year in the practice of obstetrics and gynecology.

c. He or she has assisted a registered medical practitioner (RMP) in at least 25 cases of MTP of which at least 5 have been performed independently in a hospital established or maintained, or a training institute approved for this purpose by the government.
   i. This training would enable the RMP to do only first-trimester terminations (up to 12 weeks of gestation).
   ii. For terminations up to 24 weeks, the experience or training as prescribed under subrules (a), (b), and (d) shall apply.

ca. RMP shall have the following experience and training for conducting termination of pregnancy up to 9 weeks of gestation period by medical methods of abortion, (incorporated in amendment 2021), namely:
   i. Experience at any hospital for a period of not <3 months in the practice of obstetrics and gynecology.
   ii. Has independently performed 10 cases of pregnancy termination by medical methods of abortion under the supervision of RMP in a hospital established or maintained, or a training institute approved for this purpose by the government.

TABLE 1: Period of gestation, category and number of registered medical practitioners.

Period of gestation	*Category of practitioners*	*Number of practitioners*
Up to 9 weeks of gestation period by medical methods of abortion	(a), (b), (c), (ca), (d)	One
Till 12 weeks of gestation by surgical method	(a), (b), (c), (d)	One
Beyond 12–20 weeks	(a), (b), (d)	One
Beyond 20–24 weeks	(a), (b), (d)	Two (Form E)
Beyond 28 weeks	(a), (b), (d)	Two practitioners will perform the termination based on the decision of Medical Board

d. In case of a medical practitioner who has been registered in a State Medical Register and who holds a postgraduate degree or diploma in gynecology and obstetrics.

For MTP beyond 24 weeks gestation period the opinion shall be given by a Medical Board duly constituted by the respective State Government or Union Territory Administration at approved facilities and two RMPs eligible under clauses (a), (b) and (d) shall perform the termination of pregnancy based on the decision of such Medical Board.

PERIOD OF GESTATION, CATEGORY, AND NUMBER OF PRACTITIONERS

The period of gestation, category, and number of practitioners is given in **Table 1**.

MEDICAL BOARD

Medical Board's opinion is needed for the purposes of termination of pregnancy *beyond 24 weeks* of gestation for fetal malformation. Medical board is constituted by State Government or Union Territory. *The Medical Board shall consist of:* (1) a gynecologist, (2) a pediatrician, (3) a radiologist or sonologist, and (4) such other number of members as may be notified by the State Government or Union Territory. *Powers of Medical Board is* to allow or deny termination of pregnancy beyond 24 weeks of gestation period only after due consideration and ensuring that the procedure would be safe for the woman and whether the fetal malformation has substantial risk of it being incompatible with life or if the child is born it may suffer from such physical or mental abnormalities to be seriously handicapped. Medical board can co-opt other specialists and ask for any additional investigations, if required. Medical Board will give decision to allow or deny in Form D within 3 days of receiving the request for MTP. Termination procedure, when advised is to be carried out within 5 days of the receipt of the request for MTP.

Place of Medical Termination of Pregnancy

Medical termination of pregnancy can be done in hospitals that are established or maintained by the government or places approved by the government, which may be a nongovernmental establishment. The place should be well equipped as per MTP rule criteria. Beyond 24 weeks termination USG should be available.

BOX 1: Key features of the MTP (Amendment) Bill 2021.

- MTP is allowed up to 20 weeks on the opinion of just one medical practitioner
- To terminate pregnancies between 20 and 24 weeks, the opinion of not less than two practitioners are needed and this applies only to special categories of women as specified
- Terminations beyond 24-week gestations can be done by two registered medical practitioners only in case of substantial risk of fetal abnormalities based on the decision of Medical Board duly constructed by the State Government or Union Territory. In that case, there is no upper limit of period of gestation
- For terminations beyond 24-week gestations no other indication is considered except substantial fetal abnormalities. There is no provision for termination of late pregnancies arising from rape in this amendment—the only option is to writ petition in the court
- Registered medical practitioners only with experience and training in gynecology/obstetrics can perform MTP
- The MMA have been allowed up to 9 weeks (from previous 7 weeks). MTP by medical method up to 9 weeks is also allowed by the medical practitioners who have undergone 3 months training in O&G or have done 10 cases of MMA under supervision of registered medical practitioners in a hospital or training institute approved for this purpose in addition to other categories of practitioners
- In the amendment 2021, failure of contraceptive failure used by any woman or her partner as a cause of MTP is not restricted to married woman, it is any woman irrespective to marital status
- No registered medical practitioner shall reveal the name and other particulars of a woman whose pregnancy has been terminated under this Act except to a person authorized (appropriate authority) by any law for the time being in force and whoever contravenes the provisions as above shall be punishable with imprisonment which may extend to 1 year, or a fine, or both (amendment)

(MTP: Medical Termination of Pregnancy; MMA: medical methods of abortion; O&G: obstetrics and gynecology)

Key Features of the Medical Termination of Pregnancy (Amendment) Bill 2021

The key features of the MTP (Amendment) Bill 2021 are given in **Box 1**.

Consent for Medical Termination of Pregnancy

The written consent of the woman concerned is mandatory for termination of pregnancy. Husband's consent is not essential. In case of a minor girl (below 18 years of age) or mentally ill person, written consent to be taken from appropriate person. POCSO Act is to be considered in dealing with pregnancy in minor girl.

NB: The MTP Amendment Act and rule which are discussed here are for academic purpose. For medicolegal purpose one must consult the original documents of law and Act and the appropriate authority.

For more about spontaneous abortion, early pregnancy failure, and recurrent pregnancy loss consult author's Bedside Clinics in Obstetrics, 5th edition, Academic Publishers.

CHAPTER 4

Ectopic Pregnancy

Learning Objectives

- Various Sites of Tubal Ectopic Pregnancy
- Etiology, Risk Factors and Pathology
- The Fates (Termination) of Tubal Pregnancy
- Diagnosis
- Management of Ectopic Pregnancy
- Conservative and Expectant Management
- Interstitial Pregnancy
- Abdominal Pregnancy
- Cervical Pregnancy
- Ovarian Pregnancy
- Cesarean Scar Pregnancy
- Heterotropic Pregnancy
- Pregnancy of Unknown Location
- Prognosis and Outcome of Ectopic Pregnancy

INTRODUCTION

Ectopic pregnancy which is the pregnancy outside the normal uterine cavity was the leading cause of death in the first trimester till recently. Morbidity arises from intraperitoneal bleeding with immediate surgery, and blood transfusion in disturbed ectopic pregnancy. After survival, women suffering from ectopic pregnancy are at risk of further ectopic, subfertility, and chronic pelvic pain in the long run. Ectopic pregnancy is responsible for 1–2% of maternal deaths. With the availability of sensitive β-human chorionic gonadotropin (β-hCG) assay and high-resolution transvaginal sonography (TVS) and awareness among people, diagnosis has become early and both morbidity and mortality from ectopic pregnancy have been diminished.

DEFINITION

When pregnancy occurs outside the normal uterine cavity, it is called ectopic pregnancy, i.e., blastocyst implants other than normal endometrium of uterus.

INCIDENCE

The incidence varies from 1 in 150 to 1 in –500 pregnancies in developing countries. In developed countries, the incidence is higher, between 1 and 2%. The incidence has increased due to various reasons. The incidence varies with the age group of women, being more in the elder group than in the younger. 95–97% cases occur in the fallopian tube. Up to 15% of women who suffer from bleeding, pain in the abdomen, or both are ultimately diagnosed as ectopic pregnancy.

Earliest Documentation

The earliest documentation of ectopic pregnancy was done by Abulcasis, an Arabian surgeon practicing in Spain in the 11th century. The first successful laparotomy for ectopic pregnancy was performed by Robert Lawson in 1883.

TYPES

Different varieties of ectopic pregnancy with their incidences are given in **Figure 1**. The most common type of extrauterine pregnancy is *tubal pregnancy* in 95–97% cases of ectopic pregnancy.

Nontubal pregnancy may occur in ovary, cervix, broad ligament, abdominal cavity, and previous cesarean section scar pregnancy.

Ovarian pregnancy is rare and incidence is 1 in 7,000–40,000 pregnancies. The incidence of cervical pregnancy is 1 in 18,000 pregnancies. Abdominal pregnancy occurs in 1 in 50,000. The incidence of interstitial/cornual* (angular)

**N.B.:* There is a difference of opinion in the nomenclature of "cornual pregnancy." In recent view (William's obstetrics), cornual pregnancy means pregnancy in the upper lateral angle, i.e., near the cornu of the uterine cavity. The name of this variety had been given as angular pregnancy by Munro Kerr. According to Munro Kerr, "cornual pregnancy" was referred to as pregnancy in a rudimentary horn of the bicornuate uterus.

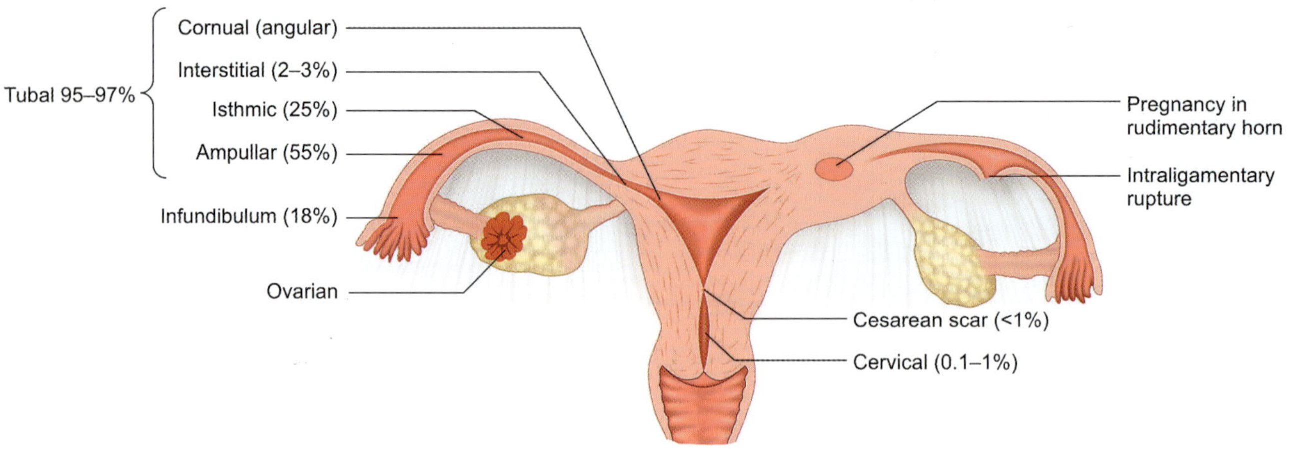

Fig. 1: Sites of ectopic pregnancy.

pregnancy is 2–3% of all ectopic pregnancies which estimates 1 in 3,000–6,000 of all pregnancies. Pregnancy in the rudimentary horn of uterus occurs in 1 in 100,000 pregnancies. The incidence of cesarean section scar pregnancy is <1%.

VARIOUS SITES OF TUBAL ECTOPIC PREGNANCY

The most common site is the ampulla (55%) followed by the isthmus (25%), then infundibulum (18%), and last interstitial variety (2%) **(Fig. 1)**. The most dangerous type is interstitial pregnancy. Interstitial rupture is most dangerous as there is a chance of rupture due to the smallest diameter of the fallopian tube. Torrential hemorrhage occurs as the utero-ovarian anastomosis (Sampson's artery) lies here and surgical management is also difficult as it lies at the utero-tubal junction.

The normal length of the fallopian tube is 10 cm. The different parts from medial to lateral are interstitial (length 1.5 cm, diameter 1 mm), isthmus (length 2.5 cm, diameter 2.5 mm), ampulla (length 5 cm, diameter 6 mm), and infundibulum (length 1 cm, diameter 3 mm). The time of tubal rupture depends on the site of implantation. Isthmic rupture mostly occurs in 6–8 weeks, ampullary pregnancy in 8–12 weeks, and interstitial rupture at 12–16 weeks.

ETIOLOGY AND RISK FACTORS OF TUBAL ECTOPIC PREGNANCY

There are various factors that may cause abnormality of tube leading to implantation of fertilized ova in tube or at another site.

The most common risk factor is previous tubal surgery, either reconstructive surgery or previous ectopic and tubal sterilization. The chance of ectopic pregnancy following a previous ectopic pregnancy is 10%. It is also not uncommon that ectopic pregnancy may occur after tubectomy, probably by spontaneous recanalization. In a previously tubectomized woman with a history of amenorrhea, pain in the abdomen and bleeding per vagina, ectopic pregnancy must be excluded. Salpingitis (chlamydial, gonococcal, tubercular) and pelvic adhesion and distortion due to any reason such as infection, endometriosis, and pelvic and abdominal surgery are risk factors of ectopic pregnancy. Attempting pregnancy in subfertility by any treatment including in vitro fertilization (IVF) and embryo transfer (ET) is likely to increase the chance of ectopic pregnancy. In previous spontaneous abortion and induced abortion, there is little increased chance of abnormal site implantation. Intrauterine contraceptive devices (IUCDs) do not increase the overall incidence, but in contraceptive failure with IUD ectopic pregnancy must be excluded as it prevents intrauterine pregnancy (IUP). The same is also true for progesterone-only contraceptive.

PATHOLOGY OF TUBAL ECTOPIC PREGNANCY

Changes in the tube: Scanty decidual changes occur in tubal mucosa and growing trophoblast penetrates to implant intramuscularly (due to lack of submucosa) resulting in hemorrhage and thinning out of muscular wall. The hemorrhage may be in the lumen, into the peritoneal cavity, or into the layers of the broad ligament. Massive hemorrhage occurs due to presence of ovarian artery at mesosalpinx.

Changes in the uterus: The uterus becomes enlarged (size not >8 weeks) due to the effects of hormones. The endometrium is transformed into a decidual membrane which may cast off either in pieces or *en bloc* (decidual cast) mimicking the shape of the uterine cavity.

Arias Stella reaction which comprise the characteristic changes in the endometrium is found in 10–15% of ectopic pregnancy due to the effect of steroid hormones. The typical histological feature is adenomatous change of the glands. These types of changes may also be found in early pregnancy, hydatidiform mole, and choriocarcinoma.

THE FATES (TERMINATION) OF TUBAL PREGNANCY

Tubal implantation may result in tubal mole, tubal abortion, tubal rupture, or spontaneous reabsorption.

Tubal mole ***(Figs. 2 and 3)****:* The specimen looks like a brown or dark-colored oval or round swelling in any part of the tube. This occurs due to choriotubal hemorrhage which separates the gestational sac from the tubal wall resulting in the death of the ovum.

Tubal abortion ***(Fig. 4)****:* Following choriotubal hemorrhage, the product of conception is expelled toward the abdominal ostium associated with hemorrhage into the peritoneal cavity. If there is excessive hemorrhage, it is collected in pouch of Douglas called *pelvic hematocele*. If the bleeding is less, an encysted collection of blood occurs around the fimbrial end of the tube which is called *peritubal hematocele*. Tubal abortion is commonly seen in ampullary implantation. If the blood is collected inside the tube with gradual distension due to partial or complete blockage of the distal end, hematosalpinx results. Abdominal pregnancy may occur (see below) if the expelled fetus through the fibmbrial end is implanted into the peritoneal cavity.

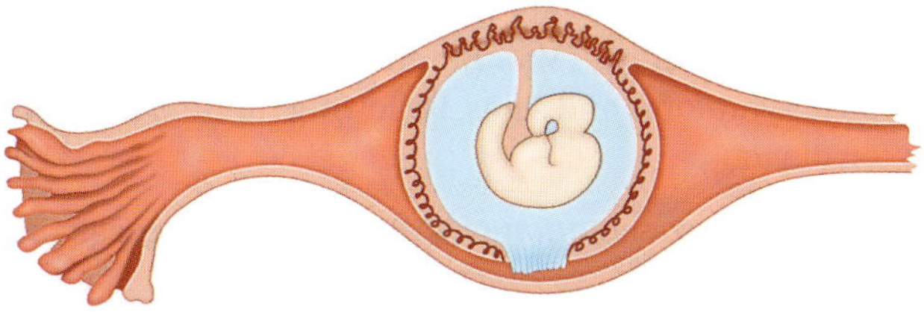

Fig. 2: Tubal mole.

Tubal rupture ***(Figs. 5 and 6)****:* Rupture occurs due to the erosion by growing chorionic villi. It is mostly seen in isthmic variety and also in interstitial variety. Rupture mostly occurs spontaneously; however, sometimes it may be precipitated by bimanual examination or coitus.

When rupture occurs on the roof or sides of the tube, *intraperitoneal* bleeding occurs and when rupture occurs in the floor of the tube in between the layers of the broad ligament *intraligamentary* bleeding (broad ligament hematoma) occurs which is commonly found in isthmic rupture. *Paratubal hematocele* is a term referred to a condition where a hematocele is formed around the ruptured site of the fallopian tube.

Spontaneous reabsorption: Death of embryo followed by spontaneous reabsorption may occur in a significant number of cases These are diagnosed recently due to the more sensitive β-hCG assay.

Secondary abdominal pregnancy or secondary intraligamentary pregnancy: The embryo with the surrounding trophoblast following rupture or abortion may be viable and implanted either in the abdominal cavity called *secondary abdominal pregnancy* (intraperitoneal) (see later) or in between the layers of the broad ligament called *intraligamentary pregnancy.*

Hematocele is the collection of the blood clots surrounded by false capsules which is formed by the lymph and covered by intestines, omentum, surface of the uterus, and layers of the broad ligament.

Reasons of Vaginal Bleeding in Ectopic Pregnancy

The bleeding is due to the shedding of decidual membrane, and blood may also come out from the site of implantation in tubal abortion.

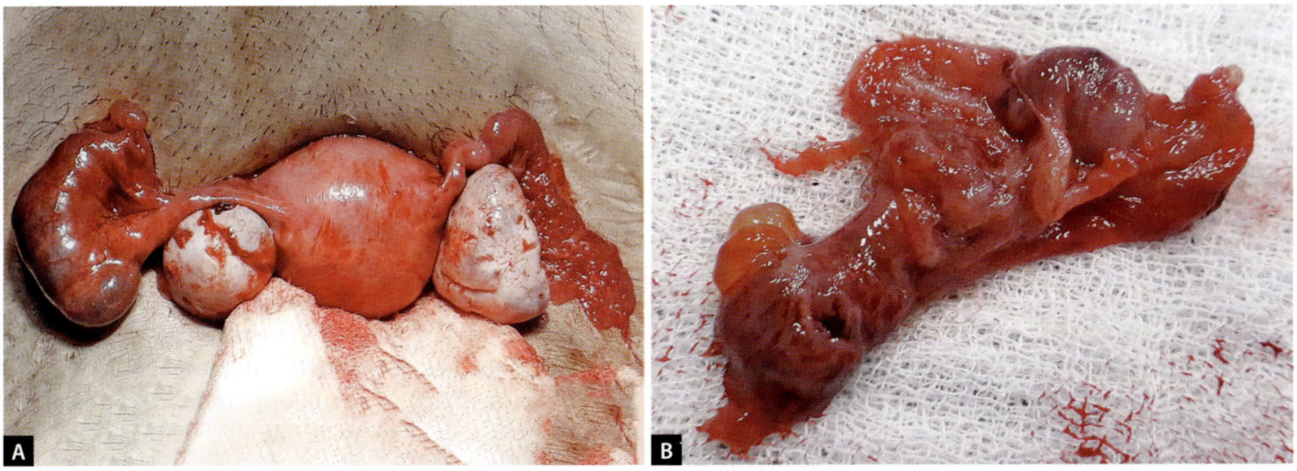

Figs. 3A and B: (A) Left-sided tubal mole. 35 years P1+1 8 weeks amenorrhea presented with bleeding P/V and pain in the abdomen. She had a history of D&C 1 week back wrongly diagnosed as incomplete abortion. (B) Excised tube containing products of conception in the same patient as in (A).
Courtesy: Dr Sumon Poddar, Dr Tanushree Mahata, Dr Anumita Chandra, RG Kar Medical College and Hospital, Kolkata, West Bengal, India.

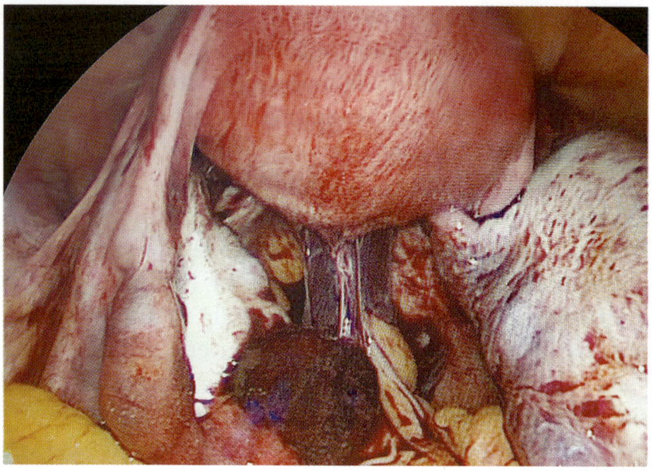

Fig. 4: Left-sided tubal abortion.
Courtesy: Dr Subhas Haldar, Consultant Gynecologist and Laparoscopic Surgeon.

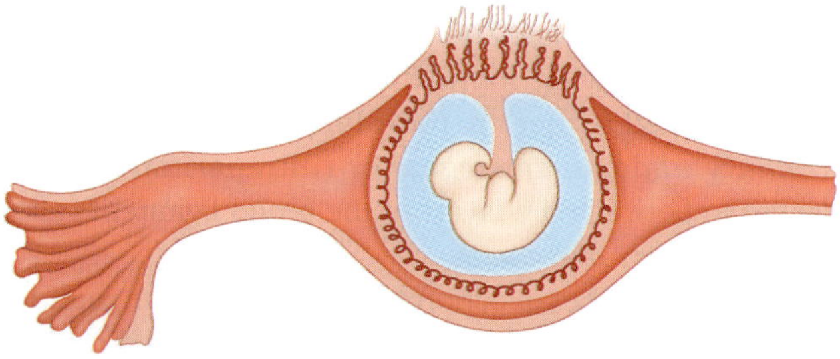

Fig. 5: Tubal rupture.

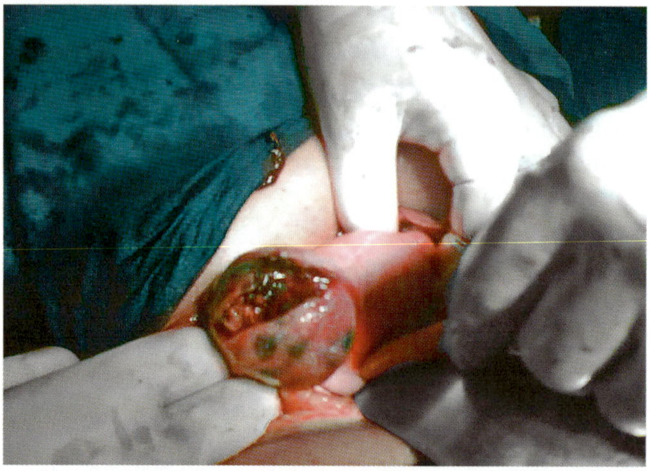

Fig. 6: Rupture tubal ectopic pregnancy.
Courtesy: Dr Pesona Grace Lucksom, Professor, Department of Obstetrics and Gynecology, Sikkim Manipal Institute of Medical Sciences, Gangtok, Sikkim, India.

Clinical Types of Tubal Pregnancy

Tubal pregnancy may be acute or chronic:

- *Acute type (30%):* It results from rapid massive hemorrhage due to tubal abortion or rupture. It is diagnosed early due to its rapid progress and being symptomatic. There is a high level of serum β-hCG and more chance of rupture.
- *Chronic type:* Due to slow oozing of blood, hematocele with a pelvic mass is formed. Death of trophoblast occurs resulting in a low level of β-hCG or nil.

CHANGING TRENDS

- *Changes in incidence and etiology:* Incidence is increasing due to the prevalence of sexually transmitted diseases (STDs), use of IUCD, tubal ligation, tubal surgery, and infertility treatment including assisted reproductive technique (ART)
- *Changing trends in presentation and diagnosis:* The patients present much earlier than before and diagnosis can also be done in the early stage due to facilities of investigations and thus diagnosed even before rupture.
- *Changing trends in management:* Recently, more conservative approaches such as medical method and conservative surgery have become possible in many cases due to earlier diagnosis.
- *Fall in case fatality:* Fatality has been decreased due to early diagnosis and rapid intervention in spite of increase in incidence.

DIAGNOSIS

Diagnosis of ectopic pregnancy is based on: (1) history-taking—symptoms and signs, (2) general examination, (3) per abdominal examination, (4) bimanual examination, and (5) investigations—urinary pregnancy test, serum β-hCG, and ultrasonography (TVS). Before rupture, there may not be typical symptoms and signs. Following rupture, diagnosis is often obvious.

Typical clinical presentation of a disturbed tubal pregnancy includes:

- Short period of amenorrhea (6–8 weeks) or just missed period
- Sudden and acute lower abdominal pain
- Vaginal bleeding
- There may be features of shock.
- History of syncope or fainting attack
- History of risk factors such as infertility, pelvic inflammatory disease (PID), previous tubal surgery

Classical triad of disturbed ectopic pregnancy includes *amenorrhea* (75%), *abdominal pain* (almost in all cases), and *vaginal bleeding* (70%). Severe vaginal hemorrhage is a typical finding of incomplete abortion, occasionally in ectopic pregnancy. Massive hemoperitoneum may irritate diaphragm resulting in shoulder pain on deep inspiration (*Danforth's sign*) which can be found in some patients.

General Physical Examination

There may be features of shock—severe pallor, tachycardia, hypotension with gradual fall of blood pressure, cold clammy skin, and sweating due to hemoperitoneum. Pallor is out of proportion to the revealed vaginal bleeding. There may not be features of shock in mild-to-moderate bleeding.

Breasts examination shows pregnancy changes of the breast.

Abdominal Examination

It may show fullness of the lower abdomen. Palpation elicits lower abdominal tenderness—muscle guard is usually not present which is obvious in septic peritonitis (differentiating feature). Shifting dullness and fluid thrill may be present. No definite mass is palpable. *Cullen's sign* (periumbilical cyanosis) is rarely found in a thin patient.

Per Vaginal Examination (Bimanual Examination)

Vagina looks pale. There is extreme tenderness on movement of the cervix (cervical motion tenderness) or palpation of the fornices. Fullness of the pouch of Douglas is seen due to collection of blood. Usually, no mass is palpable. The mass may be palpable in case of old ectopic pregnancy. The uterus is normal in size or slightly bulky due to hormone stimulation which seems to float in water. There may be vaginal bleeding and may be passage of decidual cast which sometimes may be wrongly diagnosed as miscarriage. Careful examination of the tissue and absence of villi by histopathology can confirm decidual cast.

Investigations to Confirm Ectopic Pregnancy and Other Investigations

In *disturbed* ectopic pregnancy, such as in acute rupture, diagnosis can be done mostly on clinical findings. The investigations are helpful to diagnose and to confirm the cases of tubal abortion, old ectopic, and unruptured ectopic.

The investigations are: (1) estimation of serum β-hCG or urinary pregnancy test, which becomes positive, and (2) Ultrasonography (transvaginal sonography).

Rh Anti-D Gamma Globulin

Other investigations are hematocrit, complete blood count, blood group and Rh status and routine urine analysis. *Regardless the site of ectopic pregnancy, every woman of Rh-negative blood group should receive anti-D gamma globulin.* For the first trimester, the dose is up to 50–150 μg and according to American College of Obstetricians and Gynecologists (ACOG) (2019) in later gestation the dose is 300 μg.

Ultrasonography (Transvaginal Sonography)

Findings are adnexal mass separated from the ovary with empty uterus and fluid in the pouch of Douglas. Gestational sac with fetus can be visible in adnexal mass **(Fig. 7)**. Well-defined gestational sac in the adnexal region with fetal part or cardiac activity is the definite sign of ectopic gestation which is seen in only 10–15% cases. More commonly, only a sac-like structure or complex mass associated with pelvic or general peritoneal echogenic fluid (hemoperitoneum which is characteristic of ectopic pregnancy) are the findings in ruptured adnexal ectopic pregnancy.

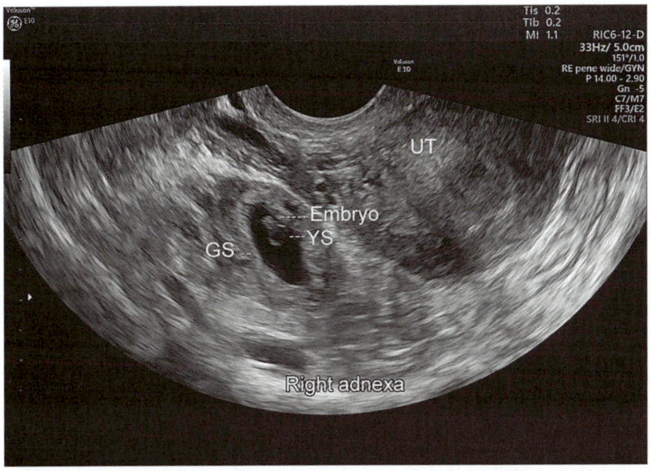

Fig. 7: USG showing right-sided unruptured tubal pregnancy. Crown–rump length (CRL) 4.5 mm, gestational age (GA) 6 weeks 1 day. *Courtesy:* Professor Kamal Oswal, Head, Department of Radiodiagnosis, Vivekananda Institute of Medical Sciences, Kolkata, West Bengal, India.

Sometimes, around the anechoic gestational sac, a hyperechoic halo is visible. If there is bleeding within the ectopic pregnancy, the adnexa looks a solid complex mass which is seen in more than half of the cases. *Ring of fire* visible by color Doppler indicates blood flow at the periphery of adnexal mass. However, a similar finding may be seen also in a corpus luteal cyst.

In case of IUP, gestational sac is evident between 4½ and 5 weeks, yolk sac at 5–6 weeks, and fetal pole with heart beat is detected between 5½ and 6 weeks in TVS, slightly later in abdominal USG.

Uterus in ectopic pregnancy: In ectopic pregnancy, the uterus becomes slightly enlarged and the endometrium becomes trilaminar. Endometrium strip thickness is not <8 mm. Anechoic fluid collection in endometrial layers which is seen early IUP may also be seen in ectopic pregnancy called *pseudogestational sac*. Here, pseudogestational sac lies in the midline of endometrial cavity whereas a normal gestational sac lies eccentrically in the endometrium (confronting to cavity shape). *Double decidual sac* (DDS) sign which is the definite earliest sign of intrauterine gestation includes two concentric echogenic rings comprising decidua capsularis and parietals separated by a hypoechoic endometrial cavity. Absence of DDS sign raises suspicion of pseudosac in ectopic gestation due to small fluid within the endometrial cavity itself.

N.B.: Sonography appearance of empty uterus, abnormal pelvic mass, and fluid in the cul-de-sac along with a positive pregnancy test is almost diagnostic of ectopic pregnancy.

Other procedures are as follows:

Laparoscopy: It is very helpful in doubtful cases. There is an added advantage of performing definitive surgery. It is performed if the patient is hemodynamically stable.

Culdocentesis: It is a safe and simple procedure. It is very useful where sonography and laparoscopy are not available. After catheterization, the posterior lip of the cervix is held by Allis tissue forceps and retracted outward and upward to the symphysis pubis to visualize the posterior fornix. The posterior vaginal wall is retracted with posterior vaginal speculum. A lumber puncture needle (18-gauge needle) fitted with syringe is punctured through the posterior fornix and on aspiration, the drawing of nonclotting blood denotes the presence of blood in the peritoneal cavity. If the aspirated blood sample clots, it indicates vessel puncture or excessive fresh hemorrhage from the rupture ectopic.

Laparotomy: It confirms the diagnosis. Negative laparotomy is better than missing and leaving behind an ectopic pregnancy only on clinical ground.

Serial hemoglobin and hematocrit estimation is essential to measure the degree of hemorrhage, especially concealed intraperitoneal hemorrhage.

Serum β-hCG Estimation—Physiological Basis and Implication of Diagnosis in Ectopic Pregnancy

β-hCG, a glycoprotein, is produced by placental trophoblast. In early pregnancy, the β-hCG level doubles every 1.4–2 days. Thus, it rises to 1,000 mIU/mL by 5 weeks, 2,500 mIU/mL by 6 weeks, and 13,000 mIU/mL by 7 weeks. A doubling of β-hCG concentration over 48 hours is often used to predict viability of fetus. Below this level, there may be disturbed uterine pregnancy or ectopic pregnancy, which can be discriminated by TVS. The minimum expected rise in its level in 2 days for a viable IUP should be at least 53%. A single measurement of β-hCG is not very helpful as there may be an overlapping of serum β-hCG level ranging from 100 to >50,000 mIU/mL in both ruptured and unruptured pregnancies.

Discriminatory Level of β-hCG

Because the exact gestational age is often unknown, corroboration of β-hCG level with USG findings is done to diagnose ectopic pregnancy. *Discriminatory level is the absolute concentration of serum* β-hCG *at which a viable pregnancy should be detected by USG scan.* With a serum β-hCG level of ≥6,500 mIU/mL, a gestation sac should be visible in the uterus by transabdominal ultrasonography in IUP and the sac should be absent in ectopic pregnancy. The level is ≥1,500 mIU/mL with TVS and in others' opinion, it is ≥2,000 mIU/mL.

Value of Serum Progesterone Assay in Diagnosis of Ectopic Pregnancy

Serum progesterone level measurement is not considered accurate enough to diagnose ectopic pregnancy. It is helpful if the level is very high or very low. When serum β-hCG and TVS are inclusive, the progesterone value may be of help. The level is much higher in viable IUP than in ectopic pregnancy or in miscarriage. A serum progesterone value of >25 ng/mL is suggestive of live IUP and <6 ng/mL is likely to be nonviable pregnancy.

Role of Endometrial Sampling as a Diagnostic Modality of Ectopic Pregnancy

It is used as a confirmatory test for disturbed IUP and thus excludes ectopic pregnancy in a case with low β-hCG or progesterone level and TVS with indeterminate findings, as it can rule out an ectopic with a small chance of interrupting a potentially viable IUP. Ectopic pregnancy is excluded if chorionic villi are obtained. If there are no villi and β-hCG level does not fall or increase, the chance of ectopic pregnancy is likely. But dilation and curettage (D&C) should not be recommended as a diagnostic modality for ectopic pregnancy because it is an invasive procedure and many cases of miscarriage can be managed successfully by conservative management without endometrial sampling. Few groups advice D&C before methotrexate therapy to identify absence of trophoblastic tissue.

DIFFERENTIAL DIAGNOSIS OF ACUTE ECTOPIC PREGNANCY

- Miscarriage
- Salpingitis
- Twisted ovarian cysts
- Rupture of chocolate cysts
- Appendicitis
- Renal stone
- Cystitis
- Ovarian apoplexy (ruptured corpus luteum cysts)

Pain in the lower abdomen is almost a common symptom in all the cases. Presence of bleeding may help to exclude the surgical causes including urinary tract infection (UTI).

The features of *ovarian apoplexy (ruptured corpus luteum cysts)* simulate the presentation of ectopic pregnancy except negative β-hCG. However, management is similar to disturbed tubal pregnancy, i.e., surgical exploration.

MANAGEMENT OF ECTOPIC PREGNANCY

Management of ectopic pregnancy depends on the site, gestational age, patient's condition at diagnosis, future desire of childbearing, and the place of management.

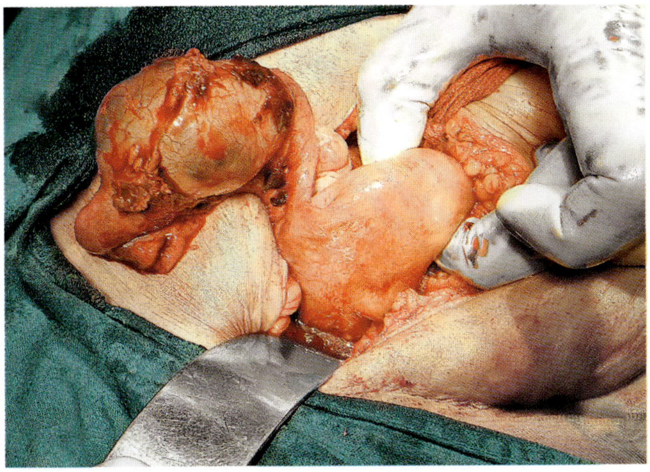

Fig. 8: Right-sided tubal ectopic pregnancy. A 36-year-old woman P1+2 with history of wrongly attempt of dilation and evacuation (D&E) twice for medical termination of pregnancy (MTP) admitted with pain in the lower abdomen and bleeding per vaginum (PV).
Courtesy: Dr Tanushree Mahata and Dr Anumita Chandra, RG Kar Medical College and Hospital, Kolkata, West Bengal, India.

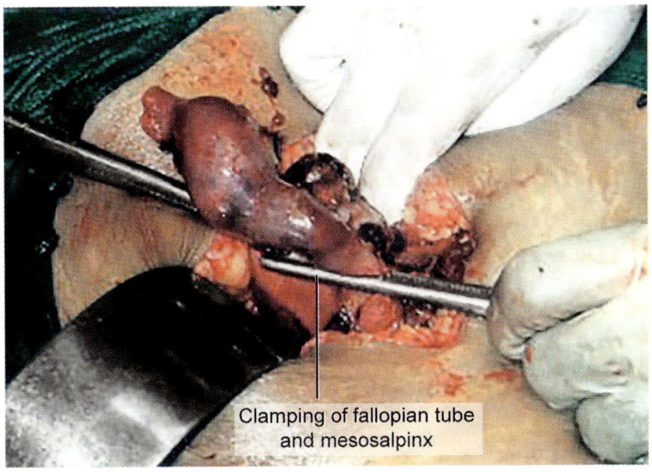

Fig. 9: Salpingectomy (laparotomy). One clamp medial to the ectopic side and another on the mesosalpinx applied laterally.

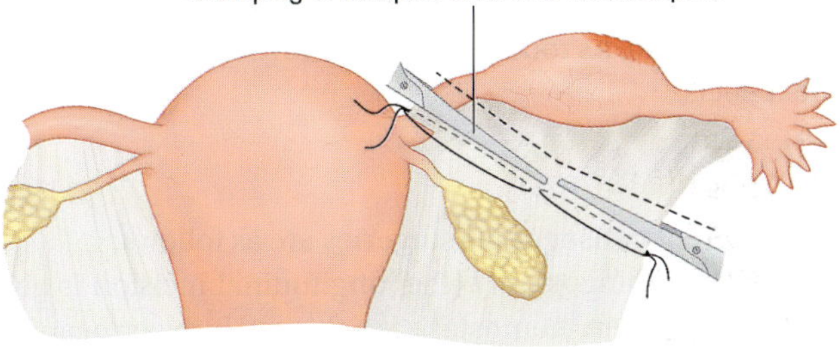

Fig. 10: Salpingectomy. One clamp medial to the ectopic side and another on the mesosalpinx applied laterally.

Regardless of the site of ectopic pregnancy, every woman of Rh negative blood group should receive anti-D gamma globulin as stated above.

MANAGEMENT OF A CASE OF DISTURBED TUBAL PREGNANCY

Immediate *hospitalization*, quick *resuscitation*, and simultaneous arrangement for *laparotomy* followed by definitive surgery, commonly salpingectomy, are the three basic steps of management **(Figs. 8 to 11)**. Other than salpingectomy, *conservative surgery* (described below) is also done.

STEPS OF MANAGEMENT OF ECTOPIC PREGNANCY

Resuscitation with Ringer's solution and arrangement for blood transfusion are done. Surgery can be done by laparotomy (open surgery) or by laparoscopy [minimal invasive surgery (MIS)].

Steps of Laparotomy

The patient is placed in supine position and general usually anesthesia is administered. After urinary bladder catheterization and antiseptic dressing and draping, an infraumbilical longitudinal skin incision is given to open the abdomen. The uterus is grasped and drawn with hands. Both the tubes and ovaries are inspected one by one to locate the site of ectopic pregnancy. Salpingectomy is done by giving one clamp medial to the ectopic site and another on the mesosalpinx applied laterally **(Figs. 8 to 10)**. Blood from the peritoneal cavity is sucked out, clots are removed, and peritoneal toileting is done. The abdomen is closed in layers. The excised specimen is sent for histopathological examination.

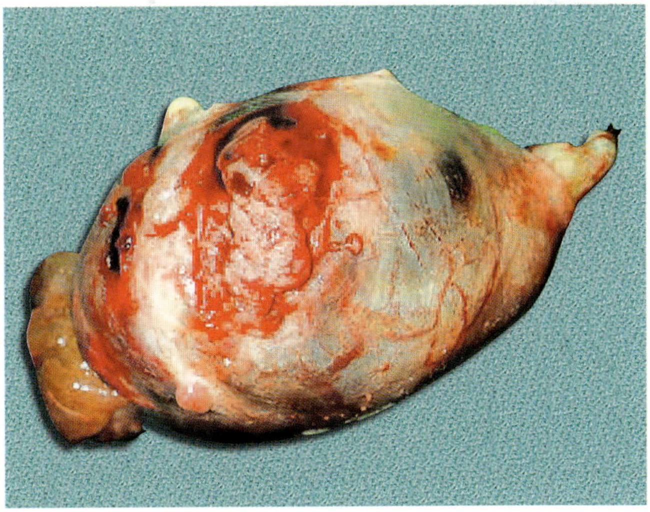

Fig. 11: Excised tube containing ectopic pregnancy.
Courtesy: Dr Avishek Bhadra, Assistant Professor, Medical College, Kolkata, West Bengal, India.

On histological examination, the *structure* of trophoblastic tissue is the usual finding; however, in true ectopic pregnancy, the resected tube may be devoid of trophoblasts which may be expelled during rupture of tubal abortion.

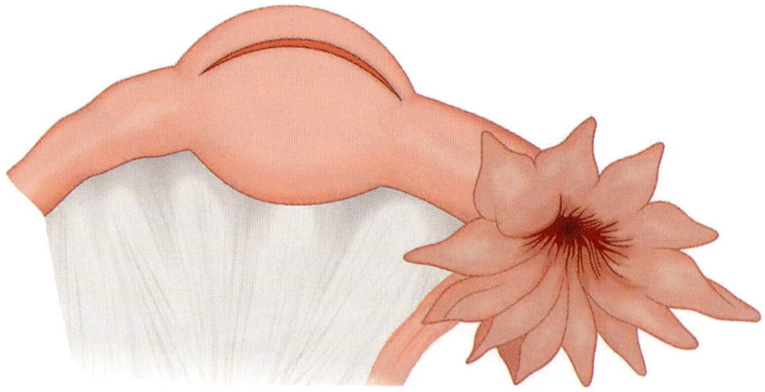

Fig. 12: Linear salpingostomy or linear salpingotomy (see text)—before removal of product.

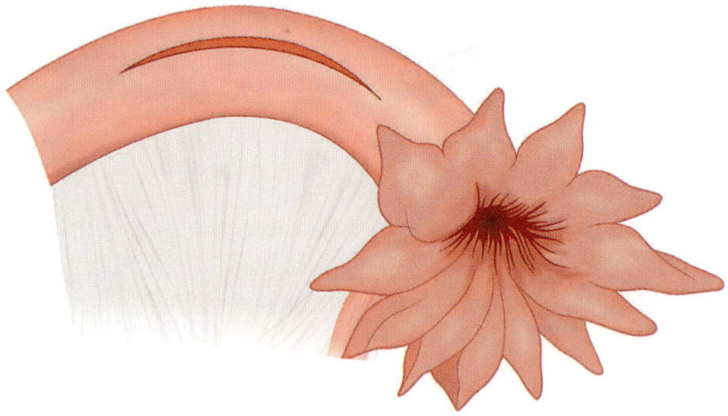

Fig. 13: Linear salpingostomy or linear salpingotomy—after surgery.

Autotransfusion

Autotransfusion is a procedure by which hemorrhagic blood from the peritoneal cavity is collected and mixed with sodium citrate solution, which is filtered through the sterile gauge and transfused to the patient. It is done where donated blood is not available. Its routine use is not advocated because of its side effects.

Conservative Surgery

The different conservative surgeries are as follows:
- Linear salpingostomy (the longitudinal incision is given and kept open, hemostasis is achieved by electrocautery) **(Figs. 12 and 13)**
- Linear salpingotomy (the incision is closed with sutures 7-0 vicryl suture)
- Segmental resection and anastomosis
- Fimbrial expression

This procedure is done either microsurgically following laparotomy or through laparoscopy (see below). The conservative surgery is indicated when the patient desires future pregnancy and the ectopic pregnancy is of small length, usually <2 cm.

Laparoscopy in Ectopic Pregnancy

Laparoscopy is done for (1) diagnostic purpose and (2) definitive surgery, where the patient is hemodynamically stable.

The advantage is that the diagnosis and management can be done in the same sitting and no laparotomy is needed. There is less blood loss, less analgesic requirement, shorter hospital stay, rapid recovery, and quick resumption to work.

Which route is preferred for surgery of ectopic pregnancy—laparotomy or laparoscopy (MIS)?

Skilled laparoscopic surgeons with the help of modern instrument prefer to do laparoscopic surgery. Shorter operative time and quick hemorrhagic control are both advantages of laparoscopy even if there is hemoperitoneum. A hemodynamically unstable patient, in general, is considered as a contraindication of laparoscopic surgery. Many experienced surgeons feel safe to do rapidly with safety. But pneumoperitoneum-associated lowered venous return and cardiac output must be taken into consideration in making decision of laparoscopic surgery in an unstable patient. With more experience, laparoscopy has become the preferred surgical approach for ectopic pregnancy in expert hand.

Types of surgery done in laparoscopy are:
- *Definitive—salpingectomy* **(Figs. 14 and 15)**
- *Conservative surgery—salpingostomy* **(Figs. 16 and 17)**
- Others such as laparoscopic loop ligation and excision of the loop

Two trials compared the two methods between salpingectomy and salpingostomy as far as reproductive outcome is concerned. One is ESEP (The European Surgery in Ectopic Pregnancy) trial and the other is DEMETER trial (2013). There was no difference in two methods to achieve future IUP by both these trials. Salpingectomy is a reasonable treatment when the contralateral tube appears normal as it avoids persistent or recurrent ectopic pregnancy (5–8%) in the same tube. Laparoscopic salpingostomy is indicated when the other fallopian tube is damaged or absent and the woman strongly desires fertility and the woman is hemodynamically stable.

Salpingectomy can be done by (1) electrosurgical coagulation of the tube and mesosalpinx **(Figs. 14 and 15)** or (2) endoscopic suture-loop (Endo-loop) ligation and excision of the loop.

In salpingostomy **(Figs. 16 and 17)**, following 1–1.5 cm incision (using monopolar needle, bipolar needle, scissors, or harmonic scalpel) on the antimesenteric surface, the ectopic tissue is flushed and removed with blunt and hydrodissection meticulously so that no trophoblast is retained which may cause invasion and bleeding. Dilute vasopressin is injected into mesosalpinx for hemostasis before incision. Finally, hemostasis is secured by electrocoagulation and the wound is kept open to unite spontaneously. Weakly monitoring of serum β-hCG following salpingostomy is suggested to detect persistent trophoblast, and additional surgical or medical therapy is sometimes needed in case of increasing or static level of serum β-hCG.

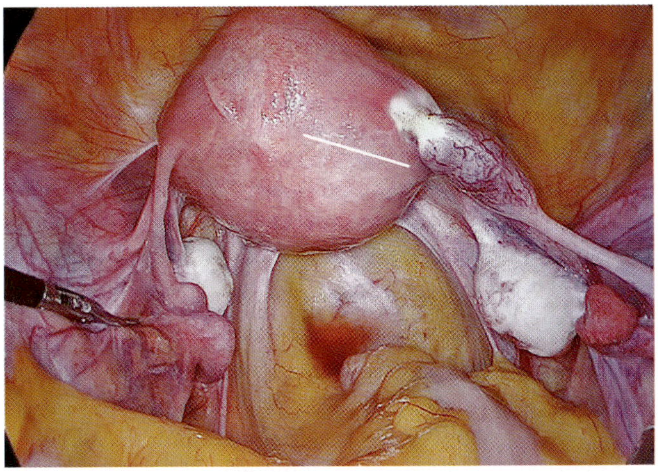

Fig. 14: Laparoscopic approach in a right-sided cornual ectopic pregnancy.

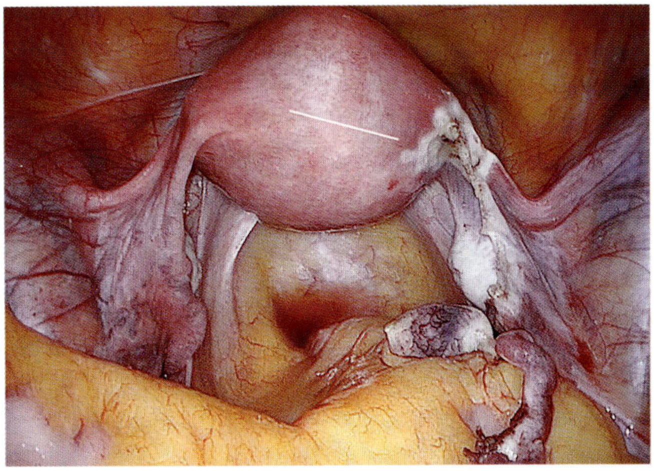

Fig. 15: Following laparoscopic salpingectomy in the case as in Figure 14.
Courtesy: Dr Subhas Haldar, Consultant Gynecologist and Laparoscopic Surgeon.

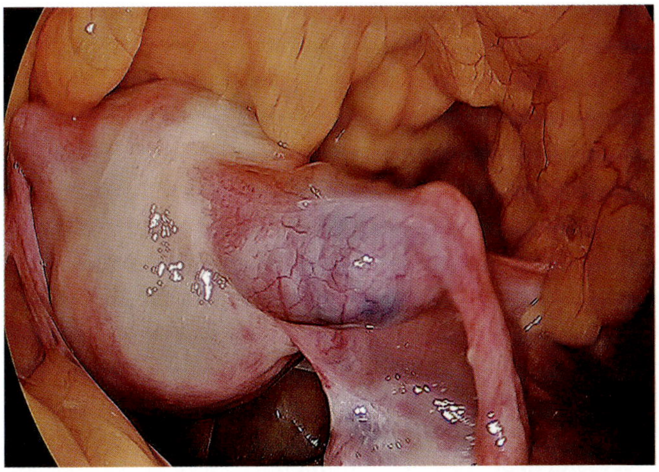

Fig. 16: Laparoscopic view of unruptured ectopic pregnancy.
Courtesy: Dr Abhinibesh Chatterjee, Consultant Gynecologist and Laparoscopic Surgeon.

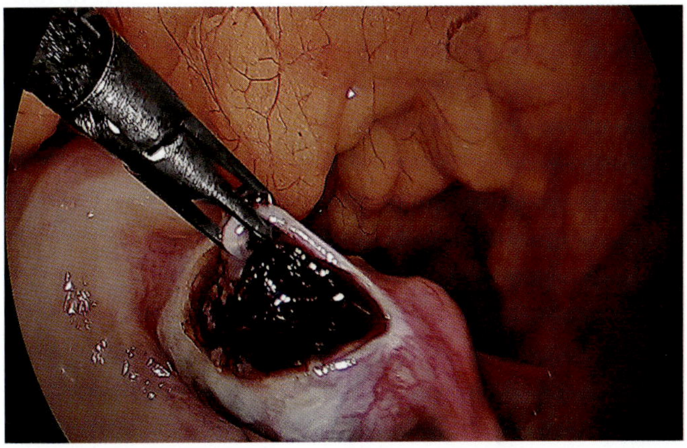

Fig. 17: Laparoscopic salpingostomy of unruptured ectopic in the case in Figure 16.
Courtesy: Dr Abhinibesh Chatterjee, Consultant Gynecologist and Laparoscopic Surgeon.

Using fallopian tube stripping forceps (FTSF) can be a better conservative method for distal fallopian tube ectopic where bleeding and recurrence are less.

Laparoscopic method is discussed in detail in Chapter 23.

CONSERVATIVE MANAGEMENT OF ECTOPIC PREGNANCY

- Medical management
- Conservative surgery as described

Medical Management of Ectopic Pregnancy

Using cytotoxic drug for treatment of ectopic pregnancy without surgical intervention in selected cases of undisturbed ectopic pregnancy is called medical management. Methotrexate is used systemically (IM or oral) or locally by directly injecting into sac, either by laparoscopy or transvaginally or by culdocentesis. It is the preferred choice if criteria are fulfilled and the patient has access to attend in emergency.

Criteria for Medical Management

- No hemodynamic instability
- No tubal rupture
- Desires fertility
- Gestational sac $\leq$3.5 cm
- Serum β-hCG <5,000 mIU/mL—best prognostic indicator
- No cardiac motion on USG
- Asymptomatic, ability, and willingness to comply with follow-up

Drugs Used and Regimen and Monitoring for Medical Therapy in Ectopic Pregnancy

Antimetabolite methotrexate, a folic acid antagonist, is used. The mechanism is blocking the transformation of dihydrofolate to tetrahydrofolate, active form of folic acid. It works against proliferative trophoblast. Preoperative laboratory investigations such as renal function test, liver function test, and complete blood count are essential.

Single dose: Methotrexate 50 mg/m^2 IM is administered without leucovorin.

Multiple dose: Methotrexate 1 mg/kg daily IM on D1, D3, D5, D7 and leucovorin (folinic acid) 0.1 mg/kg daily IM on D2, D4, D6, D8. Multiple doses are more effective than single dose. Leucovorin is administered as its action is like folic acid and prevents side effects by allowing purine and pyrimidine synthesis.

Monitoring in Case of Medical Management

For *single dose:* Serum β-hCG is measured on D1 (starting day), D4, and D7. The difference between D4 and D7 levels should be at least 15%. The dose should be repeated if the difference between D4 and D7 levels is <15% or fetal cardiac activity is present on D7. It is repeated weekly until undetectable (usually it takes 4 weeks to occur). The overall success rate is 87%.

For multiple dose: The serum β-hCG level is checked every alternate day until it is decreased to 15% in 2 consecutive days. Then weekly serum β-hCG estimation is done until undetectable.

Side effects of methotrexate Minor side effects are nausea, vomiting, diarrhea, gastritis, abnormal liver function test (LFT), stomatitis, transient pneumonia, and bone marrow depression. Rare but serious side effects are neutropenia, pneumonitis, and alopecia. These are more common with multiple dose therapy.

Counseling and Follow-up in Medical Management

The patient should be informed that the failure rate is at least 5–10%. In failure cases, surgical intervention is needed. There is chance of tubal rupture during treatment requiring emergency laparotomy; hence, symptoms and signs of tubal rupture should be explained to the patient. Close follow-up is mandatory.

Contraindications of Methotrexate

These are tubal rupture, IUP, immunosuppression, liver, kidney and hematological disorders, breast feeding, active lung disease, peptic ulcer, and hypersensitivity to methotrexate.

During methotrexate therapy, the patient should be advised to avoid nonsteroidal anti-inflammatory drugs (NSAIDs) as these delay renal clearance, alcohol which can increase liver enzyme, folic acid-containing substance that causes reduction of methotrexate efficacy, coitus as it may aggravate rupture ectopic, and sunlight to prevent skin infection. Methotrexate is teratogenic causing skeletal and craniofacial abnormality. It is secreted in breast milk.

EXPECTANT MANAGEMENT OF ECTOPIC PREGNANCY

It is a fact that spontaneous resolution occurs in few cases of ectopic pregnancy without any treatment. With this idea, only observation can be done in women with early, unruptured ectopic pregnancy and with low serum β-hCG level with close follow-up.

The criteria for expectant management in ectopic pregnancy are:

- Patient is asymptomatic and hemodynamically stable
- Small adnexal mass (3 cm diameter)
- Low serum β-hCG level <1,000 mIU/mL or falling serum β-hCG level
- Woman willing to accept the risk of tubal rupture
- <100 mL fluid in PO
- No evidence of intraperitoneal bleeding or rupture.

Follow-up and Counseling of Expectant Management

Women with expectant treatment should be followed up twice weekly with serum β-hCG and weekly by TVS to ensure rapid decrease in serum β-hCG level and a reduction in the size of the mass by 7 days. Then weekly serum β-hCG level and TVS are advised until the serum β-hCG level becomes <20 IU/L. Expectant treatment should be undertaken only in appropriately selected and counseled patients who have easy access to hospitals. Expectant management becomes successful in 50–70% of the women.

INTERSTITIAL PREGNANCY (FIGS. 18 TO 21)

Pregnancy occurs in the portion of the fallopian tube that traverses the uterine wall. In addition to other risk factors, prior ipsilateral salpingectomy is specific to this pregnancy. Pregnancy may grow up to 8–16 weeks following which rupture takes place. It is the *most dangerous type* of ectopic pregnancy as torrential hemorrhage occurs due to dual supply by both uterine and ovarian arteries and mortality is high.

Diagnosis is very difficult and confused with IUP implanted near cornu. As it is diagnosed late, the scope of conservative method with medical therapy is less.

Ultrasound criteria of diagnosis are: (1) endometrium lies 1 cm away from the sac, (2) uterus is empty, (3) there is very thin uterine myometrium surrounding the sac, and (4) an echogenic line extends from the gestational sac to the uterine cavity, called "interstitial line sign." MRI and 3D sonography are helpful to diagnose in dilemmas. Majority are diagnosed on laparoscopy/laparotomy and currently can be diagnosed by USG **(Fig. 21)** before rupture. Laparoscopically a swelling

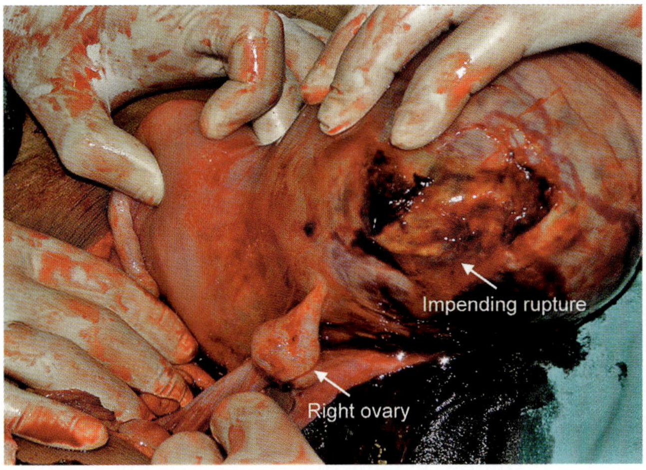

Fig. 18: Interstitial pregnancy (impending rupture) on the right side at 21 weeks in 2nd gravida woman who presented with pain in the abdomen and managed by conservative surgery without sacrificing the uterus (part of the uterine tissue, right fallopian tube, sac containing a live fetus, and placenta removed).
Courtesy: Dr Sanjib Dutta, Sagar Dutta Medical College, West Bengal, India.

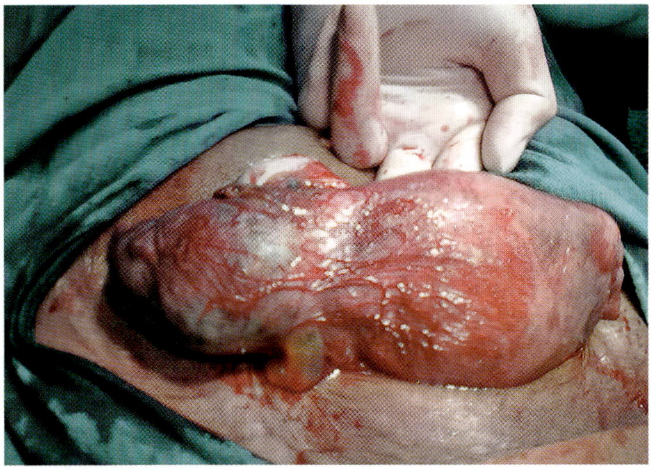

Fig. 19: Unruptured interstitial pregnancy.

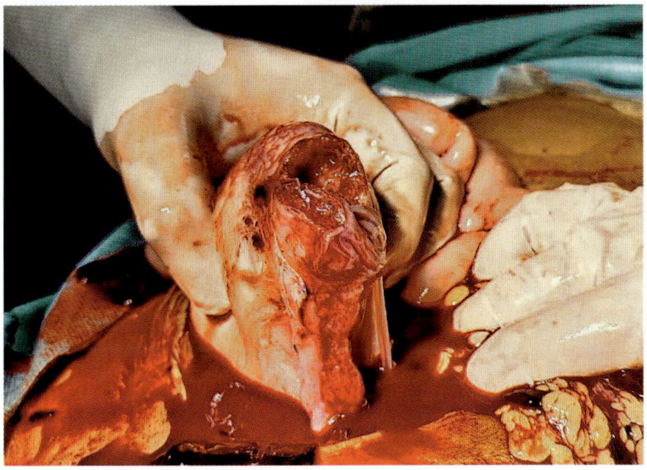

Fig. 20: Ruptured interstitial pregnancy with torrential bleeding.
Courtesy: Dr Prabhat Mondal, Associate Professor, Bankura Sammilani Medical College and Hospital, Bankura, West Bengal, India.

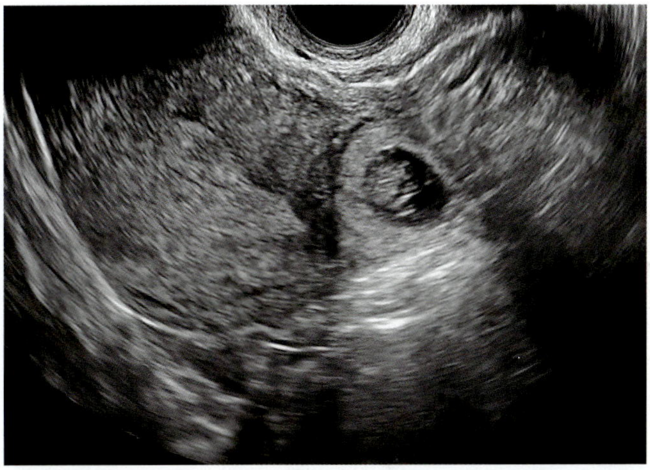

Fig. 21: Interstitial pregnancy—left side.
Courtesy: Professor Kamal Oswal, Head, Department of Radiodiagnosis, Vivekananda Institute of Medical Sciences, Kolkata, West Bengal, India.

is found lateral to the insertion of round ligament, tubes, and ovary looking normal.

Treatment is cornual resection (cornuectomy) or cornuostomy by laparotomy. The laparoscopic approach is also feasible depending upon the patient's condition and availability of an expert laparoscopic surgeon. The entire fallopian tube is removed to prevent tubal ectopic. Hysterectomy is rarely needed in cases, where there is irreparable rupture and uncontrolled bleeding.

Cornual resection: A wedge resection of the gestational sac with adjacent myometrium is done; then hemostasis is secured by interrupted sutures or electrocoagulation. Myometrial bed is closed by interrupted or continuous delayed absorbable (Vicryl) suture. Intraoperative local vasopressin injection is infiltrated for hemostasis and ligation of ascending uterine arteries may be helpful. In case of severe hemorrhage after excision, the base of the cornu is clamped by two clamps, followed by salpingectomy. Then myometrium in each clamp is sutured with transfixing stitch. Interrupted sutures are given for complete hemostasis.

Cornuostomy: In this technique, the sac is enucleated after incision instead of excision. The rest of the procedure is same.

Chemoembolization is a combined method where methotrexate infusion is given followed by uterine artery embolization (UAE). Only medical management can be done following early diagnosis either by single or multiple methotrexate regimen. Anticipating the rupture in subsequent pregnancy, the ACOG suggests cesarean delivery after $37^{0/7}$ weeks.

Cornual Pregnancy (Angular Pregnancy)

Implantation at lateral angle of the uterine cavity just medial to uterotubal junction is called cornual pregnancy. Munro Kerr described it as *angular pregnancy. Cornual pregnancy* was meant to term "pregnancy in rudimentary horn." In true sense, it is not a variety of ectopic pregnancy but may be confused with interstitial pregnancy. The relation with round ligament can differentiate the two. In interstitial pregnancy, the round ligament usually lies medial to it. Once pregnancy is detected at one cornu of the uterus by early scan, it is very essential to do serial ultrasonography with close follow-up of the patient. As it grows inside the uterus medially (true cornual or angular pregnancy) it becomes intrauterine, but when it grows inside the interstitial part of tube (laterally), it becomes interstitial pregnancy which is very dangerous to be ruptured at 12–16 weeks.

Pregnancy in Rudimentary Horn (Figs. 22 to 25)

Pregnancy occurs in a blind rudimentary horn of a uterus bicornis unicollis (bicornuate uterus). Transabdominal migration of sperm to an ipsilateral ovary results in a blastocyst implanting in the rudimentary horn. This was also referred to as "cornual pregnancy" by Munro Kerr. Rupture is common during the second trimester with massive hemorrhage. Prerupture diagnosis and management are possible with routine ultrasonography in first-trimester pregnancy. Treatment is operative removal of the horn along with the products of conception.

ABDOMINAL PREGNANCY (FIGS. 26 TO 30)

When pregnancy occurs inside the peritoneal cavity, it is called abdominal pregnancy. Tubal, ovarian, and intraligamentous pregnancy are not included in abdominal

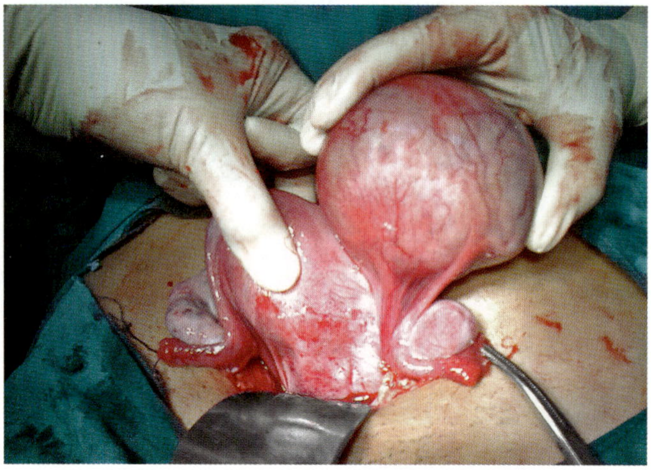

Fig. 22: Pregnancy in rudimentary horn—left side.

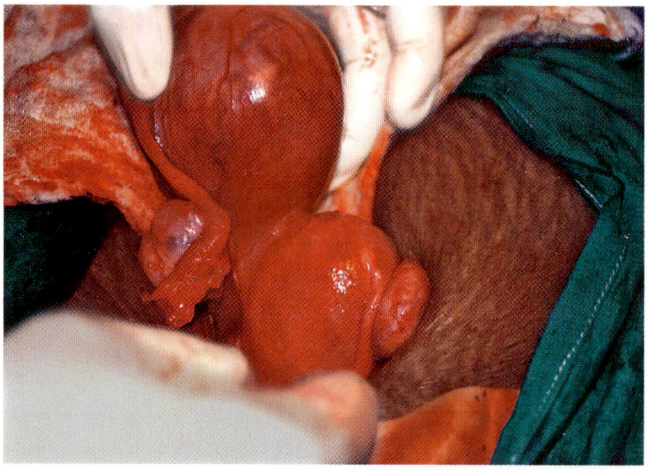

Fig. 23: Pregnancy in rudimentary horn (cornual pregnancy)—right side. *Courtesy:* Dr Nilotpal Roy, Assistant Professor, North Bengal Medical College and Hospital, West Bengal, India.

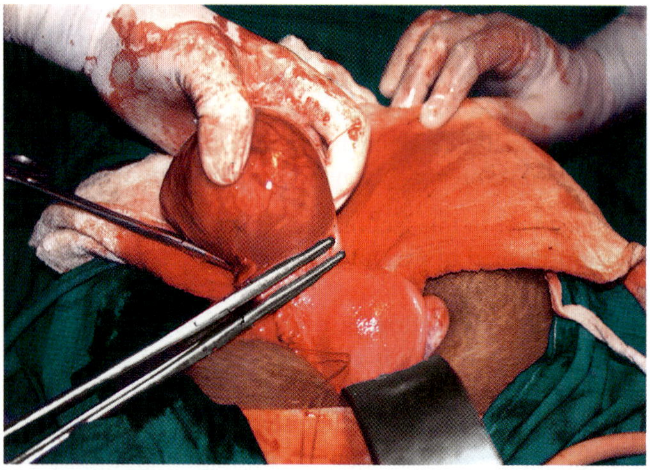

Fig. 24: Clamp given to excise rudimentary horn as the case in Figure 23.

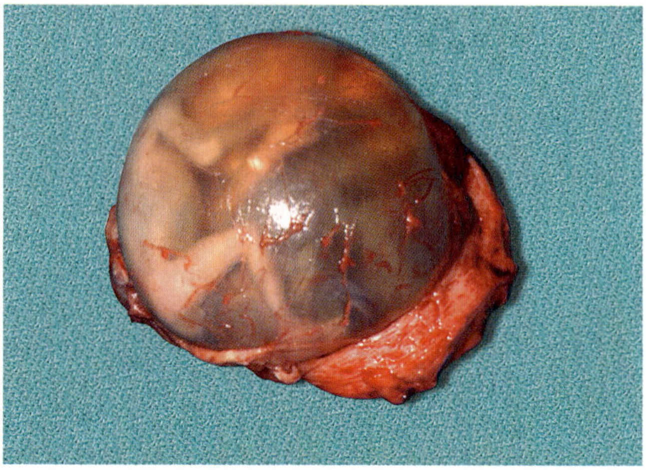

Fig. 25: Excised horn to cut open to show the pregnancy sac with the fetus inside as in Figure 24.

pregnancy. Primary abdominal pregnancy is very rare and difficult to prove. Studdiford criteria (1942) for primary abdominal pregnancy are: (1) normal looking fallopian tubes and ovaries, (2) absence of uteroperitoneal fistula, (3) pregnancy is solely related to peritoneal surface, and (4) there is no evidence of secondary implantation following tubal pregnancy. Abdominal pregnancies are mostly secondary because these result from tubal abortion or rupture. The growing embryo becomes implanted into the peritoneal cavity, and around the amnion a false membrane is formed which is made up of deposition of lymph and pregnancy grows in the new site following attachment of the placenta with the neighboring structures and a newer vascular connection is established. The incidence of abdominal pregnancy is very rare, only 1 in 50,000.

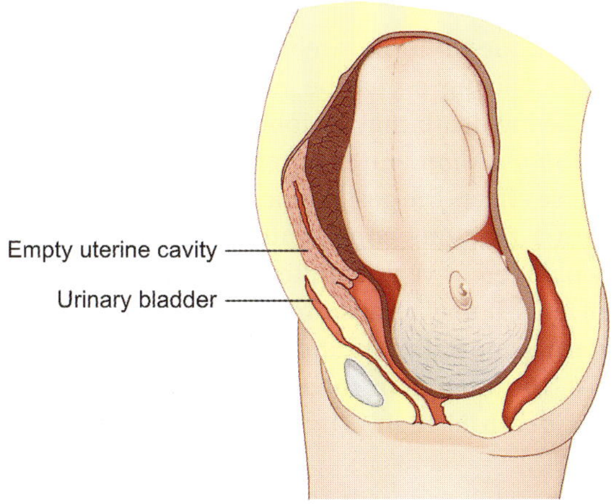

Fig. 26: Schematic diagram of abdominal pregnancy. The baby is outside the uterine cavity.

Diagnosis

There may not be any symptom, may be vague pain in the abdomen or history of features of ectopic pregnancy in early months. Pregnancy symptoms may be exaggerated. In advanced gestation on abdominal examination, *Braxton Hicks contraction* is absent, uterine contour is not well

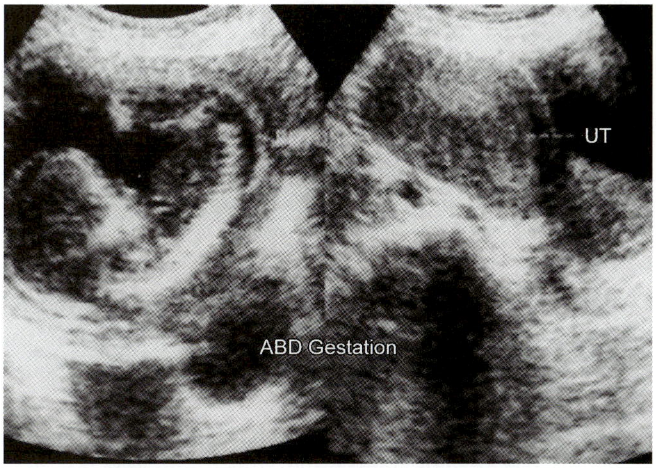

Fig. 27: USG showing abdominal pregnancy.

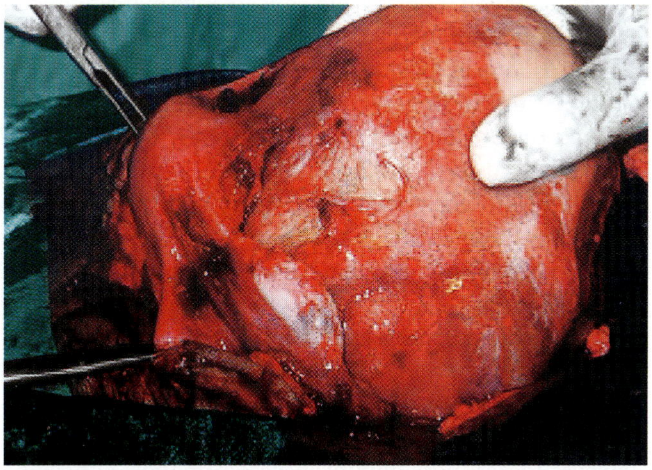

Fig. 28: Laparotomy done in abdominal pregnancy at term. Baby is outside the uterine cavity behind the uterus is separately seen.

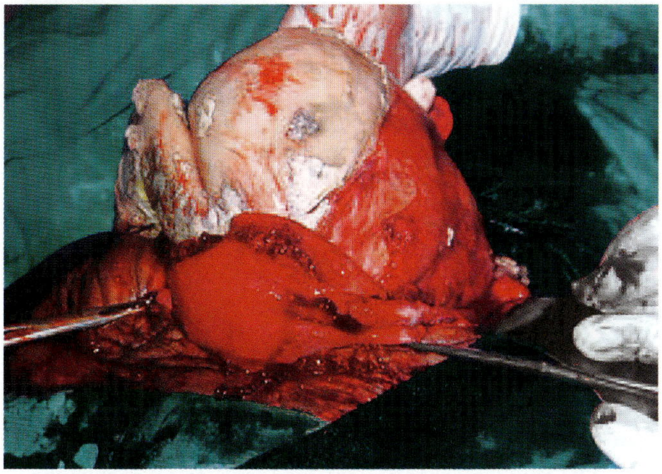

Fig. 29: Baby is being delivered from the abdominal cavity.

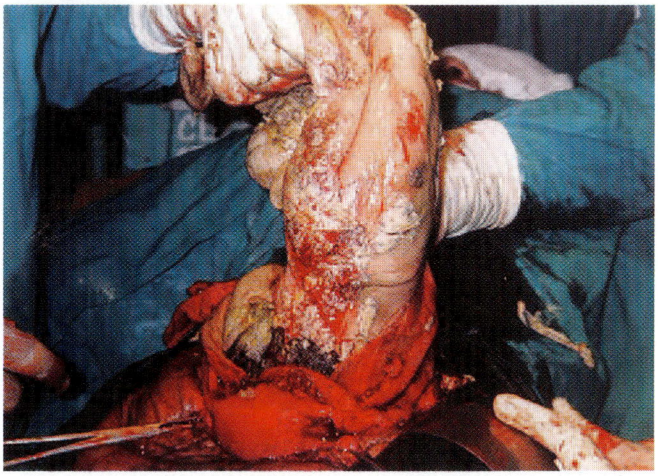

Fig. 30: Baby is almost delivered. In abdominal pregnancy at term (a stillborn baby was delivered).

defined, and fetal parts are palpable superficially. On vaginal examination, the cervix is displaced and uterus may not be palpable separately always.

Sonography **(Fig. 27)** may help in diagnosis but cannot diagnose in all the cases. The uterus may be separately seen; there is absence of myometrium between the fetus and maternal parieties or bladder. Gestational sac is found to be surrounded by intestinal loops. Abnormal fetal position and eccentric placental location along with above findings are suspicious. Oligohydramnios is common. MRI is helpful to diagnose and also to visualize the placental attachment with other structures. Maternal serum alpha-fetoprotein levels are raised. Repeated failure of induction can be suspicious of abdominal pregnancy.

Management

Surgical removal of the fetus following laparotomy **(Figs. 28 to 30)** with proper arrangement for blood transfusion is the treatment as torrential hemorrhage may occur after placental separation. It can be life-threatening. Waiting to age of viability has been reported, but conservative management is discouraged for potential complications and intervention is justified as soon as diagnosed. A skilled surgeon accustomed to retroperitoneal surgery is essential to tackle these cases.

Ligation of placental vessels prior to their removal is advisable due to possibility of massive hemorrhage, especially during removal of the placenta for which sometimes the placenta is not removed. Over-enthusiastic exploration is avoided. If the placenta is attached to a vital organ, it is better to leave the placenta after cutting and tying the umbilical vessels. Aseptic autolysis of placenta occurs taking months to years, and follow-up is done by serial serum β-hCG estimation and Doppler ultrasound or MRI. Methotrexate may be given in the postoperative period. However, there is possibility of abscess formation, adhesions, intestinal obstruction, thromboembolic manifestations, and abdominal wound dehiscence on leaving the placenta in situ. Before or after the delivery of fetus, embolization of placental vessels may be beneficial.

Different Fates

It may continue till term rarely **(Figs. 28 to 30)**. The fetus may be dead, living, or may be malformed in 20% cases. The fetus following death may become mummified or calcified to form *lithopaedion* and may retain for long time without any adverse effect. The gestational sac following an infection may form a fistulous communication with the intestine, urinary bladder, or vagina. In the early stage, following the death of fetus, it may be absorbed.

Maternal mortality in abdominal pregnancy is much higher, 8–10 times than tubal pregnancy. The chance of neonatal death is high. The fetus may have congenital anomaly.

CERVICAL PREGNANCY (FIGS. 31 TO 35)

When blastocyst implants within the endocervical canal, it is called cervical pregnancy. Anatomically placenta fully or partly lies below the level of uterine vessels' entry or below the level of peritoneal reflection of the anterior uterine wall. Cervical pregnancy rarely goes beyond 20 weeks.

The incidence of cervical pregnancy is 1 in 18,000. Cervical pregnancy is increasing due to ART. D&C in previous pregnancy is one important risk factor.

Diagnosis

Only a high degree of clinical suspicion can be used for diagnosis because it mimics spontaneous abortion on the way of expulsion. Painless vaginal bleeding occurs in nearly 90% cases. In one-third of the cases, massive hemorrhage occurs. Vaginal examination shows ballooning of cervix with partly dilated os with slight bulky uterus which is less than the size of the cervix or less than that. Vaginal examination

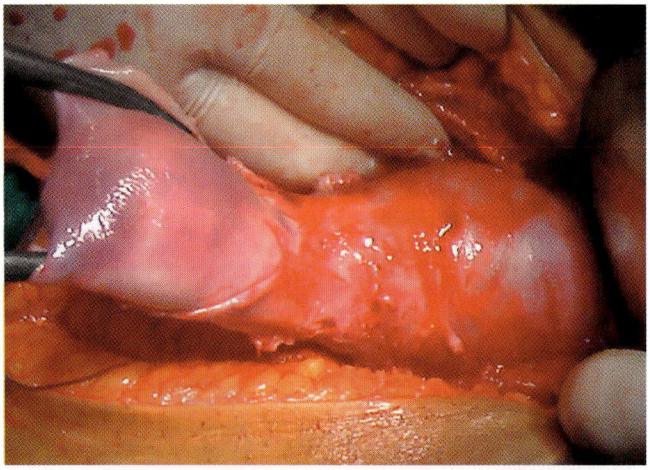

Fig. 31: Cervical pregnancy—laparotomy findings of uterus and enlarged cervix.

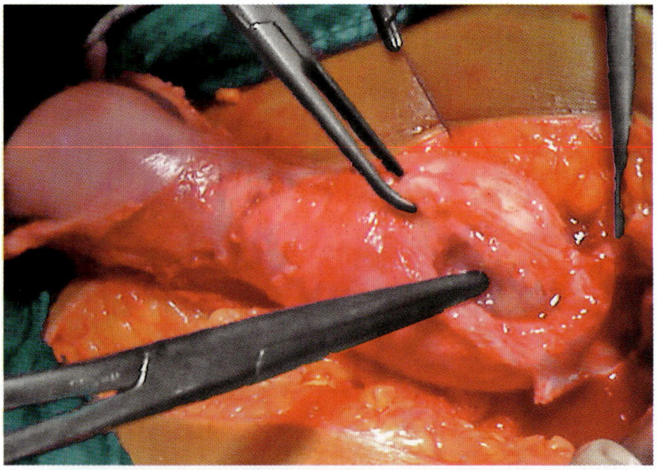

Fig. 32: Cervical pregnancy—enlarged cervix to cut open to show product of conception.

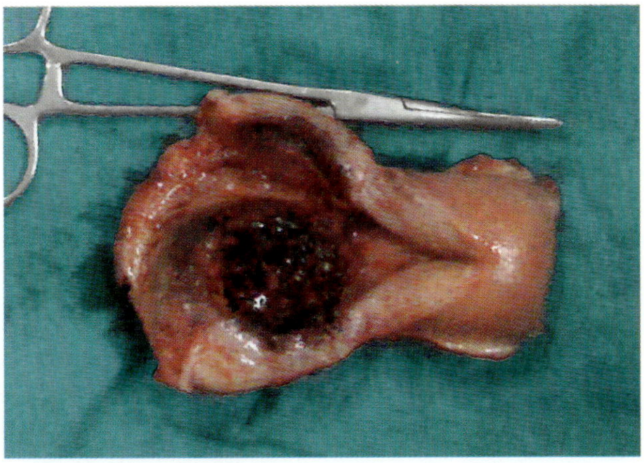

Fig. 33: Cervical pregnancy—specimen of hysterectomy with enlarged cervix to cut open to show product of conception.
Courtesy: Dr Pradipto Sanyal, RG Kar Medical College and Hospital, Kolkata, West Bengal, India.

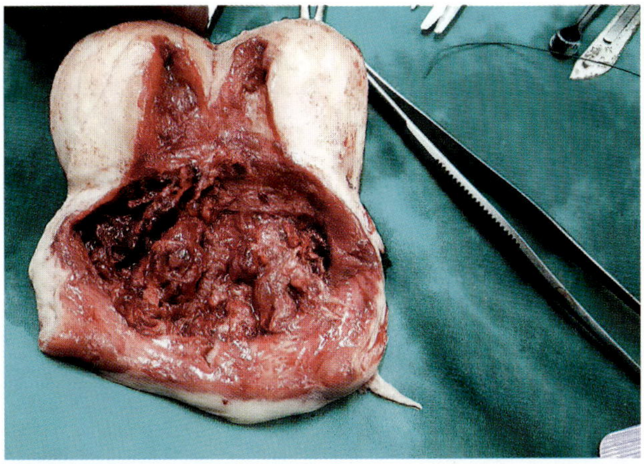

Fig. 34: Specimen of uterus to cut open to show cervical pregnancy. 34 years P2+0 L-I2 complaint of bleeding P/V following amenorrhea for 7 weeks was admitted as inevitable abortion. Torrential hemorrhage started on attempt of evacuation. Hysterectomy done.
Courtesy: Dr Prabhat Mondal, Associate Professor, Bankura Sammilani Medical College and Hospital, Bankura, West Bengal, India.

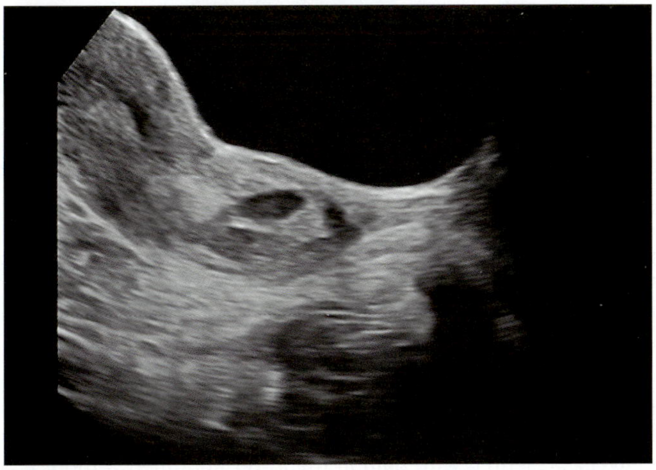

Fig. 35: Ultrasonography of cervical pregnancy.
Courtesy: Professor Abhijit Rakhsit, RG Kar Medical College and Hospital, Kolkata, West Bengal, India.

should be done very gently as it may precipitate brisk hemorrhage.

Sonographic findings (transvaginal) show hourglass uterus with empty uterine cavity, distended cervix, a gestational sac/tissue in cervical canal, and a part of cervical canal in between endometrial cavity and gestational sac/tissue. "Sliding sign" (movement of gestational sac with pressure over cervix by vaginal probe) is negative. Color Doppler shows increased vascularity. 3D sonography and MRI are useful for diagnosis.

Differential diagnoses includes spontaneous abortion, cancer in the cervix, degenerated cervical polyp, cervical fibroid, and placenta previa.

Criteria for diagnosis of cervical pregnancy as suggested by Paalman and McElin, 1959:

- Amenorrhea followed by painless bleeding
- Softened and disproportionately enlarged cervix at least to the size of uterine corpus
- Products of conception are entirely confined and firmly attached to the endocervix
- A close internal os and a partially open external os

Criteria for diagnosis of cervical pregnancy on hysterectomy specimen (Rubin 1911):

- Opposite placental attachment, there must be cervical glands.
- Placental attachment must be below the entrance of uterine vessels or below the peritoneal reflection of both anterior and posterior surfaces of the uterus.
- Placental attachment to the cervix must be intimate.
- Fetal elements must not be present in the corpus uteri.

Management

The options are as follows:

- Medical method with methotrexate in a hemodynamically stable patient, systematically in single dose or multidose regimen or locally 50 mg methotrexate along with feticidal potassium chloride into the gestational sac
- Chemoembolization
- Suction evacuation with or without UAE, intracervical vasopressin injection, cervical cerclage at the level of internal os to reduce the blood loss
- Suturing the descending cervical branches on two lateral aspects of cervix at 3 and 6 o'clock positions vaginally is a very effective method for hemostasis.
- Foley's catheter placement inflated the balloon with 30 mL fluid intracervically for 24–48 hours after suction evacuation is a good option.
- The last but not the least option is hysterectomy which is needed in uncontrolled bleeding in conservative

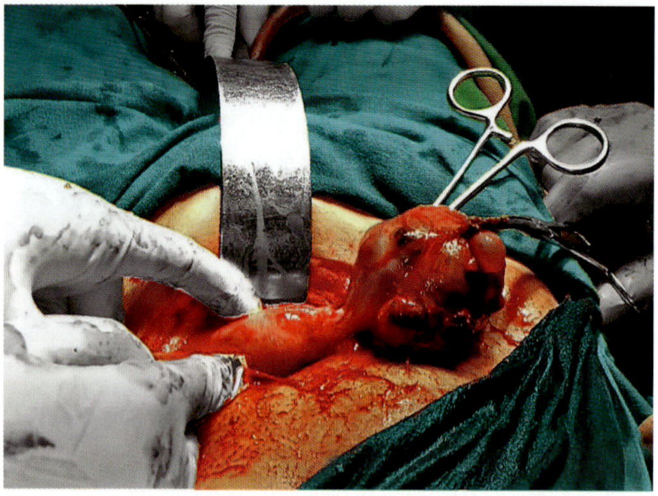

Fig. 36: Operative finding showing right-sided ovarian ectopic pregnancy.

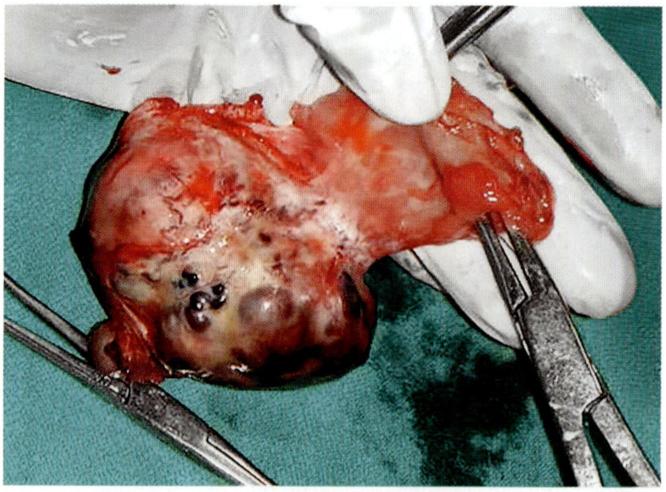

Fig. 37: Salpingo-oopherectomy in the ovarian pregnancy as in the patient in Figure 36.

methods, especially in advanced gestation. One should be careful about ureteric injury during hysterectomy as the cervix becomes distended in cervical pregnancy.

OVARIAN PREGNANCY (FIGS. 36 TO 38)

If an ectopic pregnancy is implanted within the ovary, it is termed ovarian pregnancy.

Ovarian pregnancy is diagnosed by *Spiegelberg's criteria.* Spiegelberg in 1878 suggested four criteria for diagnosis of primary ovarian pregnancy. The criteria are:

1. The tube on the affected side must be intact and will be away from the ovary.
2. The fetal sac must occupy the position of the ovary.
3. The ovary must be connected to the uterus by the ovarian ligament.
4. Definite histological evidence of ovarian tissue must be present in the sac wall.

The incidence is 1 in 7,000–40,000. ART and IUCD increase ovarian pregnancy. Risk factors associated in tubal pregnancy also play here.

Presenting symptoms and signs are similar to those of tubal pregnancy. Rupture may occur at any time in early pregnancy. USG shows an echogenic area surrounded by an echogenic ring around which there is cortical tissue. Diagnosis is mostly confused with corpus luteal hemorrhage (ovarian apoplexy) even during surgery.

Management of ovarian pregnancy is always surgical, either by laparotomy or by laparoscopy. If the patient is hemodynamically stable and there is a suitable service provider, laparoscopy is preferred. Wedge resection or excision of the mass leaving behind the healthy tissue in case of a small lesion with minimal bleeding is done. Ovariectomy is performed in case of larger size and excessive bleeding. When ovarian tissue is preserved, serum β-hCG is monitored.

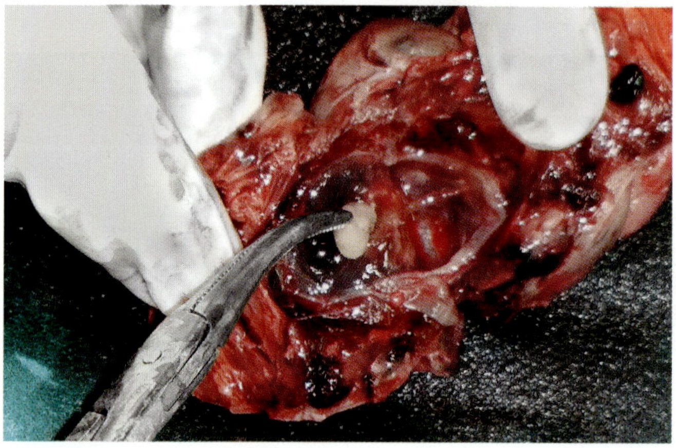

Fig. 38: Cut open to show the fetus in the specimen of ovary following ovariectomy 19 years P1+0 with previous Caesarean delivery presented with pain in the lower abdomen without any amenorrhea. Urinary pregnancy test (UPT) positive with sonographic diagnosis of right-sided tubal ectopic. Ovarian pregnancy diagnosed and both the tubes were normal.

Courtesy: Dr Bivas Mondal, Dr Anamika, RG Kar Medical College, Kolkata, West Bengal, India.

CESAREAN SCAR PREGNANCY (FIGS. 39 TO 43)

Cesarean scar pregnancy (CSP) is an entity where pregnancy is implanted into a prior cesarean delivery uterine scar and located outside the normal uterine cavity and is completely surrounded by myometrium and fibrous tissue of the scar. Larsen and Solomon reported the first case of cesarean scar pregnancy in 1978.

The incidence ranges from 1 in 1,800 to 1 in 2,000 pregnancies.

These vary in size and in many ways are similar to a placenta increta and may be more dangerous than placenta accrete spectrum (PAS). PAS and CSP are said to be spectrum of the same disorder. Invasion of myometrium early in the first trimester may lead to uterine rupture and profuse bleeding as the pregnancy advances. When the pregnancy grows inside the uterine cavity, it is called endogenic and when it grows outside through the bladder and peritoneal cavity it is called exogenic. The exogenic is more dangerous than endogenic. If CSP is not ruptured, pregnancy may progress to a viable stage and behave like PAS. Recent evidence shows that all scar pregnancies do not behave like ectopic pregnancy and conservative management is possible.

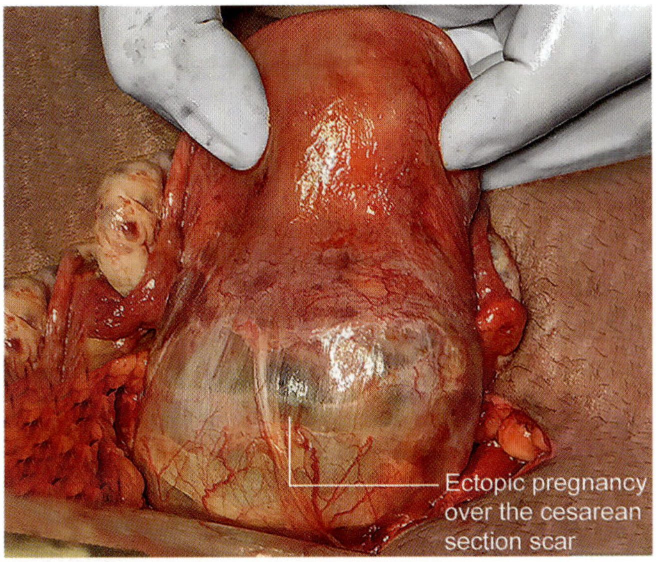

Fig. 39: *Cesarean scar ectopic:* Laparotomy finding 26 years P1+2 LI-1, lower segment cesarean section (LSCS) 4 years back followed by two miscarriages presented with missed abortion at 12 weeks. With attempt of surgical evacuation, there was torrential bleeding P/V and implantation over the scar suspected. Laparotomy is done followed by hysterectomy as a life-saving measure.
Courtesy: Professor Alok De, Dr Anindya Das, Associate Professor, NB Medical College, West Bengal, Kolkata.

Clinical Presentation

Depending on the gestational age, the clinical presentation may be asymptomatic (5–6 weeks), or there may be abdominal pain and bleeding, which may range from spotting to life-threatening hemorrhage. Women may also present with painless vaginal bleeding. Scar ectopic pregnancy is diagnosed in a significant number of asymptomatic women during routine sonography.

Imaging

Sonographic criteria **(Fig. 42)** for the diagnosis of this condition are:

- The trophoblast is located between the bladder and the anterior uterine wall.
- Fetal parts are not present in the uterine cavity.
- On a sagittal uterine view that runs through the amniotic sac, no myometrium is seen between the gestational sac and the urinary bladder as seen by the lack of continuity of the anterior uterine wall.
- Vascularity at the scar by color Doppler.

On Doppler imaging **(Fig. 43)**, (1) the sac is well perfused (in contrast to the avascular appearance of an aborting gestational sac) and (2) the negative "sliding organs sign" defined as the nondisplacement of gestational sac from its position at the level of the internal os when gentle pressure is applied by the endovaginal probe. Diagnosis is done by suspicion of the condition, clinical features, and ultrasound criteria. Attempt of medical termination of pregnancy (MTP) in a pregnancy with prior CS either by medical method or by surgical curette may result in profuse bleeding in undiagnosed CSP cases. For this reason, sonography is advisable before MTP in pregnancy with prior CS.

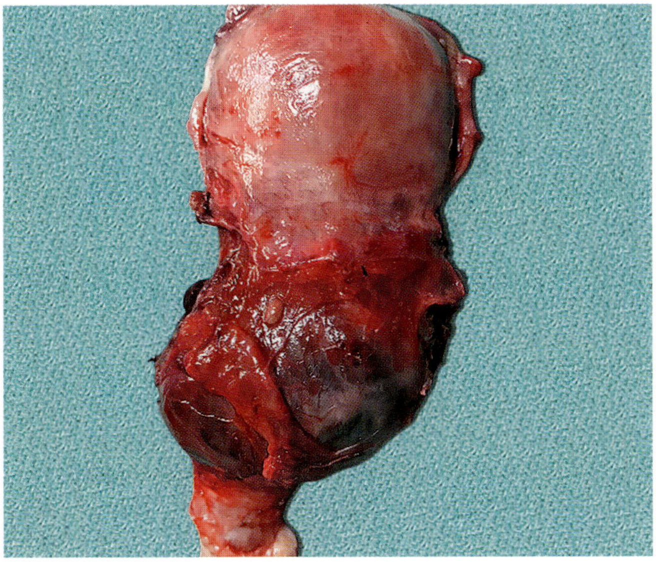

Fig. 40: Scar ectopic—hysterectomy specimen of the patient as in Figure 39.

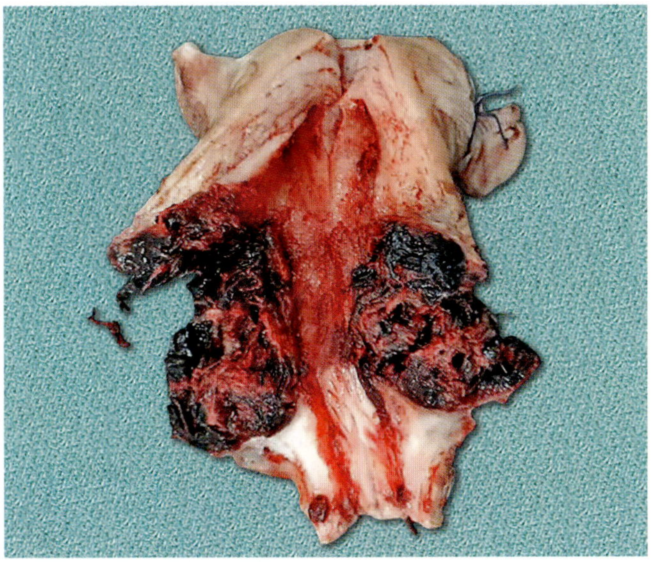

Fig. 41: Hysterectomy specimen to cut open in a scar ectopic pregnancy.
Courtesy: Dr Prabhat Mondal, Associate Professor, Bankura Sammilani Medical College and Hospital, Bankura, West Bengal, India.

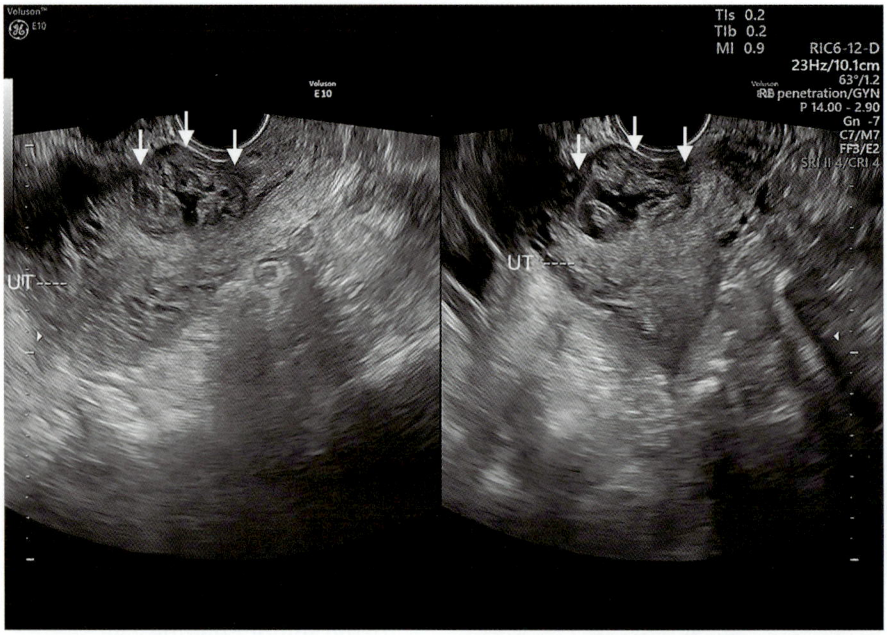

Fig. 42: Sonographic showing scar ectopic containing fetus with vascularity in a 24-year 2nd gravida, lower segment cesarean section (LSCS) 3 years back who was admitted with pain in the abdomen with a history of intake of abortifacient at 8 weeks. Laparotomy is done followed by excision of sac situated in the scar and repaired.

Courtesy: Professor Abhijit Rakshit, RG Kar Medical College; Professor Kamal Oswal, Head, Department of Radiodiagnosis, Vivekananda Institute of Medical Sciences, Kolkata, West Bengal, India.

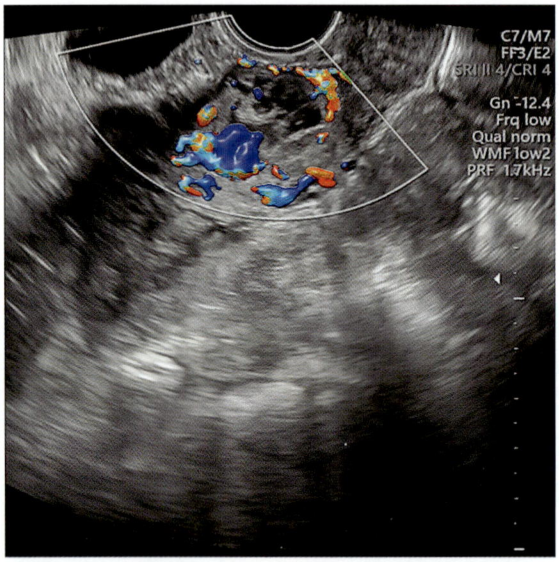

Fig. 43: Color Doppler of the same patient as in Figure 42.

Management

Once diagnosed, termination is justified for fear of bleeding, rupture, or possibility of *PAS* following continuation.

The surgical options are *uterine*-preserving wedge resection by laparotomy or by laparoscopy, hysteroscopic resection, transvaginal isthmic resection by anterior colpotomy, D&C with or without hysteroscopy following UAE or vacuum aspiration under sonographic guidance [Society for Maternal-Fetal Medicine (SMFM) 2020] without curettage.

Hysterectomy is an option in parous woman and in case of uncontrolled bleeding. Expectant management is discouraged by the SMFM (2020).

Medical management with local or systemic methotrexate has been done but with less success. In advanced pregnancy, local injection of feticidal KCL along with local methotrexate is suggested.

Use of Foley balloon catheter as tamponade is also an effective measure to control bleeding, especially when the medical method is used. Cervical ripening with a double balloon catheter is ideal to use as distal balloon helps to retain it and the proximal balloon arrests bleeding by mechanical pressure. Prognosis of future pregnancies is good with increased risk of CSP and PAS.

HETEROTROPIC PREGNANCY

When one pregnancy occurs inside the uterus and the other in any ectopic place simultaneously, the entity is called heterotrophic pregnancy. The most common combination along with IUP is tubal ampullary pregnancy. The incidence of heterotrophic pregnancies is 0.33 per 10,000 pregnancies, but with ART the incidence rises to 9 per 10,000 pregnancies. The patient usually presents with features of ectopic pregnancy. Rupture is more common in in heterotopic pregnancy as by USG attention goes to IUP and tubal ectopic is overlooked. After diagnosis, if a woman wants the pregnancy, surgery in the form of resection or aspiration of ectopic pregnancy is done. Methotrexate is avoided to save the ongoing IUP.

Twin tubal pregnancy: Both embryos in the same tube or one in each tube may also occur. *Heterotrophic cervical pregnancy*: Simultaneous cervical pregnancy and IUP may occur very rarely.

PREGNANCY OF UNKNOWN LOCATION

The term "pregnancy of unknown location" (PUL) refers to a situation when the pregnancy test is positive but there are no evidences of intrauterine or an extrauterine pregnancy by TVS. A significant number of cases is categorized in this group.

This situation may occur in (1) early IUP, (2) ectopic pregnancy, (3) early pregnancy failure, or (4) complete abortion

The management seems to be highly crucial as the pregnancy may be ectopic and late diagnosis may have serious outcome. Sonographic evaluation in addition to serial β-hCG measurements is essential to determine the location of pregnancy and managed accordingly. TVS may also need to be repeated. Serum progesterone may be done as it is the best indicator for viability. Sometimes, determination of the location of pregnancy in cases of PUL is not possible since both miscarriage and ectopic pregnancy may resolve spontaneously without any treatment. Final outcomes are categorized as *visualized IUP*, *visualized ectopic pregnancy*, *spontaneously resolved PUL*, and *persisting PUL*. Persisting PUL needs follow-up. In low-level β-hCG, ectopic pregnancy may also rupture. It is important to follow-up the patients with PUL until the serum β-hCG level comes below the negative for pregnancy threshold and the final diagnosis is concluded. High-resolution ultrasonography may reduce the PUL.

PROGNOSIS AND OUTCOME OF ECTOPIC PREGNANCY

The incidence of ectopic pregnancy has increased, but mortality and morbidity have decreased significantly. Early diagnosis with the help of serum β-hCG assay and high-resolution TVS has enabled for a more conservative approach and fertility preservation. Still, ectopic pregnancy is an important cause of morbidity and mortality in first-trimester bleeding. To diagnose ectopic pregnancy, the dictum is always "think ectopic." Ectopic pregnancy is responsible for 1–2% of maternal deaths. After survival, women suffering from ectopic pregnancy are at risk of further ectopic, subfertility, and chronic pelvic pain in the long run. Regarding fertility outcome after one ectopic (tubal) pregnancy IUP occurs in 50–70% cases and chance of recurrence is 10% for which early scan is indicated in future pregnancy. Regardless of the site of ectopic pregnancy, every woman of Rh-negative blood group should receive anti-D gamma globulin.

CHAPTER 5

Gestational Trophoblastic Disease

Learning Objectives

- Classification of Gestational Trophoblastic Disease
- Hydatidiform Mole
- Gestational Trophoblastic Neoplasia
- Invasive Mole
- Choriocarcinoma
- Placental Site Trophoblastic Tumor
- Epithelioid Trophoblastic Tumor
- Future Pregnancy

INTRODUCTION

Gestational trophoblastic disease (GTD) is a distinct type of placental tumors of wide variations, some of which have malignant potentialities and some are malignant with local and distant spreads. Characteristic peculiarities of GTD are that there is a definite tumor marker, β-human chorionic gonadotropin (β-hCG), and almost all have excellent prognosis with treatment. Fertility can be preserved in most of the cases. Though not so common, almost all obstetricians have to deal with molar pregnancies multiple times in their clinical practice. The most common GTD is hydatidiform mole (H. mole) which is of non-malignant variety.

CLASSIFICATION OF GESTATIONAL TROPHOBLASTIC DISEASE

Gestational trophoblastic disease is basically of two types on histological basis: (1) molar pregnancy and (2) nonmolar pregnancy. Molar pregnancy has the typical trophoblastic villi, whereas nonmolar GTD is devoid of structure of villi. Nonmolar GTDs are trophoblastic malignant neoplasms. Molar pregnancies are of two types: (1) hydatidiform mole, either complete or partial varieties, and (2) invasive mole. Due to the marked invasiveness to the myometrium and metastatic nature, invasive mole is considered as malignant. Nonmolar trophoblastic diseases are always malignant and are of three subtypes, namely choriocarcinoma, placental site trophoblastic tumor (PSTT), and epithelioid trophoblastic tumor (ETT), which are different in histological nature and degree of spread.

According to the modified World Health Organization (WHO) 2014, GTD is classified as follows:

- *Gestational trophoblastic disease:*
  - *Molar pregnancy:*
    - Hydatidiform mole
    - Complete mole
    - Partial mole
    - Invasive moles
  - *Trophoblastic tumors:*
    - Choriocarcinoma
    - PSTT
    - ETT
- *Gestational trophoblastic neoplasia (GTN):*
  - *GTN are all the malignant GTDs, namely:*
    - Invasive mole
    - Choriocarcinoma
    - PSTT
    - ETT

It is not always possible to diagnose the specific types of GTN as tissues for histopathology cannot be retrieved and management is done on serum β-hCG level and clinical basis.

Incidence

Gestational trophoblastic disease ranges from 1 to 2 per 1,000 deliveries, varies in countries, and is more among Asians.

HYDATIDIFORM MOLE

Hydatidiform mole is an abnormal pregnancy where the chorionic villi are changed to grape-like translucent vesicles resembling hydatid cysts.

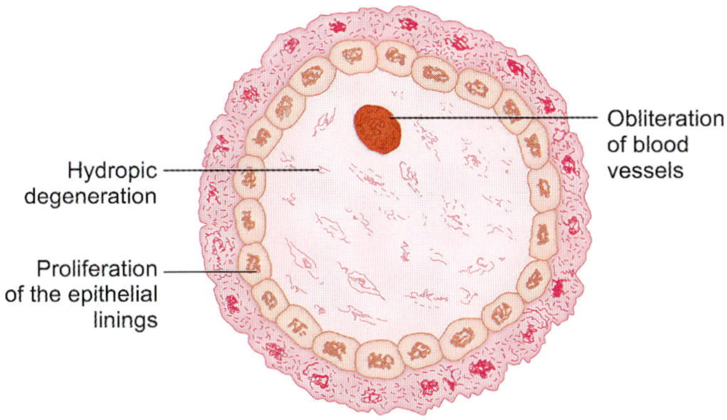

Fig. 1: Pathological changes of villi in hydatidiform mole.

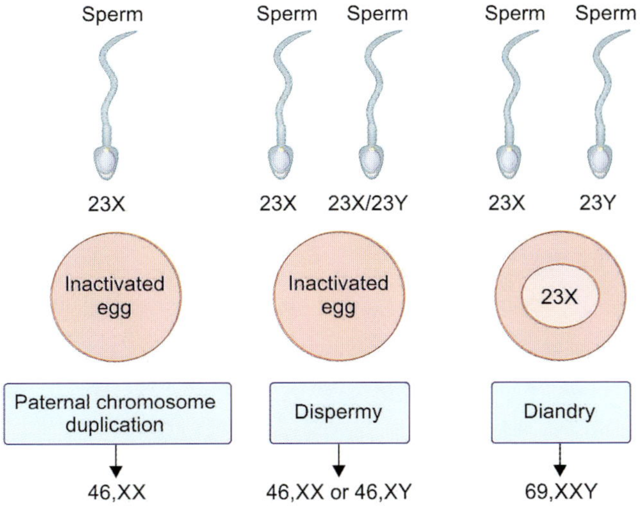

Fig. 2: Histopathology of hydatidiform mole.

Risk factors: Extremes of age are strongest risk factors for complete mole. Higher paternal age also increases the risk. History of GTD increases the chance of pregnancy in next pregnancy by 1–4% and after two molar pregnancy 20% of later conception results in molar pregnancy.

Pathology: Trophoblastic proliferation and edema of stroma of villi occur in the placenta.

Histopathology of H. mole **(Figs. 1 and 2)** is characterized by: (1) hydropic degeneration of connective tissue core of villi, (2) proliferation of the epithelial linings, (3) obliteration of blood vessels in the villus core. There is absence of fetus and amnion in complete mole. The uterus becomes enlarged more than the period of amenorrhea (POA). There is formation of theca-lutein cysts of ovary due to prolonged exposure to elevated β-hCG.

Types

Complete mole and partial mole: Chromosomal abnormalities are the characteristic features and accordingly categorized into *complete mole* and *partial mole.*

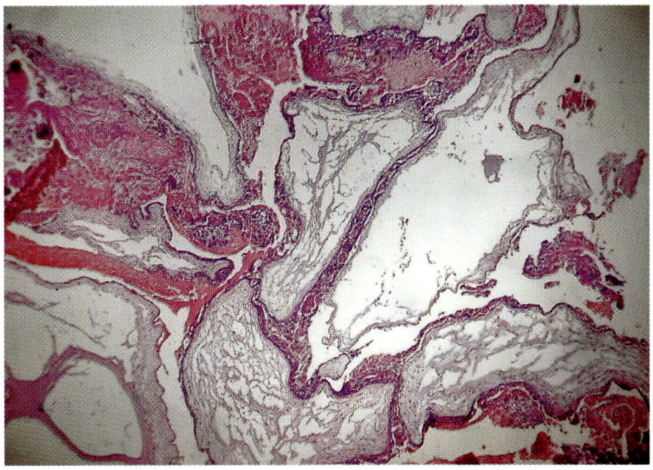

Fig. 3: Chromosomal pattern of hydatidiform mole.

The chromosomal pattern in complete mole is either 46, XX (85%) or 46, XY and that of partial mole is typically triploid, i.e., 69, XXX or 69, XXY—each of these is composed of one maternal and two paternal haploid sets of chromosome **(Fig. 3)**.

In complete molar pregnancy, 85% of the cases of chromosomal pattern is 46, XX with both chromosomes being of paternal origin. This phenomenon is called *androgenesis.* The ovum whose genes have been inactive is fertilized by haploid sperm, which then duplicates after meiosis. The ovum's own chromosomes are either absent or inactivated. At times, the chromosomal pattern composition in a complete mole may be 46, XY due to dispermic fertilization, either 23X or 23Y sperms. In both cases, the chromosomal complements are solely of paternal origin. In case of partial mole, two sperms, either 23X or 23Y, fertilize a haploid egg containing 23X which is not inactivated resulting in triploid. Hence, the chromosomal pattern in complete mole is either 46, XX (85%) or 46, XY and that of partial mole is typically triploid, i.e., 69 XXY—each of these is composed of one maternal and two paternal haploid sets of chromosomes.

In complete mole, there is complete absence of fetus or embryonic elements. In partial mole, there are partial changes and fetus or embryonic elements are present **(Fig. 4)**. The partial moles have triploid karyotype. The clinical manifestations are less in intensity. They present with signs and symptoms of incomplete or missed abortion until sonography is performed.

Differentiating features of partial mole and complete mole are given in **Table 1**.

Diagnosis

Diagnosis of hydatidiform mole is based on:

- History
- Clinical examination
- Investigation

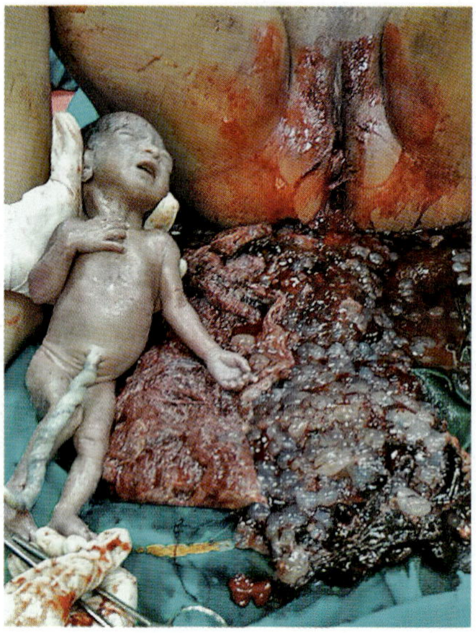

Fig. 4: Partial mole with living baby.
Courtesy: Dr Keka Mondal, RG Kar Medical College, Kolkata, West Bengal, India.

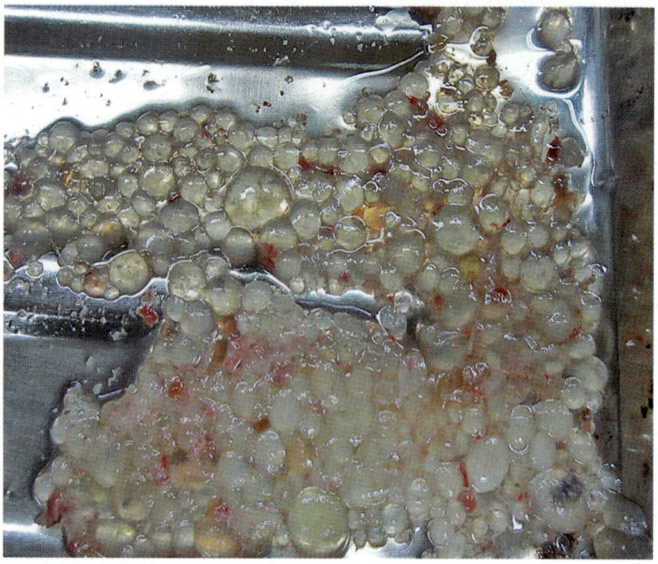

Fig. 5: Vesicle-like structures.
Courtesy: Dr Ajanta Samanta, Assistant Professor, RG Kar Medical College, Kolkata, West Bengal, India.

TABLE 1: Differentiating features of partial mole and complete mole.

Features	*Partial mole*	*Complete mole*
Karyotype	Usually 69, XXY	46, XX or 46, XY
Pathology		
• Embryo–fetus	• Often present	• Absent
• Amnion, fetal red blood cells	• Often present	• Absent
• Villous edema	• Variable, focal	• Diffuse
• Trophoblastic tissue	• Variable, focal, slight to moderate	• Variable, slight to severe
Clinical presentation		
• Diagnosis	• Missed abortion	• Molar gestation
• Uterine size	• Small for dates	• 50% large for dates
• Theca-lutein cysts	• Rare	• 25–30%
• Medical complications (preeclampsia, hyperthyroidism)	• Rare	• Frequent
• Gestational trophoblastic neoplasia	• <5–10%	• 20%

History

Salient points of history suggestive of H. mole are amenorrhea followed by brown or bloody vaginal discharge, continuous or intermittent. Bleeding is the most common symptom (90%) evident by 12 weeks. Discharge is described as "white currant in red currant juice" as it is frequently mixed with the ruptured moles. History of expulsion of grape-like vesicles per vagina **(Figs. 5 and 6)** is found in 40% cases. There is pain in the abdomen—more when moles are in the process of expulsion. Features of preeclampsia develop more than one-fourth of cases.

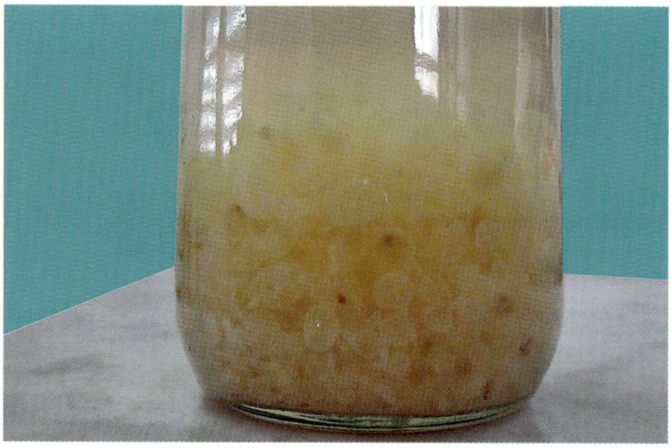

Fig. 6: Specimen of hydatidiform mole showing vesicles.

Associated symptoms are sense of ill-being, hyperemesis gravidarum, features of thyrotoxicosis (2%), and dyspnea. Thyrotoxicosis is due to liberation of chorionic thyrotrophin by trophoblast. There is no quickening in advanced pregnancy. The mode of clinical presentation has been changed from excessive bleeding and expulsion of grapes-like structure per vagina with pallor in midtrimester pregnancy (around 16 weeks or later) to early detection by routine sonography (at 8–9 weeks) and very high β-hCG.

Clinical Examination

On clinical examination, there are signs of early pregnancy, pallor, and features of preeclampsia (high blood pressure and proteinuria in half of the cases). On abdominal examination, the height of the fundus is more than POA (75% cases) due to trophoblastic proliferation, regeneration, and hemorrhage inside the uterus.

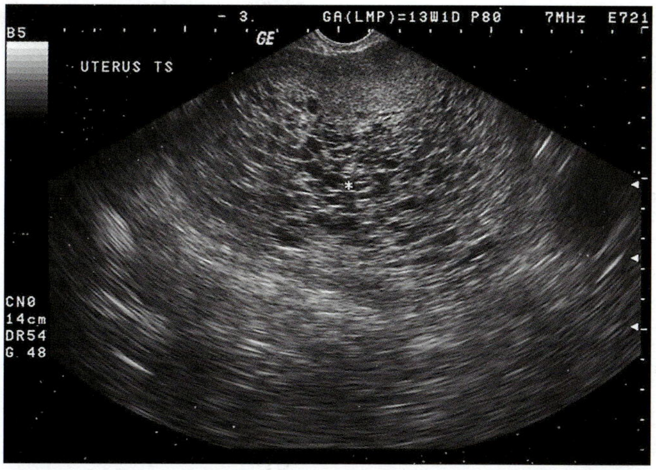

Fig. 7: Snowstorm appearance in USG—typical finding of hydatidiform mole.
Courtesy: Professor Kamal Oswal, Head, Department of Radiodiagnosis, Vivekananda Institute of Medical Sciences, Kolkata, West Bengal, India.

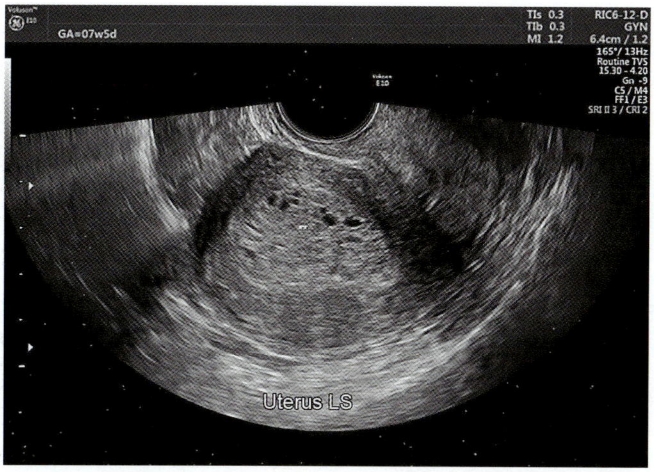

Fig. 8: Sonography showing early molar changes.

In few cases, the height may correspond to POA and rarely (10%) less than POA. Consistency of uterus feels soft cystic or doughy. Fetal parts are not palpable (except in partial mole) and fetal movements are absent. FHS is absent. Vaginal examination shows blood-stained discharge or frank bleeding, and vesicles may be seen. Cervical os may be closed or open. Internal ballottement is absent. On adnexal region palpation ovaries may be cystic and enlarged due to theca-lutein cysts.

Investigations

Ultrasonography shows intrauterine mass with multiple small echogenic spaces, typical "snowstorm" appearance, and absence of fetal parts **(Figs. 7 and 8)**.

Urinary β-hCG and serum β-hCG levels are higher than normal. The most important diagnostic tool in H. mole is sonography with an appearance of "snow storm." Snowstorm appearance may also be found in missed abortion and degenerated fibroid. Serum β-hCG and endovaginal sonography can diagnose most of the molar pregnancy within 10 weeks of pregnancy.

Hook effect: "Hook effect" is a phenomenon when the urinary pregnancy test becomes negative in spite of presence of β-hCG.

This is due to prozone phenomenon. A very large amount of β-hCG may produce this type of false-negative result in urinary immunoassay in a situation such as H. mole. The test becomes positive on dilution of urine. Serum β-hCG pregnancy tests may also be negative in a very high level of β-hCG. Hook effect is not specific of β-hCG. This phenomenon can also be found in case of ferritin, prolactin, prostate-specific antigen, CA-125, thyrotropin, and rapid plasma reagin for syphilis.

Phantom hCG: False-positive serum β-hCG elevation may be detected in absence of β-hCG. This is called "phantom effect." The false-positive hCG is a consequence of interference of heterophil antibodies with standard assays for β-hCG. Heterophil antibodies are human antibodies that have the capability to bind to other species' immunoglobulins. There are several strategies to clarify false-positive β-hCG detection. As the heterophilic antibodies are not renally excreted, it is unlikely that the urinary test will be false positive. Some laboratory methods can block the heterophilic antibodies with additives. Different β-hCG assays by alternate techniques can detect the absence of true β-hCG. Serial dilution of samples will dilute the serum β-hCG concentration proportionately. Phantom β-hCG assessment will remain unchanged.

Other Investigations for Hydatidiform Mole

Complete hemogram and blood grouping are done in all cases. X-ray of chest to view any metastasis in lung, liver function tests, thyroid hormones, and renal function is assessed if indicated.

Serum β-hCG level in hydatidiform mole and normal pregnancy: A single value of serum β-hCG level >100,000 mIU/mL or/and rapidly increasing titer are suggestive of H. mole. In normal pregnancy, the serum β-hCG level usually does not exceed 60,000 mIU/mL but may reach up to 100,000 mIU/mL between 60th and 80th day after the last menses and then tends to decline at 10–12 weeks and reaches at nadir by about 20 weeks.

Management

- Resuscitative measures with IV fluid containing 10 units of oxytocin in one bottle and blood requisition.
- Immediate *evacuation*, once diagnosed. Suction curettage is the treatment of choice irrespective of the uterine size.
- Follow-up

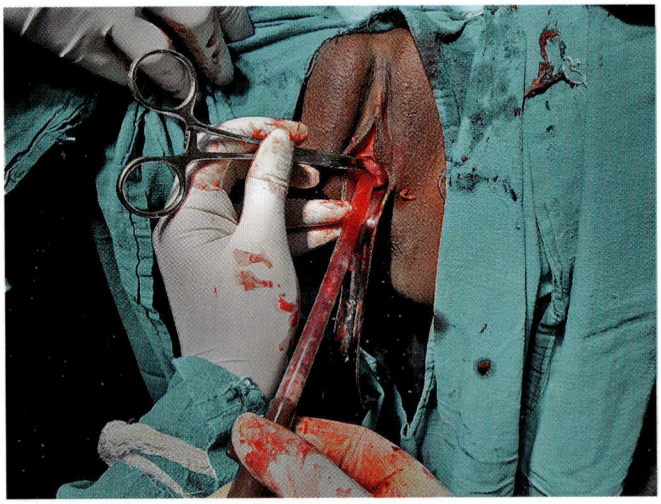

Fig. 9: Suction evacuation in hydatidiform mole.

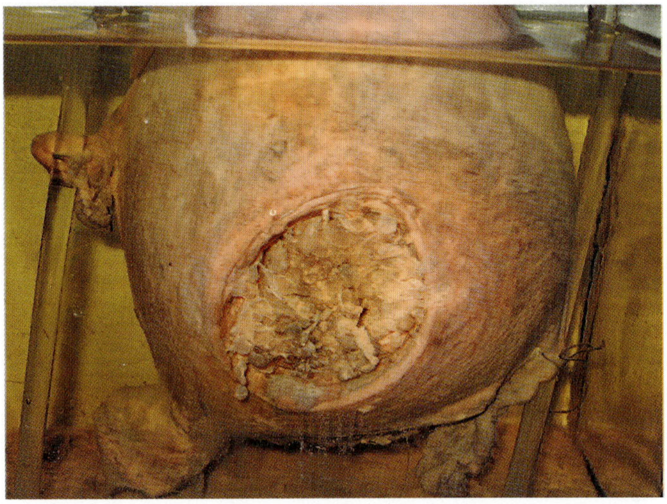

Fig. 10: Specimen of hysterectomy to cut open to show vesicles of molar pregnancy.

Steps of Suction Evacuation (Fig. 9)

Intravenous fluid crystalloids such as Ringer's solution 500 mL charged with 10 units of oxytocin are started. Blood is kept ready in hand. The patient is placed in lithotomy position; antiseptic dressing and draping are done. Under deep sedation or general anesthesia, suction evacuation is done. Cervix is dilated if it is not already dilated. Suction evacuation with a larger cannula (10–12 size) is done with a negative pressure of 200–250 mm Hg. Following completion of evacuation, the uterine cavity is curetted very gently as there is a chance of perforation of the soft uterine wall. The product of conception is sent for histopathological examination. Ploidy status and immunohistochemistry staining for P57 may help in distinguishing partial and complete moles.

Anti-D prophylaxis is required following evacuation of a molar pregnancy in an Rh-negative mother. Routine curettage is not mandatory as there is chance of perforation. If it is done, it should be done very gently. Curettage after 1 week of evacuation as practiced previously is not encouraged nowadays.

Evacuation of H. mole by the medical method is better to be avoided due to theoretical possibility of embolism and dissemination of trophoblastic tissue through the venous system with potent oxytocic. Using mifepristone and misoprostol for evacuation is not well studied.

In case cervix is tubular and os is seen closed, dilatation of the cervix is done first, which is followed by suction evacuation. Slow dilatation of cervix with laminaria tents is not so popular nowadays. Prostaglandin (PGE1—misoprostol) administered vaginally 3–4 hours before suction evacuation is a better option. It makes the cervix soft and ripe and suction evacuation becomes easier. However, prostaglandin is still not universally accepted for this purpose. Prolonged cervical preparation with prostaglandins should be avoided to reduce the risk of embolization of trophoblastic cells [Royal College of Obstetricians and Gynaecologists (RCOG)].

Role of Hysterectomy in H. Mole as a Treatment (Fig. 10)

Hysterectomy is not the usual treatment for H. mole. It is rarely indicated and virtually not needed. Torrential vaginal bleeding with unfavorable cervix not controlled by any method is the only indication. In a patient of age >40 years and family completed, hysterectomy may be considered. Hysterectomy does not eliminate persistence of trophoblastic tumor but reduces the chance of recurrent disease. GTN is seen in 3–5% cases following hysterectomy. Hence, routine follow-up should always be done also in hysterectomy cases.

Complications

- Hemorrhage that may lead to shock
- Perforation of the uterus
- Preeclampsia and eclampsia
- Infection
- Coagulation failure
- Pulmonary embolism following evacuation
- Choriocarcinoma 3–4%, persistent trophoblastic tumor in 15–20% cases
- Recurrence 1–4%

Follow-up

Because of its complications like malignant transformation (GTN), follow-up is mandatory. About 3–5% cases of H. mole develop choriocarcinoma and 15–20% cases become locally invasive. Hence, the main purpose of follow-up is to detect the feature of malignancy at the earliest.

Follow-up Parameter

Following evacuation, serial measurement of serum β-hCG is the gold standard for monitoring development of GTN. However, clinical parameters and other investigations are also considered. The monitoring parameters are history, clinical examination, β-hCG estimation, and other investigations such as X-ray of chest.

History such as lack of sense of well-being, irregularity of vaginal bleeding, dyspnea, cough, and hemoptysis are suggestive of development of GTN.

During clinical examinations in follow-up bleeding per vagina, size of the uterus and its involution process, size of the ovary and presence of any metastasis, especially on anterior vaginal wall are noted.

Standard Protocol of Serial β-hCG Estimation

Serum β-hCG is done every 2 weeks till it becomes negative, then monthly for 6 months, and then follow-up is discontinued and pregnancy may be allowed. Usually, the serum β-hCG level becomes negative in 4–6 weeks. A rise or persistent plateau of β-hCG demands evaluation and treatment.

Regarding the optimum period of follow-up following a diagnosis of GTD, the follow-up schedule is individualized. If hCG becomes normal with 8 weeks of pregnancy event, follow-up is done 6 months from the date of evacuation. If hCG does not return to normal within 8 weeks of pregnancy event, then follow-up will be for 6 months from the normalization of the β-hCG level.

Pregnancy Following H. Mole

Pregnancy is avoided for 1 year. However, there is no contraindication of pregnancy 6 months following negative β-hCG. Though chance of further molar pregnancy is low, the patient should be counseled. In more than 98% cases, there will be no molar pregnancy.

Following chemotherapy, women are advised not to conceive for 1 year after completion of treatment.

Contraception

Estrogen–progesterone contraceptives or DMPA can be used. Use of combined pill has a slight risk of developing GTN. Combined pill is started once hCG is normalized. IUCD should not be used until hCG levels are normal to reduce the risk of uterine perforation.

Twin Pregnancy with One Molar and Other Normal

In twin pregnancy, one fetus may be chromosomally normal and the other may become complete molar pregnancy. This situation is to be differentiated from the single partial mole with its abnormal fetus. Other differential diagnoses are chorioangioma, mesenchymal dysplasia, and subchorionic hemorrhage. Chorionic villus sampling (CVS), amniocentesis, and fetal cord blood sampling with fetal karyotyping determination may be needed to differentiate. If the pregnancy is continued, then survival of the normal fetus is unpredictable as the effect of molar pregnancy may cause comorbidity. Besides, development of pregnancy complications due to twin gestation such as preeclampsia, hemorrhage, and thyrotoxicosis may need preterm delivery. Development of GTN is another risk factor. For those reasons, many women opt for termination of pregnancy.

Ectopic Molar Pregnancy

Ectopic GTD is extremely rare. Surgical removal is the treatment followed by histopathological confirmation.

Indications of Prophylactic Chemotherapy of H. Mole

The role of prophylactic chemotherapy is controversial. It is considered in high-risk complete moles, particularly if serum hCG testing is unavailable or follow-up is impossible.

The high-risk group of patients include women who are more than 45 years of age, three or more previous births, previous history of molar pregnancy, initial serum β-hCG >100,000 mIU/mL, uterine size larger than 20 weeks, and theca-lutein cysts larger than 6 cm.

GESTATIONAL TROPHOBLASTIC NEOPLASIA

Gestational trophoblastic neoplasia includes all the malignant GTDs: (1) Invasive mole, (2) choriocarcinoma, (3) PSTT, and (4) ETT. Its origin takes place from any type of pregnancy.

It is not always possible to diagnose the specific types of GTN as tissues for histopathology cannot be retrieved and management is done on the serum β-hCG level and clinical basis. Management is done in the similar line. Aggressiveness and prognosis differ.

Origin

As stated, GTN always arises from some type of pregnancy, the most common (50%) from H. mole, 25% either from spontaneous abortion or from ectopic pregnancy. Others, though uncommon, develop from pregnancy either term or preterm.

Chance of GTN in Complete Mole and Partial Mole

In complete mole, there is 20% chance of GTN. But in case of partial mole, the chance is <5%. Following normal pregnancy, the chance of GTN is very less. The need for chemotherapy following a complete mole is 15% and that after a partial mole is 0.5%.

Diagnostic Criteria of Postmolar GTN

- Plateau of serum β-hCG level (±10%) for four measurements during a period of 3 weeks or longer—days 1, 7, 14, 21.

- Rise of serum β-hCG >10% during three weekly consecutive measurements or longer during a period of 2 weeks or more—days 1, 7, 14
- The serum β-hCG level remains detectable for 6 months or more.
- Histological criteria for choriocarcinoma

Staging (Anatomical) of GTN (International Federation of Gynecology and Obstetrics)

- *Stage I:* Disease confined to the uterus
- *Stage II:* GTN extends outside of the uterus but limited to the genital structures (adnexa, vagina, broad ligament)
- *Stage III:* GTN extends to the lung, with or without known genital tract involvement
- *Stage IV:* All other metastatic sites

Anatomical staging is done by pelvic examination, chest X-ray, and CT scan of abdomen and pelvis. CT scan of chest and head is done if chest X-ray is found abnormal.

Diagnosis

Gestational trophoblastic neoplasia is primarily diagnosed by the persistent elevated serum hCG.

Usually, no tissue is available for pathological study in most of the cases.

Invasive Mole (Fig. 11)

In invasive mole, there are excessive trophoblastic overgrowth and extensive penetration by the trophoblastic cells including whole villi. These penetrate into the myometrium **(Fig. 11)**, sometimes involving the peritoneum, parametrium, or vaginal vault. These are locally invasive and chance of widespread metastasis is less. Invasive mole almost develops from mole—partial or complete variety.

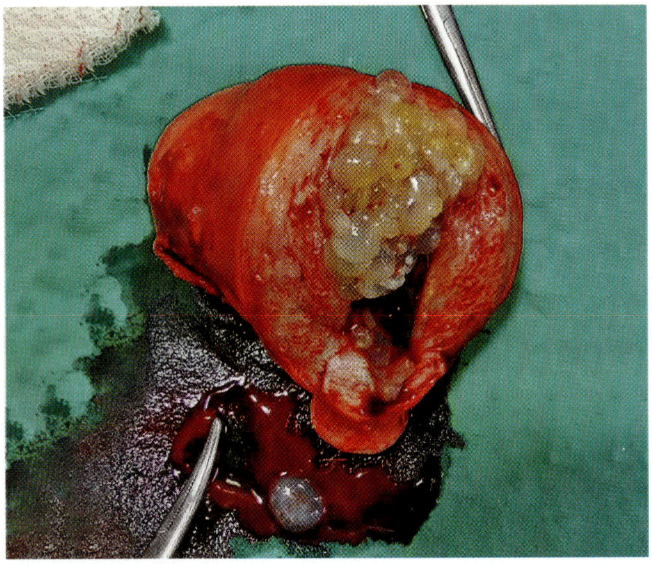

Fig. 11: Hysterectomy specimen showing the invasive mole. 41-year-old multigravida with living issue 3 presented with torrential hemorrhage with severe anemia.
Courtesy: Dr Rupali Modak, Assistant Professor, RG Kar Medical College, Kolkata, West Bengal, India.

Gestational Choriocarcinoma (Figs. 12 to 14)

Gestational choriocarcinoma is an extremely malignant form of GTN and carcinoma of the chorionic epithelium. It mostly develops from molar pregnancy but may develop from nonmolar pregnancy. The incidence of development of gestational choriocarcinoma is 1 in 30,000 nonmolar pregnancy.

Macroscopically, the uterus becomes bulky. Both the ovaries enlarge due to theca-lutein cyst **(Figs. 12 and 13)**.

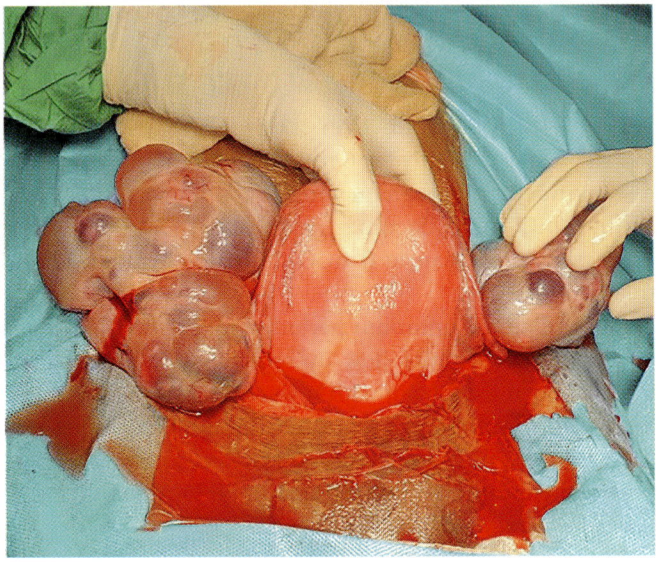

Fig. 12: Laparotomy finding showing bulky uterus and bilateral enlarged ovaries due to theca-lutein cysts. A 38-year-old P2+0 patient, living issue 2 was admitted with recurrent excessive vaginal bleeding.

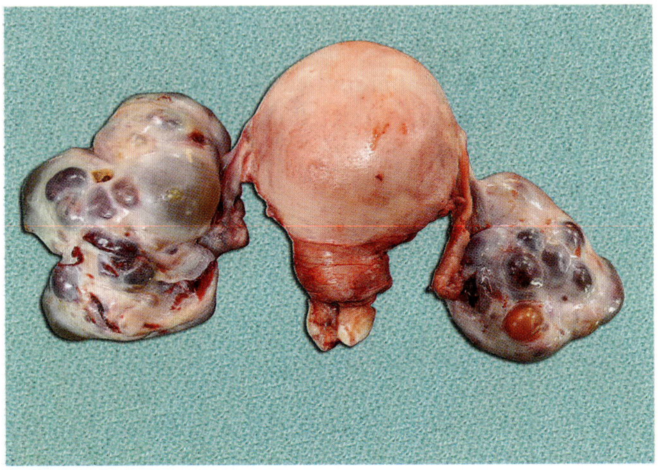

Fig. 13: Hysterectomy specimen of the patient as in Figure 12. Decision of hysterectomy is taken as there was uncontrolled bleeding. Initially, the patient was tried with conservative treatment.
Courtesy: Dr Anirban Mondal, Associate Professor; Dr BC Kameswari, Senior Resident, Bankura Sammilani Medical College, Bankura, West Bengal, India.

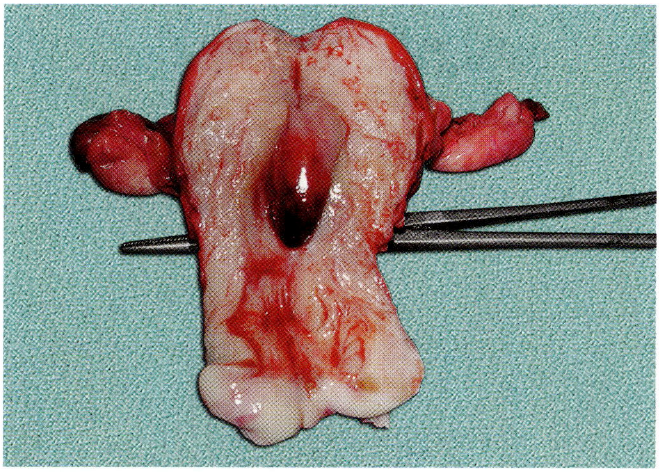

Fig. 14: Choriocarcinoma.
Courtesy: Dr G Kamilya, Professor, Institute of Postgraduate Medical Education and Research, Kolkata, West Bengal, India.

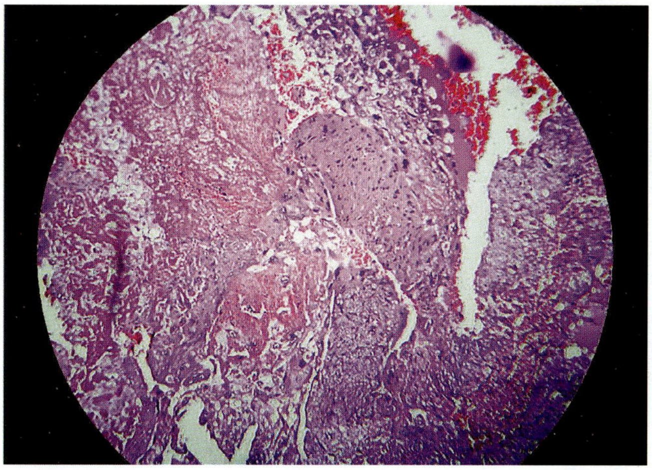

Fig. 15: Microscopical features of choriocarcinoma—intermediate trophoblast, multinucleated syncytiotrophoblast, large areas of necrosis, and hemorrhage.
Courtesy: Dr Anup Boler, Associate Professor, Pathology.

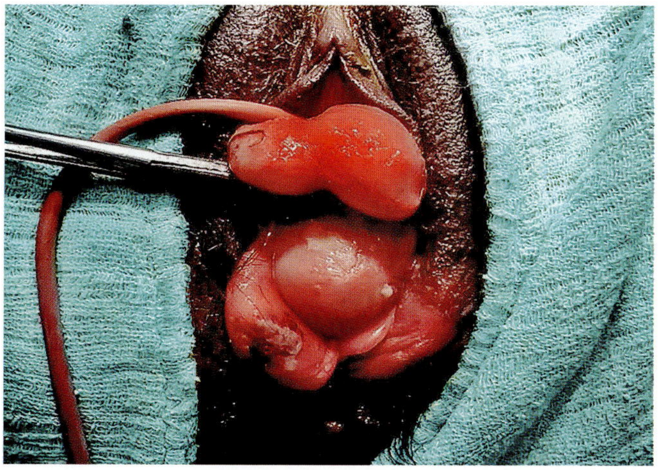

Fig. 16: Placental site trophoblastic tumor (PSTT) metastasis in vagina.
Courtesy: Professor Chandana Das, Head, Department of Gynecology and Obstetrics, Nil Ratan Sircar Medical College and Hospital (NRSMC&H), Kolkata, West Bengal, India.

There may be a large mass inside the uterine cavity invading both myometrium and blood vessels. In case of involvement of the endometrium, sloughing and infection of the surface occur. The tumor is dark red or purple and ragged or friable. Microscopically, columns and seeds of trophoblastic cells penetrate the muscle and blood vessels, and cellular anaplasia may be present. There are presence of intermediate trophoblast, multinucleate syncytiotrophoblast with hemorrhage and necrosis **(Fig. 15)**.

The important diagnostic feature of choriocarcinoma is *absence of a villous pattern* which is present in H. mole or invasive mole.

Metastasis occurs early and is usually bloodborne. The common sites are lungs (75%) and vagina (50%). The other sites are vulva, kidneys, liver, ovaries, brain, and bowel. There is direct spread to peritoneum, tubes, and ovaries.

Diagnosis of choriocarcinoma is done keeping possibility of this condition in mind, presence of unusual bleeding after term pregnancy or abortion, serum β-hCG measurement, and chest X-ray.

Treatment is chemotherapy. For a low-risk patient, a single-agent drug is given. For high-risk women, multiple agents chemotherapy are prescribed. Hysterectomy reduces the total dose of chemotherapy. Sometimes, radiotherapy may be needed in a condition such as brain metastasis.

Placental Site Trophoblastic Tumor

This trophoblastic neoplasia arises from the placental implantation site following term pregnancy, abortion, ectopic pregnancy, or molar pregnancy. It is an uncommon (1–2% of all GTN) but important variant of choriocarcinoma.

Histologically, there are predominantly cytotrophoblastic cells which arise from invasive intermediate trophoblast.

Placental site trophoblastic tumor primarily remains inside the uterus; it is locally invasive and rarely metastasizes in very advanced cases to the lungs, liver, or vagina **(Fig. 16)**.

Bleeding is the main symptom. The serum β-hCG level may be normal to elevated and produces a small amount of hCG (<300) and human placental lactogen. A uterine arteriovenous fistula **(Fig. 17)** may be present.

Hysterectomy is the most efficacious treatment for nonmetastatic variety as it is less sensitive to chemotherapy and if the ovaries are healthy, these are not removed. Aggressive combined chemotherapy is given in metastatic variety. Radiation can also be given. 10-year survival is 70% but in advanced stage of IV it is much less.

Epithelioid trophoblastic tumor: Epithelioid trophoblastic tumor is a rare variety of trophoblastic tumor. It may

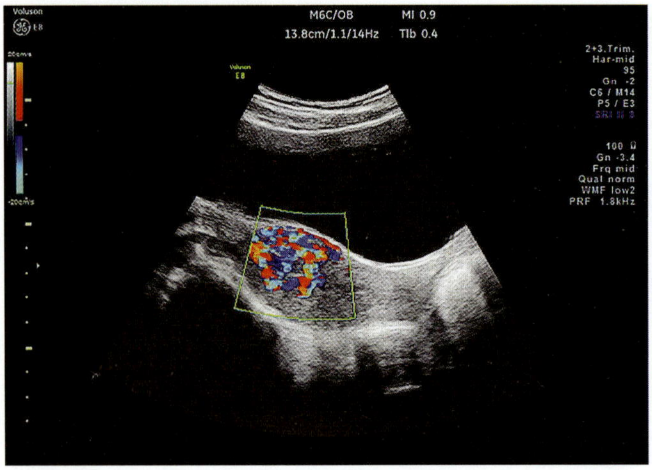

Fig. 17: Color Doppler study shows arteriovenous malformation in uterine fundus.
Courtesy: Professor Kamal Oswal, Head, Department of Radiodiagnosis, Vivekananda Institute of Medical Sciences, Kolkata, West Bengal, India.

TABLE 2: Modified WHO prognostic scoring system as adapted by FIGO.

FIGO Scoring	***0***	***1***	***2***	***4***
Age in years	<40	≥40	–	–
Antecedent pregnancy	Mole	Abortion	Term	–
Interval months from end of index pregnancy to treatment	<4	4–6	7–12	<12
Pretreatment serum β-hCG in mIU/L	$<10^3$	$<10^3$–$<10^4$	$<10^4$–$<10^5$	$\geq 10^5$
Largest tumor size, including uterus (cm)	<3	3–<5	≥5	–
Site of metastases	–	Spleen, kidney	Gastro-intestinal	Liver, brain
Number of metastases	–	1–4	5–8	>8
Previous failed chemotherapy	–	–	Single drug	Two or more drugs

(ETT: epithelioid trophoblastic tumor; FIGO: International Federation of Gynecology and Obstetrics; hCG: human chorionic gonadotropin; PSTT: placental site trophoblastic tumor)

develop many years after pregnancy. Usually, a patient of the reproductive age group presents with abnormal vaginal bleeding. It develops from chorionic-type intermediate trophoblast by neoplastic transformation.

Macroscopically, it presents as a discrete, hemorrhagic, solid, and cystic lesion located in either the fundus, lower uterine segment, or endocervix. Microscopically, it is seen as uniform population of mononuclear intermediate trophoblastic cells forming nests and solid masses.

Histologically, ETT is close to cervical squamous cell carcinoma (SCC). But ETT is positive for CK18 and human leukocyte antigen G, and cervical SCC is not.

It metastasizes in <25% cases and 10% became fatal. Diagnosis is done by endometrial biopsy.

Hysterectomy is the treatment due to chemoresistance. Metastatic type is treated by multiagent therapy.

Modified WHO Prognostic Scoring System as adapted by International Federation of Gynecology and Obstetrics (FIGO): The prognostic scoring system is described in **Table 2**.

90% patients are of low risk and 10% belong to high risk.

Treatment

Treatment is done by either single-agent therapy or multiagent therapy depending on the *FIGO scoring system*. The scoring parameters of GTN are given in **Table 2**.

- Women with score ≤6 are at low risk and treated with single-agent intramuscular methotrexate on alternate day with folinic acid for 1 week followed by 6 rest days.
- Women with score ≥7 are at high risk and are treated with multiagent chemotherapy which includes methotrexate, actinomycin-D, etoposide, cyclophosphamide, and vincristine (EMACO).
- In all cases, treatment is continued until the β-hCG level comes normal and then further 6 consecutive weeks.
- Cure rate is 100% in low-risk group and 95% in high-risk group.

Chemotherapy for GTN Based on the FIGO 2000 Scoring System

- Women with score ≤6 are at low risk and are treated with single-agent intramuscular methotrexate 50 mg on day 1, 3, 5, and 7 with tablet folinic acid 15 mg orally 24–30 hours after methotrexate on day 2, 4, 6, and 8. Chemotherapy is repeated every 2 weekly. After hCG returned to normal, consolidation with two to three more cycles of chemotherapy is needed to reduce chance of recurrence (FIGO 2015).
- Alternatively, single-agent actinomycin D can be used in low-risk group. If a single agent fails, a combined regime is used.
- Women with score ≥7 are at high risk and are treated with multiagent chemotherapy which include methotrexate, actinomycin-D, etoposide, cyclophosphamide, and vincristine (EMACO).
- In high-risk cases, treatment is continued until the hCG level comes normal and then further 6 consecutive weeks.
- Cure rate is 100% in low-risk group and 95% in high-risk group.

- Adjuvant hysterectomy reduces the total dose of chemotherapy.
- *Role of surgery:* Hysterectomy is considered in the following conditions:
  - When there is primary treatment failure of PSTT, epithelioid trophoblastic tumor, and other chemo-resistant cases, in cases of uncontrolled vaginal or intra-abdominal bleeding as an emergency procedure.
  - Hysterectomy reduces the total dose of chemotherapy in low-risk cases. Disease persistence after hysterectomy in GTN is about 3–5%. Residual lung metastasis persists in 10–20% cases.
- *Radiotherapy* is used for brain metastasis.

Dose of EMACO Regime (BAGSHWE Regime)

E = Etoposide (100 mg/m^2 IV infusion in saline over 30 minutes)
M = Methotrexate (100 mg/m^2 IV infusion over 12 hours)
A = Actinomycin D (0.5 mg IV stat)
C = Cyclophosphamide (600 mg IV in saline)
O = Vincristine (oncovin) (10 mg/IV stat)

Role of Radiotherapy

- *Patient with brain metastasis:* Whole brain radiation of 3,000 cGy over 10 days
- High-dose intrathecal methotrexate used to prevent hemorrhage and for tumor shrinkage
- Interventional radiotherapy (hepatic artery ligation or embolization) or whole liver radiation (2,000 cGy over 10 days) for liver metastasis

Other Surgery

Lung resection and craniotomy in lung and brain metastases.

Survival Rate in GTN

In stages I, II, and III, survival rate is 100%.

Long-term Outcome of Women Treated for GTN with Chemotherapy

Women are likely to have an earlier menopause. Women who receive multiagent chemotherapy may have increased risk of developing secondary cancers.

FUTURE PREGNANCY

Fertility following H. mole is not impaired and outcome is also good. As there is chance of recurrence, early pregnancy sonography is always advisable. Fertility and pregnancy outcome following GTN and chemotherapy, in general, is good. Adverse outcomes and spontaneous abortion have been reported if pregnancy occurs within 6 months. Pregnancy outcome within 12 months following chemotherapy for GTN is favorable and it is best to conceive after 12 months as relapse occurs within 1 month.

CHAPTER 6

Cervical Incompetence and Cervical Cerclage

Learning Objectives

- Etiology
- Diagnosis
- Management
- Cervical Cerclage—Indications, Steps, Complications
- Emergency or Rescue Cerclage
- Transabdominal Cerclage, Laparoscopic Cerclage

INTRODUCTION

Cervix is the lower part of the uterus 2–3 cm in length with an endocervical canal which remains closed during pregnancy to keep the contents of uterus in situ till the onset of labor at term when it becomes dilated for the passage of fetus and afterbirths. When the function of the cervix is impaired due to the intrinsic defect, midtrimester abortion or preterm labor may supervene. This is called cervical insufficiency or previously known as cervical incompetence. Cervical insufficiency is characterized by painless cervical dilation in the second trimester **(Fig. 1)**. The idea of cerclage is to reinforce the strength of cervix to maintain its competence.

ETIOLOGY

The exact etiology is not known. There may be: (1) congenital and/or (2) acquired defect.

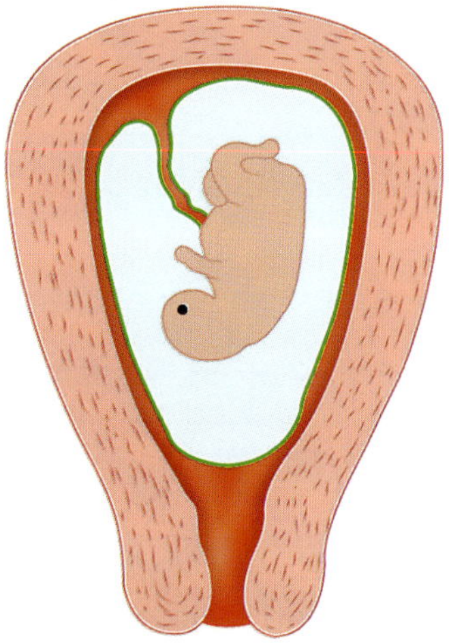

Fig. 1: Incompetent cervix.

Congenital

Inherent Genetic and Intrinsic Defects

Cervix has three components, namely smooth muscle 5–25% (less in lower part), collagen, and connective tissue containing glycosaminoglycans (dermatan sulfate and hyaluronic acid). During pregnancy, structural and biochemical changes occur which include increased water content, increased glycosaminoglycans, increased collagen solubility, and decreased stromal stiffness. During ripening, smooth muscle has little role. There is a decrease in collagen and protein concentration during ripening. Collagen decreases due to proteolytic digestion by the action of collagenase. The relative amount of dermatan sulfate and hyaluronic acid is changed near term and ripening occurs. Whether the congenital defect of the components of cervix or certain genes, namely *Has2* or *Has1*, or genes related to collagen metabolism are associated remains unclear. One-fourth of women suffering from cervical insufficiency is found to have a first-degree relative with the same disorder.

Müllerian Anomaly and Cervical Insufficiency

It is a common observation that women with uterine anomalies such as bicornuate and unicornuate uterus **(Fig. 2)** are likely to deliver preterm. Short cervix, cervical intrinsic defect, and uterine distension are implicated as causes for preterm delivery. Cervical cerclage is claimed to improve the outcome; however, routine cerclage is not recommended in uterine anomaly.

Diethylstilbesterol exposure to female fetus: Diethylstilbesterol (DES) exposure has been reported to be associated with uterine anomaly as well as cervical insufficiency from 1978.

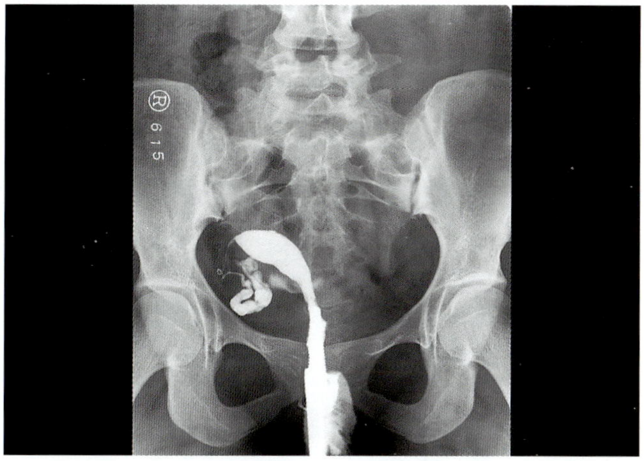

Fig. 2: Hysterosalpingography (HSG)—unicornual uterus. Banana-shaped uterus.
Courtesy: Professor Kamal Oswal, Head, Department of Radiodiagnosis, Vivekananda Institute of Medical Sciences, Kolkata, West Bengal, India.

Whether cervical cerclage improves the outcome of pregnancy is uncertain.

Marfan syndrome and Ehlers–Danlos syndrome which are multisystemic disorders primarily affecting the soft connective tissues are associated with an increased risk of cervical insufficiency.

Acquired Causes

Cervical conization, cervical amputation, forceful dilation and curettage (D&C), dilation and evacuation (D&E), and forceful delivery in undilated cervix are alleged to be important acquired factors for cervical insufficiency. Though conflicting results reported by different workers, cold-knife conization or loop electrosurgical excision procedure (LEEP) are considered to be significant increase risk of preterm birth. One large study showed a fourfold increase of pregnancy loss before 24 weeks in women with a previous history of conization. National Institute for Health and Care Excellence (NICE) guideline (2020) recommends prophylactic cervical cerclage for women with short cervix diagnosed during sonography, and who have had either preterm premature rupture of membranes (P-PROM) in a previous pregnancy *or* a history of cervical trauma. Cervical trauma means physical injury to the cervix including surgery such as previous cone biopsy (cold knife or laser), large loop excision of the transformation zone [(LLETZ) any number], or radical diathermy. Women with pregnancy termination by surgical evacuation are at an increased risk of cervical incompetence.

DIAGNOSIS

History

Repeated pregnancy loss in midtrimester in 16–24 weeks is suggestive of cervical incompetence. Typical history is painless cervical dilatation in midtrimester of pregnancy

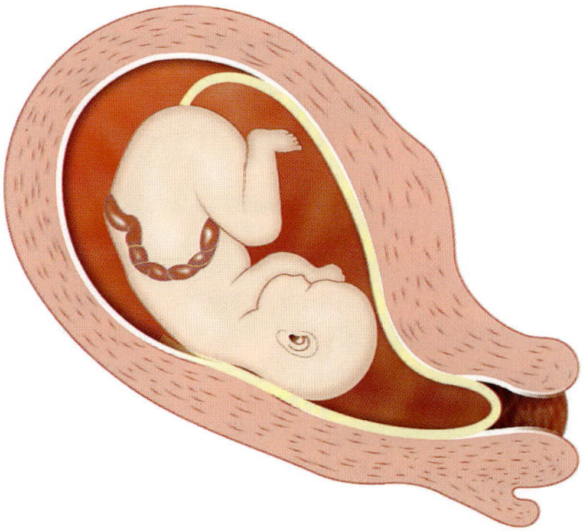

Fig. 3: Dilatation of cervix with herniation of membranes.

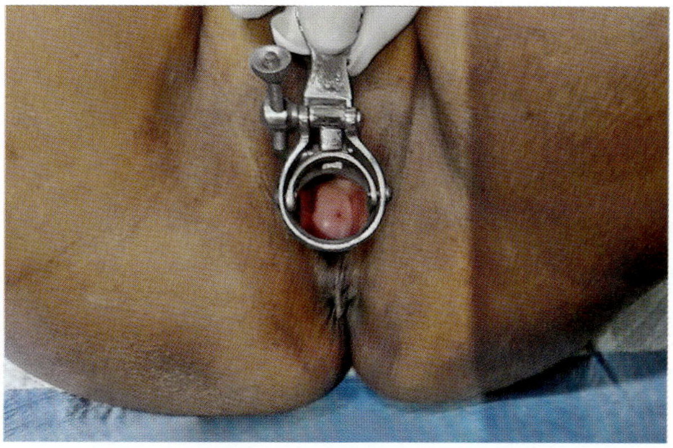

Fig. 4: Direct visualization of cervix by Cusco's speculum.

followed by ballooning and prolapse of the amniotic sac and then membranes rupture following which delivery of fetus occurs **(Fig. 3)**. Usually, the fetus remains alive at the time of delivery. This typical event may be repeated in future pregnancies. Cervical incompetence does not cause first-trimester miscarriage.

In nonpregnant conditions, Hegar's cervical dilator of 8 size may be easily negotiated through the internal os; however, it is not a reliable test. Hysterocervicography may show funneling of the cervical canal at the premenstrual period in a nonpregnant condition.

During pregnancy on weekly speculum examination from 10 weeks onward **(Fig. 4)**, dilatation of the cervix with herniation of membranes **(Fig. 3)** can be seen on inspection.

Ultrasonography

Cervical incompetence can be diagnosed by ultrasonography **(Figs. 5 and 6)** at 14 weeks of pregnancy. The length of the cervical canal becomes <30 mm (normal 35–40 mm), diameter of the internal loss becomes >20 mm, and there is funneling of the internal loss. Short cervical length is defined as ≤25 mm measured between 16 and 24 weeks of gestation. The length of the cervix below 25 mm is associated with a high risk of preterm delivery.

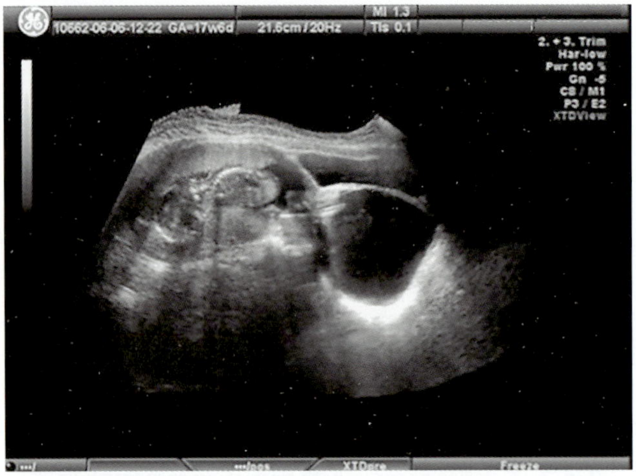

Fig. 5: Cervical incompetence at 17 weeks' gestation.
Courtesy: Professor Kamal Oswal, Head, Department of Radiodiagnosis, Vivekananda Institute of Medical Sciences, Kolkata, West Bengal, India

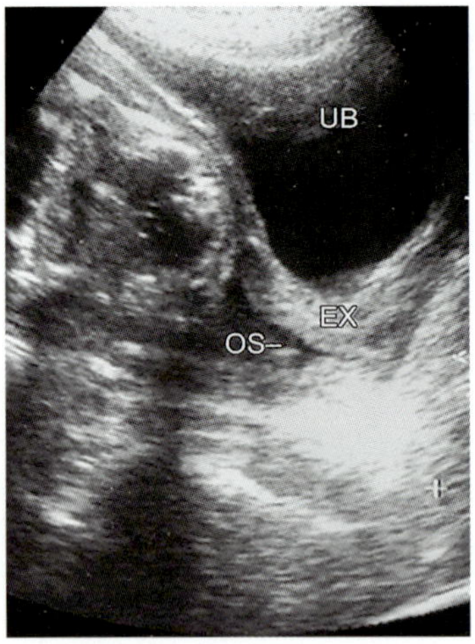

Fig. 6: Cervical incompetence with breech presentation at 14 weeks.

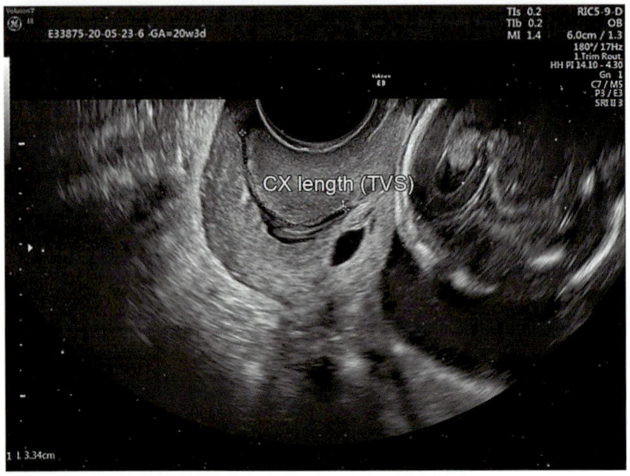

Fig. 7: Endocervical length measurement by transvaginal sonography (TVS) for screening at 20 weeks for preterm labor.
Courtesy: Professor Kusagradhi Ghose, Institute of Fetal Medicine (IFM), Kolkata, West Bengal, India.

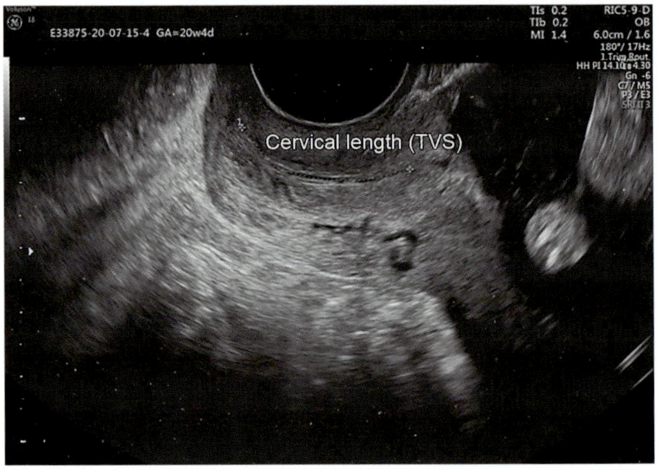

Fig. 8: Transvaginal sonography (TVS) screening of cervical length in the same patient as in Figure 7.

Transvaginal ultrasound is preferred to the abdominal method because in the latter, full bladder is necessary where the length of the cervix is increased and the internal os may be closed giving a false impression. Serial ultrasonography is helpful to diagnose cervical incompetence.

Cervical Length Screening (Figs. 7 and 8)

Cervical length screening is now recommended in women with prior preterm birth. Between 16 and 24 weeks, sonographic cervical measurement is done every 2 weeks.

The role of universal cervical length screening is controversial and not approved as it has not been shown to be cost effective. If performed, it should be done transvaginally by a qualified ultrasonologist. Cervical length screening is now recommended in women with prior preterm birth. As per American College of Obstetricians and Gynecologists (ACOG 2021) guideline, serial endovaginal ultrasound measurement of cervical length is recommended starting at $16^{0/7}$ weeks of gestation and repeated every 1–4 weeks, depending on individual patient risks and findings until $24^{0/7}$ weeks of gestation for a woman with a singleton pregnancy and a prior spontaneous preterm birth. If ultrasound monitoring detects a cervical length of 25 mm or less, options for intervention include cerclage or vaginal progesterone. Vaginal progesterone is recommended for asymptomatic individuals without a history of preterm birth with a singleton pregnancy and a short cervix. The ACOG (2021) guideline suggests for the anatomy assessment of the cervix at the $18^{0/7}$ - $22^{6/7}$ weeks of gestation in individuals without a prior preterm birth, with either a transabdominal or an endovaginal approach.

MANAGEMENT

- Progesterone
- Cervical cerclage

Currently, prophylactic progesterone, mostly in the vaginal route, has become the recommended treatment for prevention of preterm labor in addition to cervical cerclage.

Prophylactic vaginal progesterone or prophylactic cervical cerclage is recommended to women who have both a history of spontaneous preterm birth (up to 34^{+0} weeks of pregnancy) and mid-trimester loss (from 16^{+0} weeks of pregnancy onward), and the transvaginal ultrasound scan shows a short cervix (cervical length of 25 mm or less) carried out between 16^{+0} and 24^{+0} weeks of pregnancy by NICE (2020) and ACOG (2021) guidelines. Vaginal progesterone is started between 16^{+0} and 24^{+0} weeks of pregnancy and is continued until at least 34 weeks. The Food and Drug Administration (FDA) has approved only 17-hydroxyprogesterone caproate (17-OHP-C) to prevent recurrent preterm birth, which is not beneficial in short cervix. Prophylactic cervical cerclage is also considered (NICE 2020) for women when the transvaginal ultrasound scan carried out between 16^{+0} and 24^{+0} weeks of pregnancy shows a cervical length of 25 mm or less, and who have had either P-PROM in a previous pregnancy *or* a history of cervical trauma. Society of Obstetricians and Gynaecologists of Canada (SOGC) (2020) recommends vaginal progesterone as an effective and potentially superior alternate therapy (strong/moderate) if a cerclage is being considered in patients with a singleton pregnancy and a previous spontaneous preterm birth or a cervical length ≤25 mm between 16 and 24 weeks in the current pregnancy.

Cervical Cerclage

Surgery of cervical insufficiency consists of application of a cerclage either vaginally or abdominally. A transabdominal cerclage is done either by open surgery or by laparoscopic or robotic surgery.

G Ernest Hermann described cervical cerclages first in 1902 which were placed through the vaginal route. Shirodkar (1955) and McDonald (1957) described the methods in two different ways. Vithal Nagesh Shirodkar (1899–1971) **(Fig. 9)** from Goa, India, introduced this operation using fascia lata. Ian McDonald (1922–1990) originally did this operation using silk suture (from Australia) in a more simplified form than that of Shirodkar's cerclage operation. The McDonald method is commonly preferred due to its simplicity.

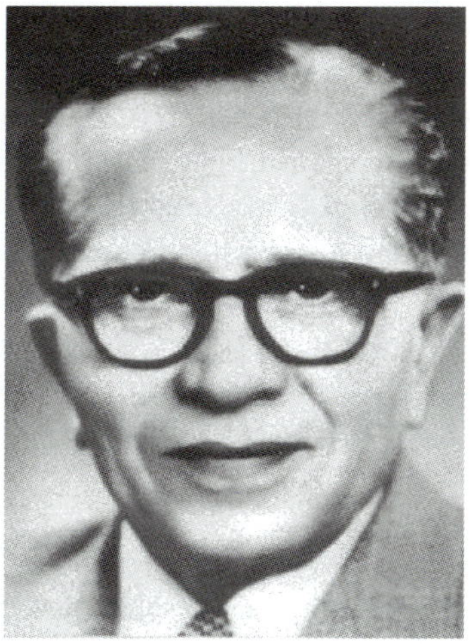

Fig. 9: Vithal Nagesh Shirodkar (1899–1971).

Indications of Cerclage

The indications of cerclage are: (1) prophylactic cerclage (history—indicated), (2) ultrasound-indicated cerclage with prior preterm birth, (3) ultrasound-indicated cerclage without prior preterm births, and (4) rescue cerclage.

Prophylactic cerclage means when cerclage is given in women with history suggesting cervical insufficiency. Ultrasound-indicated cerclage is given in shortening of cervix with or without prior preterm birth. Rescue cerclage or emergency cerclage is applied when the cervix is dilated and the membrane is visible or bulges during the second trimester provided inevitable abortion or preterm labor is excluded. Cervical cerclage is not recommended for prevention of preterm birth based solely for multiple gestation (ACOG 2021).

To sum, the indications are as follows:

- There is a history of preterm delivery before 34 weeks or midtrimester loss from 16 weeks' pregnancy onward.
- In a singleton pregnancy, a cervical length of <25 mm between 16 and 24 weeks by transvaginal sonography (TVS). Benefit with cerclage in women with short cervix only and without history of preterm delivery is uncertain.
- Emergency or rescue cerclage—when the cervix is dilated, effaced, or both (exposed unruptured fetal membranes) in the absence of contraction.

Contraindications of cerclage are preeclampsia, chorioamnionitis, preterm labor, active bleeding, rupture membranes, multiple pregnancy, and preferably not after 24 weeks.

Time of Application of Cerclage

Prophylactic cerclage before dilatation is usually placed between 12 and 14 weeks' gestation.

Preoperative Evaluations

Indication is justified. There should not be any bleeding, contractions, or ruptured membranes. Before doing cerclage, sonography is essential to confirm that the baby is living and there is no other anomaly of the uterus. Aneuploidy and other malformation screening are done. Tests for chlamydial and gonorrhea infection are done. If positive, treatment is given. Pap smear screening is done. The efficacy of prophylactic tocolysis is not proved.

Steps of Shirodkar's Operation (Figs. 10 to 13)

The patient is placed in standard dorsal lithotomy position. Regional anesthesia is suitable for cerclage. The cervix

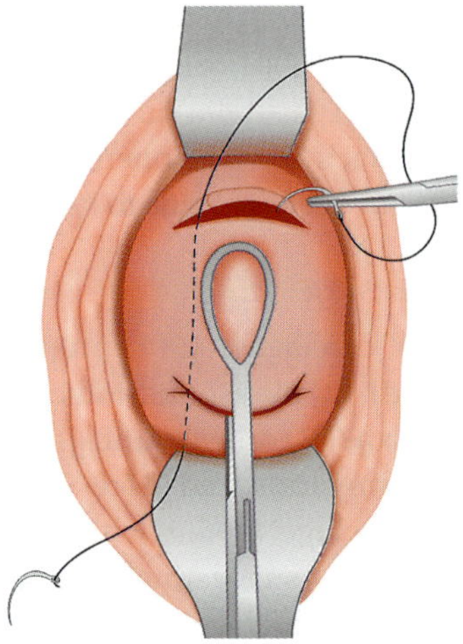

Fig. 10: Steps of Shirodkar's cerclage operation—incision and thread placement.

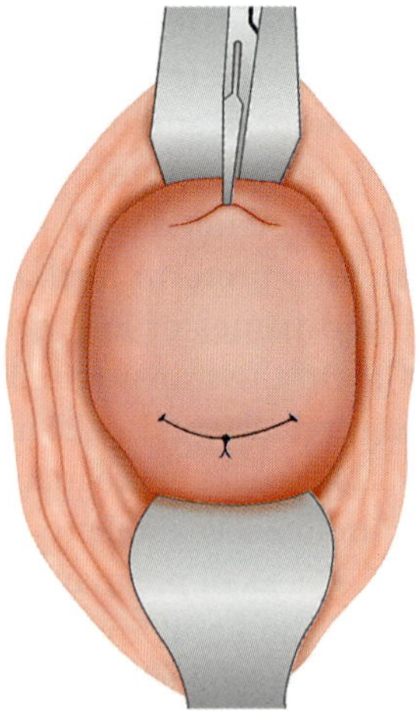

Fig. 11: Steps of Shirodkar's cerclage operation—two ends of thread tied posteriorly.

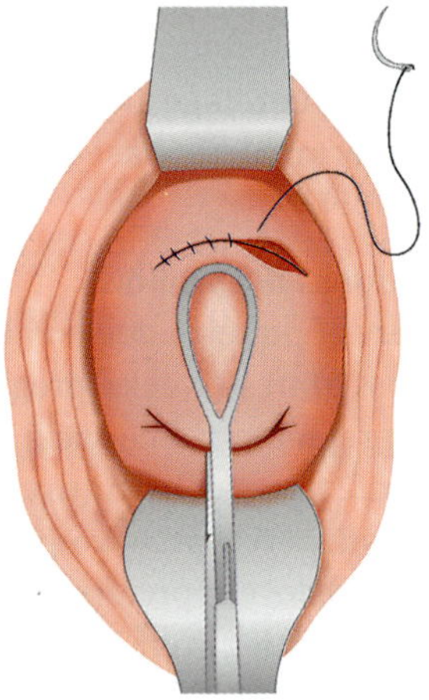

Fig. 12: Steps of Shirodkar's cerclage operation—anterior and posterior incisions closed with stitches.

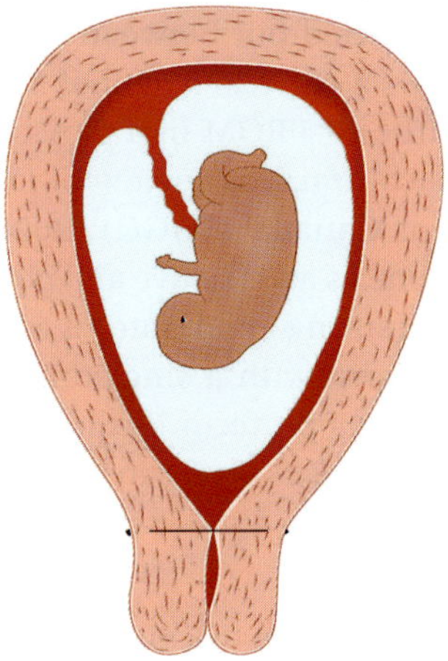

Fig. 13: Following Shirodkar's cerclage.

is exposed by retracting the posterior vaginal wall with Sims speculum or Auvard speculum. Another Landon retractor (right angle) may be used anteriorly or laterally to expose the vagina well. Both the lips of the cervix are held with two sponge-holding forceps separately. A small transverse incision is made at the cervicovaginal junction below the base of the bladder (2 cm above the external os). The bladder is pushed up with blunt dissection as far above as possible avoiding injury to bladder. A small vertical incision or transverse incision is made on the posterior wall of the cervix at the cervicovaginal junction.

A nonabsorbable suture—silk, Mersilene tape (5 mm) or nylon (1 or 2) or polypropylene monofilament suture—is passed from the anterior to the posterior aspect submucosally using a large, curved, and round body needle or Shirodkar's needle. This is done on both sides. The two ends of the suture are tied posteriorly, a tail of the cerclage suture is kept long and visible for removal later **(Fig. 11)**, and the anterior and posterior incisions are closed with interrupted catgut stitches.

Steps of McDonald's Operation (Figs. 14 to 19)

The patient is placed in dorsal lithotomy position. Regional anesthesia is preferred. The cervix is exposed with Sims speculum. Both the lips of the cervix are held with two sponge-holding forceps separately. A nonabsorbable suture such as silk, Mersilene tape (5 mm), or nylon (1 or 2) or polypropylene monofilament suture is passed from anterior to posterior and then from posterior to anterior like a purse string suture all around the cervix as high as possible taking successive deep bites (four to six bites). Two ends of the suture are tied anteriorly and kept long for removal later. No incision is needed in this operation and bladder mobilization is not done.

The success rate is the same (75–85%) as Shirodkar's operation and there is less blood loss. The chance of cervical scar formation is also less.

Complications of Cerclage Operation

Complications of cerclage are PROM, infection, onset of uterine contraction and hemorrhage, and later fibrosis

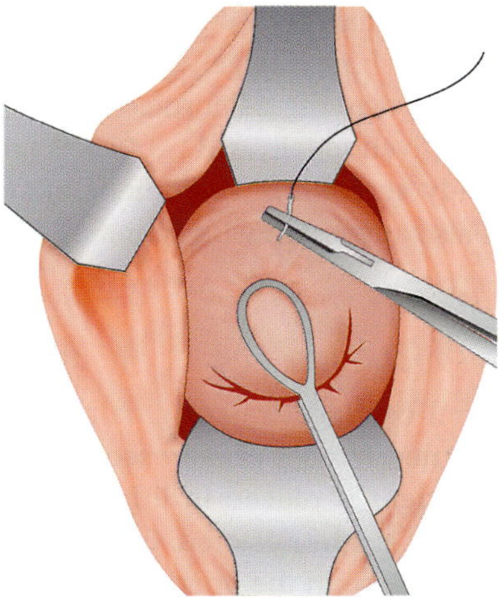

Fig. 14: Steps of McDonald's operation—needle introduction.

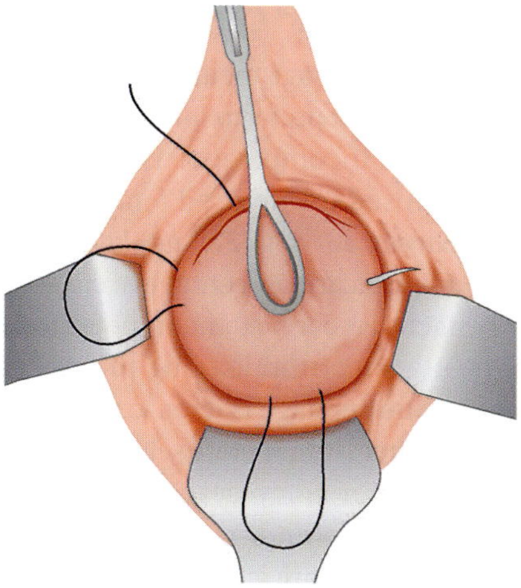

Fig. 15: Steps of McDonald's operation—suture placement.

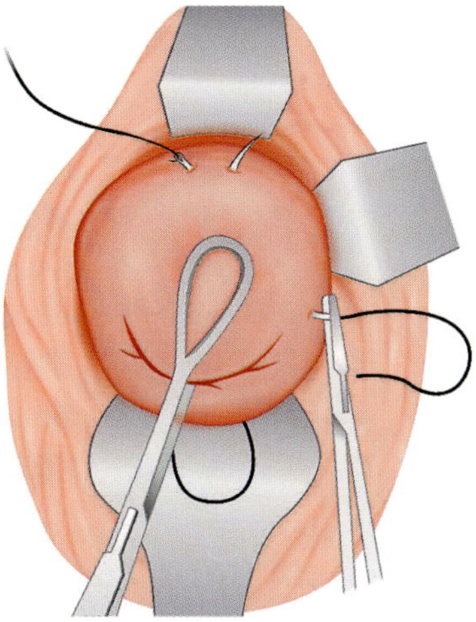

Fig. 16: Steps of McDonald's operation—suture placement like purse-string suture.

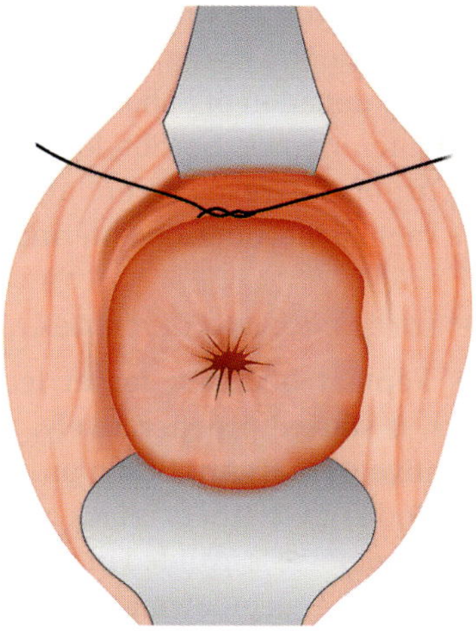

Fig. 17: Steps of McDonald's operation—two ends tied anteriorly.

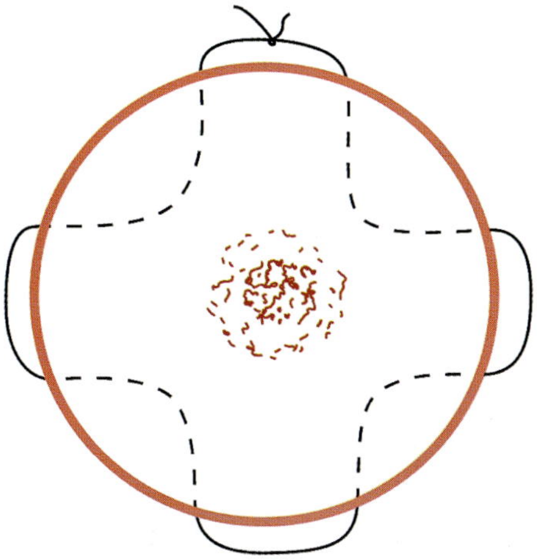

Fig. 18: Following McDonald's operation—look in transverse section.

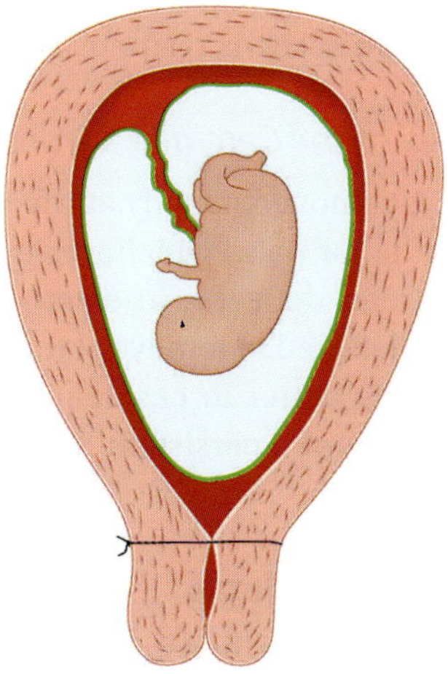

Fig. 19: Following McDonald's operation—look in sagittal section.

leading to cervical dystocia. Cervical laceration following suture displacement is one complication and occurs mostly in an unattended case of onset of labor with cerclage in situ. Cerclage removal is urgent after labor onset to avoid cervical injury and uterine rupture. Bladder and ureteral injury followed by fistula formation are other rare but serious injuries. These are uncommon during prophylactic cerclage.

Emergency or "Rescue" Cerclage

Emergency or rescue cerclage means emergency application of cerclage in threatened preterm labor before or at the limit of viability if cervical incompetence is recognized (cervical dilatation and exposed unruptured fetal membranes). It is considered in *between* 16^{+0} *and* 27^{+6} *weeks of pregnancy*. This is successful in a significant percentage of cases. The concept is based on the fact that cervical incompetence and preterm labor are part of a spectrum leading to preterm delivery. Emergency or rescue cerclage is a reasonable approach and should be offered after proper counseling.

Placement of emergency cerclage is difficult due to thinned dilated cervix with a risk of membranes rupture and tissue tearing. There are various methods to repose the prolapsed membranes. It should be done very gently and membranes can be pushed with a moist wide sponge stick. Other methods are traction on cervical edges and insertion of Foley catheter inside the cervix, inflation to deflect the sac first, followed by deflation of balloon with simultaneous cerclage suture tightening over the tube, followed by removal.

Contraindications of rescue cerclage are signs of infection, active vaginal bleeding, and uterine contractions.

Postoperative Care Following Cerclage Operation

The patient is kept at bed rest for at least 48 hours. Tocolytic agents, if started preoperatively, are continued in the postoperative period. Antibiotic prophylaxis in the perioperative period is given (there is lack of evidence of the benefit). Sexual intercourse is avoided in the initial period.

At the time of discharge following a cerclage operation, the patient must be warned that she must attend hospital immediately in case of abdominal pain. If there is onset of labor pain, the stitch must be removed, otherwise there will be tear and laceration of cervix resulting in profuse bleeding.

Time of Removal of the Cerclage Sutures

Cerclage suture is removed usually at the end of 37 weeks or at the onset of labor pain, whichever is earlier for both vaginal and cesarean delivery. In elective plan cesarean delivery, it can be deferred to remove at the time of cesarean delivery. Removal is better in cesarean delivery to avoid the rare complication of a persistent foreign body, such as vaginal erosion.

Transabdominal Cerclage

Durfee and Benson described transabdominal cerclage in 1965. Later, laparoscopic and robotic methods were introduced.

Indications of Transabdominal Cerclage

Cerclage through the abdominal approach is done in selected cases, e.g., previous failure of cerclage through the vaginal approach (scarring), cervicitis, severe defects of cervix (congenitally short or hugely amputed), and persistent nonhealing wound over vaginal fornices.

It should be given ideally at 11–14 weeks of pregnancy after aneuploidy screening. Placement of suture before conception is also advocated with similar results and is also practical.

Steps of Transabdominal Cerclage (Figs. 20 and 21)

Transabdominal cerclage was originally started through laparotomy, but now it is done laparoscopically or by robotic surgery. The patient is placed in lithotomy position and general anesthesia is administered. Cerclage is given in the cervicoisthmial region. In the open method, a Pfannenstiel incision is sufficient. A small transverse incision is made on the uterovesical fold of peritoneum and the bladder is retracted downward to expose uterine isthmus. A window

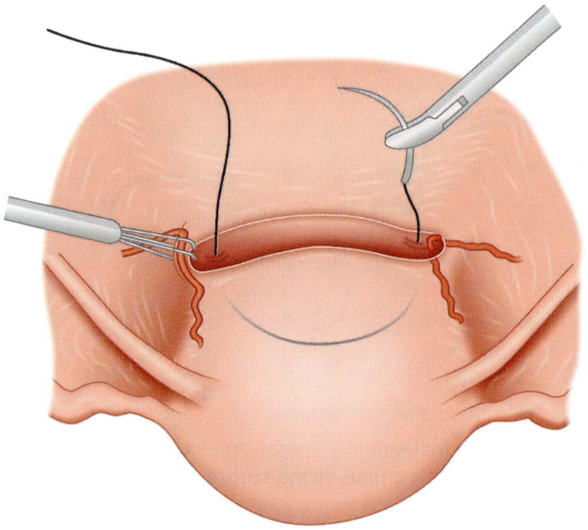

Fig. 20: Steps of transabdominal cerclage.

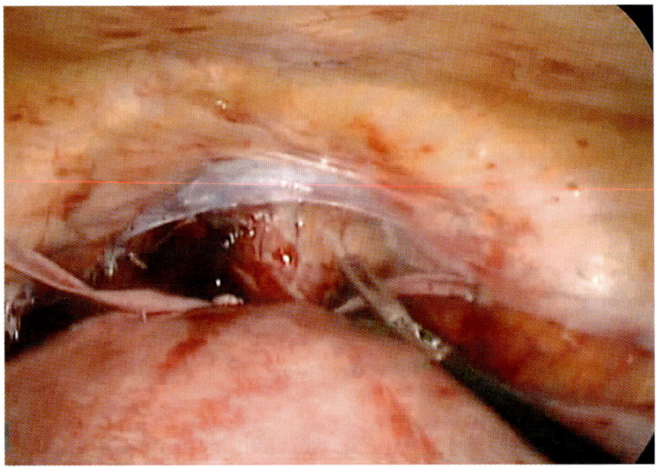

Fig. 21: Laparoscopic cervical cerclage.
Courtesy: Dr Aloke De, Professor, NB Medical College, West Bengal, India.

is made at the level of internal os in free space just medial to uterine vessels on each side. Mersilene tape with needle is usually used. The suture is passed either anterior to posterior or posterior to anterior taking care not to include or injure the ureter which lies posterior and lateral. The knot is tied anteriorly and the cut peritoneum is closed with absorbable suture. The knot can also be tied posteriorly, behind the uterus. The landmark of needle placement is 1.5 cm above and 1 cm lateral to the insertion of each uterosacral ligament. This landmark is particularly useful for the laparoscopic approach. The procedure can also be done without using needle avoiding the accidental vessel puncture with needle. Instead, a long Kelly clamp is used for passing the Mersilene tape in open method.

The cerclage is kept till the child-bearing is completed. Cesarean delivery is done. The conception rate is 70–80% with the cerclage in situ. In spontaneous abortion, D&E can be done with the stitch in place.

Use of Cervical Pessary

Cervical pessary is a promising noninvasive additional therapy to prevent preterm delivery in short cervix. Silicon rings, such as Arabian pessary, are used. It is not FDA approved for prevention of preterm birth due to conflicting results. Hans Arabian from West Germany designed this round cone-shaped pessary made of flexible silicone in the late 1970s. The idea is to increase the uterocervical angle, thus preventing the direct pressure by the fetal head over the cervix.

CHAPTER 7

Invasive Prenatal Testing and Fetal Therapy

Kusagradhi Ghosh
MD DNB FICOG FRCOG RCOG/RCR PG Diploma in Advanced Fetal Ultrasonography
Professor (Obs and Gyne)
VIMS/RKMSP Hospital, West Bengal University of Health Sciences
Director, Institute of Fetal Medicine, Kolkata, West Bengal, India

Learning Objectives

- Fetal Invasive Diagnostic Procedures
- Cordocentesis
- Other Invasive Diagnostic Procedures
- Fetal Therapeutic Procedures
- Fetal Blood Transfusion
- Procedures in Complicated Monochorionic Multiple Pregnancy
- Fetal Reduction in Complicated Monochorionic Pregnancy
- Fetal Shunt Procedures
- Fetal Endoscopic Tracheal Occlusion
- Fetal Cardiac Therapy
- Other Closed Fetal Invasive Therapeutic Procedures
- Fetal ex-utero Intrapartum Therapy
- Open Fetal Surgery
- Future of Fetal Therapy

INTRODUCTION

Invasive fetal testing started as an extension of fetal diagnostic ultrasonography (USG) to confirm or exclude genetic causes of an abnormal USG finding. With rapid development of biochemical screening for fetal aneuploidy, procedures such as amniocentesis and CVS increasingly became common to exclude trisomy 21 in the fetus. Since then, fetal invasive testing has been extended to diagnosis of single gene disorders (eg thalassemia), congenital infections, and syndromic conditions.

The first documented fetal therapy was intrauterine fetal blood transfusion by Sir William Liley (1963). Open fetal surgery was largely developed through the pioneering work of Dr Michael Harrison (1982). Since then, it has become safer and is now firmly established in certain fetal conditions. Fetal surgery is now a multidisciplinary specialty involving fetal medicine specialists, pediatric surgeons, anesthesiologists, cardiologists and others. With the advent of endoscopic surgery through the fetoscope the horizon is ever expanding. Fetal stem cell therapy is the new kid on the block.

FETAL INVASIVE DIAGNOSTIC PROCEDURES

Amniocentesis

Amniocentesis is the procedure of taking out amniotic fluid sample from amniotic sac for carrying out various diagnostic tests of the fetus. Around 10–20 mL of fluid is taken out, depending upon the test required. Amniotic fluid contains floating fetal cutaneous cells and amniocytes which can be harvested after centrifuging the sample. Amniocytes are exfoliated amniotic membrane cells which are genetically identical to the fetus. Both types of cells can be subjected to testing by cytogenetics or molecular genetics, as appropriate.

Indications

Indications for amniocentesis are:

- High risk on aneuploidy screening.
- Previous history of aneuploid babies.
- Structural abnormality of fetus on ultrasound (USG).
- History of single-gene disorders in family like thalassemia/spinal muscular atrophy (SMA)/Duchenne muscular dystrophy (DMD).

- *History suggestive of perinatal infections:* TORCH (*T*oxoplasmosis, *O*ther agents, *R*ubella, *C*ytomegalovirus, and *H*erpes simplex), parvovirus, varicella, etc.

The most common indication for amniocentesis is for confirmation or exclusion of fetal aneuploidy where there is high-risk report on aneuploidy screening. Screening for fetal aneuploidy is done either biochemically (first-trimester combined test, second-trimester quadruple test, etc.) or genetically (noninvasive prenatal testing, also called NIPT).

First-trimester combined test is done between crown-rump length (CRL) 45–84 mm (11–13 weeks, 6 days usually). Quadruple screen is done between 15 and 20 weeks usually when biparietal diameter (BPD) is 32–52 mm. NIPT can be done from 10 weeks onward and theoretically there is no upper limit. Results of all these screening tests may come "low risk" or "high risk". High-risk patients are counseled and offered further invasive testing, either amniocentesis or chorionic villus sampling (CVS). Low-risk patients are usually counseled and offered to continue pregnancy without any further invasive testing. High-risk screen test does not mean the fetus has Down syndrome. Low-risk screen report likewise does not mean zero risk. After counseling, some high-risk patients may decline invasive test for fear of miscarriage (0.1–0.3%) and some low-risk patients may opt for invasive testing for 100% guarantee. Individualization is important.

Counseling

Before taking consent for amniocentesis proper counseling is important. Counseling is directed toward allaying anxiety and discuss alternatives to amniocentesis, if any. Discussion regarding procedure-related miscarriage rate (0.1–0.3%) is recommended. Provision of DNA-storage from the sample for further tests in future, if required, is to be discussed. Turnaround time (TAT) is the time interval between taking of the sample and delivery of the report to the couple. Discussion of TAT is important, as the couple may choose to have medical termination of pregnancy (MTP) when amniocentesis report is abnormal. Chance of resampling is rare (0.1%), and is usually due to slow growth of amniocytes in the amniotic fluid sample, bacterial contamination or maternal cell contamination during the process of taking the sample. Option to discuss with support groups is mentioned in case the couple cannot take a decision. Option to opt out has also to be mentioned.

Emergency contact number needs to be given to the patient in case there is any subsequent bleeding, leaking, or pain in abdomen. Discussion regarding availability of MTP services in case of abnormal report also needs to be discussed.

Procedure

Basic USG assessment is performed before amniocentesis. Number of fetuses, fetal heartbeat, placental location, subjective amniotic fluid volume, internal os, cervical length, any myomas or ovarian cyst or subchorionic bleed, if any, are documented. Cleaning of abdomen is done with Savlon or Betadine. USG probe is covered by encasing it in either sterile powder-free surgical glove or in commercially available sterile probe covers. Local lignocaine infiltration is optional. 22G spinal needle, 10 cm long is inserted under real-time USG guidance using free-hand technique (without biopsy guide) **(Figs. 1 and 2)**. Initial 2–3 mL of aspirated fluid is discarded to avoid maternal contamination. 10 mL sterile single use plastic syringes are used for taking sample for the laboratory. Usually, 10–20 mL is aspirated depending upon the test required. There is no evidence for administering postprocedure antibiotics, and they are not prescribed routinely. Mother is usually discharged after 2 hours of bed rest.

Processing of the Sample

The sample needs to be checked by naked eye inspection for any obvious maternal blood cell contamination (called bloody tap). Amniotic fluid is transferred from the aspiration syringe to 10 mL gamma sterilized plastic tubes with screw caps. Individualized identification code of sample **(Fig. 3)** is ensured. Bar coding is mandatory to avoid mixing up of samples. Ideally, a sample needs to be transported to genetic laboratory within 24 hours.

Tests that can be done from amniotic fluid sample are as follows:

- *Cytogenetic testing (cell based):* FISH (fluorescence in situ hybridization) for rapid report of chromosomes 13, 18, 21, or 23 and karyotype for acute lymphoblastic leukemia (ALL) chromosomes.
- *Molecular genetics (DNA based, where cells are lysed, DNA extracted, and amplified by genetic techniques):*

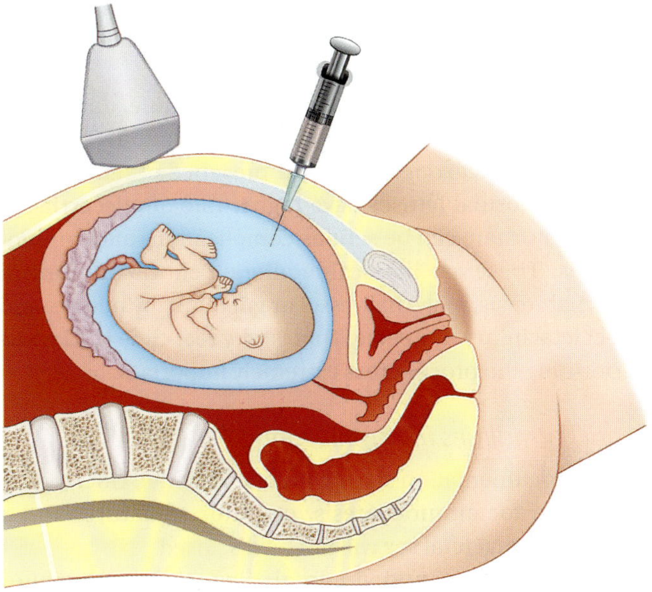

Fig. 1: Amniocentesis.

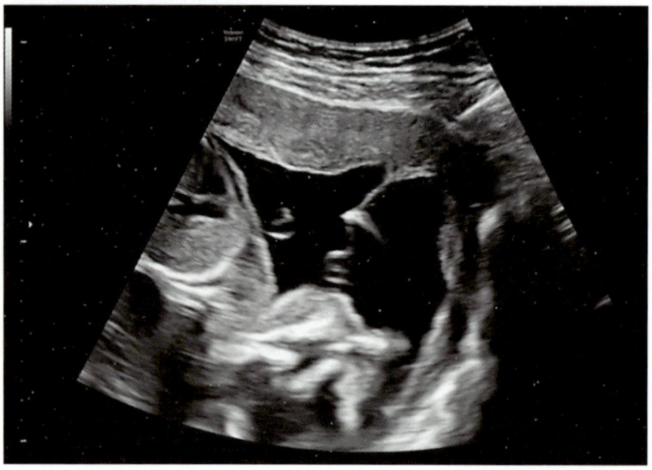

Fig. 2: Amniocentesis under sonographic guidance.

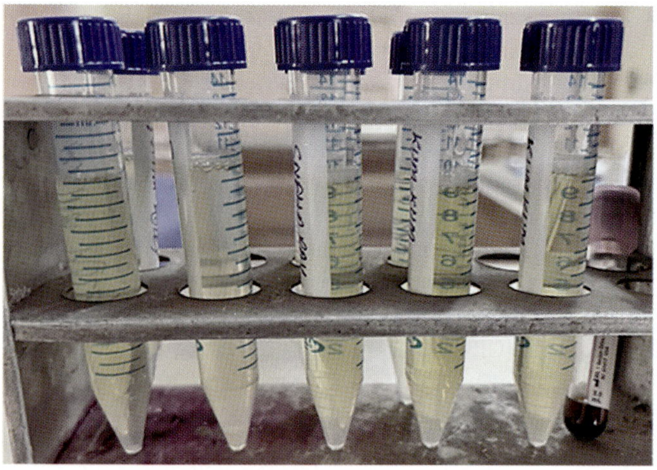

Fig. 3: Sterile plastic capped test tubes containing amniotic fluid sample after amniocentesis.

Quantitative fluorescent-polymerase chain reaction (QF-PCR) for rapid report of chromosomes 13, 18, 21, or 23.

Chromosomal microarray (CMA) for ALL chromosomes: CMA looks at microdeletions or duplications at greater resolution than possible by karyotype alone.

Apart from chromosomal aberrations amniocentesis is also performed for single-gene disorders such as thalassemia/DMD/SMA. Sanger testing/next-generation sequencing (NGS) exome testing/multiplex ligation-dependent probe amplification (MLPA), etc. are the genetic testing methods that can be performed for these genetic aberrations which cannot be picked by CMA.

Risks of Amniocentesis

Risks of amniocentesis are preterm prelabor rupture of the membranes (PPROM), infection, vaginal bleeding, pain, rhesus alloimmunization in Rh-negative pregnancy, mother-to-child transmission (MTCT) of communicable viral infections, and miscarriage (0.1–0.5%).

Miscarriage rates vary in the world literature, depending upon operator skill, gestation age (early gestation <16 weeks has higher miscarriage rate) and presence of fetal abnormality (abnormal fetuses have higher rate of miscarriage). Very rarely, there can be serious complications after amniocentesis. These are lignocaine allergy, chorioamnionitis, maternal sepsis, maternal vessel or gut injury by needle, and direct fetal injury by needle. That is why real-time USG while performing the procedure is extremely important.

Legal Formalities for Amniocentesis

Proper documentation starts with referral letter, USG report, indication for amniocentesis, operator signature, and a declaration that fetal sex will not be disclosed.

Preconception and prenatal diagnostic techniques (PC-PNDT) forms, which are mandatory to be filled up before amniocentesis, are: (1) Form F (for all pregnancy USGs), (2) Form G (for all ultrasonography-guided invasive procedure in pregnancy), and (3) Form E (for all cases where fetal sample is sent to genetic laboratory for testing).

The original forms are to be kept in the center and a copy has to be sent to the PC-PNDT department of the state department of health.

Amniocentesis in Twins

Amniocentesis in twins can be quite challenging. Accurate mapping of the fetuses as twin A and twin B is required. If one of the reports come abnormal, couple may want selective reduction of the abnormal fetus. The fetus close to the cervix or on the left of the mother is by default designated as twin A and the other as twin B. Determination of chorionicity is the next step. In dichorionic diamniotic (DCDA) twins both the sacs need to be sampled, whereas in monochorionic diamniotic (MCDA) twins sampling one of the sacs is usually enough. In twin pregnancy, amniocentesis is preferred over CVS especially when the two placentae are adjacent to each other.

Early amniocentesis: Amniocentesis before 16 weeks is called early amniocentesis. Early amniocentesis is avoided as it has a higher rate of miscarriage (1%). Amniotic fluid sample volume and fetal cells thereof is generally inadequate and there is higher chance of culture failure as well. There is higher false negative rate (due to inadequate DNA) and delay in reporting. Oligohydramnios in ongoing pregnancy and higher incidence of talipes in fetus have been reported.

Late Amniocentesis: In newly diagnosed fetal abnormalities in third trimester sometimes amniocentesis is done. However, there is higher rate of culture failure as the fetal skin becomes keratinized and cell yield is low. There is possibility of maternal blood cell contamination and preterm labor. In India, third trimester MTP is permitted only under judicial discretion.

Chorionic Villus Sampling

Chorionic villus sampling is the procedure of sampling early placental tissue (called chorion) for carrying out various diagnostic tests of the fetus. Around 3–5 mg of chorionic tissue is taken out, depending upon the test required. About 10 mg sample is required, if DNA storage has to be done. Chorion frondosum is the portion from where the sample is taken. Chorion frondosum and adjacent decidua basalis forms the future placenta. It is important to avoid decidua basalis while sampling, so as to avoid maternal cell contamination. The sample taken out consists of fronds of villi which can be seen with naked eye when suspended in normal saline in a petri dish placed over a light source. Cells in these chorionic villi can be subjected to testing by cytogenetics or molecular genetics, as appropriate.

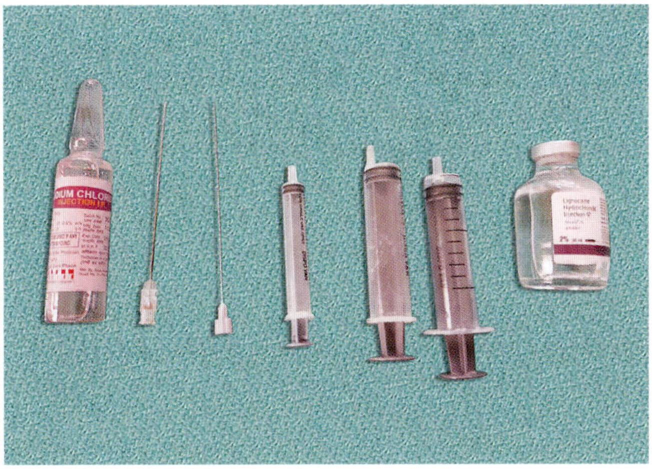

Fig. 4: Trolley set up for chorionic villus sampling (needle, syringe, lignocaine, and normal saline ampoule).

Indications

Indications for chorionic villus sampling are almost similar to that of amniocentesis. CVS can be done from 11 weeks onward and can help in early diagnosis of conditions compared to second-trimester amniocentesis, which is done after 16 weeks. CVS performed after 20 weeks is sometimes called placental biopsy. Essentially CVS and placental biopsy, the same procedure at different gestation ages. Technically CVS is more challenging than amniocentesis and has a steeper learning curve. Chance of decidual contamination is more in early phase of the learning curve. Confined placental mosaicism (1%) is a condition not seen with amniocentesis, but sometimes found in CVS. Confined placental mosaicism is a condition, where chromosomal mosaicism is present in a localized area of chorion frondosum and the fetus does not have this mosaicism. This is rare but possible. In cases where CVS shows mosaicism, sometimes amniocentesis is done to confirm or exclude it, before any clinical decision is taken. In amniocentesis, all cells are of fetal origin, so the possibility of confined placental mosaicism does not arise.

Miscarriage risk of CVS in experienced hands as reported in large studies are similar to amniocentesis (0.1–0.3%).

Counseling for CVS is done almost in the same lines as amniocentesis.

Procedure

Basic USG assessment is performed before CVS. Number of fetuses, chorionicity in multiple pregnancy, fetal heartbeat, location of the chorion frondosum (placenta), subjective amniotic fluid volume, internal os, cervical length, any myomas or ovarian cyst or subchorionic bleed, if any, are documented. Sampling can be done by transabdominal approach (more common) or by transvaginal approach.

Figure 4 shows CVS trolley which includes syringe, needle with stylet, lignocaine, and normal saline ampoule.

Transabdominal Chorionic Villus Sampling

Localizing the chorion is important so that point of entry of the needle can be decided upon. Anteriorly located chorion (placenta) in the upper part of uterus is easiest to sample. Chorion in lower segment is sometimes difficult to approach because of bladder anteriorly. Options are to do such cases by the transvaginal approach, or schedule for amniocentesis later on. When chorion is located at fundus, one has to go through thick myometrium to approach the sampling site and transient uterine cramps are possible. In laterally located chorion, one has to be careful to avoid the uterine vessels and branches.

Cleaning of abdomen is done with Savlon or Betadine. USG probe is covered by encasing it in either sterile powder-free surgical glove or in commercially available sterile probe covers. Contrary to amniocentesis, 2–3 mL of local lignocaine infiltration is a must as a wider bore spinal needle (18G or 20G) is used for CVS. Real-time USG guidance using free-hand technique is commoner than that using a biopsy guide. Following placement of the needle within the placental substance under USG guidance, the stylet is taken out and a 10 mL syringe containing 2–3 mL normal saline or any media (e.g., Ham's F10) is attached to the hub of the needle. Negative suction is created by pulling the plunger of the attached syringe. Chorion sample is obtained by few repeated to-and-fro movements of the needle. At the end of the procedure, the syringe-needle combo is taken out and the fluid inside the needle (containing the villi) is flushed onto a petri dish containing normal saline/media. Postprocedure antibiotics to mother is optional. Mother is usually discharged after 2 hours of bed rest.

Transcervical Chorionic Villus Sampling (Fig. 5)

Preprocedure basic USG assessment is similar to transabdominal route. Bladder is usually kept half full, legs are put up on stirrup in supine position. Vagina is cleaned with povidone-iodine. Vaginal speculum is used to visualize the cervix. Tenaculum is usually not used. Assistant holds the transabdominal USG probe over the suprapubic area. A specially designed olive-tip malleable metal cannula is used for sampling. The vaginal operator mentally maps the placenta as anterior, posterior, right or left lateral, and bends the first few centimeters of the malleable cannula near the tip into a smooth curve in that direction. The cannula is then inserted through external os, till the tip can be seen on USG screen. The tip is then further inserted under USG guidance into the placental substance **(Fig. 6)**. Sampling is done as in transabdominal technique by few to-and-fro motion with negative suction. Processing of the sample is same as in transabdominal technique. Postprocedure antibiotics is operator's preference.

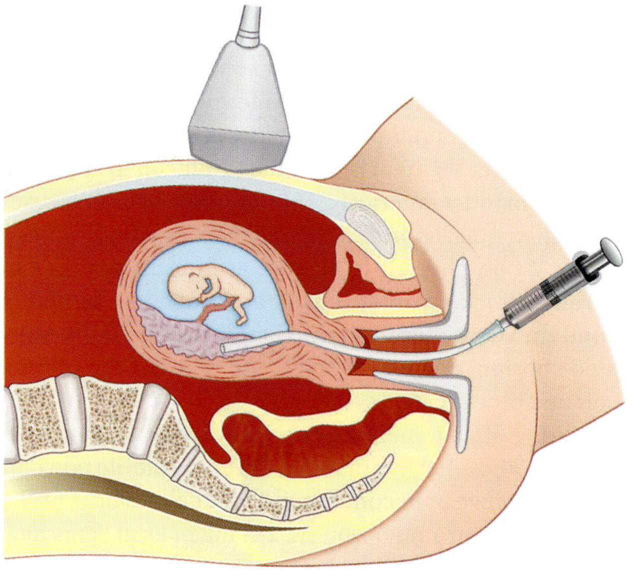

Fig. 5: Transcervical chorionic villus sampling.

Transvaginal technique may not be preferred by all patients. The rate of postprocedure vaginal spotting is slightly more compared to transabdominal method; however, the miscarriage rates are similar. Transvaginal method is especially suitable when placenta is low lying. Quantity of chorion tissue obtained is more compared to transabdominal method and uterine cramping is less. Transcervical method is not suitable for placentae situated in upper segment. Chance of multiple insertions is more common in transcervical method to obtain adequate sample. The choice of technique mostly depends upon operator's preference and patient choice.

Processing of the Sample

The fluid flushed from the aspiration syringe into the petri dish contain aspirated chorion sample. The petri dish is placed over a light source and fronds of villi can be seen floating within the flushed fluid in the petri dish **(Fig. 7)**. The villi are picked up under naked eyes with the help of a small nontooth forceps and transferred into a 10 mL gamma sterilized plastic tube with screw caps. The test tubes have transport media to prevent degradation of DNA. Individualized identification code of sample is ensured. Bar coding is mandatory to avoid mixing up of samples. Ideally, sample needs to be transported to genetic laboratory within 24 hours.

Tests that can be done from CVS sample are similar to that of amniocentesis.

Complications of Chorionic Villus Sampling

Complications of CVS are vaginal bleeding, subchorionic hematoma, uterine cramping, infection, rhesus alloimmunization in Rh-negative pregnancy, MTCT of communicable viral infections, and fetal limb reduction defects, if done before 10 weeks. It affects fingers or toes.

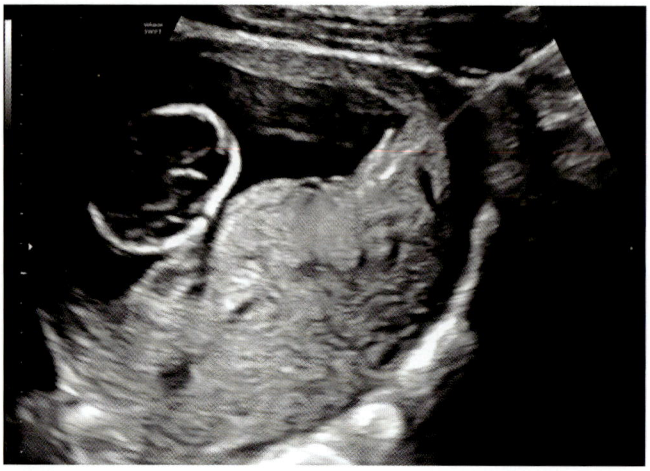

Fig. 6: An 18-gauge spinal needle in placental tissue during the procedure of chorionic villi sampling under ultrasound guidance.

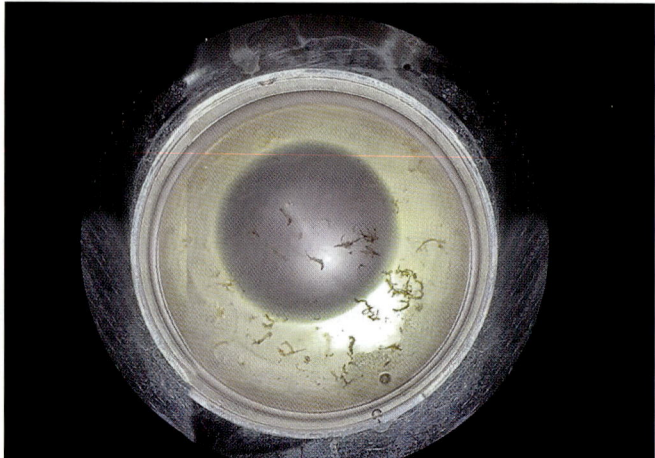

Fig. 7: Chorionic villi as seen in naked eye in a petri dish containing normal saline following aspiration by chorionic villus sampling.

Few cases of oromandibular hypoplasia have been reported but the association is not clear. Miscarriage rate is 0.1–0.5%. Miscarriage rates vary in the world literature, depending upon operator skill (0.3–0.5%).

Serious complications are rare. These are lignocaine allergy, chorioamnionitis, maternal sepsis, maternal vessel or gut injury by needle, or direct fetal injury by needle. That is why real-time USG while performing the procedure is extremely important.

Legal formalities for CVS are similar to that of amniocentesis.

Chorionic Villus Sampling in Twins

In MCDA twins, there is single placental mass with T-sign. In such cases, one sampling is enough because both the fetuses are genetically same (except in very rare cases).

In DCDA twins, where the placental masses are separate, sampling of both the placentae are necessary by two different entries using separate set of needle and syringe. The challenge is in DCDA twins with adjacent placenta masquerading as a single placental mass. It is difficult to decide where one placenta ends and the other starts. Performing CVS in such cases is not advisable, and patients are usually counseled for twin amniocentesis after 16 weeks.

CORDOCENTESIS

Cordocentesis is a needle procedure, whereby a sample of fetal blood is taken from the umbilical vein of the fetus under real-time USG guidance. Cordocentesis is also known as PUBS (percutaneous umbilical blood sampling). Cordocentesis just for diagnostic purpose is going out of fashion, as most fetal diagnostic tests can be done much earlier by CVS or amniocentesis. Furthermore, CVS and amniocentesis are easier to perform and also has less procedure-related miscarriage rate compared to cordocentesis. In current obstetric practice, cordocentesis is mostly performed as a step leading to fetal therapy in the same sitting.

Indications

Cordocentesis is mostly done after 24 weeks of gestation. Indications for cordocentesis are:

- Assessment of fetal anemia in rhesus alloimmunized pregnancy.
- History suggestive of perinatal infections: TORCH, parvovirus, varicella, etc.
- Chromosomal and genetic testing (rare)
- Injecting agents for fetal therapy (e.g., fetal arrhythmias, stem cell transplant).

The most common indication for diagnostic cordocentesis is rhesus incompatibility. Cordocentesis, purely for diagnostic purpose, was previously used to measure fetal hemoglobin and hematocrit to decide whether the fetus needed blood transfusion or not. Cordocentesis is an invasive test with potential miscarriage rate (1%). Hence, diagnostic cordocentesis for assessment of fetal anemia has been replaced by noninvasive measurement of middle cerebral artery (MCA)-peak systolic velocity (PSV) by color Doppler.

Currently, diagnostic cordocentesis is done as a first step to measure fetal hematocrit before fetal blood transfusion (FBT), to decide the "volume" of blood transfusion needed. The requisite blood volume is then transfused in the same sitting through the same cordocentesis needle. After FBT is complete, a further sample of fetal blood is drawn through the same needle to assess the post-transfusion hemoglobin and hematocrit.

Diagnostic cordocentesis is also done in suspected cases of perinatal infections in the mother to confirm fetal infection, if any. Placental infection may not be associated with fetal infection. Hence, positive PCR for TORCH and other infections in fetal blood are more specific than positive PCR in CVS or amniotic fluid sample.

Counseling

Before taking consent for cordocentesis, proper counseling is important. Counseling has to focus on why the procedure is necessary, how it will be done, potential complications, and alternative options, if any. Emergency contact number needs to be given to the patient in case there is any subsequent bleeding, leaking, or pain in abdomen.

Procedure

The procedure is discussed under the heading of fetal blood transfusion later on in this chapter. **Figure 8** shows sonographic-guided introduction of needle within umbilical vein. HemoCue apparatus (portable hemoglobinometer) is used for testing hematocrit in the fetus.

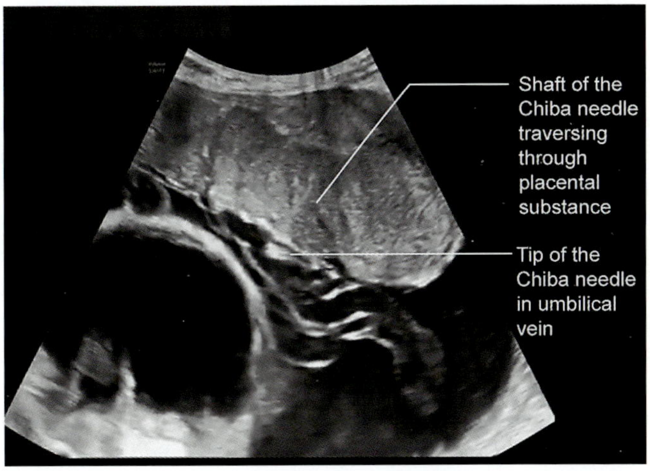

Fig. 8: Cordocentesis: Chiba needle entering the umbilical vein under ultrasound guidance.

Processing of the Sample

When cordocentesis is performed for perinatal infections or for genetic testing, the blood sample is transferred to ethylenediamine tetraacetic acid (EDTA) tube and transported to the laboratory. 2–5 mL of blood is usually sufficient.

Risks of Cordocentesis

Potential complications of cordocentesis are PROM, vaginal bleeding, pain, fetal exsanguination from cord puncture site, chorioamnionitis, rhesus alloimmunization in Rh-negative pregnancy, and MTCT of communicable viral infections. Miscarriage (1%) is operator dependent and depends upon sampling site and less common with anterior placenta. Echogenic bowel of fetus is due to swallowed blood in amniotic fluid in case, there is leakage of fetal blood from puncture site into the amniotic sac.

Legal Formalities for Cordocentesis

Same as for other invasive fetal interventions. Specific license for cordocentesis is required.

OTHER INVASIVE DIAGNOSTIC PROCEDURES

Other invasive diagnostic procedures are:
- Coelocentesis (abandoned)
- Fetal skin biopsy and fetal muscle biopsy (rare)
- Fetal pleural effusion fluid sampling (for CMA and TORCH)
- Fetal urine sampling before vesicoamniotic (VA) shunting.

FETAL THERAPEUTIC PROCEDURES

Multifetal Pregnancy Reduction

With the advent of assisted reproductive technologies (ART), multiple pregnancy, especially higher order multiple pregnancy (triplets or more), is on the rise. Multifetal pregnancy reduction (MFPR) is the procedure by which higher order multifetal pregnancy (HOMP) is reduced to twins. Sometimes reduction is done from twins to singleton. The aim is to sacrifice one or two fetuses to increase the salvageability of the remaining fetuses. Selective reduction is usually referred to reduction of an abnormal fetus in multiple pregnancy. MFPR can be done abdominally or by transvaginal route. Most common substance used is intracardiac potassium chloride (KCl) to achieve cardiac asystole in the target fetus. Fetal intracardiac lignocaine has also been used. Gas embolism by injecting intracardiac air into fetal heart is associated with high rate of failure and has been largely abandoned. Fetal reduction in monochorionic (MC) pregnancy cannot be done by these substances, as there is vascular connection between MC fetuses. Radiofrequency ablation, interstitial laser photocoagulation, or bipolar cord occlusion techniques are used for reduction in MC pregnancy.

Indications

Indications for MFPR are:
- HOMP: Triplets or more
- Twins to singleton (maternal request)
- Selective reduction of abnormal fetus on USG
- Selective reduction after discordant genetic report (Down syndrome, thalassemia, monogenic diseases)
- Reduction in complicated MC pregnancy.

Why Multifetal Pregnancy Reduction?

Higher order multifetal pregnancy is associated with disproportionate maternal and perinatal complications. Miscarriage, fetal anomaly, stillbirth, and preterm delivery in pregnancy with triplets are more than three times compared to pregnancy with single fetus. In HOMP infants, cerebral palsy and neurodevelopmental delay are significantly higher. Maternal complications like abdominal discomfort, shortness of breath, gestational diabetes mellitus (GDM), severe preeclampsia, antepartum hemorrhage (APH), postpartum hemorrhage (PPH), and maternal mortality are significantly more. Reduction of these complications are achieved by MFPR. Studies have however shown that perinatal morbidity of spontaneous twin pregnancy is less than triplets reduced to twins. The procedure-related miscarriage rate of MFPR is around 5% and is justified in HOMP.

Multifetal Pregnancy Reduction from Twins to Singleton

Multifetal pregnancy reduction from twin to singleton is debatable. Most studies have not found statistical difference in take-home baby rate between reduced and unreduced twin pregnancy. The advantages of twin reduction, namely late miscarriage, prematurity, and maternal complications, are balanced by procedure-related miscarriage rate (5%) of twin MFPR. Couple may request twin reduction due to financial reasons of bringing up two babies, or they may already be having one previous baby. Preprocedure counseling of such couple regarding pros and cons of twin MFPR is important.

Procedure

Trolley setup for MFPR is shown in **Figure 9**.

Selection of the Target Fetus

Selection of the target fetus is important. A thorough USG is done to assess early fetal anatomy. The target fetus is selected based on multiple parameters. CRL length, presence of any anomaly, and approachability are the important ones. The fetus with the smallest CRL or the one with an abnormality is chosen. The parameters may always not concur, for example, the fetus with the smallest CRL may be in a location where approach is difficult. So, individualization is important.

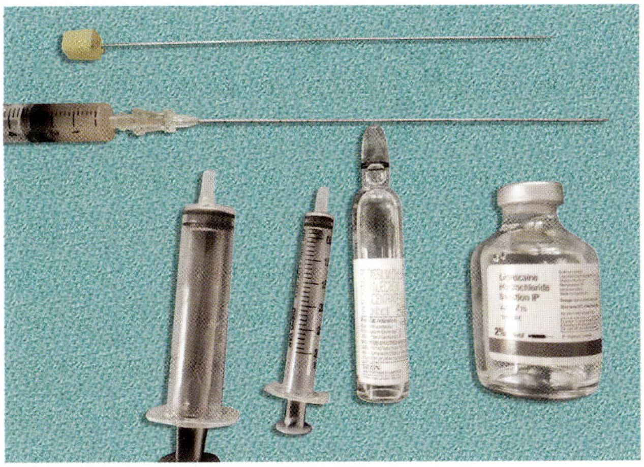

Fig. 9: Trolley set up for selective fetal reduction.

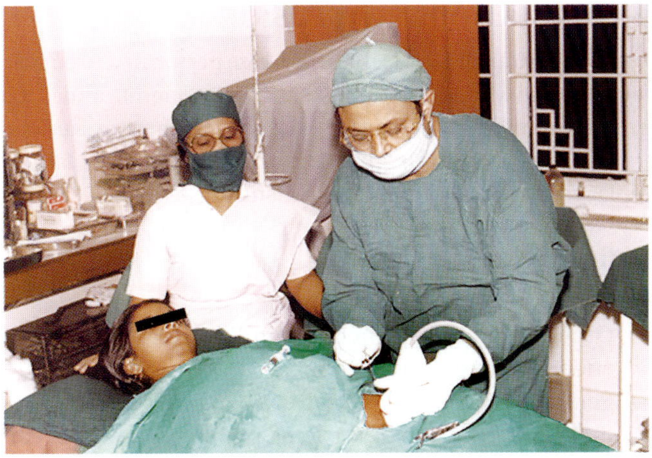

Fig. 10: Selective fetal reduction (transabdominal route) under ultrasound guidance.

Transabdominal Multifetal Pregnancy Reduction

Transabdominal MFPR is usually done between 11 and 13 weeks. **Figure 10** shows approach of selective fetal reduction (transabdominal route) under USG guidance. A thorough USG examination of all the fetuses is done to rule out obvious anomaly. Nuchal translucency (NT) is measured. Some operators wait for first-trimester screening report of Down syndrome before performing MFPR. The fetus near the internal os is avoided as there is higher chance of miscarriage. The point of entry is then selected, so that the needle does not pass-through other sacs. The sides of the uterus are avoided for the uterine vessels; fundal entry cause more cramps. Entry near midline is usually attempted. After antiseptic dressing and draping of maternal abdomen, local lignocaine injection is given. 20G or 22G spinal needle is used and after intracardiac placement of the tip, 1–2 mL of KCl is injected under USG guidance **(Fig. 11)**. The needle is taken out after ensuring cardiac asystole. Antibiotic injection antibiotic is usually given; injection anti-D is given to rhesus negative women. These women are discharged same day.

Transvaginal Multifetal Pregnancy Reduction

Here a transvaginal USG probe is used. Trans-forniceal needle entry is achieved with a biopsy guide. The entry is almost similar to oocyte pickup in in vitro fertilization (IVF). The needle is usually passed into the lower sac as this approach is easier in transvaginal route (contrary to transabdominal method where the lower sac can be avoided). Transvaginal MFPR is usually done around 10 weeks or even earlier. The earlier it is done, more is the chance of missing anomalies. Furthermore, autoreduction can sometimes occur in earlier gestation. So, most fetal medicine centers prefer to wait up to 11–12 weeks before attempting MFPR. IVF specialists usually tend to do at earlier gestation through transvaginal method, since the procedure is similar to oocyte retrieval.

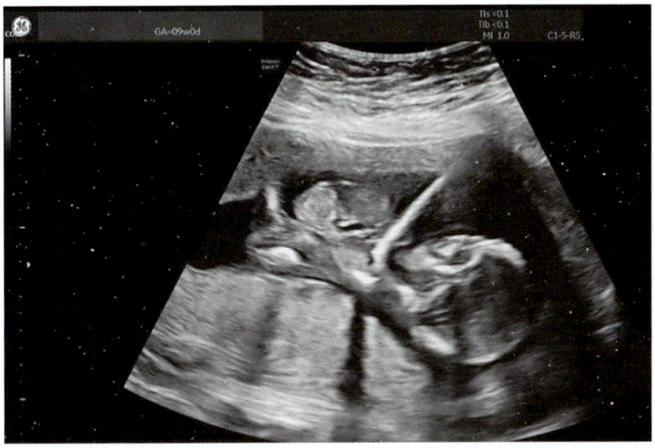

Fig. 11: Dichorionic diamniotic pregnancy: Intracardiac injection of potassium chloride through 20G spinal needle during selective fetal reduction of the fetus with exomphalos.

NB: In transvaginal CVS, the needle entry is transcervical through external and internal os.

Risks of Multifetal Pregnancy Reduction

Risks are uterine cramping, infection, injury to uterine vessels, failure (may have to be repeated), rhesus alloimmunization in Rh-negative pregnancy, and MTCT of communicable viral infections. Average miscarriage is 0.1–0.5%, may be as high as 5%.

Complications are high after 14 weeks.

Legal Formalities for Multifetal Pregnancy Reduction

The legal formalities are same as in other fetal invasive procedures. MFPR is not considered MTP, as the pregnancy as such is not terminated.

FETAL BLOOD TRANSFUSION

Fetal blood transfusion is the procedure performed to correct fetal anemia when the fetus has significant anemia and is too premature to be delivered. Previously intraperitoneal fetal transfusion used to be given, but now it has been largely replaced by intravascular fetal transfusion.

Indications

- Rhesus alloimmunized pregnancy
- Other blood group incompatibilities leading to fetal anemia (K and L blood groups)
- Perinatal infections (parvovirus)
- Platelet transfusion in the fetus [immune thrombocytopenic purpura (ITP) of mother].

The most common indication for FBT is rhesus incompatibility. When a rhesus negative mother develops rhesus antibodies, she becomes indirect Coombs test (ICT) positive, and is said to be alloimmunized. If the fetus is rhesus positive, there is a risk of hemolytic anemia in the fetus. Severity of alloimmunization is assessed by determining severity of fetal anemia. Currently, assessment of fetal anemia is by noninvasive measurement of MCA-PSV by color Doppler. When MCA-PSV multiples of the median (MoM) value is >1.5 for a particular gestation, the fetus has significant anemia. If prematurity precludes early delivery, the fetus is given in utero blood transfusion.

Portable hemoglobinometer **(Fig. 12)** is used for testing pretransfusion and post-transfusion hematocrit in the fetus.

Counseling

Counseling has to focus on the indication as to why FBT is needed. Option of early premature delivery in a center with neonatal intensive care unit (NICU) facility versus intrauterine FBT as an attempt to prolong gestation has to be discussed. The total procedure takes time and the mother has to lie supine, in left lateral position for 20–30 minutes. All preparations are made in the operation theater (OT) before the mother is asked to lie on the table. Potential complications are discussed and emergency contact number needs to be given to the patient in case there is any subsequent bleeding, leaking, or pain in abdomen. Some patients may like to have video recording of the procedure.

Procedure

A trolley containing injection atracurium is made ready **(Fig. 13)**.

Basic USG assessment is performed before FBT. Estimated fetal weight and MCA-PSV are measured. Both are needed to calculate the blood volume to be transfused. FBT is given with O-negative packed cell (hematocrit >85%) **(Fig. 14)**. The donor blood is irradiated (to prevent graft-versus-host reaction), relatively fresh (collected within last 7 days) and has to be cytomegalovirus (CMV) negative. Umbilical vein is usually sampled at placental insertion site. Placental-site cordocentesis is easier with anterior or lateral placenta wherein the needle goes through the placental substance toward the cord insertion site. In posterior placenta cordocentesis, needle has to go transamniotic to reach the cord insertion. The alternative is to do FBT into the intrahepatic segment of the umbilical vein soon after it enters fetal liver. For such FBT in posterior placenta, fetal paralysis is required. Fetal paralysis is usually done by injection artacurium 0.1 mg/kg body weight of the fetus. 22G spinal needle is used for fetal paralysis, artacurium is injected into the gluteal or the thigh muscle of the fetus, and the needle is taken out. Paralysis takes 5–10 minutes. During that time, the blood bag is attached to a blood transfusion set, which is connected to a three-way tap.

Local infiltration is done with 2–3 mL 2% lignocaine. 15 cm long 20G (or 22G) cordocentesis needle is used. A needle is advanced using free-hand technique under real-time USG guidance **(Figs. 15 and 16)**. The needle is

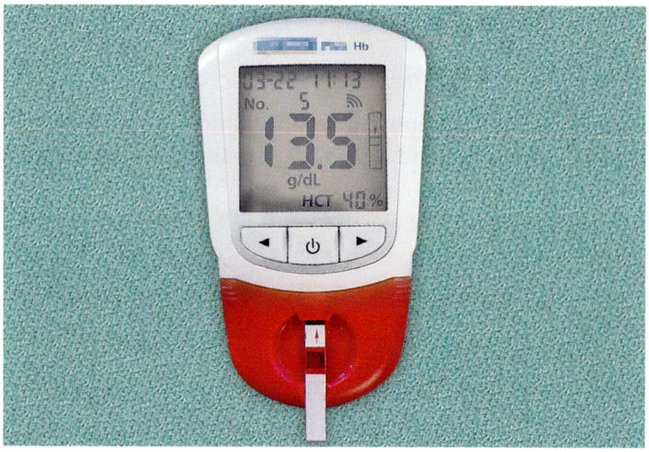

Fig. 12: Portable hemoglobinometer used for testing pretransfusion and post-transfusion hematocrit in the fetus.

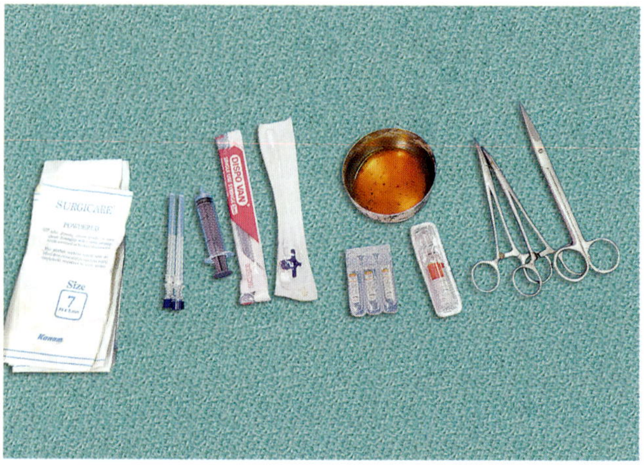

Fig. 13: *Fetal blood transfusion:* Trolley set up with injection atracurium.

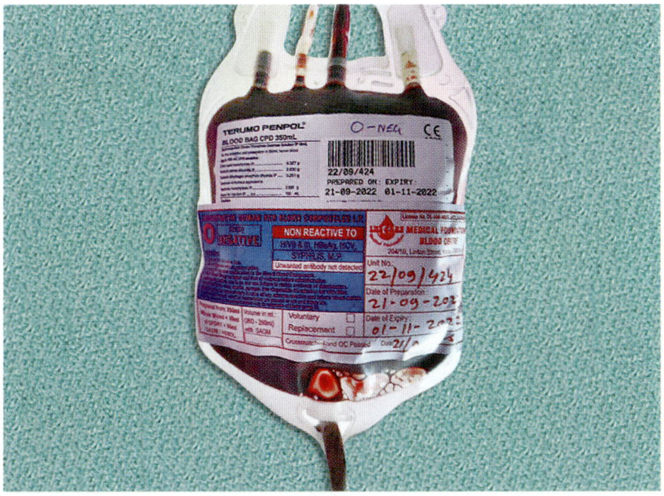

Fig. 14: O-negative irradiated leukodepleted plasma reduced blood unit for fetal transfusion.

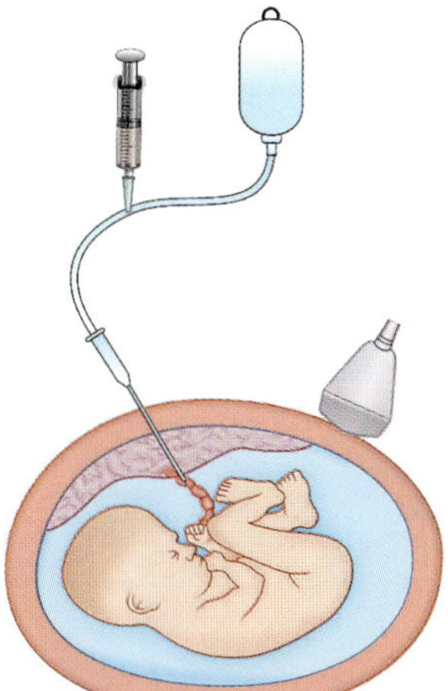

Fig. 15: Intrauterine transfusion.

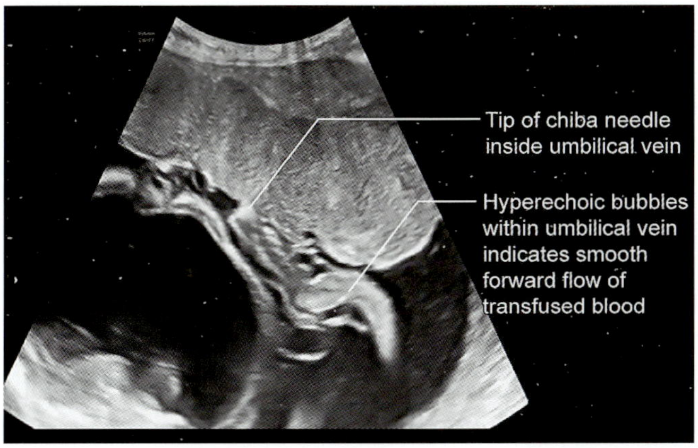

Fig. 16: 20-gauge Chiba needle inside the umbilical vein under ultrasound guidance during intrauterine blood transfusion in a case with anterior placenta.

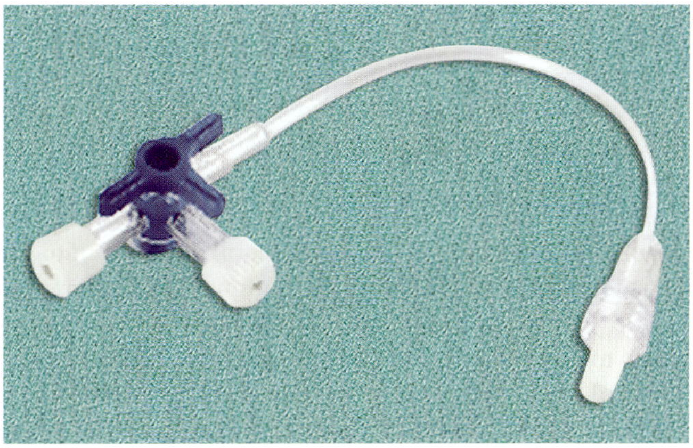

Fig. 17: Three-way cannula used in intrauterine transfusion.

echo-tipped and has echogenic markings over the shaft at 1 cm intervals. This makes the needle visible on USG examination. Desired needle placement inside umbilical vein is confirmed by flushing with normal saline and visualization of microbubble flow on 2D USG. 2 mL heparinized syringe is used to draw blood sample. Immediate hemoglobin and hematocrit measurement is possible by hand-held HemoCue apparatus. Volume of blood to be transfused is calculated using online formula available at perinatology.com. The parameters required are estimated fetal weight, pretransfusion fetal hematocrit, and hematocrit of the donor blood.

One end of the three-way tap **(Fig. 17)** is connected to the hub of the cordocentesis needle. A 10 mL disposable syringe **(Fig. 18)** is attached to the third tap. The syringe is used to draw blood from the bag and push it through the cordocentesis needle using the taps appropriately.

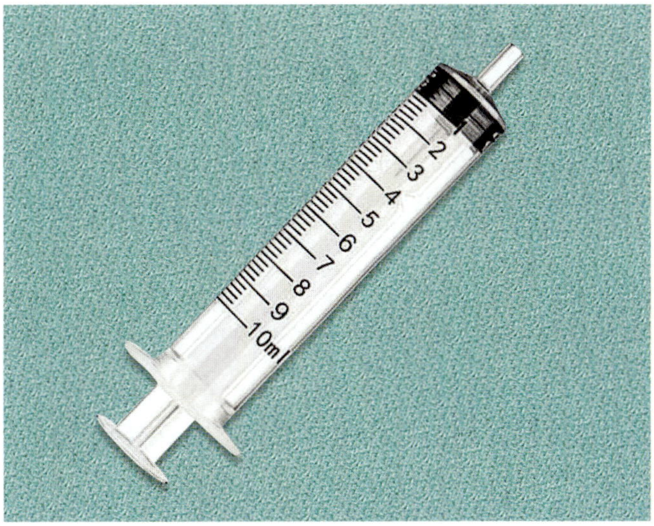

Fig. 18: 10 mL disposable syringe.

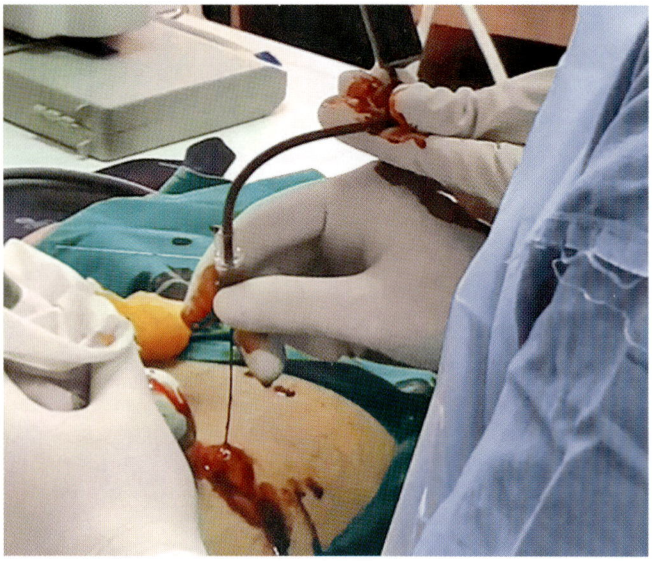

Fig. 19: Procedure of intrauterine fetal transfusion in a case of fetal anemia in Rh-negative pregnancy.

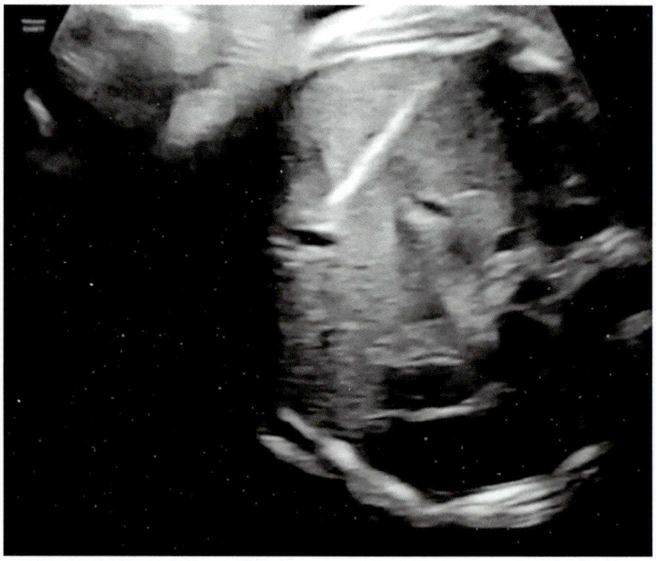

Fig. 20: Chiba needle entering the intra-abdominal umbilical vein under ultrasound guidance during intrauterine blood transfusion in a case of posterior placenta where cord insertion site is not approachable.

Procedure of intrauterine fetal transfusion in a case of fetal anemia in Rh-negative pregnancy is shown in **Figure 19**.

Requisite volume of FBT is completed and postprocedure blood sample is drawn for hemoglobin and hematocrit measurement. Post-FBT documentation of fetal heart rate and MCA-PSV is important. Sometimes, Chiba needle needs to enter the intra-abdominal umbilical vein under USG guidance during intrauterine blood transfusion, in case of posterior placenta where cord insertion site is not approachable **(Fig. 20)**.

Risks of Fetal Blood Transfusion

The risks of fetal blood transfusion are that of cordocentesis. However, complications rise with duration of transfusion, amount of blood transfused, and whether multiple entries were needed or not. Miscarriage rate (3–5%) is operator dependent and depends upon sampling site and less common with anterior placenta.

Preterm prelabor rupture of the membranes, fetal exsanguination from cord puncture site, and chorioamnionitis are more common than PUBS.

Echogenic bowel of fetus may occur few weeks after FBT. This is due to swallowed blood in amniotic fluid, in case there is leakage of fetal blood from puncture site into the amniotic sac.

Legal Formalities for Fetal Blood Transfusion

Same as for other fetal invasive procedures. License for cordocentesis must be there. Facility for inpatient admission and emergency care facility should be there. Consent for emergency operation should be taken in case of complications. PC-PNDT forms F and G are signed.

PROCEDURES IN COMPLICATED MONOCHORIONIC MULTIPLE PREGNANCY

Laser Photocoagulation in Twin-to-Twin Transfusion Syndrome

Twin-to-twin transfusion syndrome (TTTS) (or feto-fetal transfusion syndrome) is a complication seen in MC twin pregnancy, due to chronic unbalanced circulation from one fetus to the other through vascular connections in the shared placenta. It occurs in around 10–15% of MC twins. This results in hemodynamic overload of the recipient twin and exsanguination of the donor twin. The recipient twin develops hypervolemia, hyperdynamic circulation, polyhydramnios, polycythemia, macrosomia, and signs of cardiac overload evident on Doppler examination. The donor twin develops hypovolemia, fetal growth restriction (FGR), oligohydramnios, small urinary bladder volume [low glomerular filtration rate (GFR)], and fetal hypoxia evident on Doppler examination. The vascular anastomotic channels can be arteriovenous, venoarterial, arterioarterial, or venovenous. The latter two are usually present on the surface of the placenta and are bidirectional. The other two dip from the surface into the cotyledon, anastomose within the placental substance, are unidirectional and are the culprits. These dipping vessels are photocoagulated before they dip and become invisible.

Quintero has classified TTTS into four stages. Fetal intervention becomes necessary when fetuses cannot be delivered due to extreme prematurity and stage II has been reached. Previously, serial amnioreduction of the polydramniotic sac used to be done to balance pressure between the two sacs and reduce respiratory distress of the mother with the aim of prolonging the pregnancy. The actual pathology of vascular anastomosis is, however, not addressed by this management. The perinatal results were not satisfactory. Serial amnioreduction has largely been replaced by laser photocoagulation of the intertwin vascular anastomotic channels through a fetoscope.

Indications

Indications for laser photocoagulation are:

- MC twins
- TTTS
- Premature fetuses 18–28 weeks
- Quintero stage II or above.

Counseling

Counseling regarding choice between antenatal laser photocoagulation and premature delivery in a center with NICU facility is to be discussed. Procedure-related miscarriage, PPROM, and premature labor (10–15%) need to be mentioned. Operator expertise is very important. The donor twin (hypoxic) usually has poorer survival, especially when it becomes stuck-twin, due to severe oligohydramnios. Studies show stuck-twins have more neurological problems in childhood, probably related to brain ischemia. When the recipient twin develops evidence of cardiac compromise/cardiomegaly, it has poorer prognosis. Laser photocoagulation is usually done under local infiltration anesthesia as daycare procedure, however, facility for inpatient admission should be available. Emergency contact number needs to be given to the patient, in case there is any subsequent bleeding, leaking, or pain in abdomen.

Procedure

Laser photocoagulation is done through fetoscope **(Fig. 21)** under USG guidance. The entry is into the recipient sac. It is relatively easy to do when placenta is posterior as the fetal surface of the placenta can be visualized directly through a straight fetoscope. With anterior placenta, curved scope has to be used, and is challenging. The telescope is 3 mm in diameter with a side channel through which the laser fiber is passed. The assembly is passed through the maternal abdomen and into the amniotic cavity through a 3.5 mm trocar under USG guidance by direct trocar entry or by the Seldringer technique. The laser can be diode laser or Nd: YAG laser with a wavelength of 400–600 µm. The vascular equator is identified. This is few cm away from where the intertwin membrane is inserted on the placental surface. The vascular equator can be seen on the placental surface of the recipient sac. The anastomotic channels on the placental surface are identified. The red dot of the laser light is focused

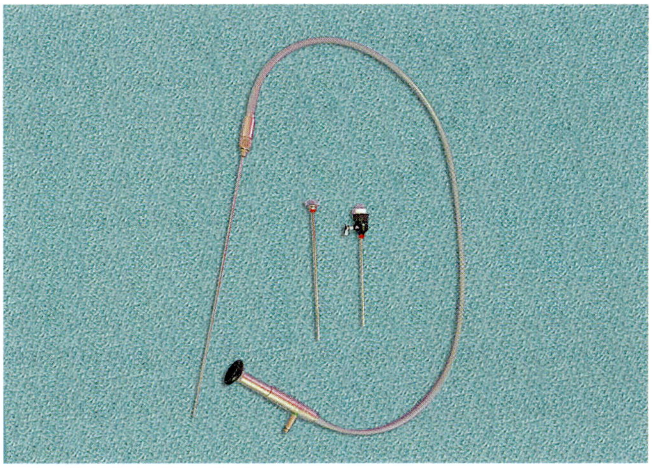

Fig. 21: Fetoscope sheath with lens attachment with insertion trocar and cannula.

on a vessel and the laser foot pedal is activated for few seconds. The vessel is coagulated and become white. All the anastomotic channels are dealt with one by one. Any leftover smaller unidentified anastomosis may lead to subsequent TAPS (twin anemia polycythemia sequence). Therefore, the surface of the placenta connecting the coagulated vessels is also photocoagulated as there can be smaller anastomotic vessels there. This is called Solomon technique. TAPS can only be diagnosed by MCA-PSV Doppler study as the oligopoly sequence disappears after laser treatment of TTTS. That is why follow-up Doppler study is essential after laser photocoagulation.

Risks of Laser Photocoagulation

Apart from the complications common for all fetal invasive procedures, the following deserve special mention.

These are PPROM, preterm labor (10–15%), subsequent development of TAPS, intra-amniotic bleed, and laser burn to fetus. Operator expertise is very important.

Legal Formalities for Laser Photocoagulation

Legal formalities are same as for other fetal invasive procedures. License for fetoscopy must be there.

FETAL REDUCTION IN COMPLICATED MONOCHORIONIC PREGNANCY

Indications of fetal reduction in MC multiple pregnancy:

- Twin reversed arterial perfusion (TRAP) syndrome
- One fetus abnormal in MC twins
- Higher order MC pregnancy.

Principle of Interstitial Fetal Reduction

In dichorionic twins, fetal reduction of the target fetus is done by intracardiac KCl injection under USG guidance as has been discussed before. In MC twins, this procedure cannot be used as there are vascular communications between the placentae and KCl can readily pass to the other fetus. For fetal reduction in MC twins, vascular coagulation of feeding vessels of the target fetus is done by interstitial vascular coagulation "within" the body of the target fetus. These interstitial procedures are performed through needles under USG guidance where fetoscope is not required. This is different from photocoagulation of communicating vessels in TTTS.

Vascular occlusion is achieved by thermal effect. The principle is similar to that of diathermy used in open or endoscopic surgery. The controlled heat generated coagulates the proteins of the vascular wall and occludes the blood flow. Occlusion of feeding vessels lead to hypoxia of the target fetus and eventual asystole after some time. Interstitial vascular occlusion of the target fetus can be done by using laser (interstitial laser photocoagulation), or by using radiofrequency (radio frequency ablation or RFA) **(Figs. 22 to 24)**.

In TRAP syndrome, the acardiac fetus is subjected to interstitial laser or RFA **(Fig. 25)**. Laser console is used in fetal therapy (for vascular occlusion in TTTS or for interstitial photocoagulation for fetal reduction in MC twins) **(Fig. 26)**.

Figure 27 shows sonographic monitoring of laser fiber just below insertion of umbilical cord.

Figure 28 shows the team performing interstitial laser for fetal reduction.

Principle of Bipolar Cord Occlusion

This is a method of selective reduction in MC twins, where a loop of umbilical cord is held within the prongs of a bipolar forceps and vascular occlusion of umbilical vessels is achieved by using bipolar thermal forceps. This is not interstitial coagulation as the coagulation occurs "outside" the fetal body. Specially designed bipolar needle forceps is used under USG guidance to hold a loop of umbilical cord of the target fetus. This is a needle procedure and fetoscope is not necessary.

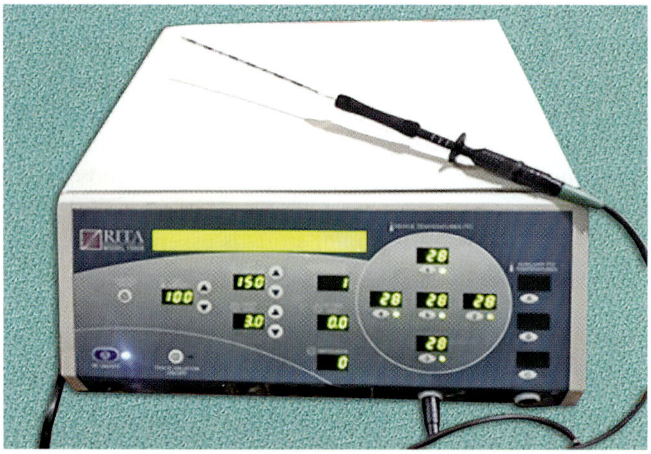

Fig. 22: Radiofrequency ablation system used for selective fetal reduction in monochorionic multifetal gestation.

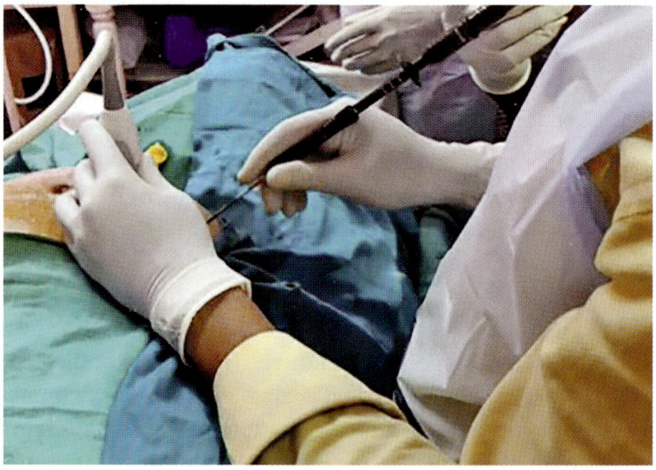

Fig. 24: Needle electrode of radiofrequency ablation system in selective fetal reduction in monochorionic multifetal gestation.

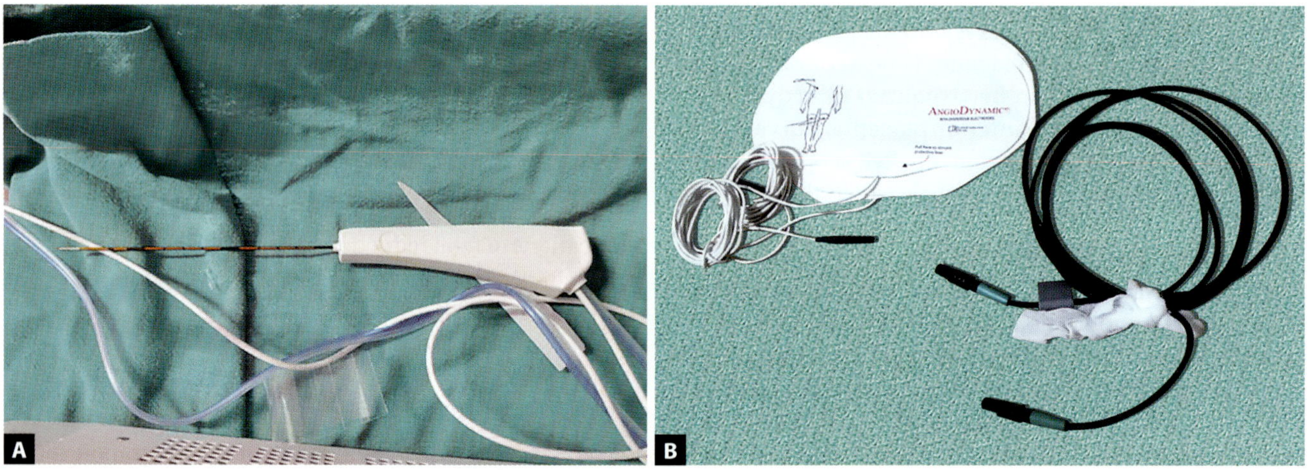

Figs. 23A and B: (A) Radiofrequency needle electrode used to coagulate umbilical of fetus to be reduced in selective fetal reduction in monochorionic twins; (B) Patient pad (elctrode) and connecting cord of the RFA system.

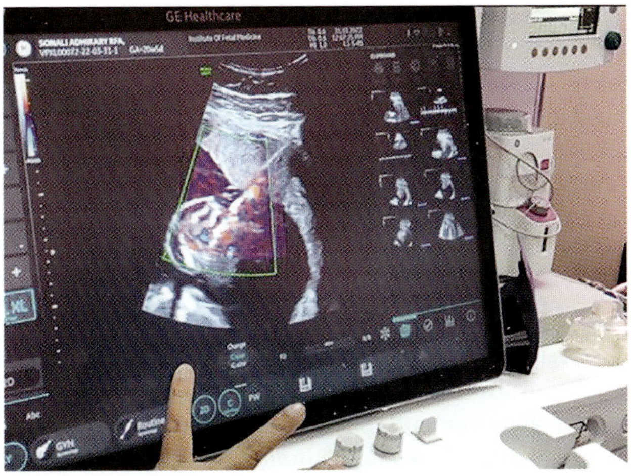

Fig. 25: Radiofrequency ablation of acardiac fetus in twin reversed arterial perfusion syndrome.

FETAL SHUNT PROCEDURES

Fetal shunts are temporary procedures to drain fluid from fetal hollow organs (urinary bladder or pleural cavity) to relieve pressure effect on vital organs (kidneys or lungs, respectively).

Vesicoamniotic Shunt

Vesicoamniotic shunt procedure is done for LUTO (lower urinary tract obstruction) of the fetus. This is a temporary procedure done to drain the overfilled bladder into the amniotic cavity through a double-pigtail catheter. VA shunting is done under USG guidance whereby one end of the shunt is placed within the urinary bladder and the other end in the amniotic cavity. The purpose of VA shunt is to relieve secondary backpressure on fetal kidneys due to LUTO of the fetus.

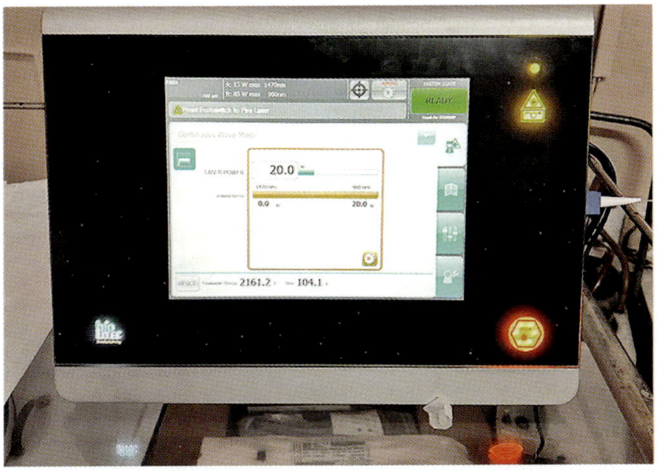

Fig. 26: Laser console used in fetal therapy (for vascular occlusion in twin-to-twin transfusion syndrome or for interstitial photocoagulation for fetal reduction in monochorionic twins).

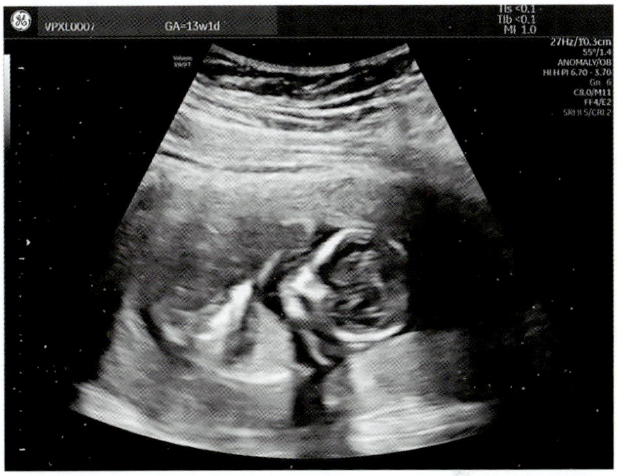

Fig. 27: Sonography shows laser fiber just below insertion of umbilical cord.

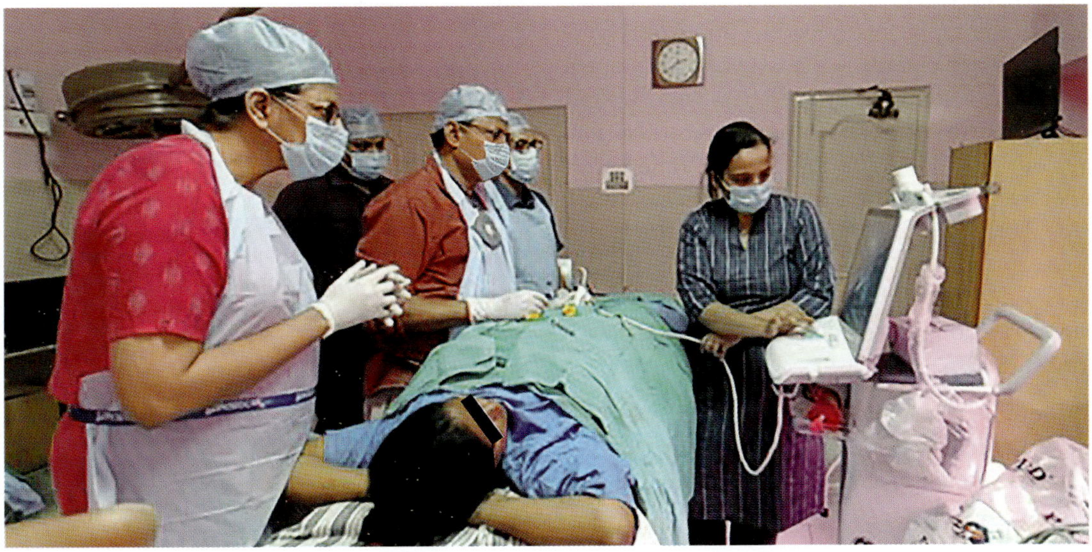

Fig. 28: Interstitial laser in a case of fetal reduction in dichorionic triplets. 15 cm 18G needle has been placed near the converging umbilical arteries of one of the monochorionic fetuses before they come out of the umbilicus of the fetus.

Indications

Indications for VA shunting are:

- Confirmed LUTO of fetus
- *Exclude irreversible backpressure effect on fetal kidneys:* Bilateral multicystic dysplastic kidneys/thin renal cortex/ severe hydroureteronephrosis
- *Exclude other structural anomalies:* Cloacal and lower gut, cardiac
- *Exclude genetic anomalies:* CMA.

The first suspicion of LUTO is dilated urinary bladder of the fetus (megacystis). Posterior urethral valve is more common in male fetuses, whereas urethral atresia occurs in both. Urethral atresia is usually associated with cloacal abnormalities and in such cases prognosis is poor. Bilateral hydroureteronephrosis due to backpressure effect is a constant finding. Absence of fetal urinary drainage results in oligohydramnios/anhydramnios and if not relieved, results in secondary pulmonary hypoplasia and talipes deformities of the fetus. Once LUTO is diagnosed other fetal anomalies need to be excluded. Amnioinfusion is sometimes necessary to improve the acoustic window for optimum scanning. Irreversible secondary renal dysplasia due to backpressure is excluded by sampling the fetal urine (vesicocentesis) and doing urinary biochemistry. Abnormal urine biochemistry has poor prognosis. Fetal chromosomal anomaly is excluded by performing placental biopsy and performing CMA. It is difficult to do amniocentesis in LUTO, due to associated severe oligohydramnios and hence placental biopsy is done.

Counseling

Patients need to be explained that VA shunting is purely a temporary procedure and definitive treatment will be required after birth. Backpressure effect on the kidneys cannot be reversed, however further damage may be halted. Possibility of shunt coming out of the bladder due to fetal body movement and arm movements is a possibility, and repeat shunting may be necessary. Option to discuss with support groups is mentioned in case the couple cannot take a decision. Option to opt out has also to be mentioned. Emergency contact number needs to be given to the patient in case there is any subsequent bleeding, leaking, or pain in abdomen.

Procedure

Fetal shunting can be done as a single procedure or as a two-step procedure.

First step: Thorough counseling, amnioinfusion, detailed fetal anomaly scan, fetal echocardiography, CMA/ karyotyping by placental biopsy, and urinary biochemistry by vesicocentesis.

Second step: Shunt placement is done after the reports are available. Harrison double-pigtail shunt is placed with the help of the shunt introducer under USG guidance. The whole assembly comes in a gamma sterilized disposable packet. The proximal coil of the double-pigtail shunt is first placed intravesical, the assembly is partially withdrawn, and the distal coil is then placed intra-amniotic. VA shunting is done as a day care procedure under local infiltration anesthesia. Mother is usually discharged after 2 hours of bed rest.

Risks of Vesicoamniotic Shunting

Risks associated with any fetal invasive procedure are present. Apart from those, shunt may come out (shunt expulsion) due to fetal movements. Shunt blockage may also occur due to amniotic debris. In both situations, reshunting may be necessary. If proper selection of case is not done the prognosis is good. PLUTO trial has shown immediate survival benefit of VA shunt but long-term results are not promising due to renal dysplasia. With increasing experience, we know how to do shunting. However, the decision when to do and when not to do is a big challenge, and further trials are necessary.

Thoracoamniotic Shunt (Pulmonary Artery Shunt)

Thoracoamniotic shunting is done for pleural effusion to relieve pressure effect on fetal lungs (poor alveolar development resulting in pulmonary hypoplasia) or the fetal heart (cardiac compression causing poor stroke volume, obstruction to venous and arterial flows, nonimmune hydrops). Unilateral pleural effusion can also cause these. Sometimes pleurocentesis is done as a preliminary step to see whether pleural fluid reaccumulates after drainage. If it reaccumulates, shunt is performed. Advantage of pleurocentesis is analysis of pleural fluid can be done for biochemistry and chromosomal analysis, and to see whether fluid reaccumulates or not.

Causes of Fetal Pleural Effusion and Indications of Pulmonary Artery Shunt

- *Chylothorax:* Abnormal lymphatic drainage into pleural space
- *Infection:* TORCH/parvovirus
- Cardiac anomalies causing congestive cardiac failure
- *Structural fetal anomalies*: Congenital pulmonary airway malformation (CPAM), congenital diaphragmatic hernia (CDH)
- *Genetic:* Trisomy 21
- Alloimmunization due to blood group incompatibilities.
- Nonimmune hydrops.

Procedure and Complications

Pulmonary artery (PA) shunt can be done with the same double-pigtail catheter as the VA shunt. The usual site of insertion is the side or the back of the fetus. Doppler is used to avoid going through any vessel. With anterior insertion shunt-expulsion is more due to fetal arm movements. Pericardial effusion is sometimes confused with pleural effusion. While shunting, left pleural cavity care is taken to avoid cardiac structures. As with LUTO, it is a day care procedure. Complications are similar to VA shunting. Possibilities of shunt-expulsion, shunt-blockage, and reshunting are there. Prognosis is better for isolated pleural effusion and in nonhydropic fetuses.

Legal Formalities for Shunt Procedures

Same as other fetal invasive procedures as already detailed before.

FETAL ENDOSCOPIC TRACHEAL OCCLUSION

Fetal endoscopic tracheal occlusion (FETO) is done for CDH of the fetus. CDH is more common on the left side, 70% occur through the posterolateral foramen of Bochdalek. Herniation of small intestinal loops and/or stomach into the fetal thorax occurs, resulting in mediastinal shift. Abnormal location/axis of the fetal heart and/or absence of stomach on abdominal circumference view are often the first clue for diagnosis. Polyhydramnios is also seen. Herniation of the liver or hydrops are poor prognostic signs. Lung head ratio (LHR) is used to assess prognosis. CDH may be isolated or associated with other structural abnormalities of the fetal heart. Genetic associations are also possible. Hence, a detailed anomaly scan of the fetus, fetal echocardiography, and amniocentesis for CMA are essential to make sure that CDH is indeed "isolated" and not an associated finding of a complex syndrome. FETO is done for isolated CDH.

Principle behind Fetal Endoscopic Tracheal Occlusion

Occlusion of the trachea by a balloon in the antenatal period causes obstruction of lung fluid draining into the amniotic cavity. This results in increase of intrathoracic pressure, thereby pushing the herniated contents out of thoracic cavity into the abdomen. This allows the lungs to expand and helps type II pneumocytes to develop. This is a temporary procedure that helps to prevent pulmonary hypoplasia during the antenatal period. After birth definitive repair of the diaphragmatic hernia site is done. FETO is usually done between 24 and 28 weeks under general/regional anesthesia. It may be done under local anesthesia also.

Procedure

Fetal endoscopic tracheal occlusion is done through fetoscope. Fetal paralysis is done as described under FBT. The fetoscopic puncture site is made near the fetal mouth. The fetoscope is guided through the fetal mouth into the trachea, if the fetus just proximal to its bifurcation into two bronchii (carina). A detachable balloon is then advanced under fetoscopic guidance and the balloon is placed just above the carina. The balloon is then inflated, detached, and left at that location. The fetoscope is withdrawn. The procedure is done as a day care procedure.

Removal of the Balloon

Removal of the balloon is usually done after 34 weeks as an elective procedure. Fetoscopic balloon retrieval is done after the balloon is punctured with a needle passed through the fetoscope. In case the patient goes into premature labor and emergency delivery is required EXIT (ex-utero intrapartum therapy) is done.

Risks of Fetal Endoscopic Tracheal Occlusion

Risks associated with EXIT procedure are high. PPROM, premature labor, abruption, and infection have been reported. Expertise is required and learning curve is steep. Emergency delivery facilities and EXIT facilities should be in place. Proper counseling about the procedure and prognosis is essential. Any fetal invasive procedure is there. Apart from those, shunt may come out (shunt expulsion) due to fetal movements. Shunt blockage may also occur due to amniotic debris. In both situations, reshunting may be necessary. If proper selection of case is not done the prognosis is good. PLUTO trial has shown immediate survival benefit of VA shunt but long-term results are not promising due to renal dysplasia. With increasing experience, we know how to do shunting. However, the decision when to do and when not-to-do is a big challenge, and further trials are necessary.

Legal Formalities for Shunt Procedures

Same as other fetal invasive procedures as already detailed before.

FETAL CARDIAC THERAPY

Indications

- *Valvular stenosis:* Critical aortic stenosis/pulmonary stenosis (by balloon valvoplasty of stenotic semilunar valve)
- Absent/restrictive foramen ovale resulting in hypoplastic left heart syndrome (by balloon dilation of interatrial septum)
- *Arrhythmias:* Tachyarrhythmias.

Principle of Balloon Valvoplasty

There are six connections within the fetal heart and one intracardiac fetal shunt. The three connections on each side are venoatrial, atrioventricular, and ventriculoarterial.

The intracardiac shunt is the patent foramen ovale. Abnormalities can occur when there is obstruction of blood flow from one segment to the other. In cases of critical aortic stenosis or pulmonary stenosis or atresias balloon valvuloplasty is done to dilate the respective valves. In case of absent or restrictive foramen ovale, the intact interatrial septum is perforated and/or dilated using the same principle.

Procedure

These procedures are a multiteam effort. The interventional radiologist/fetal medicine specialist/interventional cardiologist introduces the needle under USG guidance into the gravid uterus and does a transthoracic fetal entry. The needle is then advanced to the appropriate area of the fetal heart. In case of aortic stenosis, the needle enters the left ventricle, in pulmonary stenosis the needle enters the right ventricle. Through the needle a guide wire is passed across area of the constricted valve. The deflated balloon catheter is guided over the guide wire. The deflated balloon is placed at the annulus of the valve and dilated. This procedure is called intracardiac valvuloplasty.

In case of restricted or absent foramen ovale the procedure is similar. The needle enters the right atrium and perforates the interatrial septum. Gradual dilatation of the perforation site is done and a channel for blood flow from right to left atrium is created which serves the purpose of the obligatory intracardiac fetal shunt and thereby maintain fetal circulation.

Tachyarrhythmias

Fetal tachyarrhythmias that sometimes need treatment are supraventricular tachycardia (SVT), atrial flutter, atrioventricular (AV) tachycardia, and ventricular tachycardia (VT). These can result in fetal cardiac compromise resulting in nonimmune hydrops. Fetal tachyarrhythmias can be treated transplacentally by administering medication to the mother orally or intravenously. These can cause maternal side effects and so mothers need to be hospitalized. When these fail or cannot be given, direct fetal therapy by injecting these drugs to the fetus have been tried. Mode of drug delivery can be intramuscular, intra-amniotic, intraperitoneal, intraumbilical, or by intracardiac fetal injections. Drugs that have been tried are digoxin, propranolol, sotalol, amiodarone, flecanide, procainamide, etc. depending upon the specific tachyarrhythmia involved.

OTHER CLOSED FETAL INVASIVE THERAPEUTIC PROCEDURES

Amnioreduction

Amnioreduction is the procedure of taking out amniotic fluid in cases of polyhydramnios. Main indication for amnioreduction is to reduce respiratory distress of mother. Occasionally serial amnioreduction is done to prolong pregnancy in TTTS where laser photocoagulation or RFA is not available. 500 —1,000 mL is usually reduced at one sitting.

Amnioinfusion

Amnioinfusion is the procedure of injecting fluid (e.g., normal saline) into the amniotic sac. Indications for amnioinfusion are debatable. Amnioinfusion has been described for idiopathic oligohydramnios and PPROM, but the outcomes are not satisfactory. Amnioinfusion to create acoustic window for ruling out structural abnormality of fetus (especially to rule out renal tract abnormalities of the fetus), have also been described. In intrapartum meconium stained liquor, amnioinfusion has been tried to dilute the meconium within amniotic fluid to avoid complications of meconium aspiration with the aim of achieving vaginal delivery and avoid cesarean section. Benefits, however, are not proven.

Other Closed Fetal Therapeutic Procedures

Amniotic band syndrome: Fetoscopic surgery has been done to release amniotic bands that constrict a part of the fetus, usually a limb. This allows blood circulation to the part beyond the band constriction and allows the limb to grow.

Vasa previa: Laser photocoagulation has been done to the aberrant vessels between separate placental lobes, often traversing the internal os.

Chorioangioma of placenta: Laser photocoagulation to feeding vessels

Sacrococcygeal teratoma: Vascular occlusion to the tumor by RFA or laser. Intravascular coiling can also be done.

FETAL EX-UTERO INTRAPARTUM THERAPY

Fetal EXIT **(Fig. 29)** is the name given to temporary maintenance of fetal circulation and gaseous exchange after the fetus is half delivered, while other procedures are done by a different team to make the fetus suitable for neonatal life.

Principle

This is performed where there is airway obstruction of the fetus due to any cause. During fetal life gaseous exchange of fetus is maintained by placental circulation and pulmonary airways are not necessary for survival. However, for the neonate to survive, pulmonary gaseous exchange is mandatory. The switch from placental to pulmonary gaseous exchange occurs at the first breath. A patent airway is an obligatory requirement for the first breath to reach the pulmonary alveoli. In cases, where the fetus is otherwise normal but the upper airways are obstructed, EXIT procedure is done to temporarily maintain the placental

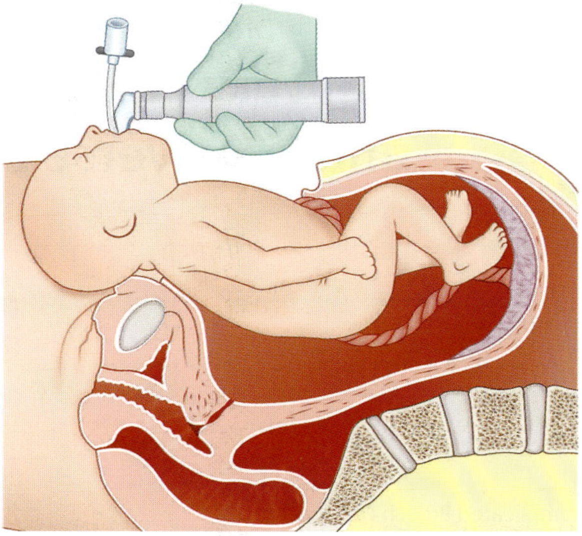

Fig. 29: Fetal ex-utero intrapartum therapy.

circulation while the fetus is half delivered, while another team works on the half-delivered fetus to establish a patent airway. Indications are endoluminal laryngeal/tracheal obstructions due to webs, polyps, etc. Congenital high airway obstruction syndrome (CHAOS) and external obstruction by neck masses, mediatinal masses are also indications for EXIT procedure.

Procedure

General anesthesia is given to the mother, temporary fetal paralysis is done. Cesarean section is done and only the fetal head/shoulder is delivered. The placenta is still attached to maintain gaseous exchange. Ecbolics are not given and uterorelaxant anesthesia is used. The mother may bleed and therefore EXIT procedures are time sensitive. The fetus is intubated and the "planned procedure" is done. Fetal tracheostomy is the most common procedure done. Operations through laryngoscope/bronchoscope can be done to remove masses. Neck masses and mediastinal masses causing obstruction to fetal airway can be removed by pediatric surgeons during EXIT. EXIT is therefore a well-planned multidisciplinary procedure done in highly equipped centers, and is still an evolving area of fetal therapy.

OPEN FETAL SURGERY

Open fetal surgery is an extension of pediatric surgery in-utero. Hysterotomy is done under general anesthesia by the obstetric/anesthetic team. Sevofluorane is used as an anesthetic agent to relax the uterus. Pfannenstiel incision or midline incision is used as appropriate. Uterine incision is planned depending upon location of the placenta. Hemostasis is secured as myometrial incision is deepened. Before opening the amniotic sac, sutures are placed on either side of proposed opening site, apposing the membranes to the myometrium. This prevents leakage of amniotic fluid/blood into extra amniotic space, as this leakage increases chance of leakage par vagina and preterm labor. Warm saline is used for irrigation once amniotic sac is opened. This helps to prevent fetal hypothermia and cord compression. Fetal paralysis is done, the operative area of the fetus is gently brought to the uterine incision.

The pediatric surgical team takes over. The fetus is stabilized by stay sutures and fetal surgery proceeds. At the end of the procedure, the hysterotomy incision is closed. Uterine relaxant and antibiotics are given. Pregnancy is continued till fetal viability. Delivery is always by cesarean section.

Indications

- Open spina bifida to protect spinal cord from toxic exposure to amniotic fluid.
- Sacrococcygeal teratoma to prevent hydrops due to hyperdynanmic fetal circulation
- Lung lesions [CPAM, bronchopulmonary sequestration (BPS)] to prevent hydrops due to cardiac compression and cardiac dysfunction resulting in fetal hypoxia.

Complications

Animal studies and limited human studies have shown up to 20% procedure-related early preterm delivery. There can be anesthesia-related complication, maternal bleeding, and infection. Open fetal surgery is still in evolving phase and can only be done after proper consent in fully equipped centers.

FUTURE OF FETAL THERAPY

The scope of fetal therapy is slowly but surely increasing. We will see more of intrauterine fetoscopic procedures like we currently see in hysteroscopic and laparoscopic surgery. Fetal medicine specialists, intervention radiologists, vascular surgeons, intervention cardiologists, pediatric surgeons, and neurosurgeons are increasingly coming together to save the fetus. Fetal anesthesia is a developing speciality. With better understanding of fetal anesthesia procedures will become safer. As centers gain experience, fetal diagnosis and therapy will become an integral part of modern antenatal care. Appropriate indications and contraindications will become clearer.

CHAPTER 8

Delivery of Breech and Transverse Lie

Learning Objectives

- Types of Breech with Frequency
- Hazards of Vaginal Breech Delivery
- Etiology and Diagnosis
- Antenatal Management
- Selection of Route of Delivery in Breech Presentation
- Indications of Cesarean Delivery in Breech Presentation
- Criteria for Planned Vaginal Breech Delivery
- Labor Management
- Complete Breech Extraction
- Complicated Breech Delivery
- Cesarean Delivery in Breech Presentation
- Transverse lie—Etiology and Diagnosis
- Risks of Transverse Lie
- Outcome of Transverse Lie Following Labor
- Management of Pregnancy with Transverse Lie
- Internal Podalic Version
- Difficulty in Cesarean Delivery in Transverse Lie
- Neglected Shoulder Presentation

BREECH PRESENTATION

INTRODUCTION

Breech presentation and delivery is strongly associated with excessive perinatal morbidity and mortality. It complicates 3–4% of all deliveries at term. Multiple factors such as prematurity, congenital anomaly, and birth injury account for the adverse perinatal outcome. To minimize the birth injury, elective cesarean delivery has been advocated by many for breech delivery. From the "Term Breech Trial" (2000) involving 26 countries and 126 centers, it was interpreted that elective cesarean delivery is the safest mode of delivery to minimize perinatal mortality and morbidity. There was no difference in maternal morbidity in abdominal and vaginal modes of deliveries. However, the interpretation of Term Breech Trial is not without controversy, and cesarean section and abdominal incision were not considered as morbid outcome in the trial. On the other hand, PREMODA study (Presentation et Mode d'Accouchement), a French prospective observational study comprising 8,000 women with term singleton breech, showed no difference in neonatal morbidity and outcome with the mode of delivery (2006) and by secondary analysis the rate of severe maternal morbidity was not different (2019) in two modes of deliveries. In reality, cesarean delivery is associated with several complications in the present and future pregnancies. Besides, many mothers come in advance labor with breech presentation when abdominal delivery does not become possible. Many patients refuse cesarean delivery, and cesarean delivery may not be available in all settings. In addition, vaginal breech delivery has been documented with highly satisfactory outcomes in properly selected cases. However, it requires technical skill, knowledge, and judgment of the accoucheur which is only possible with experience. Due to a smaller number of vaginal breech delivery, technically skilled persons are less available now and the new generations lack proper training. Medicolegal concern also has reduced the attempt of vaginal breech birth.

In the literature and textbooks published in last century and onward, there is lack of consensus on the proper technique of vaginal breech delivery; even with the same nomenclature, the procedure differs. Not all pregnancies with breech presentation need cesarean section and not every pregnancy with breech is a candidate for vaginal delivery. One must be acquainted with the vaginal breech delivery technique and also be aware of the precautions to be taken during abdominal breech delivery.

INCIDENCE

At term, the incidence of breech presentation is 3–4%. The frequency is much higher in lower gestational age. The lesser the gestational age, the more the frequency. At 34 weeks, it is 5% and at 28 weeks, it is 20%.

TYPES OF BREECH WITH FREQUENCY (FIGS. 1 TO 7)

Breech is broadly subdivided into complete breech, frank breech, and incomplete breech.

- *Complete breech* (5%) ***(Figs. 1 to 3)****:* Here, the extremities are in flexed attitude. Two buttocks, feet, and external genitalia are the presenting parts.
- *Frank breech* (65%) ***(Figs. 4 and 5)****:* Here, the thighs are flexed and legs are extended. This is the most common variety.
- *Incomplete breech* (30%): (1) Breech with knee presentation where thighs are extended but knees are flexed and (2) breech with footling presentation **(Figs. 6 and 7)**—both thighs and legs are extended.

When the head is in extreme hyperextended attitude, it is called *star gaze fetus* or *flying fetus*. In this type of breech, vaginal delivery is difficult and may result in injury to the cervical spinal cord. This is an indication for cesarean section if present after labor has begun. This is diagnosed by sonography.

In Frank breech, prognosis is best as it is a good cervical dilator and the incidence of cord prolapse is less. It is common in *primigravida*. In complete breech, prognosis is not as good as frank breech. However, as it is common in *multigravida*, the course of birth is smooth. In footling presentation, prognosis is worst for vaginal delivery.

HAZARDS OF VAGINAL BREECH DELIVERY

Hazards of vaginal breech delivery include maternal morbidity, perinatal morbidity, and mortality.

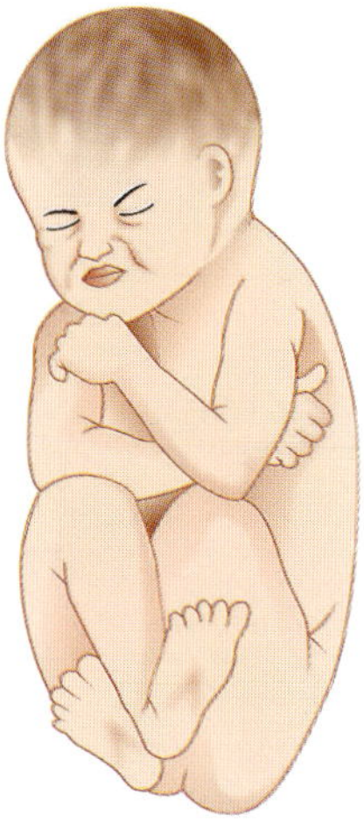

Fig. 1: Complete breech.

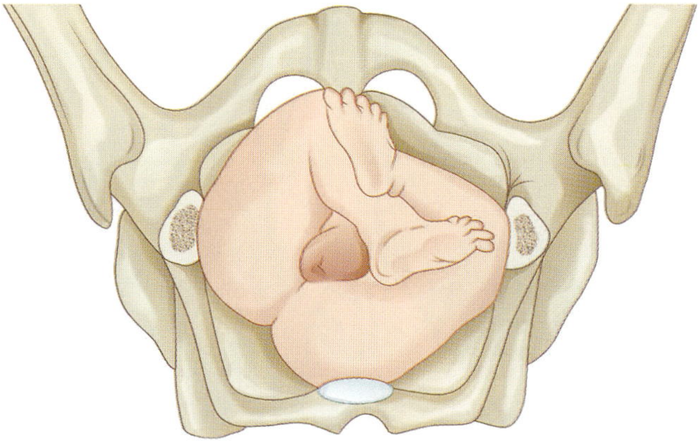

Fig. 2: Vaginal findings of flexed breech (right sacroposterior).

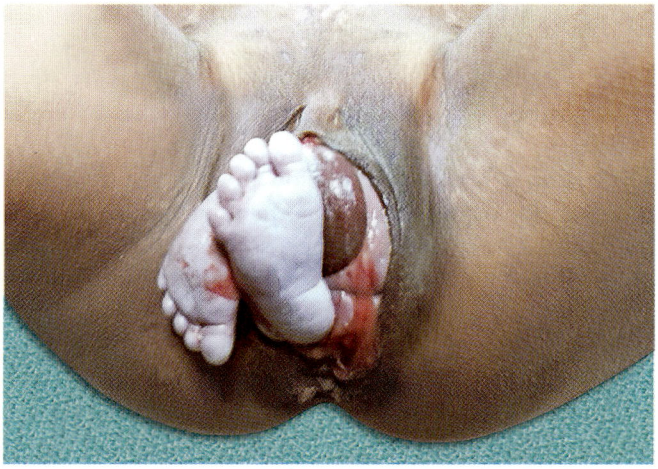

Fig. 3: Vaginal findings of flexed breech (right sacroposterior).
Courtesy: Dr Anirban Mondal, Associate Professor, Bankura Sammilani Medical College and Hospital, Bankura, West Bengal, India.

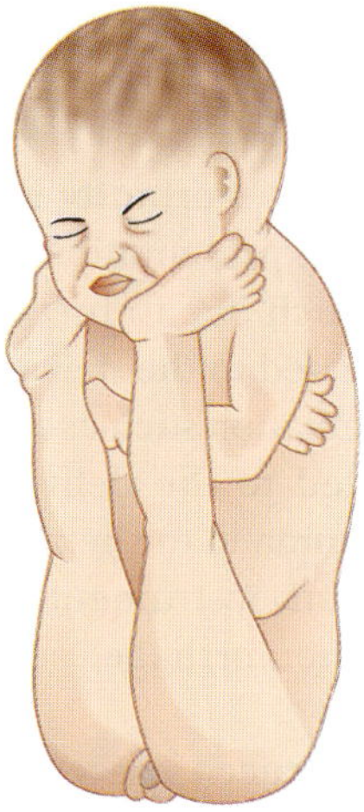

Fig. 4: Frank breech.

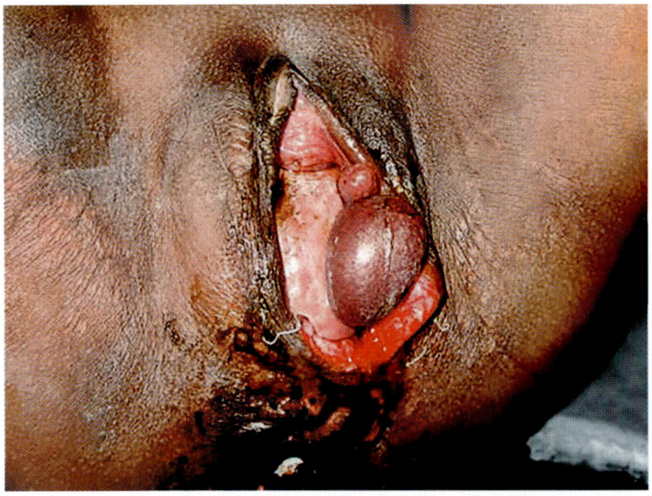

Fig. 5: Breech presentation in advance labor showing fetal scrotum.

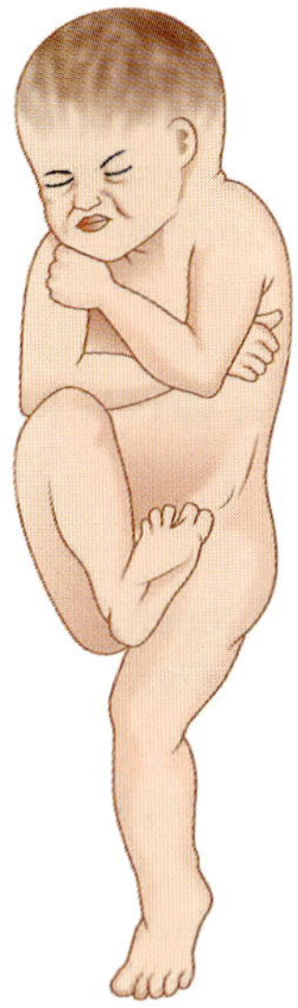

Fig. 6: Footling presentation.

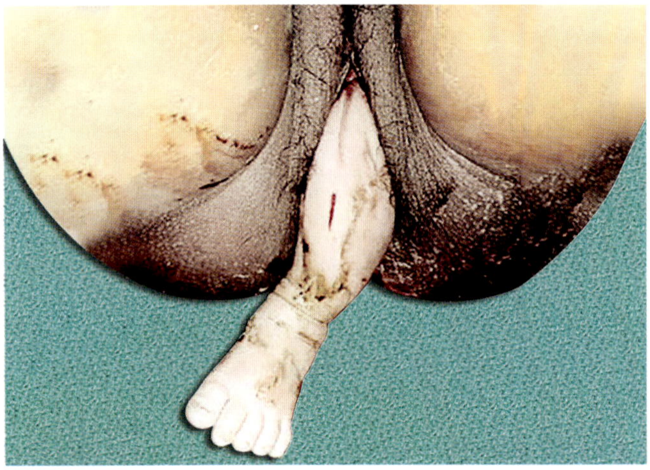

Fig. 7: Only leg is delivered (footling).
Courtesy: Dr Abhishek Bhadra, Assistant Professor, Medical College, Kolkata, West Bengal, India.

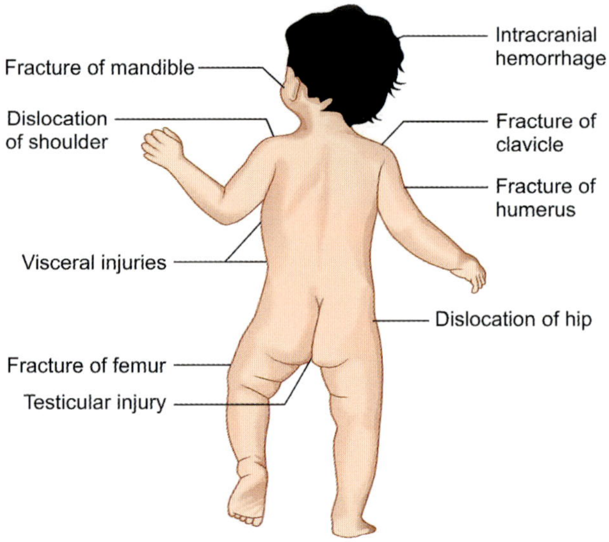

Fig. 8: Potential injuries of baby during vaginal breech delivery.

Increased perinatal morbidity and mortality are the main threats of breech presentation. There is no effect on maternal health as such due to breech presentation itself except the events related to the delivery and the etiologies causing breech presentation such as placenta previa.

The events related to the delivery causing maternal complications are trauma to the genital tract during vaginal delivery, manipulation, instrument application, cesarean section, increased hemorrhage, sepsis, and anesthetic complications.

Fetal hazards in breech presentation are due to the hazards in vaginal birth and due to inherent problems of the fetus itself such as prematurity and congenital abnormality (if any).

Fetal hazards of vaginal breech delivery **(Fig. 8)** are as follows:

- *Structural injuries* from below upward are fracture of femur, dislocation of hip, visceral injuries such as injury to testis, liver, spleen, kidney, suprarenal gland, lungs, fracture of humerus, clavicle, dislocation of the shoulder, fracture of mandible, fifth and sixth cervical vertebrae, trauma to sternomastoid muscle, and torticollis.
- *Nerve injury*: Erb's palsy—Policeman's tips (due to upper brachial plexus injury) and Klumpkey's palsy (lower brachial plexus injury)
- *Asphyxia*: Due to cord prolapse, cord compression, premature attempt at respiration, and premature separation of placenta take place.

- Hanging like death of the fetus due to sudden trauma over the medulla oblongata by the odontoid process.
- *Intracranial hemorrhage*: It occurs due to the tear of tentorium cerebelli and hemorrhage in the subarachnoid space because of the sudden compression followed by decompression during delivery of aftercoming head of breech. Premature babies are more prone to developing this problem.
- Neonatal seizure and intubation within 24 hours of birth are common among breech babies born vaginally.

Perinatal mortality in breech presentation is three to five times more than the vertex presentation. It ranges from 5 to 35 per 1,000 births.

ETIOLOGY

Common causes of breech presentation are prematurity, congenital malformation of the uterus, multiple pregnancy, placenta previa, and congenital anomaly of the fetus. Prematurity is the most common. For more details, see author's *Bedside Clinics in Obstetrics*, 5th edition, Academic Publishers.

Causes of recurrent breech are congenital malformation of the uterus and cornufundal attachment of placenta.

DIAGNOSIS AND CLINICAL EXAMINATION

Clinically, breech is diagnosed by abdominal palpation (first, second, third, and fourth Leopold maneuvers; **Figs. 9 to 12**). In the first Leopold maneuver hard, globular, ballotable head is palpable at fundus. In the second Leopold maneuver, fetal dorsum is on one side and ventral aspect is palpable on the other side of the umbilicus. By third and fourth Leopold maneuvers, the soft, broad and irregular podalic end is palpable. Lie is longitudinal. Fetal heart sound (FHS) lies above, in comparison to vertex presentation.

On per vaginal examination if the patient is not in labor, soft irregular mass is palpable through the fornix and sacrum may be palpable and if the patient is in labor ischial tuberosities, sacrum, external genitalia, and feet are palpable in case of complete breech **(Figs. 2 and 3)** whereas feet are not palpable in frank breech **(Fig. 5)**. Fetal sacrum helps to determine the position of breech. In case of footling presentation, only the feet are palpable and identified by the heels.

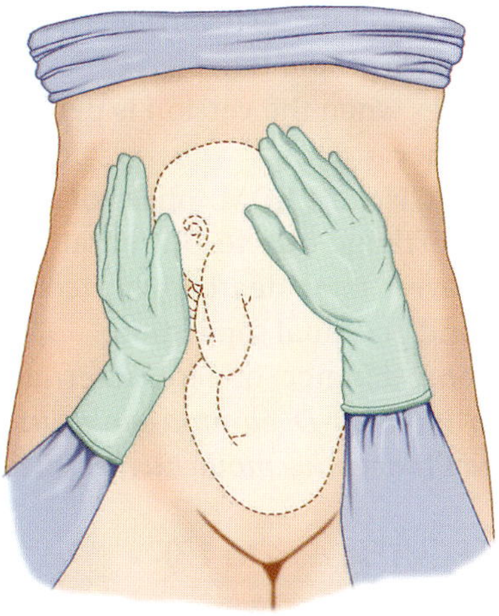

Fig. 9: Fundal grip (first Leopold maneuver).

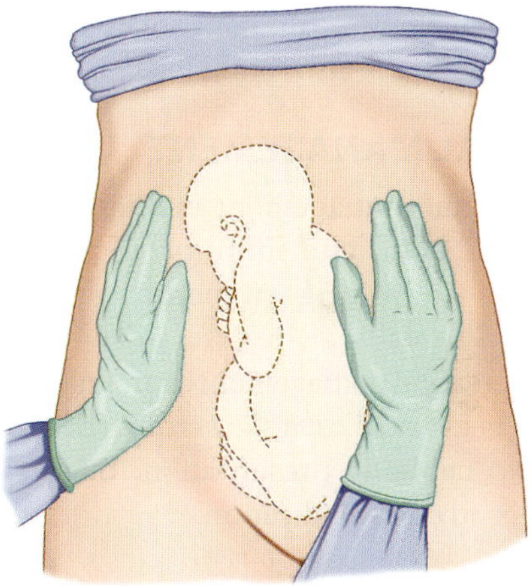

Fig. 10: Lateral grip (second Leopold maneuver)

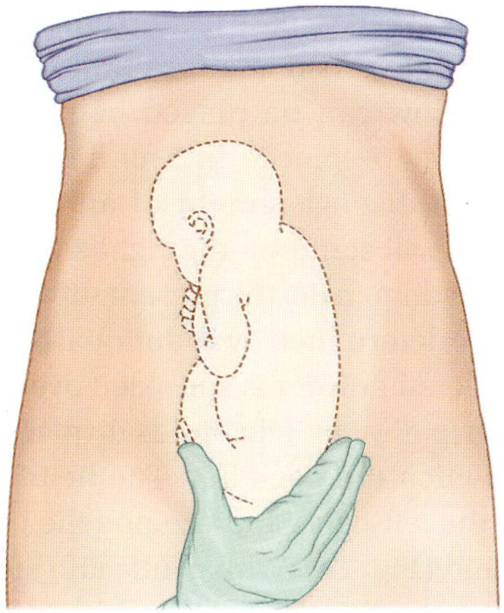

Fig. 11: First pelvic grip—Pawlik grip (third Leopold maneuver).

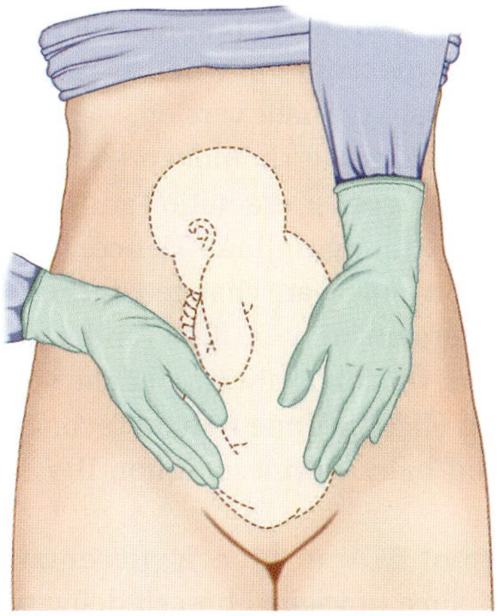

Fig. 12: Second pelvic grip (fourth Leopold maneuver).

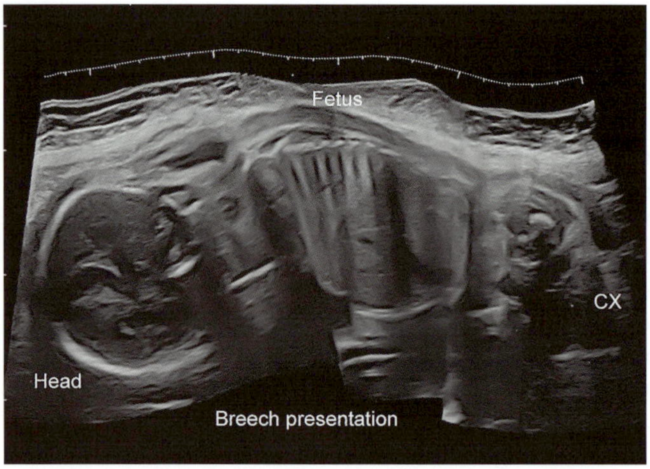

Fig. 13: Breech presentation at 32 weeks.
Courtesy: Professor Kamal Oswal, Head, Department of Radiodiagnosis, Vivekananda Institute of Medical Sciences, Kolkata, West Bengal, India.

Sonography **(Fig. 13)** confirms the diagnosis, determines the maturity of the fetus, finds out the type of breech and the attitude of head (*Star gaze appearance*), and can detect any congenital anomaly of the fetus. Presence of placenta previa is diagnosed which may be the cause of breech presentation. The amount of liquor is also estimated.

ANTENATAL MANAGEMENT

Routine antenatal management includes rest, nutritious diet, iron, folic acid, and immunization. Any obstetric complication including placenta previa must be checked for.

Specific antenatal management of pregnancy with breech presentation is *external cephalic version* (ECV). ECV makes the breech to cephalic presentation. ECV is attempted, where there is no contraindication.

External Cephalic Version

Version is an obstetric maneuver by which presentation with or without lie is changed from an unfavorable to a favorable one. In case of breech presentation, manipulation is done to make it vertex presentation whereas the lie remains the same, called external cephalic version.

In case of transverse lie, shoulder presentation is changed to either vertex or breech presentation and lie is also changed from transverse to longitudinal. Hence, in transverse lie, both presentation and lie are changed during version.

External version may be ECV and external podalic version. Internal version is always podalic version. Internal podalic version (IPV) is done only in second baby in twin. In a large-sized baby with less liquor, IPV should not be attempted.

Rationality of ECV in breech presentation is that it reduces the chance of vaginal breech delivery and also the complications arising out of it. It also reduces the cesarean section rate which is >85% in breech presentation. However, all cases are not suitable for version and contraindications are considered.

Contraindications of ECV

- Antepartum hemorrhage (placenta previa, accidental hemorrhage)
- Severe pre-eclampsia
- Contracted pelvis
- Multiple pregnancy
- Pregnancy with prior cesarean delivery
- Premature rupture of membranes (PROM)
- Congenital malformation of uterus
- Fetal factors—gross congenital anomaly, intrauterine growth restriction (IUGR), intrauterine fetal demise (IUFD)
- Other obstetric conditions—elderly primi, bad obstetric history (BOH)

Time of Version

In recent practice, ECV is done in a woman who has reached $37^{0/7}$ weeks before the onset of labor (ACOG 2020). In too early version, the possibility of reversion is more and besides, there is still a chance of spontaneous version. The possibility of failure increases when the version is performed after this period of pregnancy.

Dangers of ECV are PROM, onset of labor, chance of accidental hemorrhage due to placental separation, and fetal distress; even fetal death may occur due to cord entanglement and placental separation.

There is more chance of fetomaternal hemorrhage for which *routine anti-D gamma-globulin is given to a nonimmunized Rh-negative mother when ECV is performed.*

Procedure of ECV (Figs. 14 to 17)

External cephalic version is an outpatient department (OPD) procedure which should always be done in a well-equipped center where facility of cesarean delivery is available.

The patient is asked to pass urine. Consent is taken. The position of the patient is dorsal position with legs slightly drawn up. A pillow can be placed behind the buttocks or the patient may be placed in Trendelenburg position. This will help in disengagement of an engaged breech. The obstetrician will stand on the right side of the patient. After exposing abdomen lie, the presentation and position of the fetal back are determined by abdominal palpation. FHS is auscultated. Talcum powder is sprinkled over the abdomen. By the pelvic grip, the podalic end is displaced to one iliac fossa toward which the back lies. The head at the fundus is grasped by the left hand and the podalic pole is grasped by the right hand **(Fig. 14)**. With gentle and steady pressure, the breech is pushed to the back and head to the front of the fetus making the trunk well flexed, and this movement

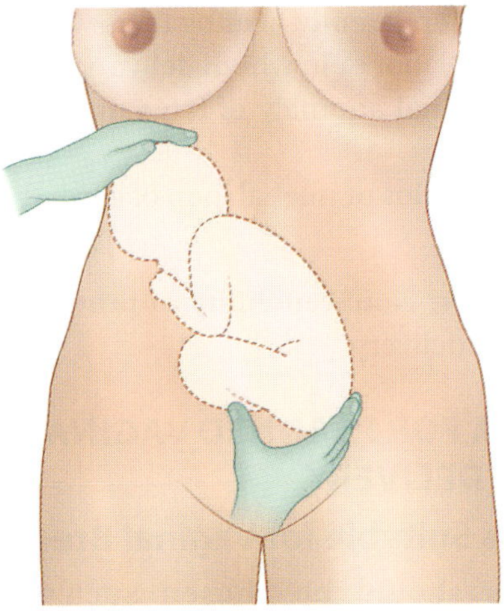

Fig. 14: External cephalic version (ECV) by forward roll—first step.

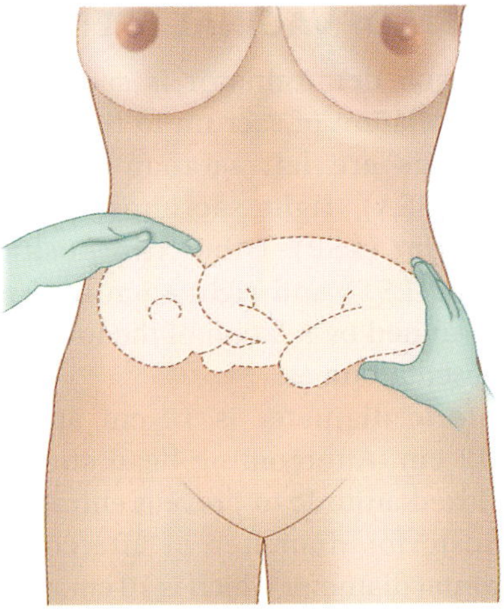

Fig. 15: External cephalic version (ECV) by forward roll—second step.

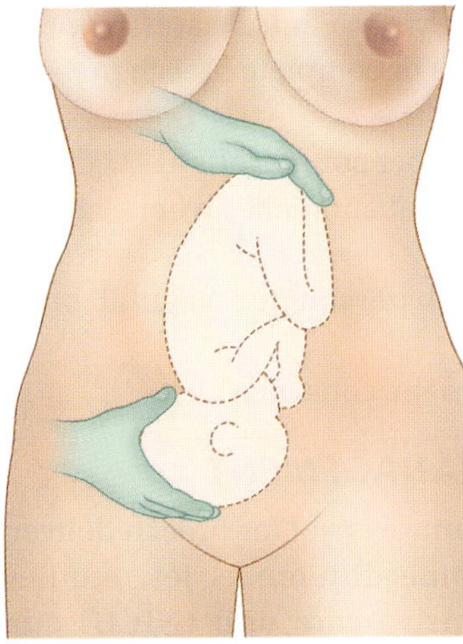

Fig. 16: External cephalic version (ECV) by forward roll—third step.

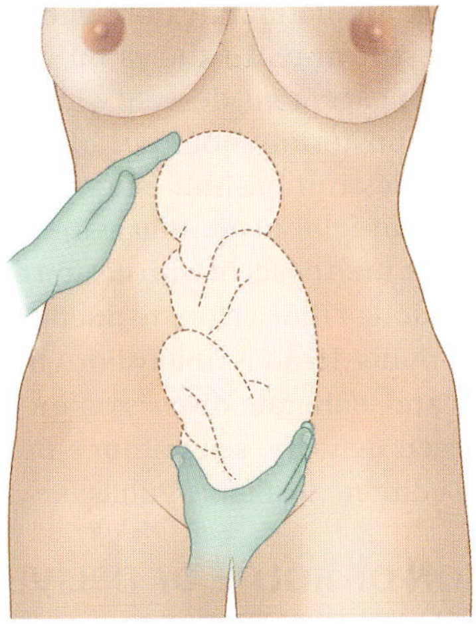

Fig. 17: External cephalic version in backward roll.

is continued until the lie becomes transverse **(Fig. 15)**. At this point, the hands are to be changed following which FHS is auscultated.

Now with the changed hands (right hand on the head and left hand on the podalic end), the head is pushed downward toward the pelvis and the breech toward the fundus to make the lie longitudinal **(Fig. 16)**. All manipulations are done in the relaxation phase. FHS is auscultated again. There may be transient bradycardia which usually passes off after few minutes. FHS is monitored at least for 30 minutes. This is *forward somersault movement* or "forward roll."

If forward roll is unsuccessful, the procedure is done in the opposite direction, which is called "backward roll" **(Fig. 17)**, but not recommended now [Royal College of Obstetricians and Gynaecologists (RCOG) 2017].

Nonstress test (NST) should be done before and after the procedure. Tocolytic drugs such as terbutaline 250 µg SC or isoxsuprine 50–100 mg IV or calcium-channel blocker (nifedipine) may be used during ECV for relaxation of uterus. However, their effectiveness is controversial.

If bradycardia does not pass off within 1 or 2 minutes, oxygen inhalation is given to the mother. If it still persists after 10 minutes' version, reversion is to be considered as there is possibility of cord entanglement. Cardiotocography (CTG) is helpful to detect any abnormality.

The *success rate* of ECV ranges from 50 to 60%, average being 58%.

If the version fails, pregnancy is continued till term. In the meantime, there is possibility of spontaneous version in few cases. In case of persistent breech presentation, it is judged on its own merit whether vaginal or abdominal delivery will be done.

Causes of failure of ECV are scanty liquor, large baby, breech with extended leg (difficult to flex the trunk due to splinting action of the limbs), uterine anomalies, obesity, and irritable uterus.

MECHANISM OF VAGINAL BREECH DELIVERY

In case of breech denominator is sacrum. Position is determined by relation of sacrum to the maternal pelvis. Various positions are left sacroanterior (LSA), right sacroanterior (RSA), right sacroposterior (RSP), and left sacroposterior (LSP). Other two positions are left sacrotransverse (LST) and right sacrotransverse (RST). Station is determined by relation of the lowermost point of buttock to the ischial spines.

Bitrochanteric diameter is 10 cm and bisacromial diameter is 12 cm. Aftercoming head should always be delivered in flexed attitude to prevent entrapment of head. The anteroposterior diameter of aftercoming head is suboccipitofrontal diameter which is 10 cm.

Delivery of the breech consists of delivery of buttocks, shoulders, and head.

Buttock is delivered by engagement in one oblique diameter of pelvic inlet, then descent, internal rotation of anterior buttock and lateral flexion with further descent followed by restitution. In the shoulder the cardinal movements are engagement, descent with internal rotation, and delivery of posterior shoulder followed by anterior shoulder. Then restitution and external rotation occur. For the delivery of fetal head engagement occurs in one oblique diameter, then descent with flexion occurs, followed by internal rotation of the occiput to put the occiput behind the symphysis pubis. Head is finally born by flexion.

For details and elaborate discussion on the mechanism of vaginal breech delivery, see author's *Bedside Clinics in Obstetrics*, 5th edition, Academic Publishers.

SELECTION OF ROUTE OF DELIVERY IN BREECH PRESENTATION

Route of delivery depends upon various maternal factors: fetal factors, maternal factors, maternal choice, amount of liquor, and availability of skill provider. Sonography is very helpful for taking the decision.

INDICATIONS OF CESAREAN DELIVERY IN BREECH PRESENTATION

Maternal factors:

- Any degree of pelvic contraction or unfavorable shape of pelvis
- Postcesarean pregnancy
- Breech with obstetric complications
- Previous history of perinatal death
- Maternal request for vaginal delivery

Sonographic findings:

- Large fetus of estimated weight >3.5 kg
- Fetus with hyperextended head
- Footling presentation
- Severe fetal growth restriction
- Preterm but apparently healthy fetus with the mother in either active labor or in whom delivery is indicated
- Congenital fetal anomaly of fetus not compatible with vaginal birth
- Oligohydramnios or nuchal loop of cord
- Nuchal arm

Provider's factor: Nonavailability of provider skilled with vaginal breech delivery

CRITERIA FOR PLANNED VAGINAL BREECH DELIVERY

Candidates Suitable for Vaginal Breech Delivery

The criteria should be chosen such that there is maximum possibility of vaginal delivery and minimizing the fetal risk. The cases suitable for vaginal breech delivery are:

- Estimated fetal weight between 2,000 and 3,500 g
- Adequate pelvis by clinical assessment
- Frank breech or complete breech presentation
- Flexed head
- Absence of other complications
- Absence of fetal anomalies where vaginal delivery is not feasible
- Experienced person for vaginal breech delivery is available
- Patient gives the consent

LABOR MANAGEMENT

Induction is controversial for breech delivery. Most studies find no outcome difference, few studies show higher neonatal intensive care unit (NICU) admission in the induction group, and some show an increased cesarean rate in the induction group. Augmentation of breech labor is also controversial. In general, progress of labor in breech presentation is slow. Many avoid augmentation. Few schools prefer to augment only in uterine hypotonicity. Others prefer amniotomy for labor augmentation.

Management of Breech Presentation in the First Stage of Labor

- History taking and examination including contraction, type of breech, FHS, dilatation of os, status of membranes, station and pelvic capacity.
- Patient should be at rest and nonambulatory to avoid early rupture of membranes.
- Monitor the fetal condition frequently, preferably with the help of CTG.
- Progress of labor is monitored.
- Oral diet is stopped; instead, intravenous fluid is given.
- Vaginal examination is done following rupture of membranes to exclude cord prolapse.

- Analgesics and sedatives
- Cesarean section is indicated in case of *uterine dystocia, prolonged labor, early rupture of membranes*, and *cord prolapse.*

Management of Breech Presentation in the Second Stage of Labor

The various options of vaginal breech delivery are:
- Spontaneous breech delivery
- Assisted breech delivery
- Total breech extraction

Spontaneous breech delivery refers to the expulsion of fetus entirely without any manipulation or even traction except support of the baby.

Assisted breech delivery in which the delivery is done with support but with minimal interference is the most preferred approach and commonly performed. In this method, the obstetrician performs maneuvers after almost spontaneous expulsion of fetal body up to umbilicus.

Complete breech extraction is the hurried delivery of baby by the obstetrician, usually under general anesthesia (GA). Indications are second baby of twin after IPV, fetal distress, and cord prolapse in the late second stage.

There is another popular term "partial breech extraction" which is used for the approach almost similar to assisted breech delivery. There is no consensus and uniformity of the terminology of various approaches of vaginal breech delivery.

Assisted Breech Delivery

Essential requirements for the assisted breech delivery are: (1) An obstetrician skilled in the art of breech delivery; (2) Presence of an anesthetist; (3) An assistant; (4) A neonatologist with baby resuscitative measures; (5) Episiotomy set; and (6) Obstetric forceps.

The principles of vaginal breech delivery are never traction from below, push the fetus through the mother's abdomen, try to keep the dorsal aspect of the fetus anteriorly, and never to be in haste.

Steps of assisted breech delivery:
1. The patient is brought to the edge of the table when buttocks are visible at the perineum. She is made to lie in lithotomy position when buttocks distend the perineum. Antiseptic dressings, draping, and evacuation of bladder are done.
2. Per vaginal examination is done to confirm full dilatation of cervix and to exclude cord prolapse. Mediolateral episiotomy is given under local infiltration of 1% xylocaine solution with or without pudendal block when the perineum is thinned out by the posterior buttock **(Figs. 18 and 19)**.
3. Legs are easily delivered if they are flexed. The anterior leg is released first, followed by the release of the posterior leg. In case of frank breech, the extended legs are delivered by abduction and flexion of the thighs with gentle pressure over the popliteal fossa **(Fig. 20)**. The ankle is grasped and the foot is delivered **(Fig. 21)**.
4. The baby is allowed to be born up to the level of the umbilicus by wait-and-watch policy **(Fig. 22)**. As soon as the umbilicus is delivered, the umbilical cord is palpated, drawn to some extent and kept in a safe position like in one sacral bay to prevent its compression.
5. If the back lies posteriorly, the fetus is rotated to bring the back to the front. Transient cessation of cord pulsation is very common at this stage. It has no effect on the outcome of the baby. The trunk of the baby is wrapped with a sterile towel. The towel will help in proper gripping of the baby and also prevent the fetus from external stimulus. The position of the arms is noted—whether they are in flexed or in extended condition.

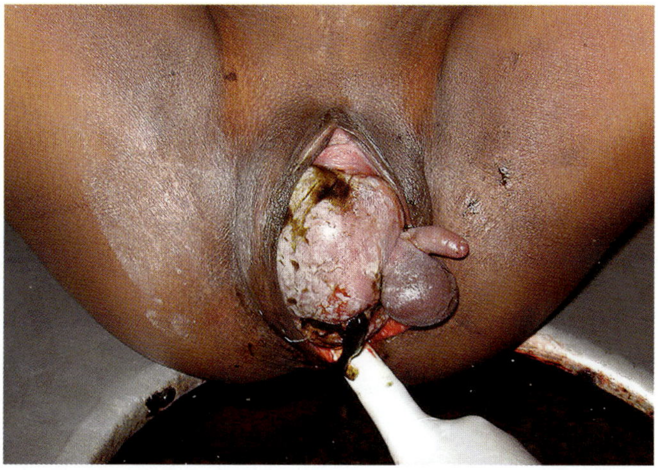

Fig. 18: Buttock is in the perineum showing fetal external genitalia.

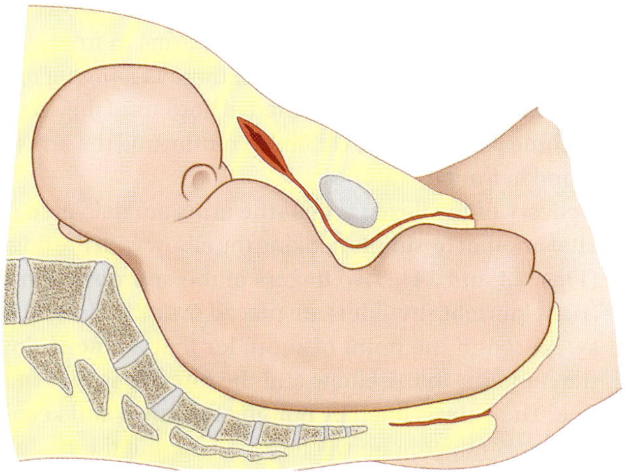

Fig. 19: Buttock is being delivered.

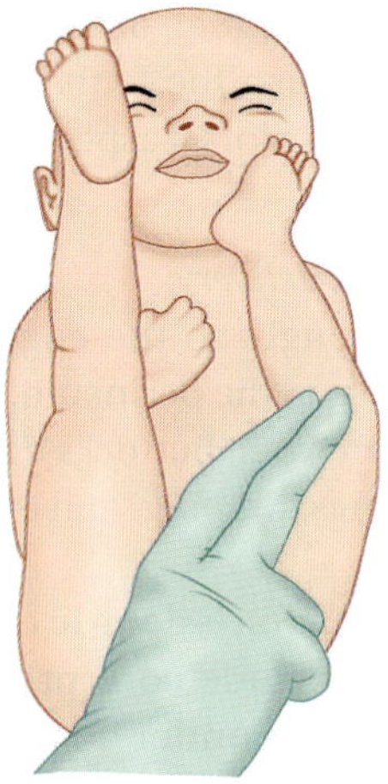

Fig. 20: Extended leg is delivered by abduction and flexion of the thigh with gentle pressure over the popliteal fossa which makes the leg flexed.

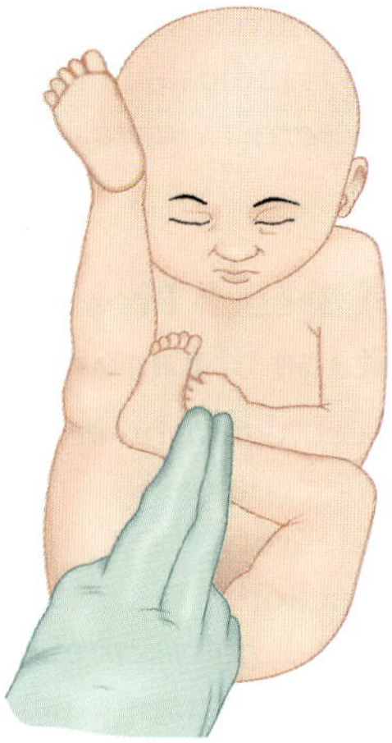

Fig. 21: Leg is delivered by grasping the ankle.

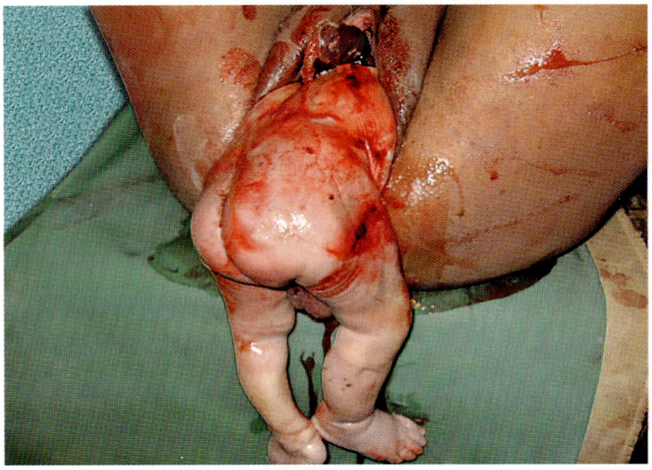

Fig. 22: Baby is born up to the level of umbilicus.

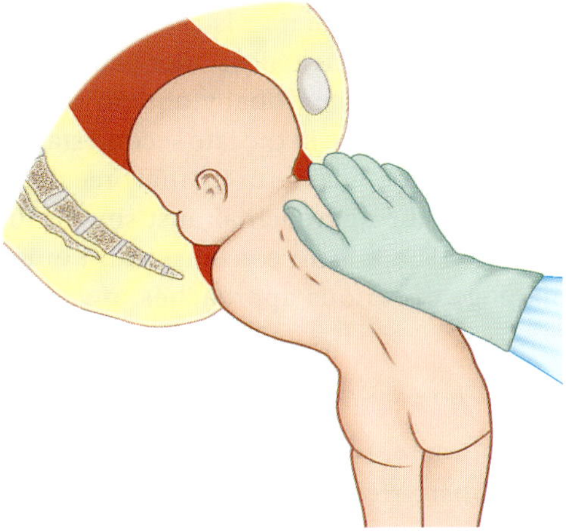

Fig. 23: Delivery of anterior arm.

6. The position of the arms is determined by two methods: (1) By palpating the medial margins of the scapula and (2) By searching for the presence of arms in front of the chest. In case of extended arms, there is *winging of the scapula*. In flexed arms, the medial borders of the scapula become parallel to the vertebral column and the arms are found in front of the chest.
7. Delivery of the flexed arms—the arms are delivered one after another by simply hooking the elbow with the fingers **(Figs. 23 and 24)**. Two fingers of the appropriate hand (right for right shoulder) are placed over the clavicle and swept round the point of shoulder that is traced down the humerus to the elbow and the forearm is thus made free. The baby is lifted by holding the ankle and keeping the index finger in between the ankles and the posterior arm is delivered in the same way. The extended arm is delivered by the classical method or Lovset maneuver

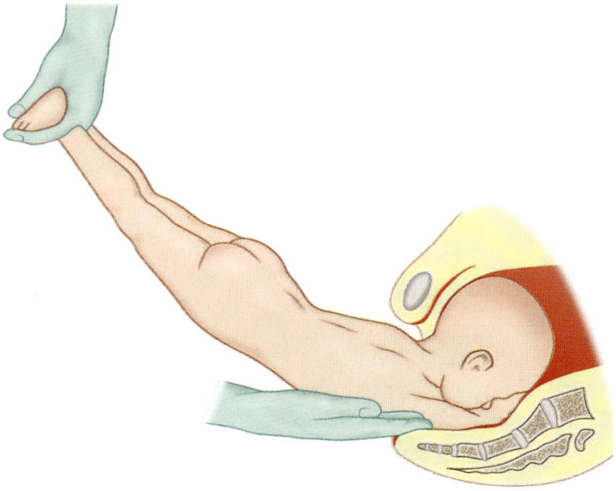

Fig. 24: Delivery of posterior arm.

described later. Lovset maneuver is employed routinely by many irrespective of the status of hand.

8. Delivery of the aftercoming head—one of the following methods is employed to deliver the aftercoming head in breech presentation:
   - Burns-Marshall technique
   - Delivery with the help of forceps
   - Malar flexion and shoulder traction method (Mauriceau-Smellie-Veit technique)

Burns and Marshall technique (1934) (Figs. 25 to 32): After the delivery of the shoulders, the baby is allowed to hang **(Figs. 25 and 26)** on its own weight for a brief period of time (1-2 minutes). In the meantime, the assistant is asked to give suprapubic pressure in downward and backward directions putting pressure more toward the sinciput so that the head is made more flexed. As soon as the nape of the neck or the hairline is visible under the pubic arch, the trunk of the baby is gradually lifted with steady traction and swung toward the mother's abdomen, making a wide arc of a circle by holding the baby's legs just above the ankles keeping a finger in between the two **(Figs. 27 to 32)**. In this method, the *pivot* should be the suboccipit and not the neck. The left hand is kept over the perineum and the face and brow is gradually delivered **(Fig. 30)**. As soon as the mouth is seen, the mouth and pharynx are sucked with mucus sucker preventing the temptation of quick delivery of the head **(Figs. 31 and 32)**. The rest of the head is delivered by depressing the trunk toward the floor.

Delivery by forceps (Fig. 33):

- *Criteria to be fulfilled*: The head should be engaged and the occiput should lie against the back of the symphysis pubis (i.e., occiput directly anterior).

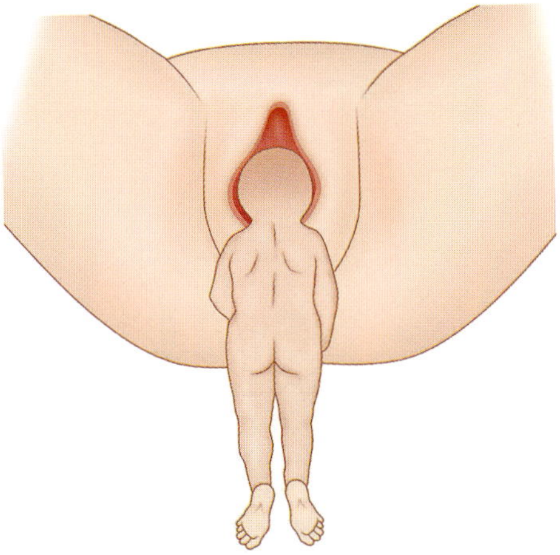

Fig. 25: Burns and Marshall technique—the baby is allowed to hang on its own weight for a brief period of time (1–2 minutes) (diagrammatic).

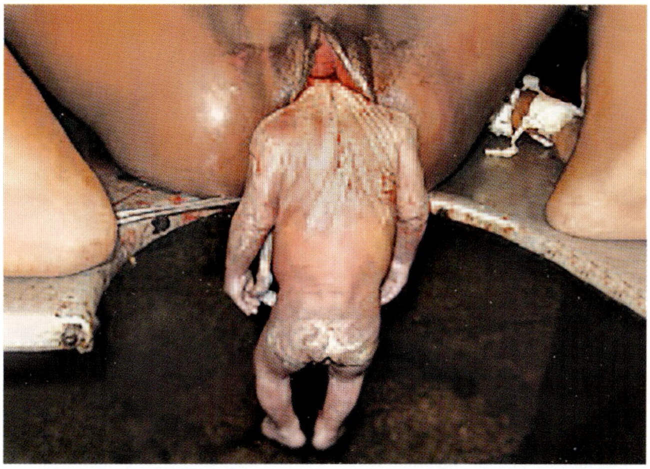

Fig. 26: Burns and Marshall technique—the baby is allowed to hang on its own weight for a brief period of time (1–2 minutes).

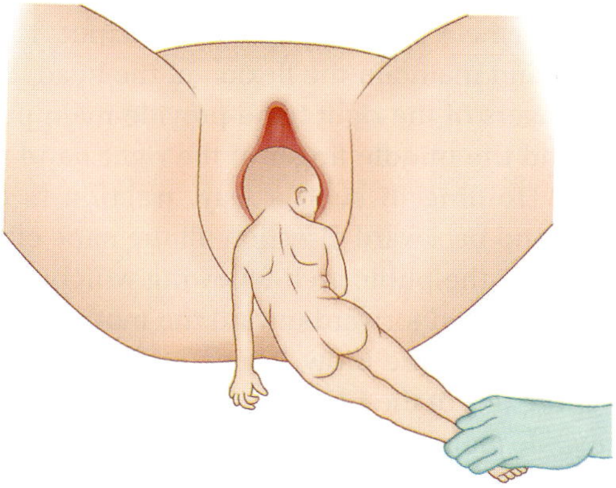

Fig. 27: Burns and Marshall technique—as soon as the nape of the neck or the hair line is visible under the pubic arch, the baby's legs are grasped just above the ankles keeping a finger in between the two.

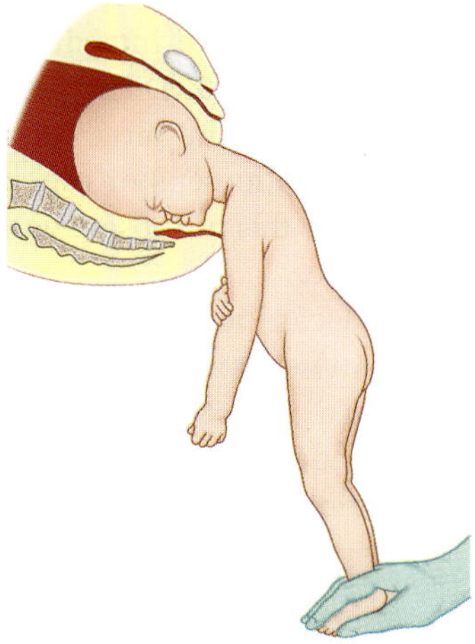

Fig. 28: Burns and Marshall technique—the trunk of the baby is gradually lifted with steady traction and swung towards the mother's abdomen.

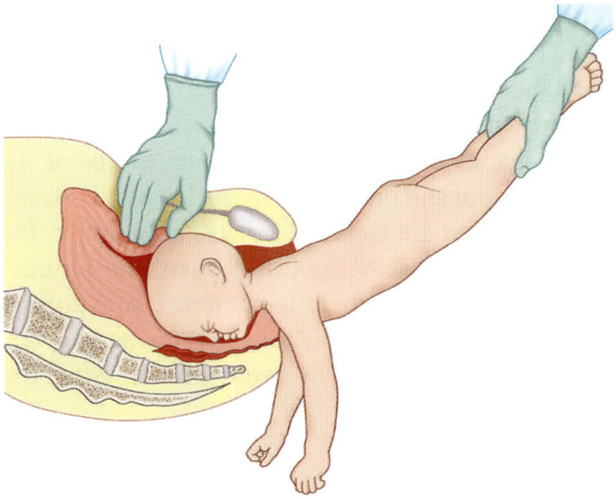

Fig. 29: Burns and Marshall technique—an wide arc of a circle is made.

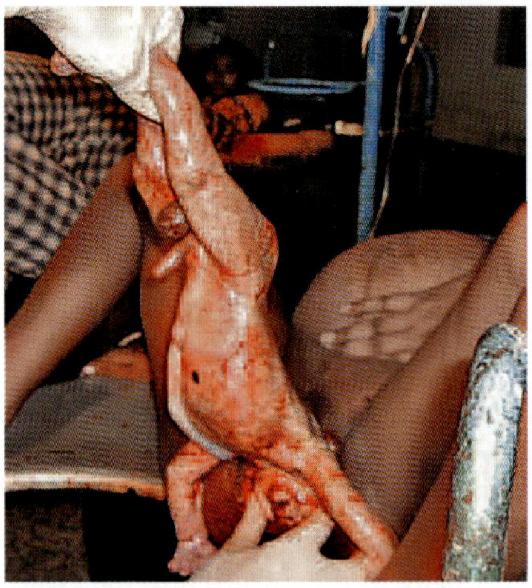

Fig. 30: Burns and Marshall technique. Baby's mouth is released.

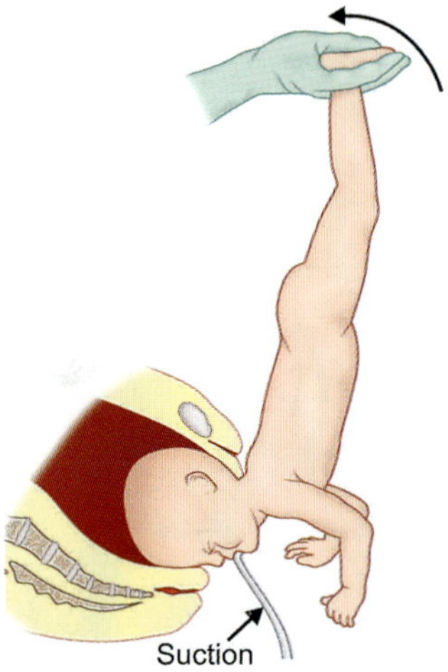

Fig. 31: Burns and Marshall technique. Baby's mouth is sucked as soon as it is released.

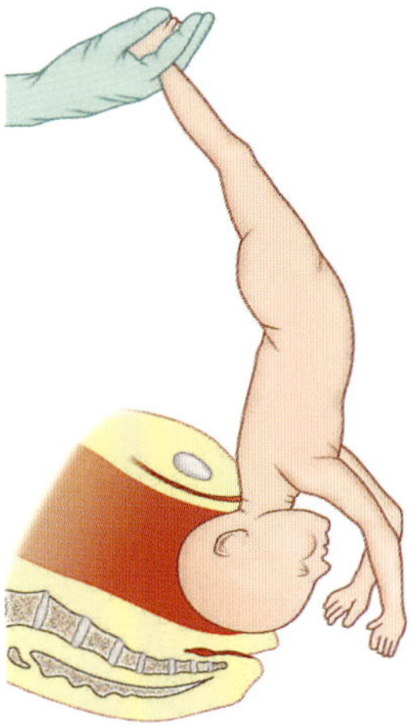

Fig. 32: Burns and Marshall technique—face is almost delivered.

- *Steps*: The assistant lifts the baby up by holding the legs, and then forceps blades are introduced from below the trunk of the baby **(Fig. 33)**. The pull of the forceps is given along the axis of the birth canal. This can be accomplished by Das's forceps or especially designed Piper forceps used for this purpose. The *Piper forceps* is devoid of pelvic curve.
- *Advantages*: Head can be delivered with controlled traction, flexion can be maintained in a better way, and head is delivered in a protective cage.
- *Disadvantages*: Rotation should be complete. Head must be at low down station.

Malar flexion and shoulder traction method (Mauriceau-Smellie-Veit technique) (Fig. 34)

*Steps **(Fig. 34)**:* Over the supinated left forearm, the baby is placed with the limbs hanging on both sides. The left index and the middle fingers are placed on either malar prominence of the baby. The index and ring fingers of the pronated right hand are forked over the shoulder on each side of the neck, and the middle finger is placed along the dorsum of the neck reaching up to the occiput. The fingers of the left hand maintain the flexion of the head, the index and ring fingers of the right hand provide main pull of the traction, and the middle finger of the right hand prevents extension. Holding in such a way, traction is given in downward and backward direction till the nape of the neck appears below the pubic arch following which the fetus is carried upward and forward toward the mother's abdomen delivering the face and brow. Then, the trunk is depressed to deliver the rest of the head. An *assistant gives suprapubic pressure* while pulling the head in the same way as Burns and Marshall technique.

Advantages: This procedure can be applied even when the head is high up and not necessarily in the anteroposterior direction

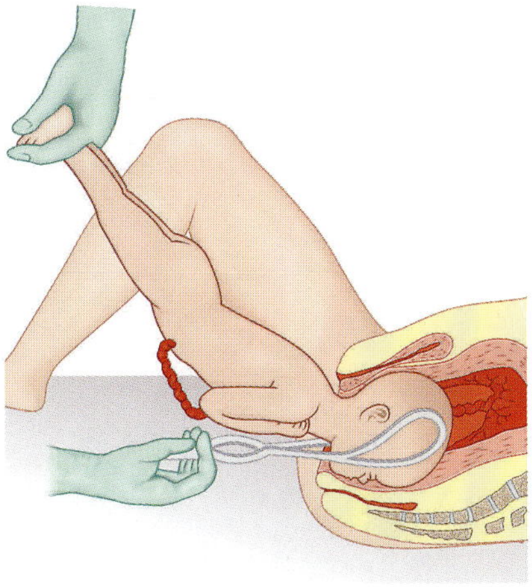

Fig. 33: Forceps in aftercoming head of the breech.

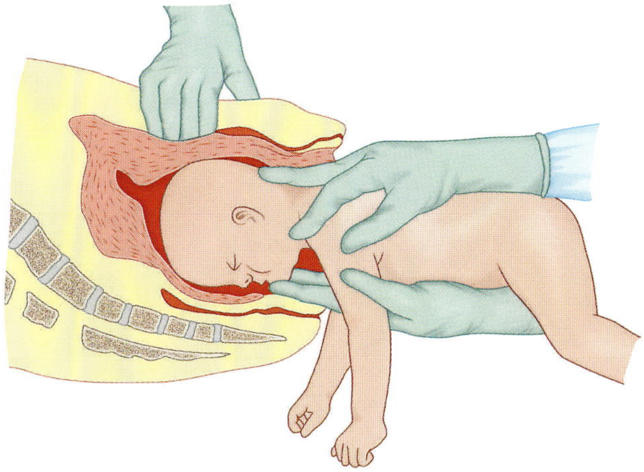

Fig. 34: Malar flexion and shoulder traction method.

(i.e., rotation is not completed). The baby may be asphyxiated and resuscitated. This method was originally known as "jaw flexion shoulder traction" where the index finger of the left hand was introduced into the mouth for hooking.

Of these three methods in delivery of aftercoming head of breech, no method is superior to other. It depends on the obstetrician's choice. When the Burns and Marshall technique fails, the head can be delivered by *malar flexion and shoulder traction* method. For forceps application, criteria must be fulfilled.

Delivery of the aftercoming head of breech is the most crucial part of delivery of the breech. Arrest of the aftercoming head of breech may result in either delivery of an asphyxiated baby or a stillborn baby. Sudden compression followed by sudden decompression during hurried delivery of fetal head may cause *intracranial hemorrhage.* Optimal time between the delivery from umbilicus and the mouth is *5–10 minutes* after which there is chance of asphyxia.

Third-stage Management in Assisted Breech Delivery

It is managed as usual. At this stage, active management of labor is done with Inj. oxytocin 10 IU IM after delivery of the fetus.

Usefulness of Episiotomy in Vaginal Breech Delivery

Episiotomy straightens the birth canal. It prevents the compression of the aftercoming head. It is essential for instrumental delivery and manipulation.

Bracht maneuver: Bracht maneuver (1935) is the delivery of breech with minimal interference. It has been described by Erich Bracht (1882–1969). The procedure involves spontaneous delivery only by supporting the baby's body against gravity during birth, without use of traction. The traction interferes with the normal mechanism of labor.

COMPLETE BREECH EXTRACTION

Hurried delivery of the baby is done by an obstetrician prior to engagement usually under GA. Groin traction is performed to deliver the podalic end. Lovset maneuver is employed routinely. Downward traction is done to bring the head in pelvis. All the stages of assisted breech delivery are done actively by the obstetrician Second baby of twin which is in transverse lie is delivered by breech extraction after IPV.

COMPLICATED BREECH DELIVERY

Arrest of Buttocks at the Perineum

The causes are weak uterine contraction, rigid perineum, large baby with extended legs, and pelvic outlet contraction.

Management if Arrest Occurs at the Perineum

It depends upon the causes. In weak uterine contraction, oxytocin infusion is started. In rigid perineum, episiotomy with groin traction is given. In breech with extended legs, groin traction is given. In case of pelvic outlet contraction, cesarean section can be done even at this stage.

Groin Traction (Figs. 35 and 36)

Indications are breech with extended legs and arrest at outlet. Types are single-groin traction and double-groin traction.

Procedure: Following episiotomy, the index finger is placed at the anterior groin and traction is given more toward the trunk than the femur. This is done during contractions. Simultaneous fundal pressure is also given. Anterior groin is manipulated at the beginning. Traction with the other index finger may also be given in the posterior groin when the buttocks are born. The traction is continued till the delivery up to the level of knee when the anterior leg is released followed by the posterior leg. Breech hook is applied only in the case of *dead fetus.* Groin traction is seldom practiced nowadays.

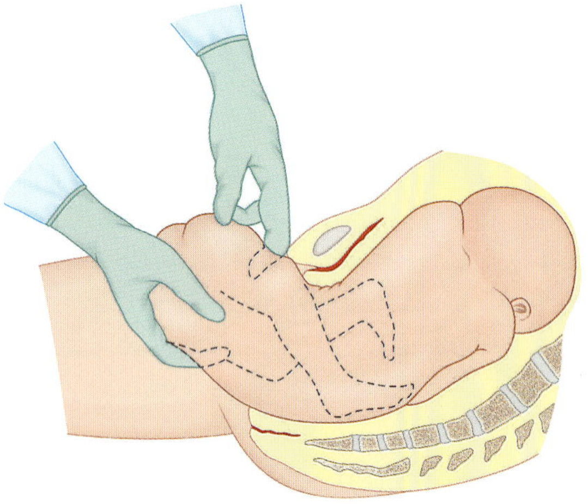

Fig. 35: Groin traction in frank breech (diagramatic).

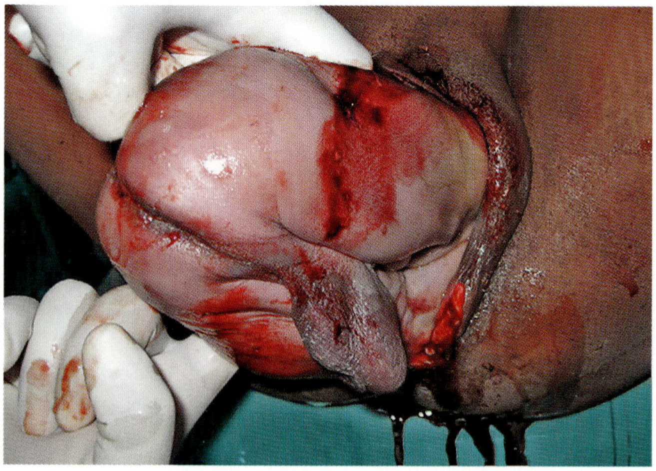

Fig. 36: Groin traction in frank breech.

Arrest of Buttocks in the Pelvic Cavity and Above

The causes are weak uterine contractions, large baby, contracted pelvis, combination of multiple factors such as extended legs, and weak uterine contractions. When buttocks in the pelvic cavity (ischial spine) and above it are usual than when cervix becomes fully dilated, buttocks should come to the perineum. If this does not occur, interference is needed. Cesarean section is the treatment of choice in this condition. However, *Pinard's maneuver* may be attempted in breech with extended legs.

Pinard's Maneuver (Frank Breech Extraction) (1889)

Indications: Breech with extended legs gets arrested in the pelvic cavity and above (groin traction is given when arrest occurs at the level of perineum).

Principle: It is the process of breech delivery which involves manipulation within the birth canal to convert a frank breech into a footling breech. It helps in bringing the fetal feet within the reach of the operator (bringing down the legs).

*Procedure **(Fig. 37)**:* The index and middle fingers are carried up to the knee (popliteal fossa); then pressure is exerted and leg is abducted. Spontaneous flexion usually occurs and then the foot is grasped and brought down. The hand is chosen in such a way that the palmer aspect will face the ventral aspect of the fetus. This procedure should be done under anesthesia.

Delay In Delivery of the Shoulder

Reasons are mainly due to extended arms with lateral or dorsal (nuchal) displacement. Extension of the arms occurs mostly due to unnecessary pulling of fetus from below during delivery. The principle "Don't traction from below but push from above" is followed to avoid extension of arms. Diagnosis is done by observing the winging of scapula and absence of the fetal arms in front of the chest of the fetus.

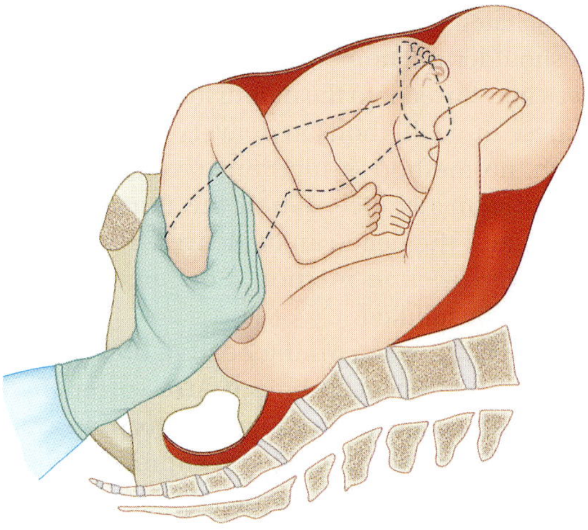

Fig. 37: Pinard's maneuver for bringing down a leg.

Management of breech with extended arms are classical method or Lovset maneuver.

Classical Method

Principle: By internal manipulation, the posterior arm is brought down first followed by the anterior one.

Procedure: General anesthesia is administered. The choice of hand to be introduced is one that corresponds to the back of the baby. The angle of the anterior shoulder is brought under subpubic angle by pulling the fetus. The baby's trunk is lifted along the ventral aspect of the baby by holding the ankles. The index and middle fingers of the selected hand are introduced along the posterior arm till the elbow is reached. Then the fingers are applied as splint to the posterior arm which is pushed over the face of the baby and then gradually pulled down. The extended anterior arm is pushed down by introducing the other arm in similar fashion while the baby's trunk is depressed toward the perineum. In case of dorsal or nuchal displacement, the baby's trunk is rotated so that the arm is made posterior and delivery is done as previously.

Lovset Maneuver (Figs. 38 to 41)

Lovset maneuver is one of the methods of bringing down the extended arms (1937) during breech delivery.

Principle: The method is based on taking advantage of configuration of pelvic architecture where the lower part of the anterior wall of pelvis is deficient. When the posterior shoulder which lies below the sacral promontory is rotated forward, it would appear below the symphysis pubis and can be delivered easily. The other shoulder can also be delivered by rotation of the trunk in reverse direction.

Prerequisites are that the inferior angle on the anterior scapula must come below the symphysis pubis before attempting the procedure. The shoulder should lie in the anteroposterior diameter of the pelvis. The posterior shoulder should lie below the sacral promontory.

Procedure

Step I: The trunk of the baby is grasped with *femoropelvic grip* keeping medial sides of the thumbs parallel to each other. The buttock is slightly elevated anteriorly at first, thus maintaining the downward pull to make lateral flexion of the trunk. This will bring the posterior shoulder much below the sacral promontory. The trunk of the baby is rotated 180° keeping the back anterior. The completion of rotation will bring the posterior shoulder to emerge below the symphysis pubis and then brought down by hooking.

Step II: The other shoulder is then delivered by rotation of the trunk in reverse direction keeping the back anterior.

Advantages are that no internal manipulation is needed, no GA is required, it can be done when the classical method is difficult, and it is safe and easy to do.

Entrapment of the Aftercoming Head of Breech

This is the most crucial condition as it causes compression of the umbilical cord, and until and unless delivered quickly the baby will be asphyxiated or will die. The causes are deflexed head, large baby, occipitoposterior position, hydrocephalus,

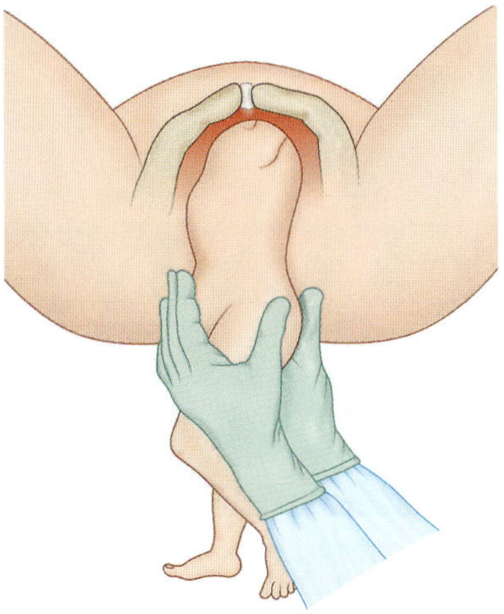

Fig. 38: Lovset maneuver. Trunk is grasped with femoro pelvic grip, slightly elevated anteriorly and then rotated 180°.

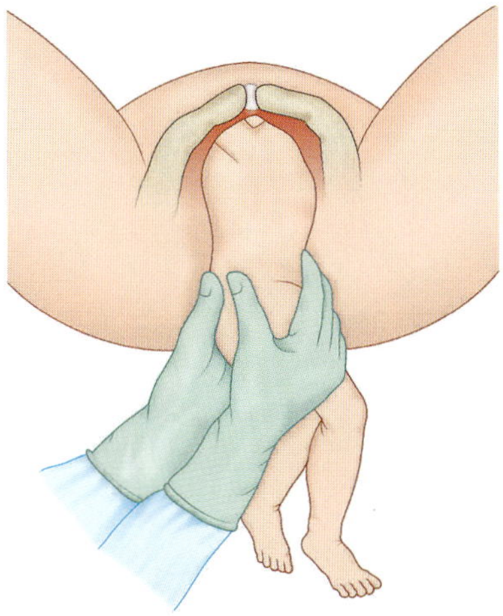

Fig. 39: Lovset maneuver. Posterior shoulder emerges below symphysis pubis as anterior.

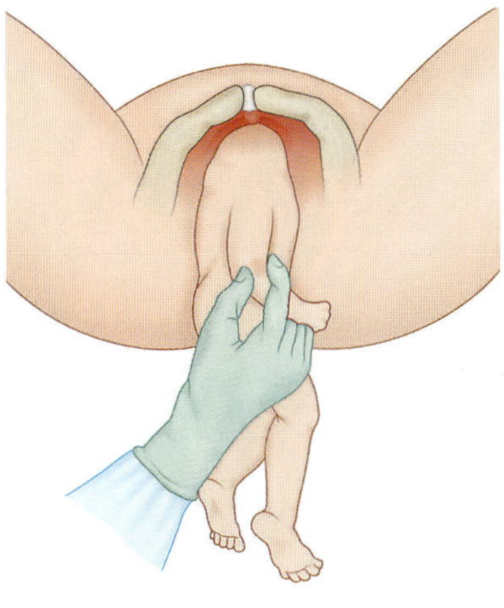

Fig. 40: Lovset maneuver. The shoulder is delivered and again trunk is rotated 180° in reverse direction.

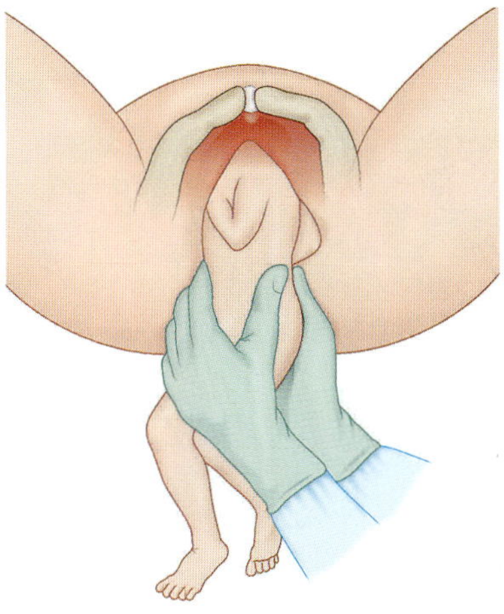

Fig. 41: Lovset maneuver. The other shoulder is delivered below the symphysis pubis.

rigid perineum, incompletely dilated cervix, and pelvic contraction.

Management depends on the cause. If it is due to rigid perineum, episiotomy is given. If needed, either forceps delivery or malar flexion shoulder traction is done depending upon the station of the head. If it is only for deflexed head if the head is in the pelvic cavity, episiotomy and forceps are given to deliver fetal head.

When head is high up, it is delivered by malar flexion and shoulder traction. If the cause is large baby, malar flexion and shoulder traction may be attempted. In occipitoposterior position, the fetal trunk and head are rotated to bring back of the fetus to anterior. If not possible (in case of premature baby), the head is delivered face to pubis by reverse jaw flexion and shoulder traction maneuver (Prague maneuver) **(Fig. 42)** or by forceps. Prague maneuver is the reversed malar flexion and shoulder traction method.

In hydrocephalus, perforation of the head is done. In incompletely dilated cervix which usually occurs in the case of small premature baby, the cervix may be manually slipped over the occiput while giving gentle traction on the fetus (shoe-horn method). **Figures 43 to 45** show arrest of aftercoming head in undilated cervix in prolapsed uterus and living baby was delivered vaginally by manual slipping over the occiput.

If this fails, *Duhrssen incisions* at 10, 2, and 6 o'clock positions are given **(Fig. 46)**. The positions are so selected that bleeding from laterally located cervical branches of the uterine artery is minimum. After delivery, the cut margins are repaired.

Contracted pelvis: Malar flexion and shoulder traction method may be tried in minor contractions. If the pelvic contraction is significant, the baby usually dies and craniotomy is done to deliver it.

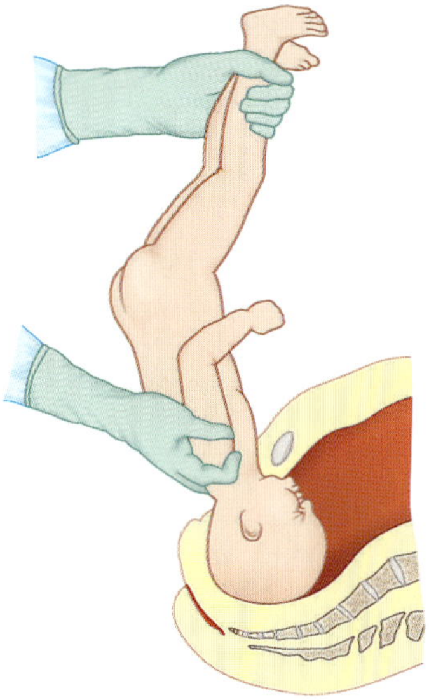

Fig. 42: Prague maneuver.

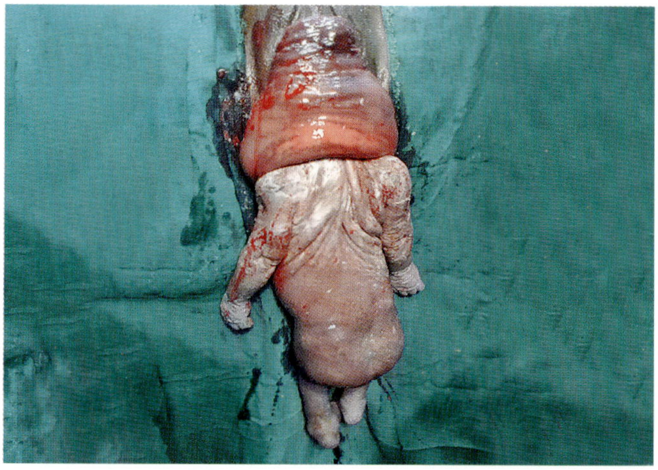

Fig. 43: Arrest of aftercoming head of breech in undilated cervix in a case of genital prolapse.

Courtesy: Dr Anirban Mondal, Associate Professor, Bankura Sammilani Medical College and Hospital, Bankura, West Bengal, India.

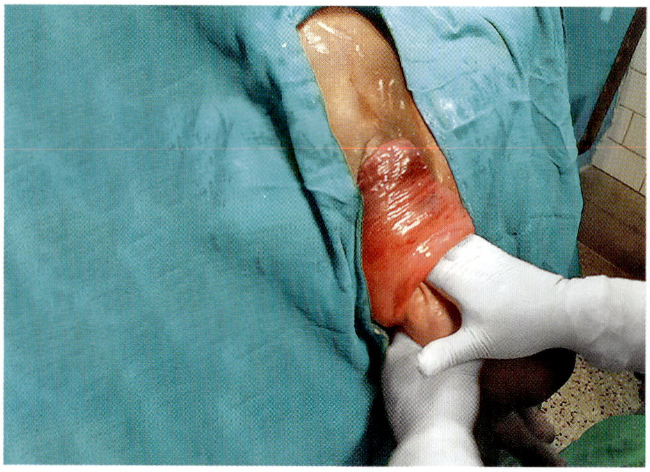

Fig. 44: Cervix is manually slipped over the occiput to deliver the aftercoming head as in the patient (Figure 43).

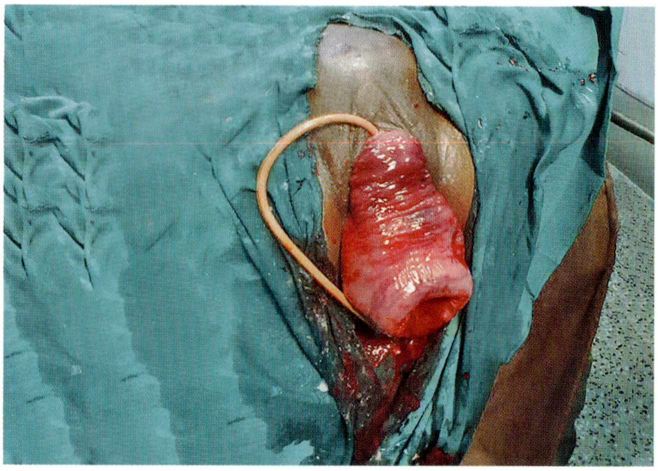

Fig. 45: Prolapsed cervix atter delivery as case in Figures 43 and 44. Look, there is no injury of cervix.

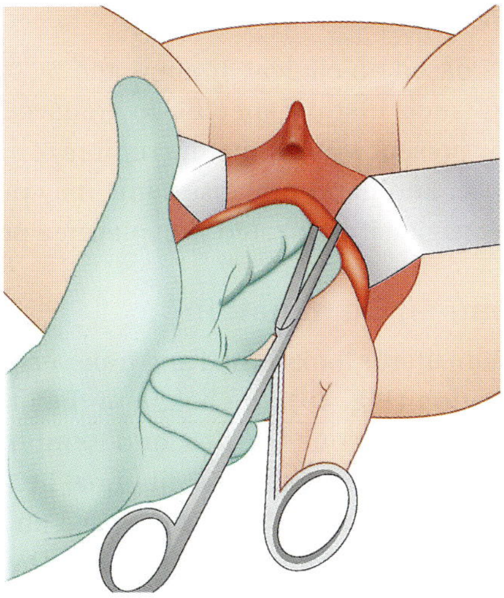

Fig. 46: Duhrssen incisions.

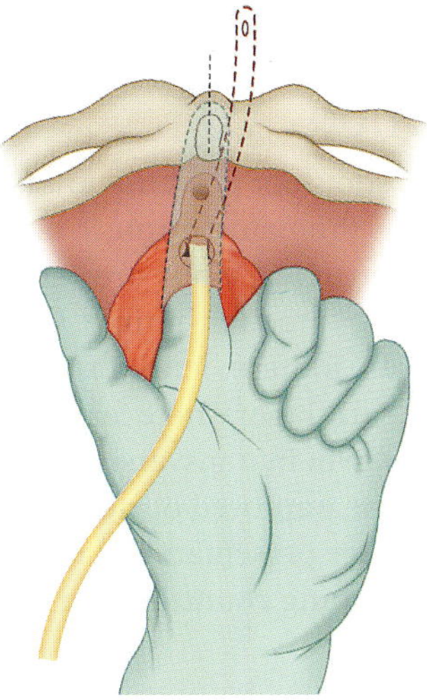

Fig. 47: Symphysiotomy—catheterization done and finger is kept behind symphysis pubis.

Symphysiotomy (Figs. 47 and 48)

Though rarely done, in case of arrest of aftercoming head of breech, symphysiotomy may be practiced deliberately to enlarge the anterior pelvis to complete the delivery. The details are given in chapter 13.

Zavanelli Maneuver

Zavanelli maneuver is a method by which the fetus is replaced into the vagina and uterus, and cesarean delivery is accomplished. It is classically practiced in shoulder dystocia.

CESAREAN DELIVERY IN BREECH PRESENTATION

Cesarean delivery in breech presentation is not without risk to the baby and the same type of injury may occur as encountered in vaginal breech delivery. Long bone fracture is common in abdominal breech delivery.

Procedures and Precautions During Cesarean Delivery

Laparotomy incision should be adequate and uterine incision should be generous.

In preterm fetus, the lower uterine segment is not well formed, especially when the patient is not in labor. If the lower uterine segment is not wide, it is better to give vertical incision than to extend by T-shaped or H-shaped incision.

In case of frank breech, buttock is lifted through uterine wound and is delivered in leg-extended condition by hooking the index finger inside groin and applying traction. Simultaneously, the back of the fetus is made anterior.

In case of incomplete breech, the feet are delivered one by one; then traction is given holding both the feet. Once the buttock comes outside, the fetus is held in femoropelvic grip by placing the fingers on iliac crest and this will protect fetal abdominal structure from compression.

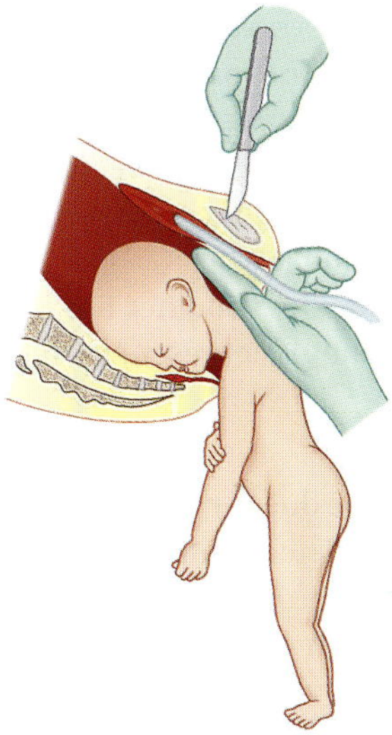

Fig. 48: Symphysiotomy—symphysis pubis is severed by scalpel.

The arms are delivered one after another by simply hooking the elbow with the fingers. Two fingers of the appropriate hand (right for right shoulder) are placed over the clavicle and swept round the point of shoulder that is traced down the humerus to the elbow and the forearm is thus made free. Arms can be delivered by rotating the trunk in Lovset maneuver fashion when hands are extended.

Aftercoming head is delivered by malar flexion and shoulder traction method (Mauriceau-Smellie-Veit technique) or by using forceps (Piper). In all cases, the neck should not be extended. Forceps are applied below the body of the fetus keeping the operator's hand inside the uterus. After articulation, head is delivered by flexion.

All manipulations should be gentle, slow, and not to be hurried avoiding mishandling of the fetus.

TRANSVERSE LIE

INTRODUCTION

Transverse lie or shoulder presentation is not uncommon in clinical practice. Premature rupture of membranes, cord prolapse, and obstructed labor are the consequences if unattended and not cared for in time. Cesarean delivery is the mode of delivery for term fetus. External version may be tried at term or in early labor where feasible. IPV can be done for second baby of twin in transverse lie provided the liquor is adequate. With the improved obstetric care, the incidence of neglected shoulder presentation has become less; still it is seen some developing countries and referred from rural areas.

The incidence of shoulder presentation is near 3 in 1,000 deliveries at term.

DEFINITION

Lie is said to be transverse when the long axis of the fetus lies perpendicular to the long axis of the maternal spine or centralized uterus. When the long axis of the fetus forms an acute angle, it results in oblique lie. In labor, the oblique lie becomes either longitudinal or transverse; therefore, oblique lie is usually transitional.

In transverse lie, the shoulder lies over the pelvic inlet; hence, it is called shoulder presentation.

ETIOLOGY

Transverse lie may be due to maternal factors and fetal factors. No obvious cause is detected in a significant number of cases.

Maternal causes are multiparity with lax abdomen—10-fold increase with four or more deliveries, contracted pelvis, placenta previa, uterine anomaly—subseptate or arcuate, hydramnios, and pelvic tumor.

Fetal causes are prematurity, multiple pregnancy, intrauterine fetal death, and fetal congenital anomaly.

DIAGNOSIS

Diagnosis is based on clinical findings and by sonography. There is no such history specific to transverse lie; few patients may present with premature rupture of membranes, cord prolapse, and hand prolapse some may present with bleeding per vagina if associated with placenta previa.

Per Abdominal Examination

On inspection, uterus looks broad and transversely oval.

On palpation **(Fig. 49)**, the height of the uterus is less than the period of amenorrhea and symphysiofundal height is less than expected in longitudinal lie. The fundal and pelvic grips are empty, head is palpated on one side of midline or obliquely on one or other iliac fossa by lateral grip and breech on the other side.

Per Vaginal Examination

(It should only be done after exclusion of placenta previa)
Patient not in labor—presenting part is at higher level from the cervix and fornix. Only some soft parts are palpable with difficulty.

Patient in labor:

- *In early stage*: There may be an elongated bag of membranes. The side of the thorax, if approachable, may be identified by the "grid iron" feel of the ribs.
- *With cervical dilatation*: Following rupture of membranes, shoulder presentation is diagnosed by the palpation of the acromion process, scapula, clavicle, and axilla **(Fig. 50)**. The position of the axilla indicates the side of the mother toward which the shoulder is situated. There may be prolapse of the hand and arm **(Figs. 51 to 53)**.
- There may be presence of cord prolapse.

Prolapsed hand may also be found in case of compound presentation like with head and breech **(Figs. 54 and 55)**.

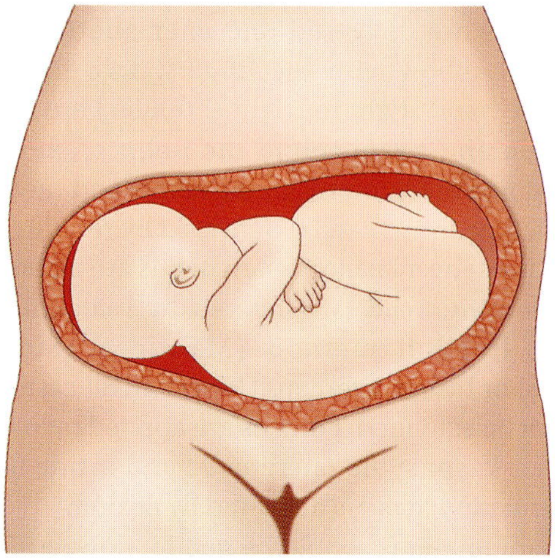

Fig. 49: Transverse lie.

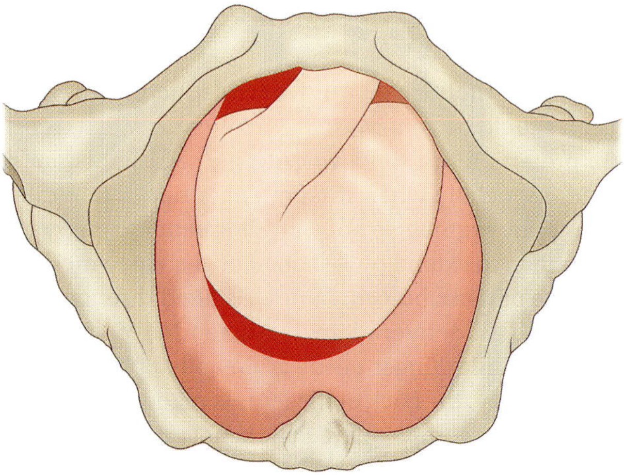

Fig. 50: Vaginal findings of shoulder presentation (Dorsoposterior).

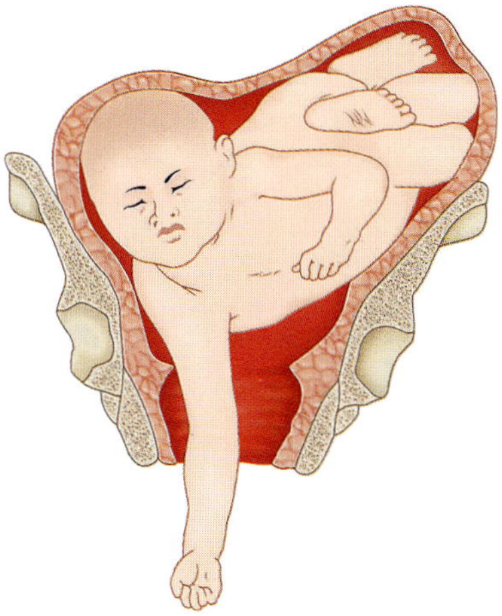

Fig. 51: Transverse lie with hand prolapse.

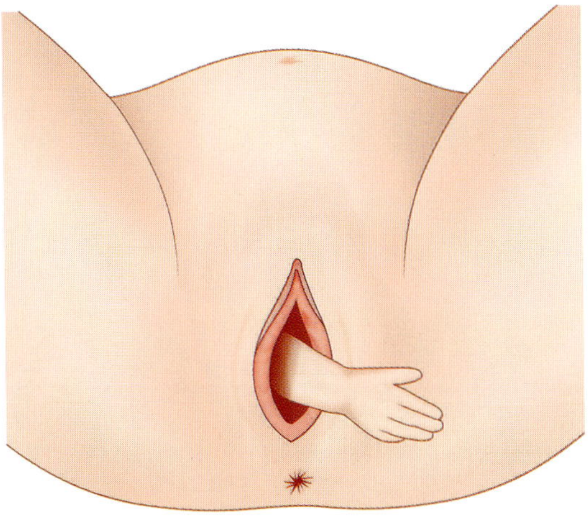

Fig. 52: Prolapsed hand visible through perineum.

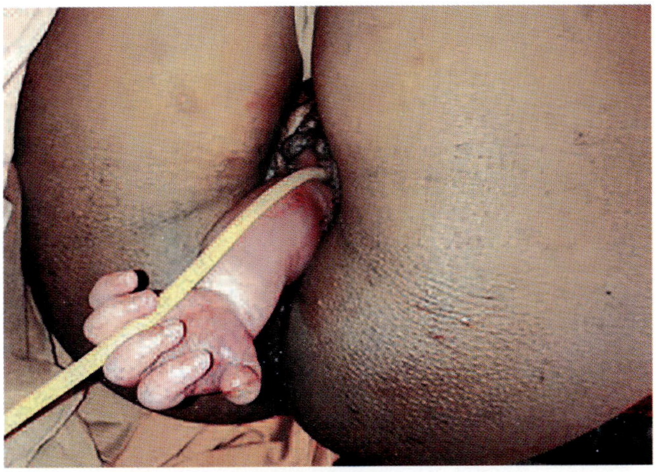

Fig. 53: Hand prolapse in transverse lie.
Courtesy : Dr Abhisek Bhadra, Assistant Professor, Calcutta Medical College, Kolkata, West Bengal, India.

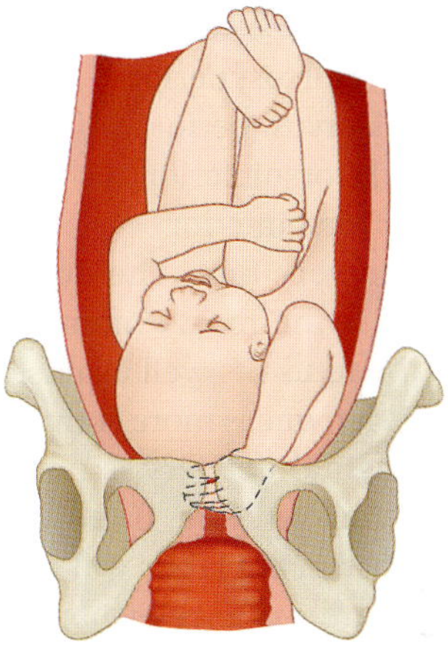

Fig. 54: Compound presentation—hand below the head.

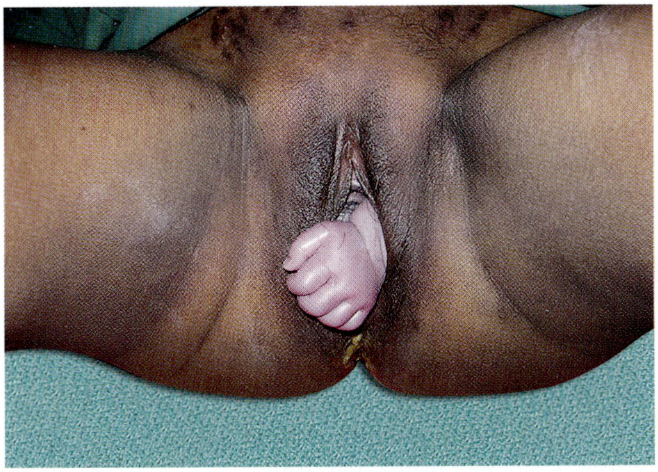

Fig. 55: Compound presentation—hand below the head.
Courtesy: Professor SL Seal, Department of Gynecology and Obstetrics, RG Kar Medical College, Kolkata, West Bengal, India.

Determination of Position of Fetal Head by the Prolapsed Hand

In outstretched hand when the palm points toward the fetal abdomen, the direction of the thumb indicates the direction of the fetal head.

Sonography

Diagnosis of transverse lie is confirmed by sonography. The other advantages of sonography are the same as in breech presentation.

MECHANISM OF LABOR IN TRANSVERSE LIE

Denominator in case of transverse lie is the back of the fetus. There may be eight positions in transverse lie:

1. (Right acromion) Dorsoanterior **(Fig. 56)**
2. (Left acromion) Dorsoanterior

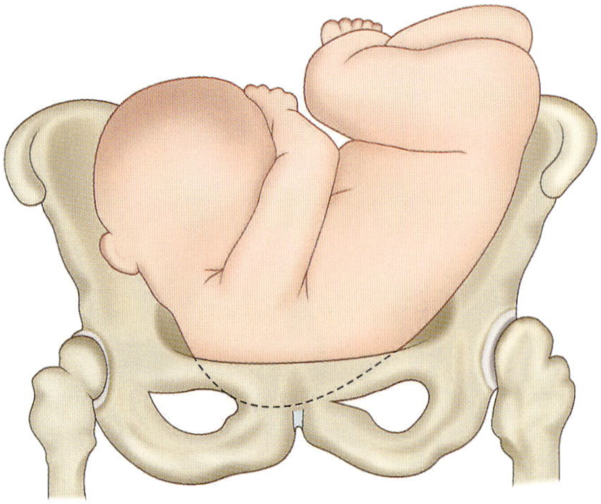

Fig. 56: Dorsoanterior (right acromion) shoulder presentation (most common).

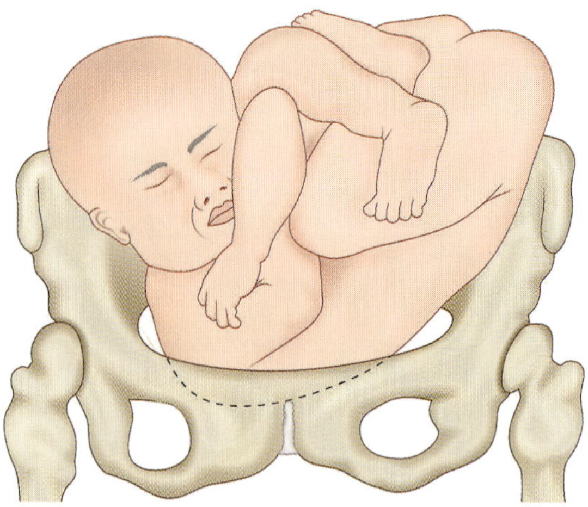

Fig. 57: Dorsoposterior (right acromion) shoulder presentation.

3. (Right acromion) Dorsoposterior **(Fig. 57)**
4. (Left acromion) Dorsoposterior
5. (Right acromion) Dorsosuperior
6. (Left acromion) Dorsosuperior
7. (Right acromion) Dorsoinferior
8. (Left acromion) Dorsoinferior

The last four are very rare. The dorsoanterior (60%), either right or left, is the most common position as the ventral aspect of the fetus fits well against the convexity of maternal spine. The left one is more common than the right.

Spontaneous vaginal delivery is not possible in case of mature fetus in transverse lie. If the labor progresses, it is inevitable that obstructed labor will occur (unfavorable outcome). In very rare instances when the fetus is small (<800 g), spontaneous delivery is possible by a special mechanism (see here).

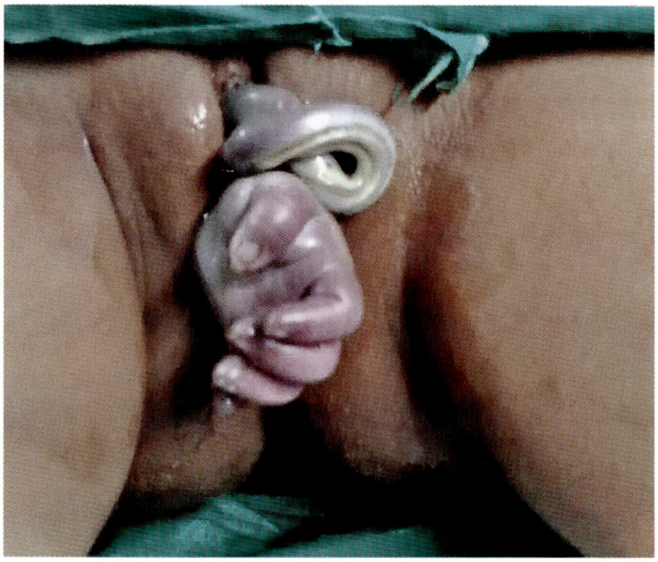

Fig. 58: Hand prolapse and cord prolapse together.

RISKS OF TRANSVERSE LIE

Risks of transverse lie are early or premature rupture of membrane, chance of cord prolapse, hand prolapse **(Figs. 53 and 58)**, and development of obstructed labor and its consequences.

Maternal risks are dehydration, ketosis, sepsis, shock, hemorrhage, chances of operative interference, and rupture of uterus.

Fetal risks are increased perinatal morbidity and mortality (25–50%) due to cord prolapse, dry labor and tonic uterine contraction, prolonged labor, and rupture of uterus.

In dorsoposterior position, the chance of fetal extension is more; hence, there is more chance of hand prolapse.

OUTCOME OF TRANSVERSE LIE FOLLOWING LABOR

If labor is allowed to continue uncared for in case of mature fetus with persistent transverse lie, rupture of membranes occurs with drainage of liquor. There may be cord prolapse → fetal shoulder is forced into the pelvis → corresponding arm is prolapsed → more descent → shoulder is arrested in the pelvic inlet with head in one iliac fossa and breech in the other → shoulder is wedged and impacted in the pelvis → vigorous uterine contraction → features of obstructed labor with formation of a pathological retraction ring → neglected shoulder presentation results **(Fig. 59)** → if left uncared for, the mother gets exhausted with dehydration, ketosis and sepsis, and the fetus usually dies → rupture of uterus occurs specially in multigravida.

FAVORABLE OUTCOME IN TRANSVERSE LIE

In a very small fetus (weight <800 g), spontaneous vaginal delivery may occur by the following:

- *Spontaneous version or rectification*: It is the sudden correction of the lie after the onset of labor where uterine contraction forces the head (rectification) or breech by

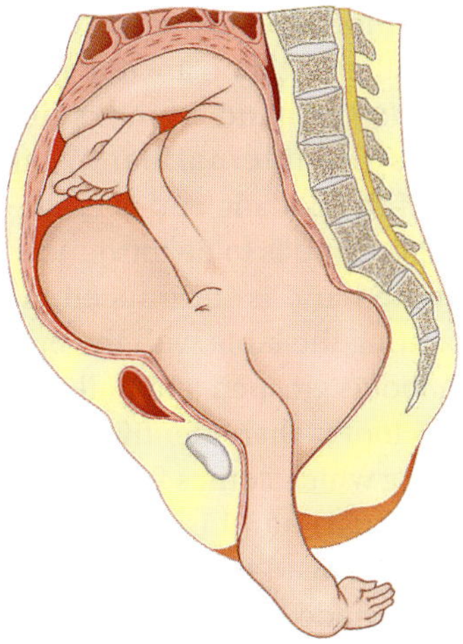

Fig. 59: Neglected shoulder presentation.

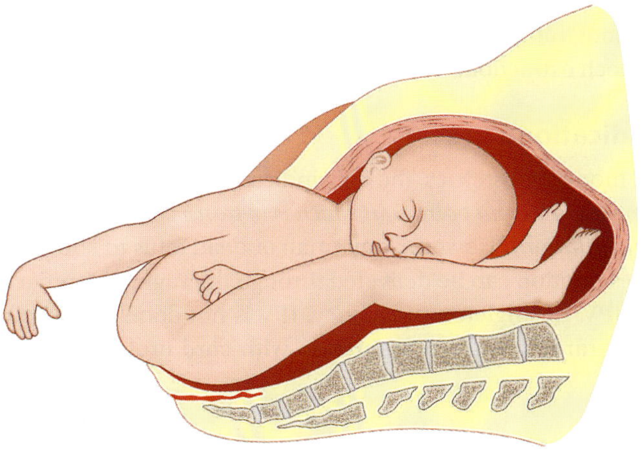

Fig. 60: Spontaneous evolution.

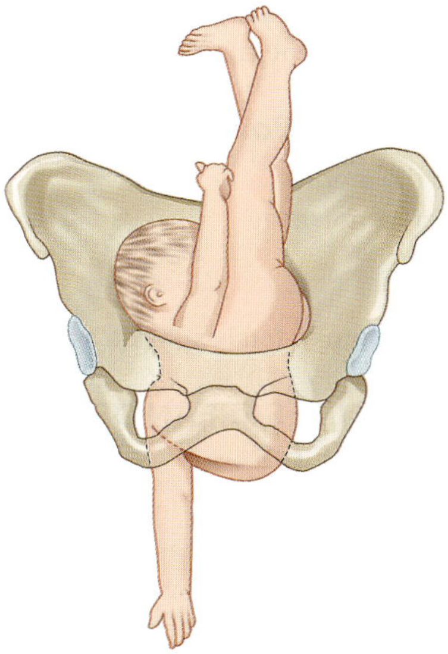

Fig. 61: Spontaneous expulsion or conduplicato corpore.

version to come into the pelvic inlet. It may occur when the liquor amount is good.

- *Spontaneous evolution* **(Fig. 60)**: When the contraction is vigorous, breech and trunk are delivered first followed by the delivery of the head.
- *Spontaneous expulsion or conduplicato corpore* **(Fig. 61)**: In this condition, the spontaneous expulsion of fetus occurs after *doubling up* at the trunk. It occurs rarely.

MANAGEMENT OF PREGNANCY WITH TRANSVERSE LIE

Definitive Management of Transverse Lie in Antenatal Period

External cephalic version is the treatment of choice after 36 weeks if there is no contraindication or co-complication.

Some prefer attempt of ECV only after 39 weeks because there is a high chance of spontaneous version if done earlier.

In case of Rh-negative mother, Rh anti-D immune prophylaxis is given.

If ECV is contraindicated or it fails, elective cesarean section is performed at term. The patient is admitted at 37 weeks. The version can be repeated before lower uterine cesarean section (LUCS) if there is no contraindication.

Transverse Lie with Mature Baby in Early Labor

When the mother is in early labor, the membranes are intact. ECV is attempted, if there is no other complication or contraindication for ECV. Following version, the head should be held in the pelvis during the next several contractions in an attempt to fix the head. If ECV fails or is contraindicated, cesarean section is performed. With ruptured membranes, delivery by cesarean section is the preferred option.

Transverse Lie with Mature Fetus in Late Labor

If the baby is alive, *cesarean section* is the most preferred method. However, if the membrane is intact, ECV may be attempted. When the cervix is fully dilated, IPV under GA is an option to deliver the baby immediately after the rupture of membranes although not preferred in case of singleton pregnancy. *In the modern-day obstetrics, the role of IPV is limited only to the second baby of twin in transverse lie.*

If the baby is dead, destructive operation, either decapitation (when neck is approachable) or evisceration (when neck is not approachable), is done. Uterine cavity is routinely explored following destructive operation. However, when the obstetrician is not well conversant with destructive operation, cesarean section is the safer method of delivery even for dead baby.

INTERNAL PODALIC VERSION

Internal podalic version is a type of version which is done through the vaginal approach, and the podalic end is drawn inside the vagina to make the presentation breech and the lie longitudinal. Following version, the baby is delivered by breech extraction.

Indications

In modern obstetrics, the only indication of internal podalic version is *second baby twin which is in transverse lie (shoulder presentation)*. However, any small or dead fetus in shoulder presentation can be delivered through the vaginal approach by IPV. In singleton pregnancy, IPV is not done nowadays. Very rarely, vertex presentation with cord prolapse IPV is done.

Criteria to be Fulfilled before Attempting Internal Podalic Version

Cervical os must be fully dilated (patient is in second stage).

There should be good relaxation of the uterus. There should be presence of sufficient liquor amnii. Membranes are immediately ruptured or attempt of IPV is done just after rupturing the membranes.

When there is no liquor, attempt of IPV will be dangerous which may result in ruptured uterus.

Fetus should be alive. Obstetrician must be experienced in this procedure.

Contraindications of Internal Podalic Version

Contraindications are neglected shoulder presentation, absence of liquor amnii, and pregnancy with prior cesarean delivery.

Procedures of Internal Podalic Version (Figs. 62 and 63)

- It should always be done at the operation theater and under GA.
- Patient is in lithotomy position. Antiseptic dressing, draping, and catheterization are done.
- *Choice of hand*: The hand which is on the side of the podalic end is the internal hand. Like in shoulder presentation, if the podalic end is on the left side of the patient, the right hand is to be introduced.
- The appropriate hand is introduced in a cone-shaped fashion separating the labia with the other hand outside the uterus. A foot is grasped and pulled down by holding the ankle. The foot is then identified by the palpation of the heel. The leg which comes first is drawn first.
- The other (external) hand is placed over the head per abdomen, and the head is pushed toward the fundus so that the fetus is made longitudinal and the leg is drawn inside the vagina with a steady traction.
- The other leg is brought down easily after the first leg. The fetus is delivered by breech extraction following IPV.
- Following delivery of the placenta, the uterine cavity is explored to exclude the rupture of uterus.

Dangers of Internal Podalic Version

- Rupture of the uterus
- Postpartum hemorrhage
- Shock
- Infection
- Fetal complications—fetal asphyxia and fetal death

DIFFICULTY IN CESAREAN DELIVERY IN TRANSVERSE LIE

As no pole lies in the lower uterine segment, *it is not well formed* and so low transverse cesarean section approach leads to the difficulty of extraction of the fetus. By grasping the legs first (podalic end), the baby is delivered as breech delivery. Transverse uterine wound may be extended by "J"-shaped incision or by inverted "T." "J"-shaped incision

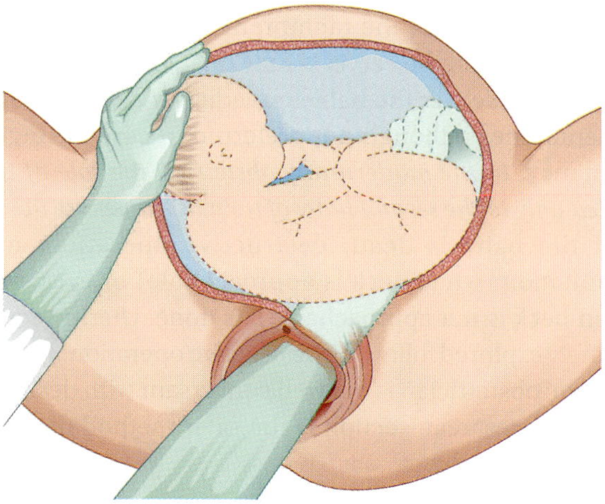

Fig. 62: Internal podalic version (IPV). A foot is grasped and pulled down by holding the ankle.

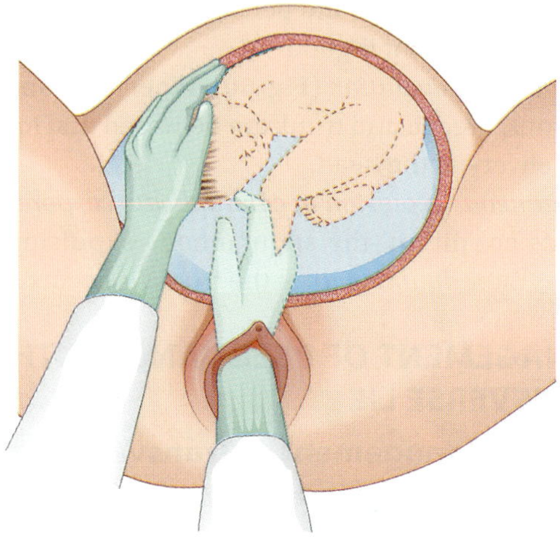

Fig. 63: Internal podalic version (IPV)—the head is pushed by outer hand towards the fundus so that the fetus is made longitudinal and the leg is drawn inside the vagina gently.

is preferred to inverted "T." Vertical incision is also preferred by many obstetricians. (See Chapter16 of Cesarean Delivery)

NEGLECTED SHOULDER PRESENTATION (FIGS. 59 AND 64)

Neglected shoulder presentation or neglected transverse lie is a situation comprising several complications that develop due to uncared for and unattended labor in a shoulder presentation. The sequences are impaction and wedging of the shoulder → obstructed labor → dehydration, ketosis, sepsis → ruptured uterus.

Management aims at prevention of the condition by managing the shoulder presentation in early labor. In established cases, first the resuscitation of mother is done with IV fluid, antibiotics, and blood transfusion followed by delivery of the baby.

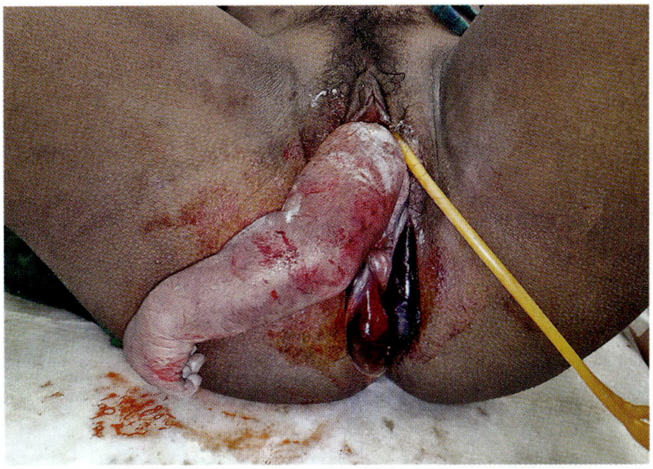

Fig. 64: Hand prolapse in neglected shoulder presentation.

Method of Delivery in Neglected Shoulder Presentation

When the baby is dead (which invariably occurs in almost all cases), destructive operation, either decapitation or evisceration (see Chapter 26 of Destructive Operation), is performed provided there is no ruptured uterus or impending rupture. In cases of suspected rupture or impending rupture or when the obstetrician is not well conversant with the procedure, laparotomy and cesarean delivery are done. Internal podalic version should never be attempted in neglected shoulder presentation.

CHAPTER 9

Twin Delivery

Learning Objectives

- Incidence of Multiple Gestations and Etiology
- Risks and Complications of Multiple Pregnancy
- Special Problems Specific to Monochorionic Twins
- Neonatal Prognosis In Multiple Pregnancy
- Embryology of Twin Gestation
- Determination of Chorionicity
- Diagnosis of Twin Gestation
- Management of Twin Pregnancy
- Time of Delivery
- Role of Induction and Augmentation
- Choice of Route of Delivery
- Indications of Cesarean Delivery
- Management of Labor in Twin Pregnancy
- Management of Some of the Common Complications Encountered during Second Stage of Labor
- Technique of Cesaren Delivery in Twin Gestation
- Twin Delivery in Pregnancy with Previous Cesarean Delivery
- Triplet or Higher Order Multiple Gestation

INTRODUCTION

Multiple pregnancy is associated with morbidity and mortality of both the mother and fetuses and neonates. Presently, the incidence of twin gestations is about 3–3.3%. Increased incidence of twin and higher order gestations is due to the infertility treatment and assisted reproductive technology (ART). Another factor is conception in advance age. Recent tendency of transfer of a smaller number of embryos ART program has decreased the triplet and higher order gestations. The rate of cesarean delivery in twin gestation has increased to >75%. There is consensus that the route of delivery of presentation in cephalic—cephalic at term is vaginal [American College of Obstetricians and Gynecologists (ACOG) 2021]. There is no improvement of perinatal outcome by cesarean delivery when first twin is cephalic. Regarding other combinations there is controversy but not all are indicated for cesarean delivery. Twin Birth Study (2013) was a large randomized trial which showed no difference of composite outcome in planned cesarean and planned vaginal delivery not considering the cesarean delivery itself a morbidity. Training and skill development for twin vaginal delivery is essential for every obstetric provider.

INCIDENCE OF MULTIPLE GESTATIONS AND ETIOLOGY

Only few decades back, the overall incidence of twin pregnancy was 1 in 80. The incidence of multiple births has increased dramatically for last few decades with 40% increase in twining rates and 3–4-fold rise in higher order multiple births mainly due to infertility therapy.

It varies with age, parity, and race. In older mothers, increased tendency of twinning is due to rise in follicle-stimulating hormone (FSH) levels. Delayed childbearing is another risk factor. Familial predisposition is explained by autosomal dominant inheritance. The incidence of monozygotic twins is relatively constant worldwide (1 in 250). However, there has been increase in monozygotic twinning also among women taking oral contraceptives and following in vitro fertilization (IVF) procedures, the cause is unknown.

Relative prevalence of dizygotic twins is two-thirds and monozygotic—one-third.

RISKS AND COMPLICATIONS OF MULTIPLE PREGNANCY

Maternal Complications of Multiple Pregnancy

Antenatal

Exaggerated pregnancy symptoms, mechanical distress, anemia, increase of preeclampsia by fourfold in multiple pregnancy than singleton pregnancy. Hydramnios especially acute hydramnios is more common in monozygotic twins. The second twin is affected most. Antepartum hemorrhage (APH), malpresentation, preterm labor, premature rupture of membranes, and obstructive uropathy are other complications. Preterm labor occurs in 50–60% cases and preterm prelabor rupture of the membrane (pPROM) in 10% cases. Latency period of pPROM is less (4 days) than that in singleton pregnancy (7 days).

Intranatal

Early rupture of membranes, cord prolapse, difficulty in delivery due to malpresentation, increased operative interference, and obstetric manipulations are the various risks. Locked twins is very rare complication. Intrapartum hemorrhage, retained placenta, and postpartum hemorrhage (PPH) are common. Uterine atonicity plays a role.

Postnatal

Puerperal sepsis, problems in lactation, and subinvolution of the uterus are increased risks in twin gestations.

Maternal Prognosis

Maternal morbidity and mortality increase due to anemia, preeclampsia, hemorrhage (APH and PPH), and increased operative and manipulative interference. It increases with the increase in number of fetuses.

Fetal Problems in Multiple Pregnancy

- *Spontaneous abortion:* More common in monozygotic twins.
- *Fetal growth restriction:* The degree of growth restriction is increased in monozygotic twins.
- Discordant growth is found in both dizygotic and monozygotic twins though the etiology is different. In monochorionic twins, discordance is attributed to placental vascular anastomosis (see below).
- *Prematurity:* Twins—50 to 60%, triplets—92%, mean gestation age in twins—37 weeks. It is the single most common cause of perinatal mortality in multiple pregnancy.
- *Congenital anomaly of fetus:* More common in monochorionic twins.
- *Intrauterine death (IUD) of fetus:* Demise of one fetus is more common than both fetuses in twin pregnancy. There is an adverse impact of dead fetus on the living one.
- Birth asphyxia and stillbirth are more common in twin pregnancy than in singleton pregnancy.
- Increase neonatal seizure, intraventricular hemorrhage, intubation, and neonatal intensive care unit (NICU) admission

DISCORDANT TWINS (FIG. 1)

Discordancy is expressed in percentage and determined from the estimated weight of each twin with the help of sonography.

$$\text{Percent} = \frac{\text{Weight of larger twin in grams} - \text{Weight of smaller twin in grams}}{\text{Weight of larger twin in grams}}$$

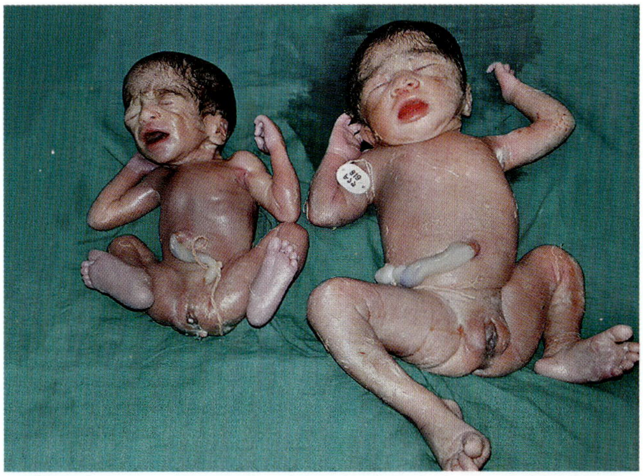

Fig. 1: Discordant twin. First twin—female 1.6 kg, second twin—female 750 g, vaginal delivery at 33 weeks
Courtesy: Dr Richa Hatila, RG Kar Medical College, Kolkata, West Bengal, India.

Discordancy >25–30% is associated with adverse perinatal outcome.

OTHER FATES OF TWIN FETUSES

- Vanishing twin (30–35%)
- Fetus papyraceous and fetus compressus **(Fig. 2)**
- Acardiac twin [twin reversed arterial perfusion (TRAP)] **(Fig. 3)**
- Twin-to-twin transfusion syndrome (TTTS)(Details are discussed in Chapter 7 of Fetal Therapy).

SPECIAL PROBLEMS SPECIFIC TO MONOCHORIONIC TWINS

- Placental vascular anastomosis resulting in twin reversal arterial perfusion (TRAP)—acardiac twin, Twin-twin transfusion syndrome (TTTS)
- Shared vascular connections resulting demise of cotwin, when one fetus dies, the living twin suffers from several problems like disseminated intravascular coagulation (DIC), neurological and renal problems.
- Cord entanglement and death, if it becomes monoamnionic.
- Conjoined twins **(Figs. 4 to 9)**

NEONATAL PROGNOSIS IN MULTIPLE PREGNANCY

Perinatal morbidity and mortality increase due to prematurity, intrauterine growth restriction (IUGR), congenital anomaly, problems during birth, etc. Perinatal mortality rate (PMR) is six times higher in twin babies than singleton baby. Monochorionic twins are at higher risk. The second baby is at higher risk than the first one. More the delay in the second twin higher is the adverse effect on second twin.

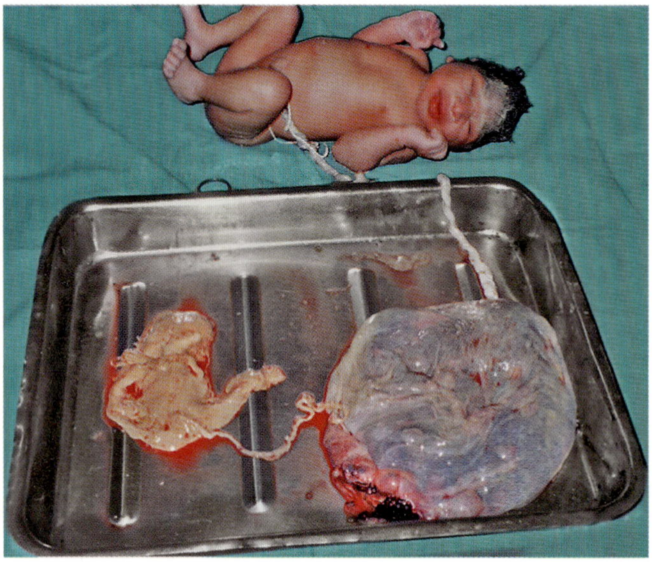

Fig. 2: Fetus papyraceous.

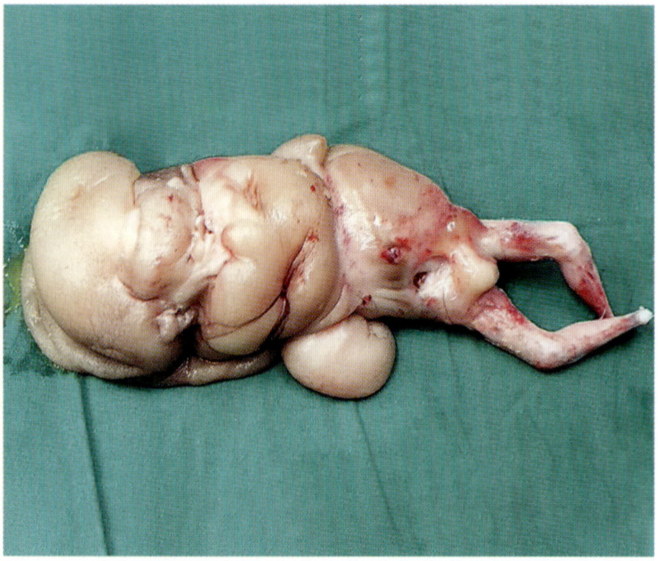

Fig. 3: Acardiac twin [twin reversed arterial perfusion (TRAP)].
Courtesy: Dr Anirban Mondal, Associate Professor, Department of Gynecology and Obstetrics, Bankura Sammilani Medical College, Bankura, West Bengal, India.

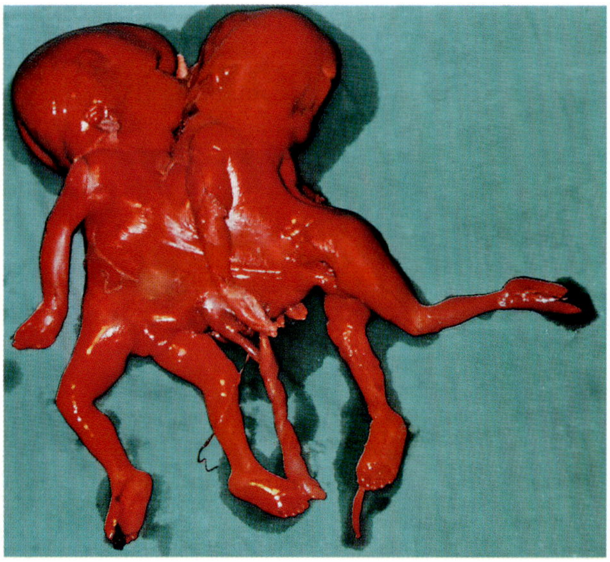

Fig. 4: Conjoined twin in early pregnancy following spontaneous abortion (thoracopagus).

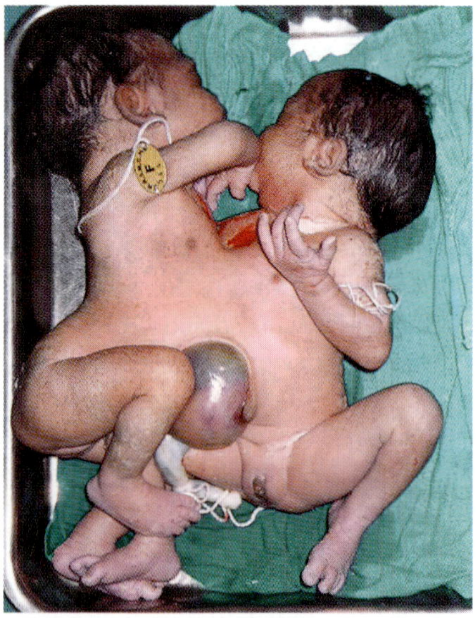

Fig. 5: Conjoined twin at late pregnancy delivered by cesarean section (thoracopagus).

EMBRYOLOGY OF TWIN GESTATION (FIG. 10)

Definition of Monozygotic and Dizygotic Twins

Monozygotic twins result from splitting of a single fertilized ovum whereas dizygotic twins arise from fertilization of two ova by different sperms. The dizygotic twins are also called binovular twins or fraternal twins whereas monozygotic twins are known as monovular twins or identical twins.

Zygosity, amnionicity, and chorionicity are the number of zygotes, amnions, and chorions, respectively, to describe the multiple gestations. Zygosity refers to the type of conception but chorionicity refers to the type of placenta. A dizygotic twin pregnancy is always dichorionic and diamnionic. However, monozygotic twins may be dichorionic diamnionic, or monochorionic diamnionic or monochorionic monoamnionic depending upon the time of division of inner cell mass following fertilization. In monozygotic twins 30% are dichorionic and 70% are monochorionic. It is the chorionicity not the zygosity which indicates the degree of perinatal risk in any individual multiple.

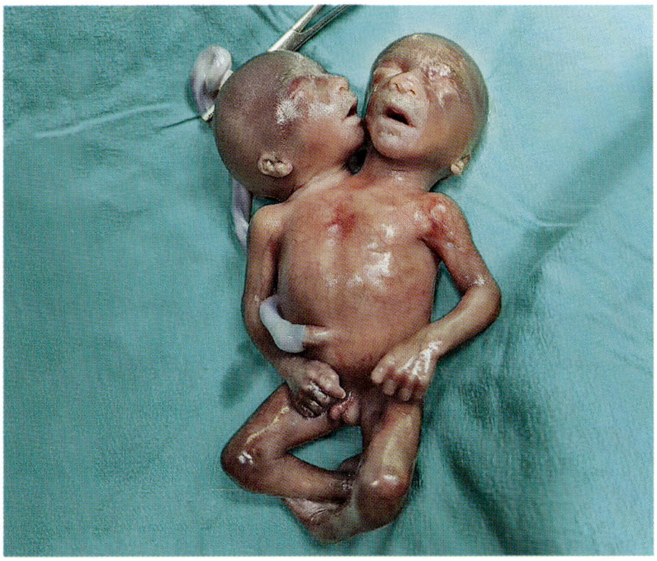

Fig. 6: Fetus with double head at 21 weeks.
Courtesy: Dr Shelly Seth, Associate Professor, RG Kar Medical College, Kolkata, West Bengal, India.

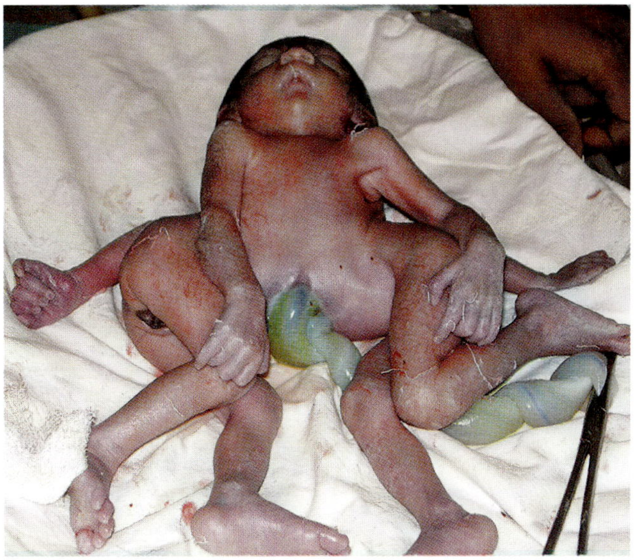

Fig. 7: Conjoined twin with single head and single thorax (cephalopagus). Presented at 30 weeks of pregnancy with preterm labor and delivered by cesarean section. Died few hours after birth.
Courtesy: Professor GS Kamilya, Institute of Postgraduate Medical Education and Research, Kolkata, West Bengal, India.

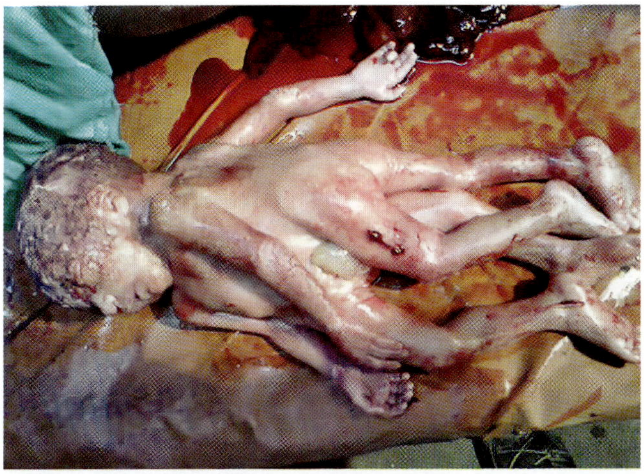

Fig. 8: Single head with multiple limbs (cephalopagus).
Courtesy: Dr Debmalya Maity, Assistant Professor, Bankura Sammilani Medical College, Bankura, West Bengal, India.

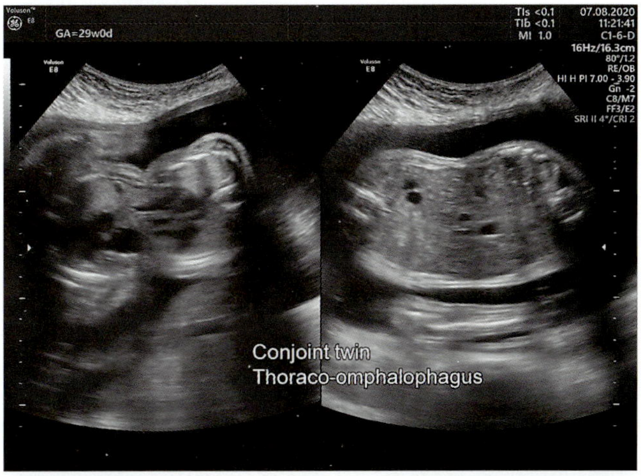

Fig. 9: Ultrasound showing conjoined twins—thoraco-omphalophagus (29 weeks).
Courtesy: Professor Kamal Oswal, Head, Department of Radiodiagnosis, Vivekananda Institute of Medical Sciences, Kolkata, West Bengal, India.

Characteristics of Amnion and Chorion of Monozygotic Twins in Relation to the Time of Division after Fertilization (Fig. 10)

Number of chorion and amnion in monozygotic twins in relation to time of division of inner cell mass:

- Within 72 hours—monozygotic, dichorionic, diamnionic twins **(Fig. 11)**. Two different placentas or a single fused placenta develops.
- Between 4th and 8th day—monozygotic, monochorionic, diamnionic twins **(Fig. 12)**.
- After 8th day—monozygotic, monochorionic monoamnionic twins **(Fig. 13)**.
- After 14th day (after the formation of embryonic disc)—conjoined twins.

DETERMINATION OF CHORIONICITY

Determination of chorionicity by ultrasound (USG) findings of number of yolk sac and number of extraembryonic coelom in very early pregnancy is less precise. It is best determined between 10 and 14 weeks gestation by observing

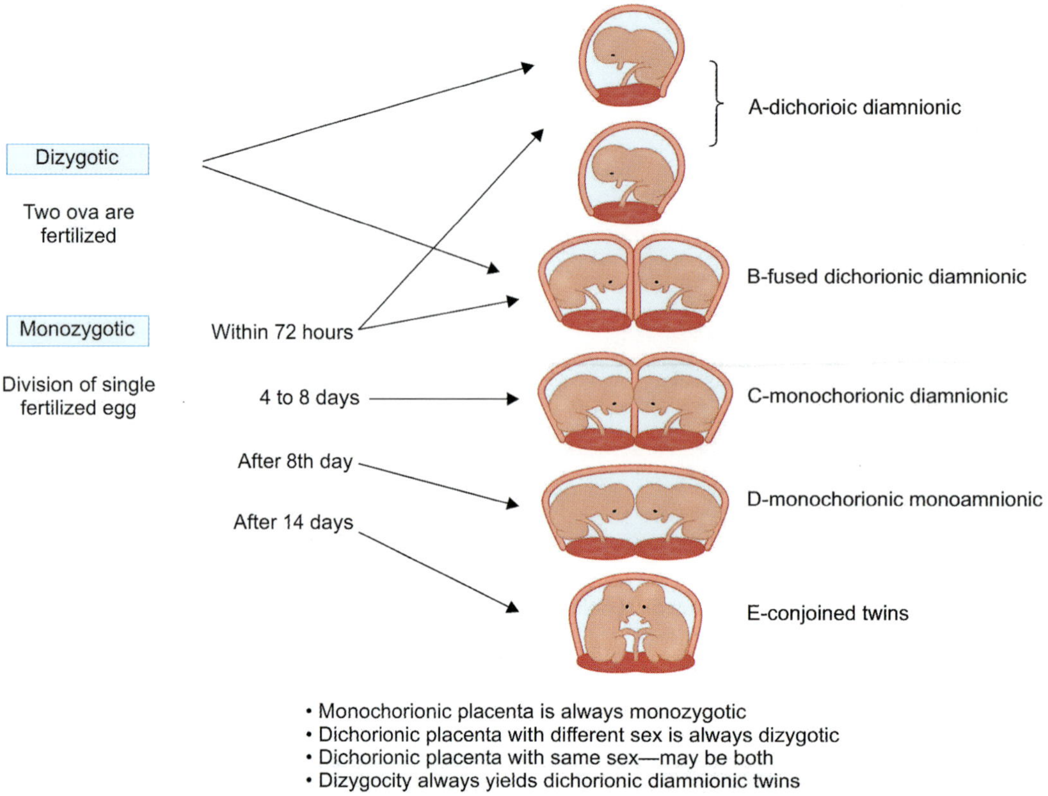

Fig. 10: Embryology of twining to show amnion and chorion of monozygotic and dizygotic twins.

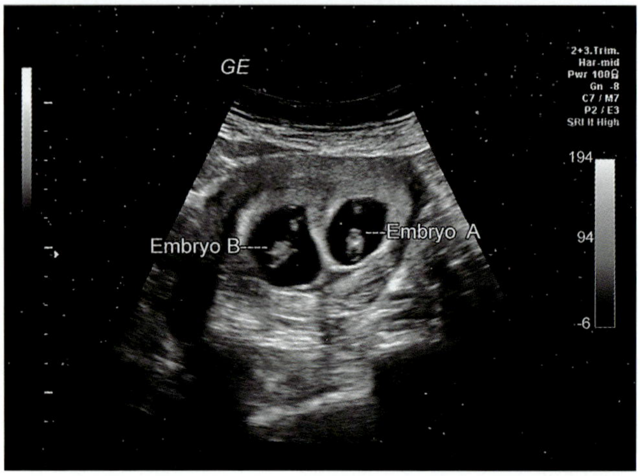

Fig. 11: Ultrasound showing dichorionic diamnionic at 8 weeks.

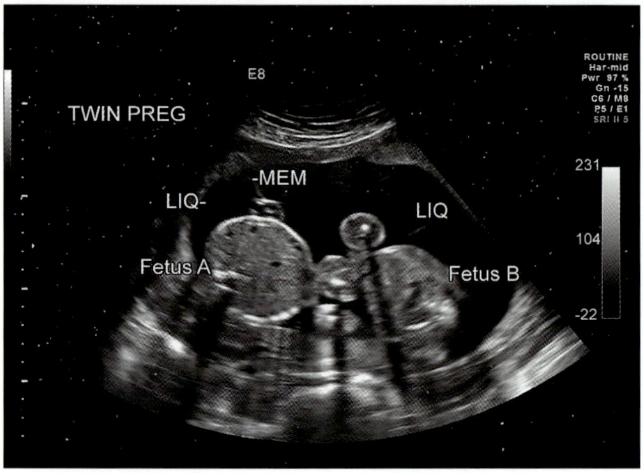

Fig. 12: Twin pregnancy monochorionic diamniotic.

the number of placental mass, number of intervening layers, thickness of intervening membranes, and presence of "twin peak" sign or "T-sign". If two placental masses are visible clearly, it indicates dichorionic twins. A single placental mass may be of monochorionic or fused dichorionic placenta.

Absence of intervening membrane means *monochorionic and monoamnionic*. In presence of membranes, the differentiating features which can be seen in high resolution USG are given in **Table 1**.

TABLE 1: Sonographic features to determine chorionicity (10–14 weeks).

USG parameters	*Dichorionic*	*Monochorionic*
Number of layers	Four layers	Two layers
Thickness	>2 mm	<2 mm
Specific sign	Twin peak sign or lambda sign **(Figs. 14 and 15)**	"T" sign **(Figs. 16 and 17)**

(USG: ultrasound)

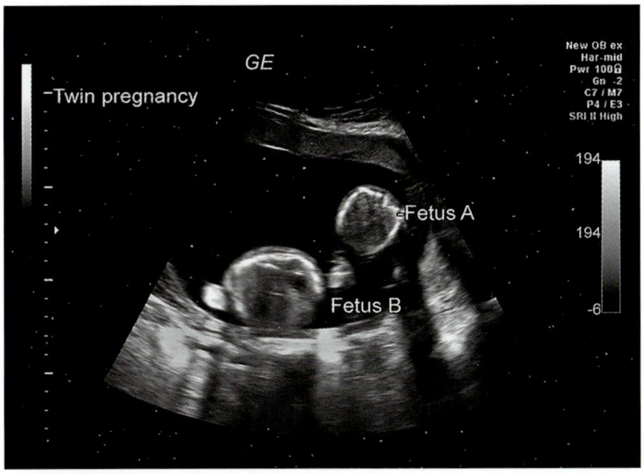

Fig. 13: Monochorionic monoamnionic twins at 20 weeks twin-to-twin transfusion syndrome.
Courtesy: Professor Kamal Oswal, Head, Department of Radiodiagnosis, Vivekananda Institute of Medical Sciences, Kolkata, West Bengal, India.

"Twin Peak" Sign

"Twin peak" sign is a sonographic finding in early weeks (10–14 weeks) where dichorionic twins are differentiated from the monochorionic twins. This sign is a triangular projection of placental tissue between the layers of dividing membrane over the chorionic surface **(Figs. 14 and 15)**. Here, the intervening membrane becomes thick (2 mm or more) and consists of four layers. "Twin peak" sign is diagnostic of dichorionic gestation. It is also known as *lambda sign (λ-sign)*. After 20 weeks, this sign may disappear.

"T-sign"

The right angle relationship between the membranes and placenta with no apparent extension of placental tissue between the dividing membrane as found in *monochorionic pregnancy* is called "T" sign. The thickness of dividing membrane is <2 mm **(Figs. 16 and 17)** and consists of two layers.

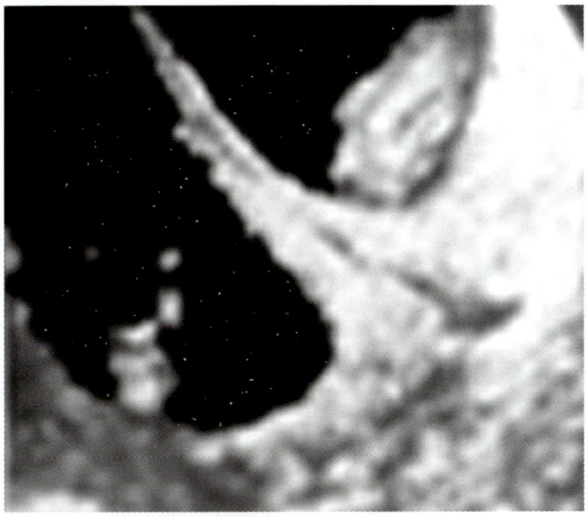

Fig. 14: Twin peak sign (lambda sign).
Courtesy: Professor Kushagradhi Ghose, Director, Institute of Fetal Medicine, Kolkata, West Bengal, India.

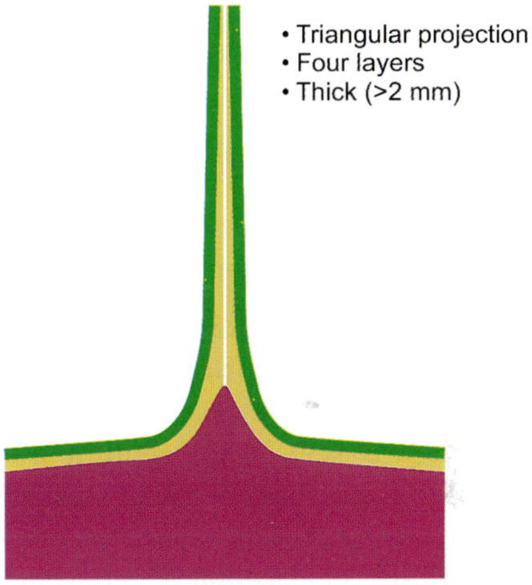

Fig. 15: Twin peak sign (lambda sign).

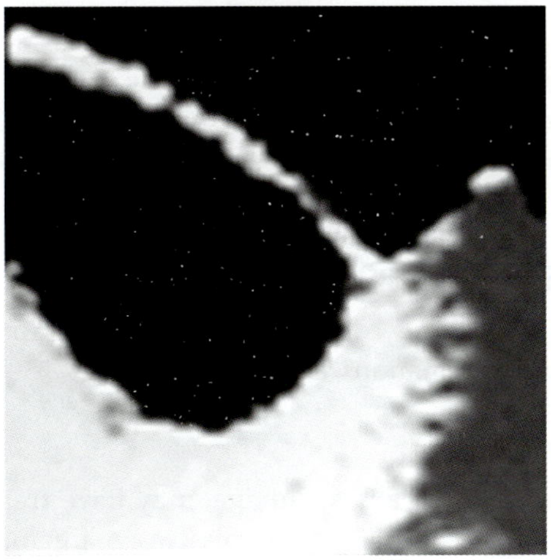

Fig. 16: T-sign.
Courtesy: Professor Kushagradhi Ghose, Director, Institute of Fetal Medicine, Kolkata, West Bengal, India.

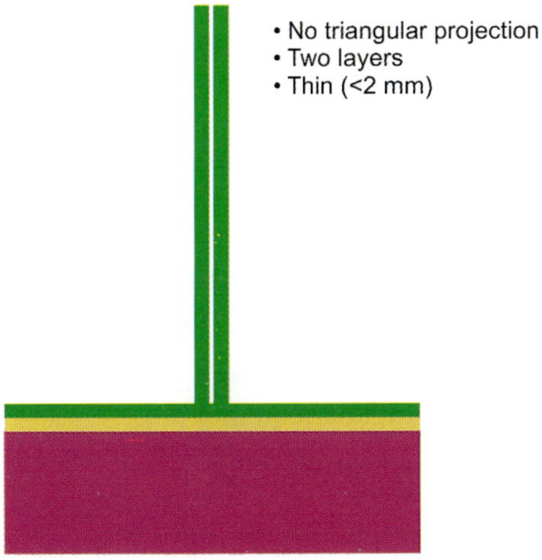

Fig. 17: T-sign.

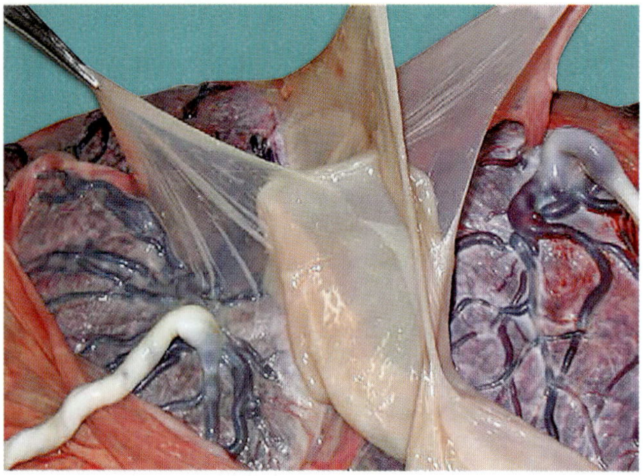

Fig. 18: Twin placenta (dichorionic diamnionic) showing intervening chorions in between two amnions.

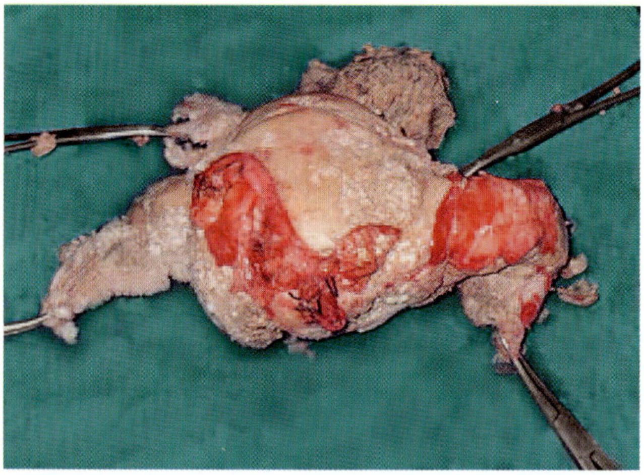

Fig. 19: Fetus in fetu.
An 8-year-old girl presented with upper abdominal lump. Computed tomography scan showed structure identical to fetal femur and spine with soft tissue. On laparotomy huge retroperitoneal encapsulated mass resembling a fetus was detected and removed. It measured 15 cm × 20 cm and weighing 585 g. It had a trunk with poorly developed four limbs with nails and there was no flat cranial bones, only there was small base of the skull covered by a scalp with hair and the body was covered with peeled off skin. Hard vertebral column was visible but heart, lung, liver, and spleen could not be identified.

Determination of chorionicity and amniocity is possible in 100% cases before 13 weeks, after which diagnosis is possible but with less accuracy. Three-dimensional (3D) USG scans are not used to determine chorionicity and amnionicity.

Following Delivery

Examination of sex: Different sex of neonates means dichorionic; same sex may be dichorionic or monochorionic.

Examination of placental mass ***(Fig. 18)****:* Two separate placental discs indicate dichorionicity. In case of single placental mass, if two layers of amnion and two layers of chorion are clearly seen in the septum, a dichorionic placenta is diagnosed. Presence of two amnions only without any intervening chorion represents monochorionic twinning. Anastomosis of placental vessels, which is present in monochorionic placenta can be diagnosed by injecting dye into placental vessels.

FETUS IN FETU (FIG. 19)

Fetus in fetu (FIF) is a rare condition where a monozygotic diamnionic parasitic twin is incorporated into the body of its fellow twin early in embryonic development and grows inside it through a vascular anastomosis with the host circulation.

Presentation in Twin Pregnancies in Order of Frequency (Figs. 20 to 26)

Most common are first cephalic and second cephalic. Combinations in order of frequency are:

- First cephalic, second cephalic (most common)—50–55% **(Fig. 20)**
- First cephalic, second breech—20% **(Fig. 21)**
- First breech, second cephalic—10% **(Fig. 22)**
- Both breech—10% **(Fig. 23)**

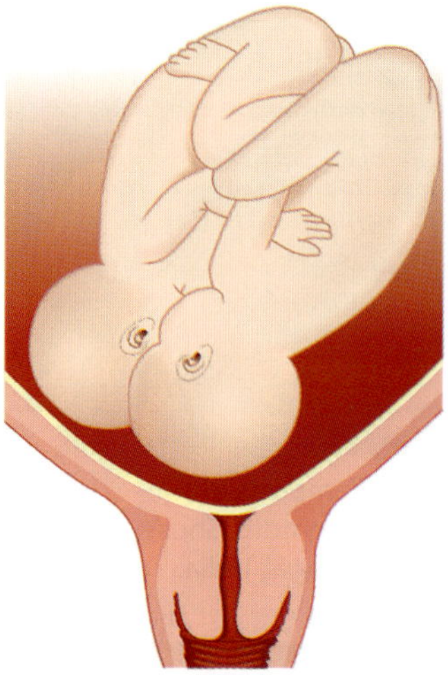

Fig. 20: Both vertex.

- First cephalic, second transverse lie—5% **(Fig. 24)**
- First breech, second transverse lie—2% **(Fig. 25)**
- Both transverse—5% **(Fig. 26)**.

DIAGNOSIS OF TWIN GESTATION

Diagnosis is done by history, physical examinations, obstetrical examinations, and sonography.

History

Mother may be of advanced age, may have treatment of infertility. She complains of excessive enlargement of the abdomen, family history of twinning, more common in maternal side. There is exaggeration of the symptoms of

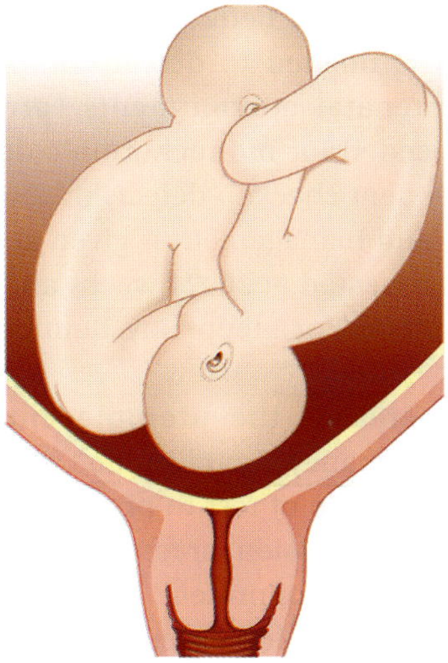

Fig. 21: First vertex, second breech.

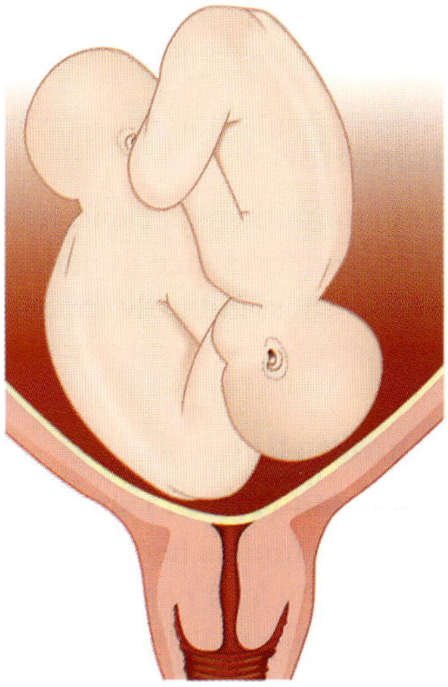

Fig. 22: First breech, second vertex.

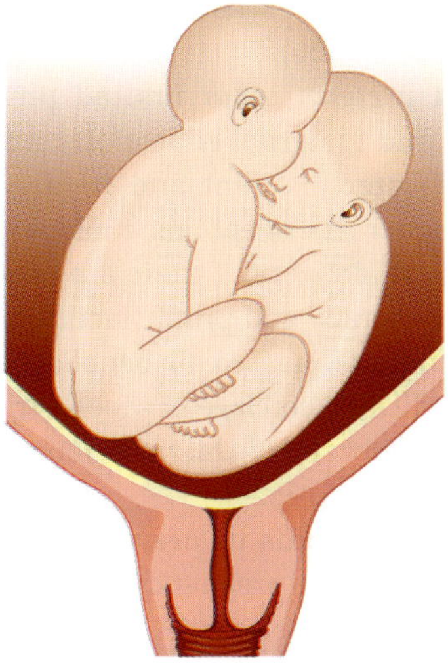

Fig. 23: Both breech.

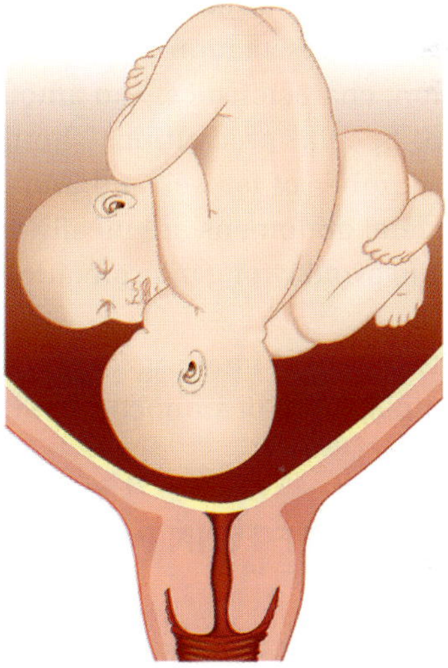

Fig. 24: First vertex, second transverse lie.

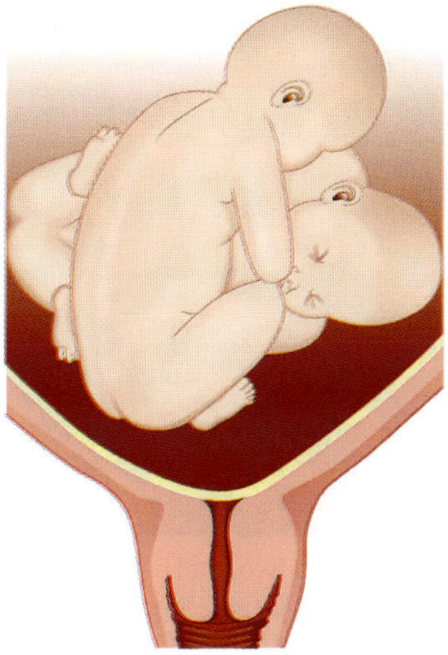

Fig. 25: First breech, second transverse lie.

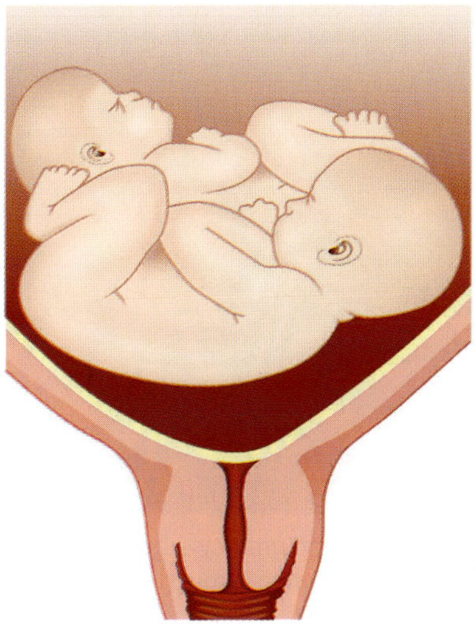

Fig. 26: Both transverse lie.

pregnancy, respiratory discomfort, palpitation, and swelling of legs.

Physical Examination

On general examination, there is rapid increase of weight during antenatal period, presence of pallor, appearance of edema legs or in other sites, and early appearance of features of preeclampsia.

Obstetrical Examination

Abdominal examination **(Fig. 27)** shows hugely enlarged abdomen, height of the fundus becomes more than period of amenorrhea, too many fetal parts, hydramnios, and two different fetal heart sounds (FHS) on different sites may be audible.

Sonography

Multiple pregnancy is confirmed by sonography **(Fig. 28)**. Fetal size, status, lie, presentation, TTTS, death of one twin, placental location, characteristics, and amount of amniotic fluid are noted. Special precautions should be taken to determine the number of fetuses and anomaly. Two fetal heads and two fetal abdomens are ideally be visualized in the same image to avoid wrong interpretation of single fetus as twins.

Magnetic resonance imaging (MRI) is helpful for diagnosis of complications of monochorionic twin including conjoined twins.

MANAGEMENT OF TWIN PREGNANCY

Prenatal Care

Antenatal complications of multiple pregnancy are many. In >50% cases preterm birth and 10% pPROM occurs. Anemia, preeclampsia, and APH are serious potential complications.

Early diagnosis offers better prognosis. Frequent antenatal checkup is needed to detect complication early. At least 11 antenatal appointments (preferably every 2 weeks) are needed for monochorionic diamniotic twin pregnancy. Frequent checkup detects the complications at an early stage, and management is given accordingly. Full blood count is repeated at 20–24 weeks and at 28th week. Prenatal test is offered for aneuploidy. Routine anomaly scan is essential.

Bed rest increases the uteroplacental perfusion, decreases the pregnancy complications, and prevents preterm labor though role of rest to prevent preterm birth is doubtful. Hospital admission for rest is not mandatory.

Calories and intake of protein, minerals, vitamins, and essential fatty acids are increased. Additional calories of 300 Kcal/day are given.

Dose of iron folic acid is increased depending on the degree of anemia. It may need to be started earlier. Women who are at high risk for preeclampsia are recommended low-dose aspirin (ACOG 2020).

To prevent *preterm labor* limited physical activity, adequate rest, and maternal education on risk of preterm labor are advocated. Patient and family members are explained of higher risk of spontaneous preterm birth and indicated preterm delivery, if there are other risk factors. Use of tocolytic therapy and prophylactic cervical cerclage, pessary, and progesterone have no beneficial effect. Physical examination-indicated cerclage in second trimester may be of benefit in dilated cervix [American Journal of Obstetrics and Gynecology (AJOG) 2020].

Use of corticosteroids to prevent lung maturity has similar effect in singleton pregnancy.

Antenatal surveillance: Evaluation of each fetus is important. Aneuplody screening is mandatory. Combined test or secondary screening is interpreted with multiple pregnancy

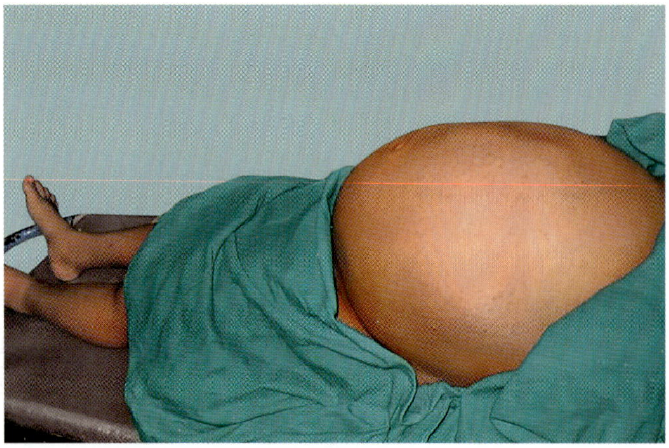

Fig. 27: Abdomen in twin pregnancy—height of the fundus is more and girth of the abdomen is much more than expected.

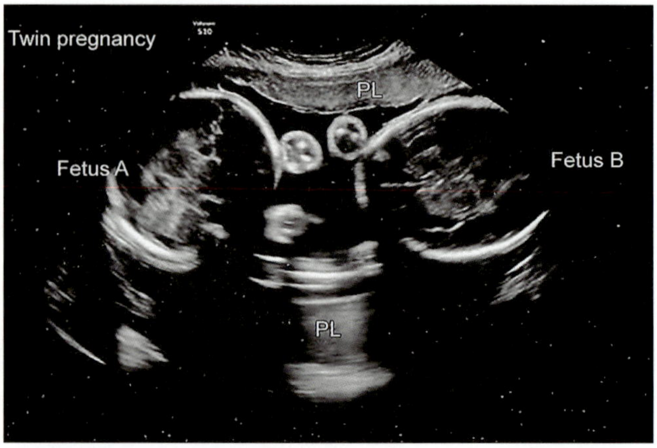

Fig. 28: Ultrasound showing two fetal heads.
Courtesy: Professor Kamal Oswal, Head, Department of Radiodiagnosis, Vivekananda Institute of Medical Sciences, Kolkata, West Bengal, India.

threshold value. Noninvasive DNA screening can be offered (ACOG 2021). Anomaly scan is performed in midpregnancy. Fetal echo is suggested in monochorionic twin. Serial USG should be performed throughout third trimester to assess growth. Nonstress test and Doppler velocimetry are employed to test the fetal well-being. As IUD is two to three folds higher, weekly antenatal surveillance is undertaken from 32 weeks in monochorionic gestation and for uncomplicated dichorion pregnancy from 36 weeks. <2 cm deepest pocket of amniotic fluid is considered oligohydramnios and >8 cm as hydramnios.

TIME OF DELIVERY

- Delivery is recommended at $38^{0/7}$ to $38^{6/7}$ weeks for uncomplicated dichorionic twin pregnancies (ACOG 2021) whereas National Institute for Health and Care Excellence (NICE) (2019) suggests planned birth at 37 weeks in an uncomplicated dichorionic diamnionic twin pregnancy.
- In uncomplicated monochorionic diamnionic twin pregnancies delivery can be undergone at $34^{0/7}$ and $37^{6/7}$ weeks as per (ACOG 2021) whereas NICE considers planned birth at 36 weeks after a course of antenatal corticosteroids.
- In uncomplicated monochorionic monoamnionic twin pregnancy delivery is recommended at $32^{0/7}$ to $34^{0/7}$ weeks (both ACOG and NICE).

ROLE OF INDUCTION AND AUGMENTATION

Routine induction of labor in a so-called uncomplicated twin pregnancy gives no maternal or fetal benefit. However, induction is indicated in cases after certain gestation age as described above and also in preeclampsia and where it will prove beneficial, if criteria for vaginal delivery are fulfilled. Oxytocin can be used safely for both induction and augmentation.

CHOICE OF ROUTE OF DELIVERY

Every case should be individualized. In uncomplicated cases when there are first cephalic, vaginal delivery is recommended while vaginal delivery may be offered in some other selected cases of first breech. Attempt of vaginal delivery is favored to avoid immediate and long-term complications of cesarean delivery.

INDICATIONS OF CESAREAN DELIVERY

Cesarean section is recommended if the first twin is not cephalic at the time of planned birth. However, cesarean delivery is indicated in following situations:

- *Obstetric indications:*
  - Placenta previa
  - Pregnancy with prior cesarean delivery—not mandatory.
  - Severe preeclampsia
  - Cord prolapses in first stage of first baby.
  - Contracted pelvis, this indication is not common as the fetuses are usually small.
- *Indications for twin itself:*
  - When the first baby is nonvertex (not mandatory)
  - Twin complicated with IUGR
  - Conjoint twins
  - When the estimated birth weight of the second twin is 500 g greater than that of first twin.
  - Nonengagement of head due to collision of fetal heads together at brim.
  - Uncontrolled bleeding following delivery of the first twin when other measures fail.
  - Problems of delivery of second twin (combined method) in some situations described below.

MANAGEMENT OF FIRST STAGE OF LABOR IN TWIN PREGNANCY

Mother is not allowed to roam in order to prevent early rupture of membranes. Oral diet is avoided as at any time there may be need for operative interference. Intravenous (IV) channel is established. Provision of blood transfusion is kept. Too much analgesics are avoided. Epidural analgesia is preferred. Maternal condition, fetal condition, and progress of labor are monitored carefully. Continuous electronic monitoring is desirable.

Per vaginal examination is done to see the progress of labor and to exclude cord prolapse after rupture of membranes.

MANAGEMENT OF THE SECOND STAGE OF LABOR IN TWIN PREGNANCY

The following are required for the management of the second stage of labor in twin pregnancy:

- Spacious operative room with cesarean facility and two baby resuscitation arrangement
- A skilled obstetrician, anesthesiologist, a double pediatric team (two pediatricians), and two neonatal nurses—one pediatric team for each infant
- IV channel with large bore needle
- Forceps, ventouse, cardiotocography (CTG) machine, and USG machine should always be available, particularly to assess the second baby following the birth of the first twin.
- Oxytocics and uterine relaxants.

Conduction of birth of the first twin:

- If the first twin is vertex, spontaneous vaginal delivery is accomplished like singleton pregnancy after giving an episiotomy. Forceps delivery can be done to avoid prolonged second stage as uterine contractile force and bearing down effort is less effective in twin gestation. Low or outlet forceps can also be applied to cut short the second stage, if criteria are fulfilled. Rarely, when the first twin presented by vertex and head is not engaged in spite of full dilation of cervical os, cesarean delivery is considered.

- If the first baby is breech, it is delivered by assisted breech delivery.
- *Prophylactic oxytocic is not given after* delivery of the first baby. The umbilical cord is clamped immediately by two clamps at both fetal and placental ends. A long cord (about 8–10 cm) is kept for intraumbilical transfusion of drug administration, if needed.
- Baby is marked as no. 1.

How will you Deliver the Second Baby of the Twin following Delivery of First Twin?

Precautions during delivery of first baby—*prophylactic oxytocic avoided, early cord clamping done,* and *a long cord preserved*

Lie, presentation, size, station, and FHS are noted by abdominal examination. Vaginal examination is done to corroborate the abdominal findings, to see the membrane status and to note the station of the presenting part.

When the lie is longitudinal—with the appearance of contraction as soon as the presenting part (vertex or breech) gets fixed at the pelvic brim and comes low down, low rupture of membrane is done. If there is delay in contraction, oxytocin drip (2.5 unit in 500 mL of 5% dextrose) is started. Cord prolapse is excluded by per vaginal examination.

- The second baby with breech presentation is delivered preferably by assisted breech delivery. If there is a delay, it is delivered by breech extraction.
- If the presentation of second baby is vertex and engaged with good descent, spontaneous vaginal delivery is awaited which becomes successful in most of the cases. If there is delay of delivery of second baby, it is delivered by forceps application when the head is low down to minimize delivery interval down.
- When second baby with vertex presentation is high up and not engaged, there is difference of opinion on procedure adapted. Oxytocin infusion is continued awaiting spontaneous delivery. Some advocates to deliver by ventouse application. Others prefer to do internal podalic version followed by breech extraction under general anesthesia (GA) (see below) **(Figs. 29A to C)**. In cases where the head is high up, possibility of cephalopelvic disproportion and hydrocephalus should be kept in mind.
- If the lie of second twin is transverse, attempt is made to make it longitudinal by external version firstly by cephalic; if it fails, then attempt is made by podalic version. If it is not possible, it is delivered by internal podalic version under GA as described in Chapter 8, Transverse Lie. Internal podalic version is most suitable option for second baby in transverse lie in twin pregnancy.

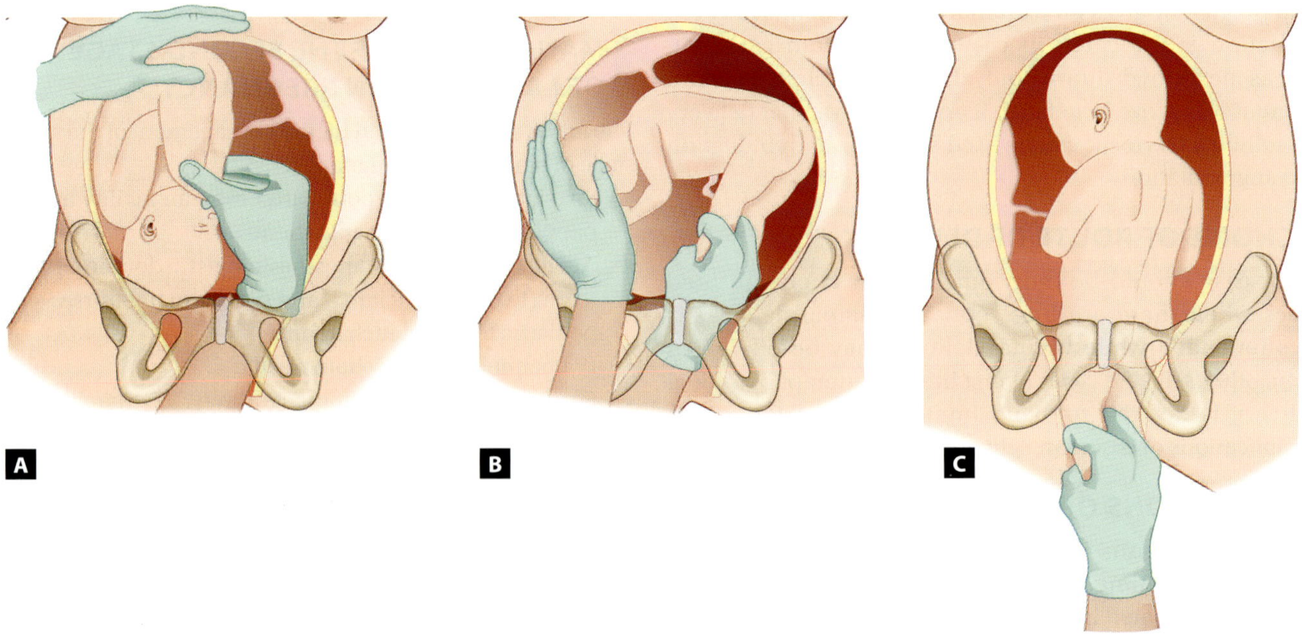

Figs. 29A to C: Internal podalic version when head is high up. (A) In case of head high up internal podalic version is attempted where right hand is introduced inside the vagina first to gasp the feet with simultaneous pushing by other hand abdominally and then fetal head is elevated away from pelvic inlet; (B) After pushing the head toward the fundus inside the upper part of uterine cavity, the feet of the fetus is drawn toward pelvic cavity by gasping; (C) The feet are drawn toward the vagina outside.

Procedure of Internal Podalic Version of Second Twin with Vertex Presentation which is High Up and Not Engaged (Figs. 29A to C)

Decision should be taken immediately, as the uterus remains relaxed immediately after delivery of first twin and membrane is still intact and no prolapse of the cord. It should only be done by experienced obstetrician.

Under anesthesia (preferably epidural) right hand is introduced inside the vagina to gasp the feet and the fetal head is elevated with simultaneous pushing the head by other hand abdominally toward lateral side away from pelvic inlet. Now the vaginal hand pushes the fetal head toward the fundus inside the upper part of uterine cavity and the abdominal hand exerts pressure to rotate the fetal head toward the fundus. Now the feet of the fetus is grasped by the vaginal hand and drawn toward pelvic cavity. The lower half of the fetal body comes out of the vaginal introitus and the trunk of the baby is held by femoropelvic grip and the baby is delivered by breech extraction, the shoulder by Lovset maneuver and the aftercoming head either by malar flexion and shoulder traction method (Mauriceau-Smellie-Veit technique) or by Piper forceps as detailed in Chapter of Breech Delivery (Chapter 8).

Optimal Time Interval between the Delivery of the First Baby and that of Second Baby

Longer the interval between the delivery of first and second twin, greater the perinatal mortality. Hence, delivery of the second twin should be accomplished as soon as possible, preferably within half an hour of delivery of the first twin. However, a good outcome can be achieved at longer interval in some cases, provided a continuous fetal monitoring is done (Longest time interval between the delivery of first and second twin as seen in literature is 143 days that is exceptional).

MANAGEMENT OF SOME OF THE COMMON COMPLICATIONS ENCOUNTERED DURING SECOND STAGE OF LABOR

Some of the common complications encountered during second stage of labor are:

- *Profuse vaginal bleeding after the birth of the first baby*: Delivery is hastened by low rupture of membranes and oxytocin drip followed by forceps when the head is low down and by internal version when the head is high up.
  In case of *breech* presentation → breech extraction
  In *transverse lie* → internal podalic version.
- *Cord prolapse in the second baby:* Baby is delivered as quickly as above and the method depends on the lie, presentation, and station.
- *In case where there is fetal distress of second baby:* Urgent delivery as outlined above. Cesarean delivery is a safer method.

Indication of Cesarean Delivery for the Second Twin after Vaginal Birth of Second Baby

Combined Delivery

Cesarean delivery for the second twin after vaginal delivery of the first baby is called combined delivery.

Combined delivery is done, if the second twin is larger or in transverse lie, there is failure to deliver vaginally by correction. Sometimes, with reformation of the cervix which becomes thickened and os closes after the delivery of the first baby, cesarean delivery is performed.

LOCKED TWINS (FIGS. 30 AND 31)

It is a very rare problem (1 in 800 twins delivered) when the chin of the aftercoming head of the first twin, presented by breech, is prevented from coming into the pelvis by the second twin presented by vertex (first breech, second cephalic). This is due to locking of the chin and neck of the second

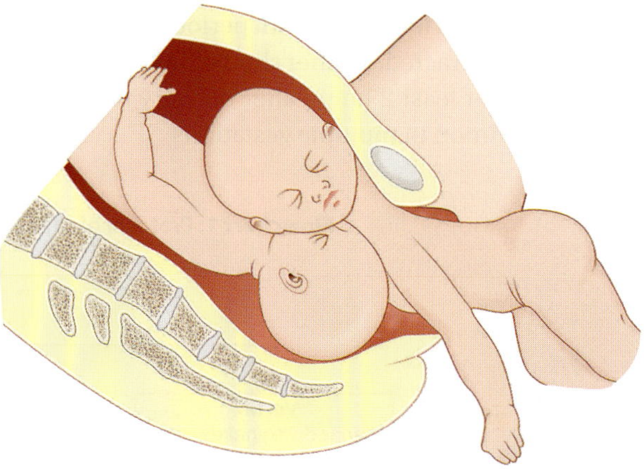

Fig. 30: Locked twin.

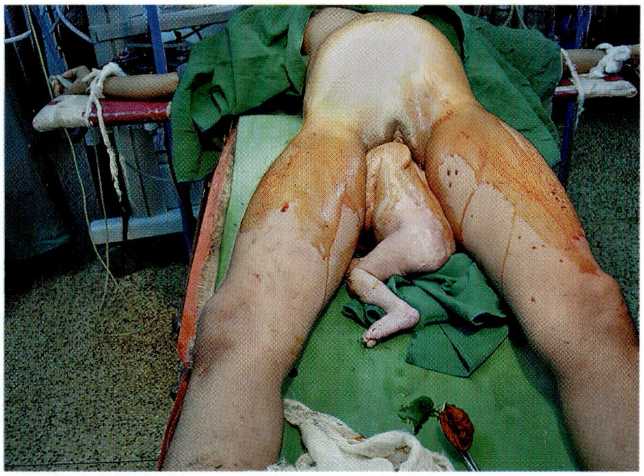

Fig. 31: Locked twin. Cesarean section was done. Second twin (living) was delivered abdominally after unlocking followed by vaginal delivery of first twin as breech.

Courtesy: Professor Subrata Lall Seal, Department of Gynecology and Obstetrics, RG Kar Medical College, Kolkata, West Bengal, India.

twin, presented by vertex. It is common in monoanionic twins or when the amniotic sac of second twin is ruptured.

Management: Delivery of the aftercoming head of first twin is done followed by pushing the head of second twin out of the pelvis. If it is not possible, then by Zavenelli maneuver the first twin is returned to pelvis and cesarean section is done to deliver both the babies. If even this is not possible, cesarean section is done and after unlocking, second twin is delivered abdominally and first twin vaginally. When first twin is severely asphyxiated or dead, decapitation of the first twin will allow its body to be delivered vaginally, followed by delivery of the second twin and finally delivery of the head of the first twin is accomplished.

MANAGEMENT OF THE THIRD STAGE IN TWIN PREGNANCY

As there is more chance of PPH, the following precautions are taken. Active management of third stage is done after delivery of second baby. Oxytocin infusion, if already started, should be continued for a significant period of time till uterus becomes well contracted. Mother should be kept under close observation for at least 2 hours after delivery remembering that PPH is common in multiple gestations.

Placenta is examined for intactness as it is large, and missing bits are common and is checked for chronicity.

TECHNIQUE OF CESAREAN DELIVERY IN TWIN GESTATION

Basically there is no difference of technique of cesarean procedure for twins and singletons pregnancy. Blood loss is more in twin gestations and is attributed mostly to atony. Short- and long-term complications of cesarean are similar to singleton pregnancy.

TWIN DELIVERY IN PREGNANCY WITH PREVIOUS CESAREAN DELIVERY

When the first twin is vertex, trial of scar [trial of labor after cesarean (TOLAC)] is not contraindicated—chance of vaginal delivery [vaginal birth after cesarean (VBAC)] of first twin is 70%.

Judicious external or internal manipulations are not contraindicated in the second twin. Rupture is a possibility. However, cesarean section is liberalized in special circumstances.

Protocol of management of mature twin pregnancy in labor is given in **Flowchart 1**.

Flowchart 1: Protocol of management of mature twin pregnancy in labor.

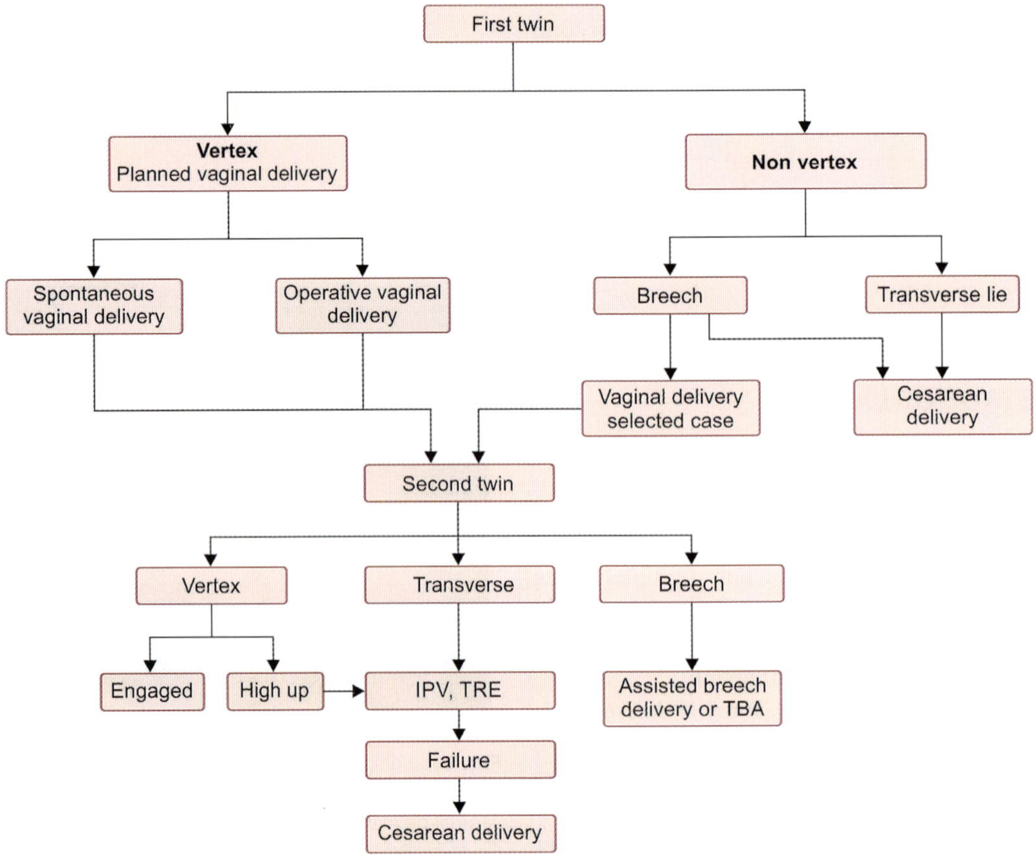

(IPV: internal podalic version; TBE: total breech extraction)

TRIPLET OR HIGHER ORDER MULTIPLE GESTATION

Increase incidence of twin and higher order gestations due to the infertility treatment and ART is now great concern. 50–60% are triplet and mostly polyzygotic. Optimal number of embryo transfer and embryo reduction are the present strategy to check the increased incidence.

Triplets may be trichorionic triamniotic, dichorionic triamniotic, dichorionic diamniotic, monochorionic triamniotic, monochorionic diamniotic or monochorionic monoamniotic. Those may be monozygotic or polyzygotic.

There is increased chance of spontaneous abortion **(Fig. 32)**. Preterm delivery is as high as 50% at 32–34 weeks. In triplet pregnancy, spontaneous birth occurs in about 75 in 100 pregnancies before 35 weeks **(Fig. 33)**. In higher order, fetus may die or may result fetus paparicious in early demise **(Figs. 34A and B)**. Growth restriction and discordance are more common.

Diagnosis is based on suspicion on history, clinical examination, and confirmed by sonography **(Figs. 35 and 36)**.

Symptoms and complications are more in comparison to twin pregnancy.

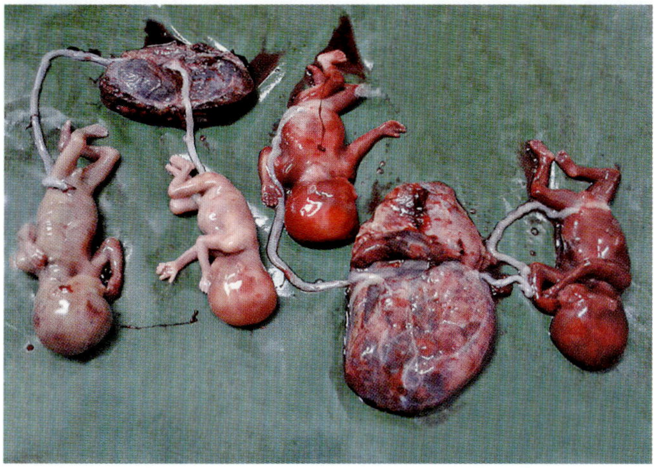

Fig. 32: Quadruplet—spontaneous miscarriage at 18 weeks.
Courtesy: Dr Anirban Mondal, Associate Professor, Department of Gynecology and Obstetrics, Bankura Sammilani Medical College, Bankura, West Bengal, India.

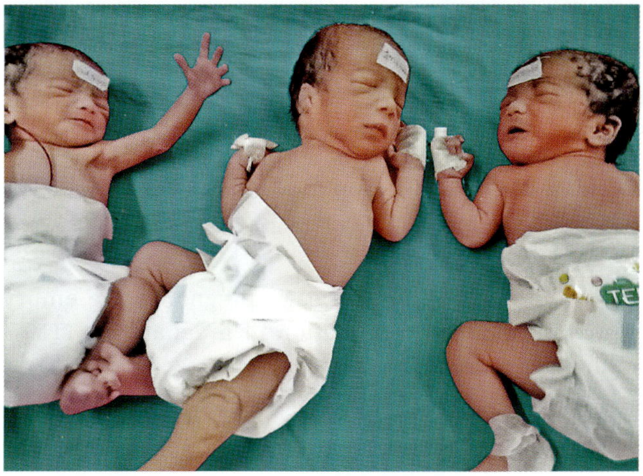

Fig. 33: Triplet pregnancy. A 22-year-old P4+0 G2 woman delivered vaginally at 33 weeks. She developed anemia and preeclampsia. She had family history of twin brother and her grandmother also had twin sons.
Courtesy: Dr Anirban Mondal, Associate Professor, Department of Gynecology and Obstetrics, Bankura Sammilani Medical College, Bankura, West Bengal, India.

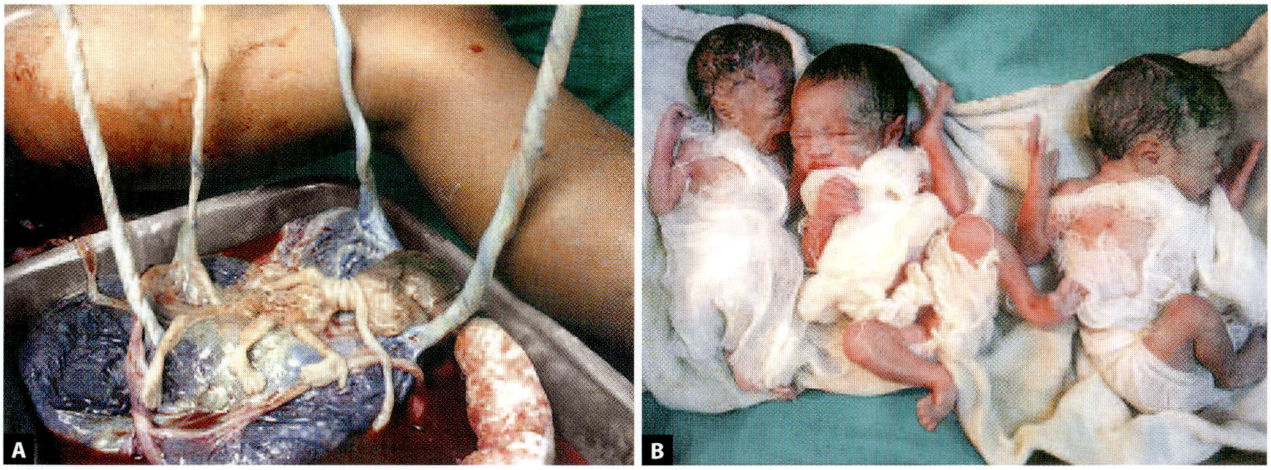

Figs. 34A and B: (A) Placenta with four umbilical cord and one fetus papyraceous; (B) three living babies. Showing quintuplet pregnancy (five). Primigravida 25–year-old woman delivered vaginally five babies, first was living male (1.5 kg), second living female (1.5 kg), third also living female (1.3 kg), and fourth was still born male weighing 900 g (not shown in the figure). The fifth was fetus papyraceous which was delivered with the placenta. Patient had no history of infertility or assisted reproductive technology treatment.
Courtesy: Professor Tanmay Mondal, Professor Dr Sudhir Adhikary, Department of Gynecology and Obstetrics, Burdwan Medical College, Burdwan, West Bengal, India.

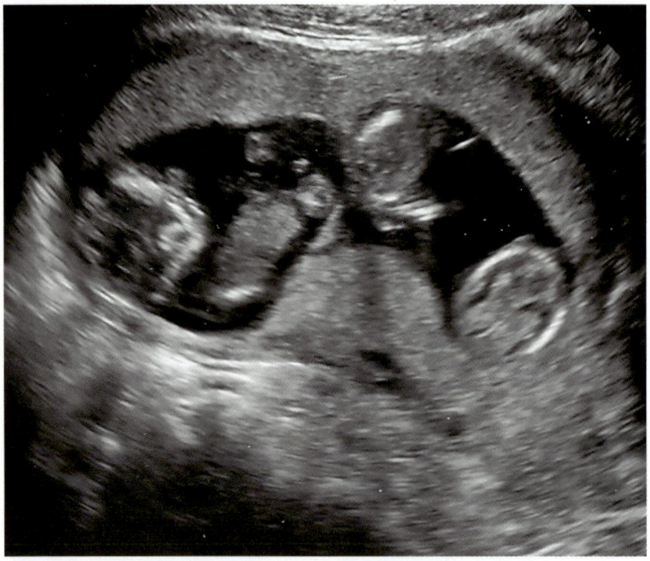

Fig. 35: Triplet pregnancy dichorionic diamniotic.
Courtesy: Professor Kamal Oswal, Head, Department of Radiodiagnosis, Vivekananda Institute of Medical Sciences, Kolkata, West Bengal, India.

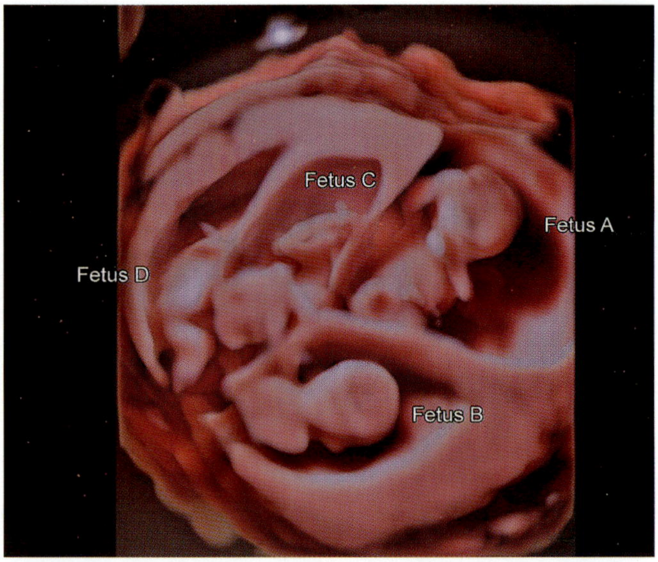

Fig. 36: Quadruplate pregnancy at 9 weeks 2 days (3D image).
Courtesy: Professor Kamal Oswal, Head, Department of Radiodiagnosis, Vivekananda Institute of Medical Sciences, Kolkata, West Bengal, India.

Management options in early pregnancy are embryo reduction, medical termination of pregnancy (MTP) or continued as such after counseling.

Delivery: Pregnancies of three or higher order are best delivered by cesarean section. However, vaginal delivery is safer in certain situations. Planned birth is recommended at 35 weeks for women with an uncomplicated trichorionic triamniotic or dichorionic triamniotic triplet pregnancy (NICE 2019).

CHAPTER 10

Placental Disorders and Hemorrhage (Abruptio Placentae, Placenta Previa)

Learning Objectives

- Vasa previa—Definition and diagnosis
- Apruptio placentae—Definition, Types, Diagnosis, Differential Diagnosis, Dangers and Management
- Placenta paevia—Definition, Classification, Grades, Difference from abruptio placentae, Dangers and Management

INTRODUCTION

Obstetric hemorrhage is the single most important cause of maternal mortality in the world. Other than postpartum hemorrhage (PPH) hemorrhagic placental disorders, namely abruptio placentae, placenta previa, and placenta accreta spectrum may cause catastrophic threat to both mother and baby. A serious concern is that incidence of both the placenta previa and the placenta accreta spectrum are on rise. Placenta accreta spectrum is written in separate chapter considering its importance in present day obstetrics (Chapter 11).

Antepartum hemorrhage (APH) is defined as the bleeding from or into the genital tract during pregnancy after the age or viability up to the birth of the baby. Previously the age of viability was considered as 28 weeks. But with the improvement of obstetric care, the definition has been changed. In UK, it is considered as 24 weeks, whereas World Health Organization (WHO) considers it to be 22 weeks. Still, in some developing countries 28 weeks is considered as age of viability. Before the age of viability, it is called abortion or miscarriage.

The vaginal bleeding during the first and second stage of labor is called *intrapartum hemorrhage*. But intrapartum hemorrhage is not separately considered in the literature and included in the definition of APH, and the bleeding during the third stage is included in *PPH*.

CAUSES OF ANTEPARTUM HEMORRHAGE

- *Causes in placenta and membranes*:
  - Placenta previa—one-third
  - Abruptio placenta—one-third
  - Vasa previa—rare
- No cause is detected—APH of indeterminate origin or unclassified—one-fourth
- *Bleeding due to local pathology (extra placental)—5%*: Cervical polyp, cervical cancer, and varicose vein of vulva and vagina.

VASA PREVIA

The umbilical cord is sometimes attached to the membranes instead of placenta, this condition is known as velamentous insertion of the cord **(Figs. 1 and 2)**. The vessels transverse through the membranes to reach the placenta. When the blood vessels while passing through the membranes incidentally lies in the lower uterine segment below the presenting part across the internal os, the condition is called vasa previa.

Vasa previa is classified into two types:

1. *Type 1:* Vessels are part of a velamentous cord insertion **(Figs. 1 and 2)**.
2. *Type 2:* Vessels span portions of a bilobed or succenturiate placenta **(Figs. 3 to 5)**.

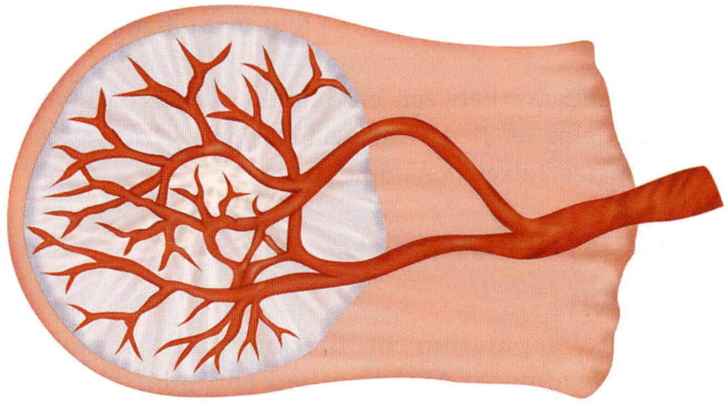

Fig. 1: Vasa previa (diagrammatic).

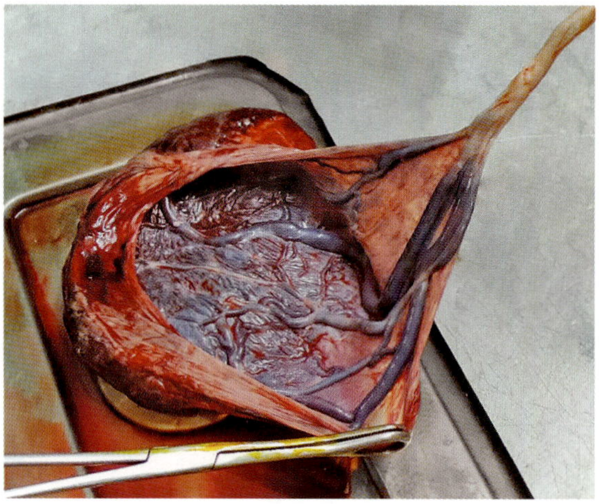

Fig. 2: Vasa previa.
Courtesy: Dr Pradipto Sanyal, Senior consultant, Obstetrics and Gynecology.

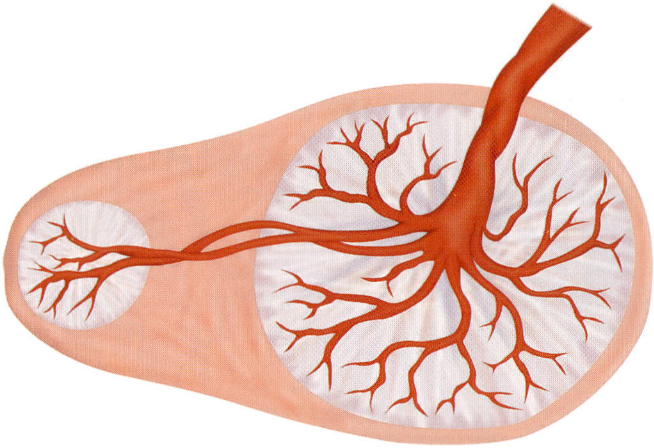

Fig. 3: Placenta succenturiata—fetal surface (diagrammatic).

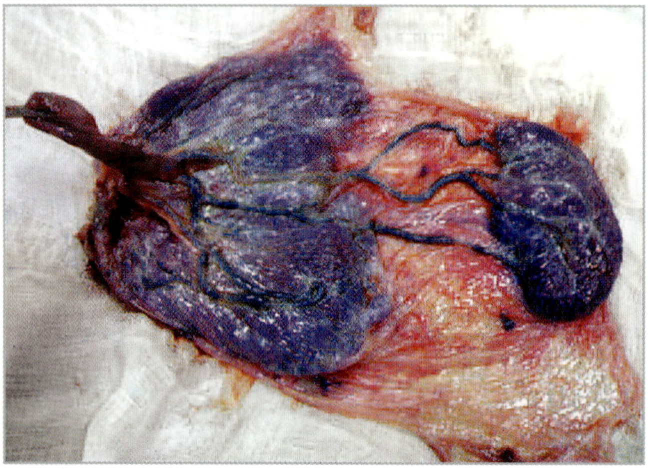

Fig. 4: Placenta succenturiata—fetal surface.
Courtesy: Professor Pesona Grace Lucksom, Sikkim Manipal Institute of Medical Sciences, Sikkim, India.

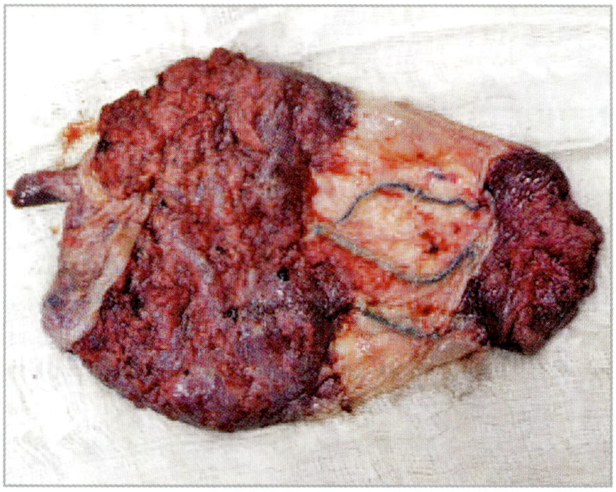

Fig. 5: Placenta succenturiata—maternal surface.
Courtesy: Professor Pesona Grace Lucksom, Sikkim Manipal Institute of Medical Sciences, Sikkim, India.

The vessels are very vulnerable to rupture, either in labor or during internal examination. It is a rare cause of APH with a high rate of fetal death with incidence 2–6/10,000 pregnancies.

In placenta previa, the mother bleeds, but in vasa previa, bleeding comes from the fetus with high fatality of fetus.

Differentiation between fetal blood and maternal blood is done by Kleihauer–Betke test (acid elution test) and Singer's test or Apt test (alkali denaturation test).

ABRUPTIO PLACENTAE

Definition

Premature separation of the normally implanted placenta leading to APH is called abruptio placentae. It excludes separation of placenta previa. The term *'accidental hemorrhage'* is popular in Great Britain. The other nomenclatures are *"abruptio placentae", "placental abruption",* or *"ablatio placentae".* In Latin "abruption" means *breaking away.*

Incidence of accidental hemorrhage is 4–2% of all pregnancies. Incidence of mild variety may be higher up to 4%.

Types and Grades of Abruptio Placentae

Abruptio placentae may be revealed type, concealed type, and mixed type. According to degree of separation it may be partial or complete. According to *Sher and Statland (1985) clinical grading grade I means which is not* recognized before delivery and usually diagnosed by presence of retroplacental clot. In *grade II (intermediate)* the classical signs of abruptio placentae are present whereas the fetus is alive. When the fetus is dead it is called *grade III (severe) which is subdivided into grade IIIa* (without coagulopathy) and grade IIIb (with coagulopathy). In another grading of hemorrhages, mild means when loss of blood is <15% of blood volume, moderate when there is 15–30% loss of blood volume, and severe when it is >30%.

Severe abruption is defined in another way (Am J OBG 2016). It is called severe abruption when one or more of the following is present: (1) presence of maternal morbidity—disseminated intravascular coagulation (DIC), shock, hysterectomy, transfusion, renal failure, and death; (2) compromised fetus—fetal growth restriction (FGR), fetal distress, or death; and (3) neonatal complication—preterm, low birth weight, or death.

Causes and Risk Factors of Abruptio Placentae

Only in few cases the cause is obvious and in most of the cases the cause is obscure. However, there are some risk factors associated with abruptio placentae.

Important causes of abruptio placentae: Causes are abdominal trauma, decompression of uterus, and premature rupture of membranes. Direct trauma to the uterus and external cephalic version (ECV) under anesthesia may cause premature separation of placenta. Rapid decompression of uterus occurs due to sudden rupture of membranes in polyhydramnios which decreases uterine volume, resulting a corresponding loss of surface area for which the placenta may shear off. There is threefold increase in the risk of abruptio placenta in preterm premature rupture of membrane (PPROM) which is managed expectantly.

Risk factors for abruptio placentae:

- With increased age and parity risk of placental abruption rises
- Hypertensive disorder of pregnancy (HDP) is the most frequent association with the abruptio placentae. In preeclampsia (PE), there is spasm of vessels in placental bed that causes anoxic damage of endothelium, which results in rupture of vessels or extravasation of blood in decidua basalis. Impaired trophoblastic invasion followed by adhesions in PE results abruption.
- Familial association has been found in some population.
- Cigarette smoking, cocaine abuse, thrombophilia, prior abruption, and uterine fibroids are associated with increased risk.

Mechanism and Pathogenesis of Abruptio Placentae

The process begins with uterine vasospasm by any cause → followed by relaxation → venous engorgement → arteriolar rupture into decidua → decidua splits with a thin layer of myometrium → decidual hematoma → enlarges to cause separation and compression of placenta by retroplacental hematoma **(Fig. 6)**.

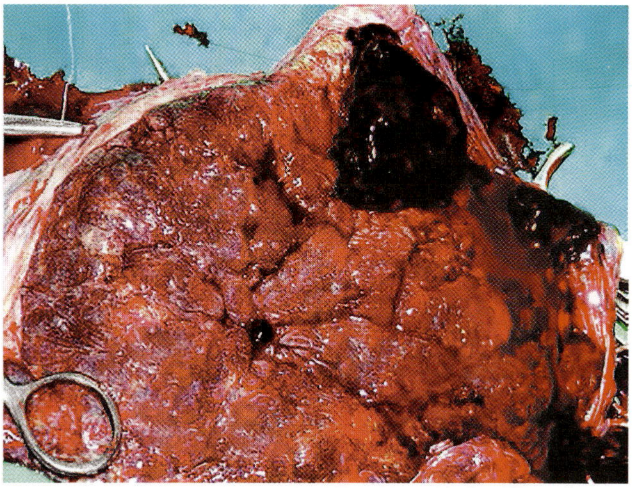

Fig. 6: Retroplacental clot—circumscribed depression on the maternal surface.

The blood may escape in the following ways:

- Blood insinuates between placenta, membranes, and uterus, and then escapes through cervix—*external* or *revealed hemorrhage* is more common **(Fig. 7)**.
- Blood collected behind the placenta which is separated up to the margin where it is adherent—*concealed hemorrhage* which causes more chance of consumptive coagulopathy **(Fig. 8)**.
- Sometimes, blood gets into amniotic sac by breaking through the membranes—*blood-stained liquor* extending inside the uterine musculature—*Couvelaire uterus* **(Fig. 9)**.

Chronic abruption-oligohydramnios sequence is called CAOS. Chronic abruption occurs when delivery does not occur for prolonged period following placental detachment. In these cases, chronic abruption may begin in pregnancy. Subsequently, oligohydramnios develops. Hemorrhage, in some cases may be arrested without delivery. Increase level of serum α-fetoprotein and placental-specific RNA may be found.

Sources of blood in abruptio placentae: Bleeding is almost always maternal. Significant fetal bleeding is seen in traumatic abruption. In traumatic abruption due to placental tears fetomaternal hemorrhage may occur, that may be profuse.

*Couvelaire uterus **(Fig. 9)**:* When there is widespread extravasation of blood into the uterine musculature and beneath the uterine serosa, the color of the uterus becomes dark port wine color, either patchy or diffuse and the uterus is called Couvelaire uterus. This is also called *uteroplacental apoplexy* and first described by Couvelaire in early 1900s.

It is found in severe form of concealed accidental hemorrhage. It is diagnosed only at laparotomy. On microscopical examination, there is infiltration of blood and fluid in between the muscle fibers which may

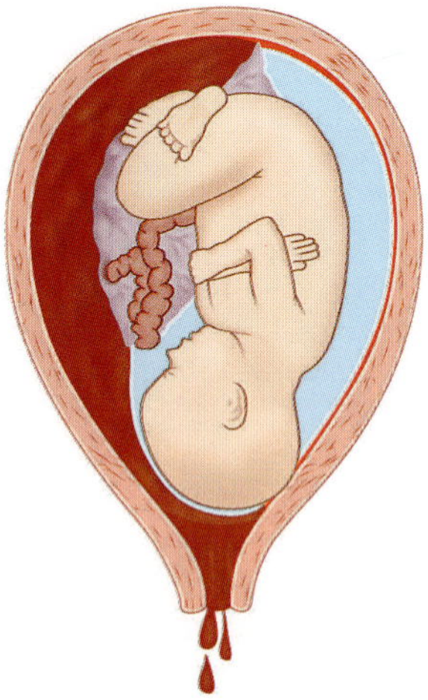

Fig. 7: Abruptio placentae—revealed type.

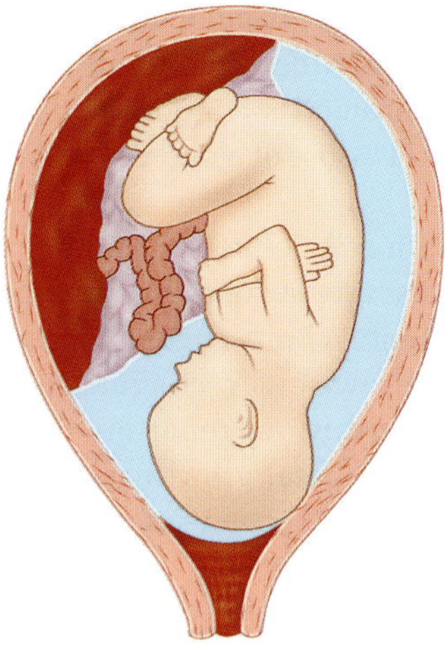

Fig. 8: Abruptio placentae—concealed type.

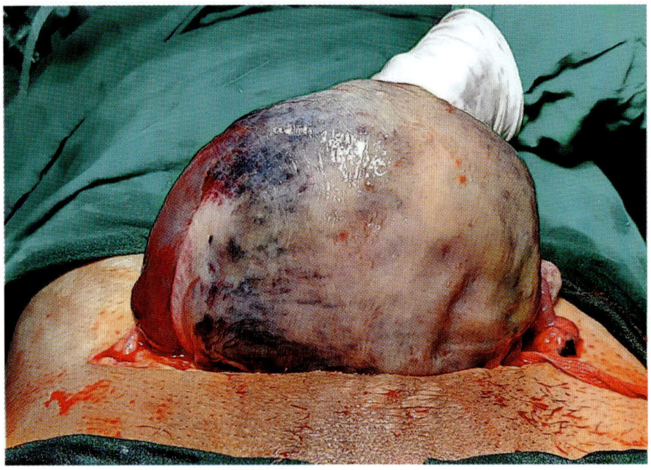

Fig. 9: Couvelaire uterus.

be necrosed. Blood effusions may also be found beneath the tubal serosa, in broad ligaments, in ovaries as well as in peritoneal cavity. The myometrial hemorrhage seldom interferes with uterine contraction and is not responsible for PPH. Couvelaire uterus itself is not an indication for hysterectomy. There is no need of specific treatment.

Symptoms and Signs of Abruptio Placenta

Symptoms and signs of abruptio placenta with differentiating features of revealed and concealed variety: The typical presentation of placental abruption is vaginal bleeding, sudden onset pain in abdomen, and uterine tenderness. However, they differ in types.

Symptoms and signs of abruptio placenta with differentiating features of revealed and concealed variety are given in **Table 1**.

Imaging

Role of sonography to diagnose abruptio placentae ***(Fig. 10)****:* Ultrasound is very helpful in diagnosing or excluding placenta previa but may not diagnose abruption placentae always, especially when blood collection is small. However, it is possible to visualize retroplacental clot with the help of a good quality machine and by an experienced sonologist, though sensitivity is poor.

Magnetic resonance imaging (MRI) is highly sensitive for abruption.

Other Investigations in Abruptio Placentae

Blood—Hb%, urine for protein, coagulation profile—clotting time, fibrinogen level, platelet count, partial thromboplastin time (PTT), fibrin degradation product (FDP), and D-dimer. These profiles are changed specially in concealed or mixed variety.

Differential Diagnosis of Abruptio Placentae

If it is associated with bleeding differential diagnosis is APH due to other causes and it is sometimes confused with rupture of uterus.

In absence of bleeding in concealed type hemorrhage, the conditions causing acute abdomen with uterine tenderness should be differentiated from rectus sheath hematoma, retroperitoneal hemorrhage, rupture of appendicular abscess, acute degeneration, or torsion of a uterine fibroid.

When bleeding is less, uterine contraction present and uterus is slightly tender, it is to be differentiated from spontaneous preterm labor.

Maternal Dangers of Abruptio Placentae

- Hemorrhage—APH and PPH. Reasons of more chance of PPH in abruptio placentae are uterine atonicity and coagulation failure.
- Shock due to hemorrhage, hypovolemia, and coagulation disorder.
- *Coagulation defect*: Consumptive coagulopathy (DIC) in 30% cases.

TABLE 1: Symptoms and signs of abruptio placenta with differentiating features of revealed and concealed variety.

Symptoms and signs	*Revealed*	*Concealed or mixed*
Pain	Slight pain or abdominal discomfort	Severe abdominal pain
Bleeding	Dark color slight to moderate	Dark color—but slight bleeding or blood-stained discharge
GC	Proportionate to external blood loss	Disproportionate to external blood loss
Features of shock	Usually absent	Usually present
Presence of preeclampsia	Irrelevant	Usually present
Fundal height	Coincides to the period of gestation	More than the period of gestation
Feel of uterus	Localized tenderness, contractions present, not so hard	Tense, tender, and woody hard (tonic contraction) Difficult to palpate
Fetal parts	Easily palpable	Usually not present, or nonassuring fetal heart rate in CTG
FHS	Present usually	
Oliguria	Normal amount of urine	Present may be abnormal

(CTG: cardiotocography; FHS: fetal heart sound; GC: general condition)

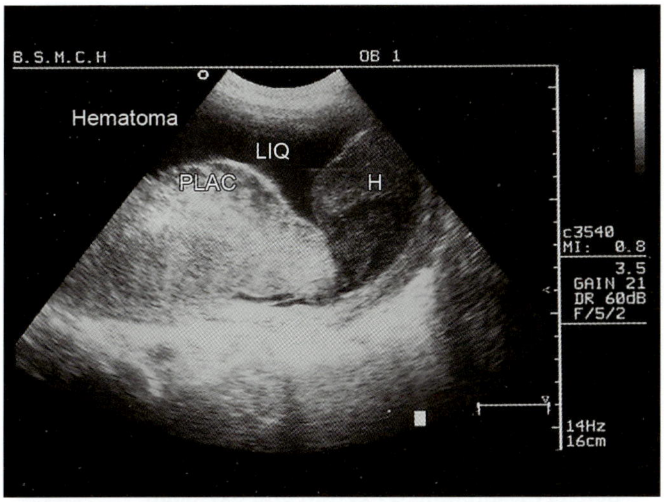

Fig. 10: Ultrasonography (USG) showing bleeding from the separated placenta and accumulated blood beneath the membranes.
(LIQ: liquor, PLAC: placenta, H: hemorrhage)
Courtesy: Dr Madan Karmakar, Professor, Department of Radiodiagnosis, Institute of Postgraduate Medical Education and Research, Kolkata, West Bengal, India.

- *Acute renal failure [acute kidney injury (AKI)]*: Inadequate treatment of hypovolemia in severe abruption may cause AKI. Blood, blood products, crystalloids, and vigorous treatment may prevent AKI, even DIC. Presence of PE increases the risk of renal injury. Most cases of AKI are reversible.
- Puerperal sepsis

Placental abruption and coagulation defect: Abruptio placentae is the most common cause of severe consumptive coagulopathy and most probably in entire spectrum of medicine. Consumptive coagulopathy is more in concealed type as due to pressure by retroplacental clot, more thromboplastin is drained into large veins. With partial abruption and live fetus severe consumptive coagulopathy is less likely.

Depletion of fibrinogen and other factors due to formation of retroplacental clot (primary pathology) and multiple small intravascular thrombi (DIC) are the secondary pathology.

There are two types of coagulopathy, *consumptive coagulopathy* and *dilutional coagulopathy*.

When there is consumption of procoagulants within the intravascular system it is called *consumptive coagulopathy*, DIC, or defibrination syndrome whereas where there is huge loss of procoagulants due to bleeding it is called *dilutional coagulopathy*.

Due to *intravascular activation of coagulation* natural hemostasis mechanism is disrupted with imbalance of natural anticoagulant mechanism which results fibrin (microthrombi) deposition leading to multiorgan failure.

Treatment with crystalloids and packed red blood cells (PRBC) in massive hemorrhage depletion of platelets and coagulation factors occur leading to dilutional coagulopathy which is indistinguishable from DIC (consumptive coagulopathy), however treatment for both is same. DIC is responsible for 25% of maternal deaths globally and associated with severe maternal morbidity like AKI.

Renal Failure in Abruptio Placentae

At the beginning, oliguria occurs due to hypovolemia and later on, serotonin liberated from damaged uterine muscle results in renal ischemia and acute tubular necrosis. In severe case, it may lead to cortical necrosis and renal failure. DIC causing microthrombi in kidney is another reason.

Fetal Dangers in Abruptio Placentae

- Fetal anoxia
- Prematurity
- More cerebral palsy among survivors
- Fetal death—death is due to (1) fetal hypoxia as a result (at least one-third of placenta is separated to cause fetal

death) of placental separation and due to (2) prematurity. Chance of fetal death in *revealed type is* 25–30% and in *concealed type is* 50–100%.

- When DIC occurs, fetus usually dies. Hence, in case of death of fetus in abruptio placentae, maternal danger becomes imminent and prompt management should be done.
- In abruptio placentae both mother and fetus are in danger. However, chance of fetal death is more in abruptio placentae than in placenta previa.

Management of Abruptio Placentae

- Patient is always managed at hospital, not at home. As soon as placental abruption is suspected, actions should be swift and decisive. Blood is sent for Hb% estimation, hematocrit, cross matching, and coagulation profile. Urine is sent for routine examination. Blood requisition is done and transfused as soon as it is available.
- Maternal and fetal condition is monitored closely. Pallor, pulse, respiration, blood pressure, and urine output are recorded. Urinary output should be at least 30 mL/h. Central venous pressure (CVP) monitoring with the help of central venous catheter is invaluable in this case, and CVP is maintained at about 4–8 cm of water. Blood coagulation profile is measured at 2 hourly intervals.
- Then definitive obstetric management for pregnancy is planned.

Definitive obstetric management of abruptio placentae: Management depends on period of gestation, type and severity of abruption, gestational age, maternal condition, and fetal status.

Immediate termination is the aim. Artificial rupture of membrane (ARM) and oxytocin are the treatment of choice for induction or augmentation.

Unlike placenta previa, the role of expectant treatment is less and the indication is when abruption is very minor and gestation is very preterm and there is no progress. These cases usually present with small painless vaginal bleeding and localized area of uterine tenderness appearing after several hours. Strict vigilance is essential. Tocolytics are contraindicated in suspected placental abruption.

When the fetus is living and viable, vaginal delivery is not imminent. Emergency cesarean section (CS) is preferred by many.

Outline of management is shown in **Flowchart 1**.

Status of Fetus and Obstetric Management

- *Fetus dead:* It signifies severe abruption (more than one-third separation) → deliver immediately → vaginal delivery allowed unless excessive uncontrolled bleeding or exsanguinated maternal condition or other obstetric contraindication for vaginal delivery.

Flowchart 1: Outline of management of abruptio placentae.

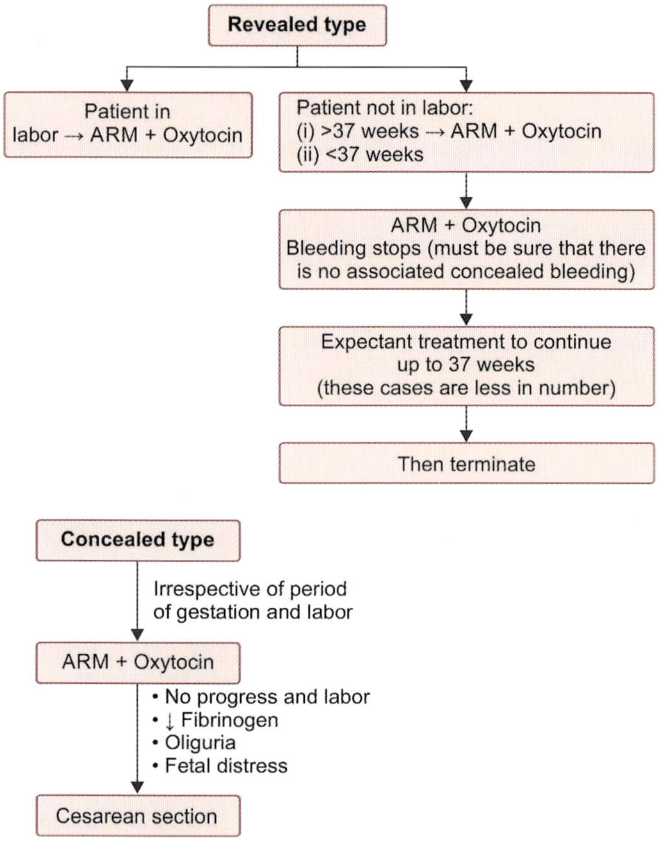

(ARM: artificial rupture of membrane)

If delayed → delivered by CS.

- *Fetus living*: Mature → delivered immediately. Vaginal delivery is attempted by ARM and oxytocin.

  If there is delay or fear of progressive concealed hemorrhage deteriorating the condition of mother CS is done. In prematurity → expectant treatment can be given in mild variety of revealed type (rarely).

Induction or augmentation: Induction or augmentation is done by ARM (amniotomy) and oxytocin. The main purpose is to hasten the onset of labor by encouraging uterine contraction, and also to reduce the uterine bleeding. ARM also helps to reduce the entry of thromboplastin and activated coagulation factor from retroplacental clot into maternal circulation. Thus, two grave complications—renal cortical necrosis and blood coagulation disorders are minimized.

Management of Labor in Abruptio Placenta

Close monitoring of labor is done, both maternal and fetal condition are closely watched. Usually labor progresses well in abruption following ARM and oxytocin. Following delivery of baby, placenta with retroplacental clot is expelled. Placenta and retroplacental clot are examined to assess the concealed blood loss. Active management of third stage of labor (AMTSL) is done. Oxytocics are used liberally to prevent PPH. Following vaginal delivery uterotonic and uterine massage are given to stimulate myometrial contraction for proper hemostasis. Sustained myometrial contraction along with blood and blood products will cause hemostasis even in presence of coagulopathy. It is the adequate fluid, blood and blood products which are more important rather than the delivery time to save the mother.

Indications of cesarean delivery in abruptio placentae:

- When cervix is unfavorable, immediate delivery is needed due to the exsanguinated maternal condition.
- Fetus is living and salvageable and vaginal delivery is not imminent. The compromised fetus is best delivered by cesarean.
- In spite of ARM, the progress of labor is delayed, general condition becomes worse, complication arises, and signs of fetal distress appear.

Cesarean delivery in abruptio placentae: Development of consumptive coagulopathy is the most danger which can be overcome by availability of adequate blood and blood components and their transfusion by assessing the degree of coagulopathy, especially levels of fibrinogen. Placenta and retroplacental clot are examined to assess the concealed blood loss **(Fig. 11)**. Couvelaire uterus itself is not an indication for hysterectomy. Attention should be given for uterine contractility and AMTSL is done with uterotonic. Anti-D immunoglobulin should be given to every Rh-negative woman within 48 hours of abruption. The usual dose is 300 μg.

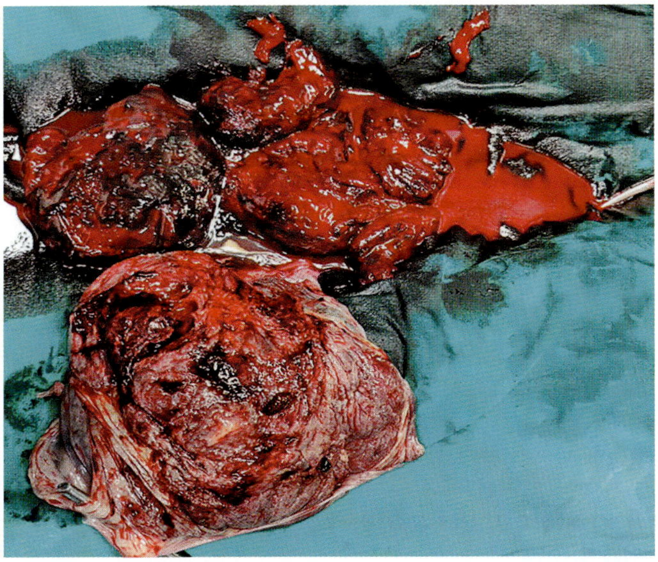

Fig. 11: Retroplacental clot with placenta-delivered following a cesarean section.
Courtesy: Dr Chandos Saha and Dr Sima Das, RG Kar Medical College, Kolkata, West Bengal, India.

PLACENTA PREVIA

Definition

Literally "previa" means in front of. When the placenta is situated partially and completely in the lower uterine segment, it is called placenta previa.

Classification

National Institutes of Health (NIH) classification: This is the latest classification.

Only two are described.

1. *Placenta previa*: The internal os is covered partially or completely by placenta.
2. *Low-lying placenta*: Placenta is implanted in the lower uterine segment and the placental margin does not cover the internal os but lies within a 2 cm wide perimeter around the os. In *marginal previa*, placenta is at the edge of the internal os but does not overlie it. The term "low-lying placenta" is applicable after 16 weeks of pregnancy.

Clinical Gradings

- Minor degree placenta previa—type I **(Fig. 12)** and type II anterior **(Fig. 13)**
- Major degree placenta previa—type II posterior, type III **(Fig. 14)**, and type IV **(Fig. 15)**

Type II posterior placenta previa: In type II posterior placenta previa, placenta lies at the level of the sacral promontory and thereby diminished resultant anteroposterior diameter prevents the engagement. Besides, placenta and umbilical cord may be compressed, resulting fetal distress. Due to nonengagement, maternal sinus lies below is not compressed and bleeding continues. For these reasons, this type is also called *dangerous placenta previa*.

Risk Factors and Associated Conditions for Placenta Previa

With increased age and parity risk of placenta previa rises. Previous uterine scar (previous CS and myomectomy) is important risk factor. Risk rises five times in pregnancy with prior cesarean delivery. The risk also increases with the increase number of prior CS. With increased placental size (twin pregnancy, placenta membranacea, placenta succenturiate, etc.), encroaching of placenta in lower uterine segment is more. Smoking by defective decidual vascularization, inflammatory or atrophic changes are the possible explanations of increase incidence of placenta previa. Assisted reproductive technology (ART) and uterine leiomyoma are the other risk factors for placenta previa.

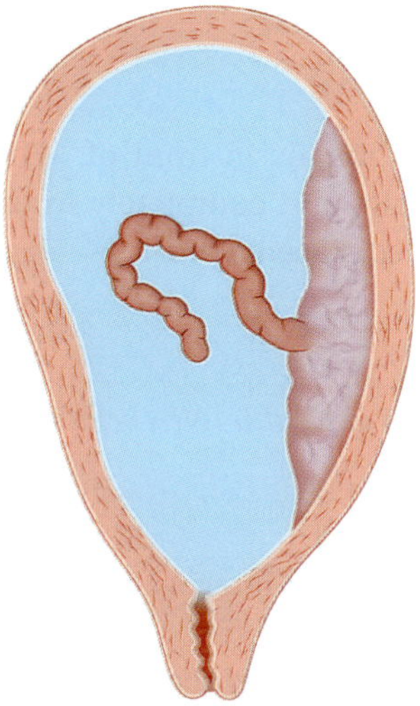

Fig. 12: Type I of placenta previa.

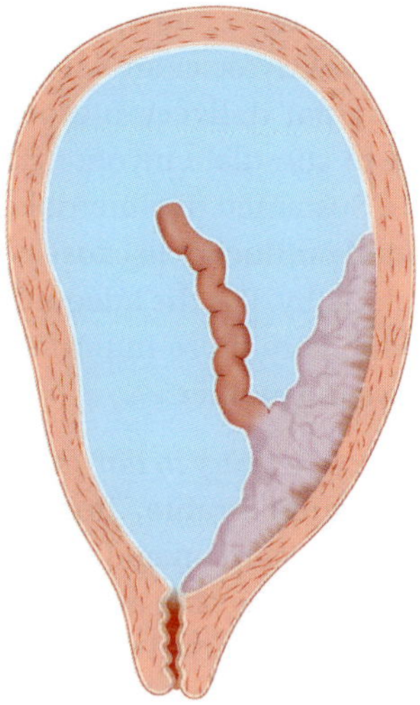

Fig. 13: Type II of placenta previa.

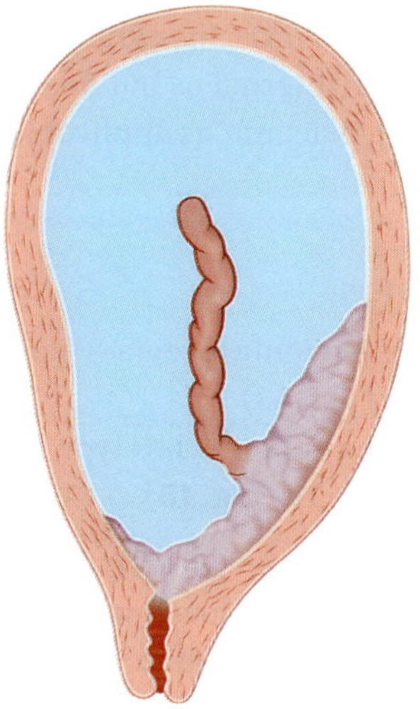

Fig. 14: Type III of placenta previa.

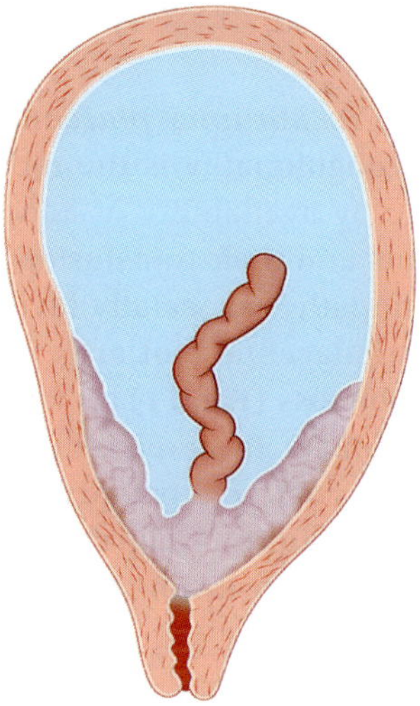

Fig. 15: Type IV of placenta previa.

Incidence of placenta previa is increasing recently due to increased rate of CS and increased incidence of multiple pregnancy and ART conception.

Placental Migration and its Role in Pathogenesis

Placental migration is the apparent movement of the low-lying placenta in relation to internal os with increased gestation. The concept comes from the fact that by ultrasonography (USG) about 5% of women have low-lying placenta but at term only 0.5% persists. In fact, the placenta does not move and term migration is misnomer. The change is due to development of lower uterine segment with advancement of pregnancy and placental growth occurs in more vascularized part of uterus, fundus, the phenomenon is known as *trophotropism*. In prior CS this migration is less likely to occur. When placenta lies within <2 cm from os, or placenta is posterior migration is also less.

A low-lying placenta identified in early pregnancy may "migrate" upward as pregnancy progresses, with formation of the lower uterine segment and expansion of the upper segment. Scar due to prior CS hampers migration due to adherence of placenta with scar and placenta previa persists.

Reasons of Bleeding in Placenta Previa

As the rate of growth of placenta is slower in comparison to the growth of lower uterine segment in last trimester and the placenta is a nonelastic structure, it gets separated from the uterine wall and thus the maternal sinuses opened resulting in bleeding. Trauma due to internal examination, coital act and ECV may also cause bleeding.

Diagnosis of Placenta Previa—Symptoms and Signs

Women with placenta previa may present with either: (1) symptomatic, (2) active antepartum bleeding, or (3) stable after one or more episodes of antepartum bleeding.

TABLE 2: Differentiating clinical features between placenta previa and abruptio placenta.

	Placenta previa	*Abruptio placenta*
1. Pattern of bleeding	1. Apparently no cause, painless, recurrent and always revealed, and bright red in color	1. May be associated with pain May be concealed or revealed Dark red in color
2. Pallor and general condition	2. Proportionate to the bleeding	2. Out of proportionate to the visible blood loss
3. Features of preeclampsia	3. No relation	3. Common association
4. Height of fundus	4. Corresponds to the period of amenorrhea	4. More than the period of amenorrhea
5. Palpation of uterus	5. Soft, relaxed	5. Tense, tender, irritable, and does not relax
6. Presentation	6. More chance of malpresentation, presenting part not engaged	6. Usually vertex and engaged
7. FHS	7. Present	7. May be absent in concealed type or revealed type when bleeding is excessive

(FHS: fetal heart sound)

Symptoms: Usual presentation is sudden onset of vaginal bleeding in second half of pregnancy which is painless and apparently causeless. There may be a P/H of vaginal bleeding in early pregnancy. No history of trauma or any precipitating factor like hypertension.

Signs: Pallor is proportionate to the amount of bleeding. Uterus—nontender, soft, and height corresponds with period of amenorrhea. Head is high floating; fetal heart sound (FHS) is well audible.

Differentiating clinical features between placenta previa and abruptio placenta are given in **Table 2**.

Time of bleeding in placenta previa in relation to period of gestation: Bleeding usually occurs before 38 weeks of pregnancy and it may occur even before 28th week of pregnancy.

Lower the placenta is situated, earlier the first episode of bleeding occurs. Hence, earlier bleeding occurs more in major degree placenta previa. However, bleeding may start even after the onset of labor also in central placenta previa. Patient may be asymptomatic and diagnosed by sonography or during CS.

In 10% cases patient remains asymptomatic, especially when the placenta is implanted near os, but not over it and bleeding start after onset of labor.

Characteristic Pattern of Hemorrhage in Placenta Previa

In an uneventful antenatal course bleeding occurs without warning (sudden in onset), not associated with pain or contractions. This is called *sentinel bleed* which is rarely so profuse to cause fatal. Blood is bright red in color and there may be recurrent episode of bleeding.

Hemorrhage occurs due to separation of placenta from lower uterine segment before onset of labor and this phenomenon is painless.

Because the separation is not a continuous process recurrent episode of bleeding occurs.

As the source of bleeding lies close to the vagina and comes out immediately after bleeding, the blood is bright red in color. In abruptio placenta, the source of bleeding is at the site of normally situated placenta and were collected for sometimes before coming out of vagina. The blood is dark red in color in placental abruption.

Categorization of the Severity of Hemorrhage in Placenta Previa (Royal College of Obstetricians and Gynaecologists)

- *Spotting*: Staining, streaking, or spotting noted on pad or underwear
- *Minor hemorrhage*: <50 mL, patient settled
- *Major hemorrhage*: 50–100 mL, with no sign of shock
- *Massive hemorrhage*: Loss is >1,000 mL and/or signs of shock

"Warning hemorrhage": The first episode of bleeding in placenta previa is very small in amount, not profuse to prove fatal and usually stops spontaneously—this is called "warning hemorrhage".

Stallworthy's sign: In low-lying placenta, when the head is pressed down in the pelvis, fetal bradycardia occurs due to compression and it becomes normal soon after the release—it is called Stallworthy's sign. However, it is not specific and may occur due to fetal head compression due to any other reason.

Imaging

Sonography scan: Scan is usually performed by transabdominal method. Transvaginal sonography is superior to transabdominal and transperineal sonography and safe. Placenta is situated on lower uterine segment and no retroplacental clot is found **(Fig. 16)**. USG can exclude

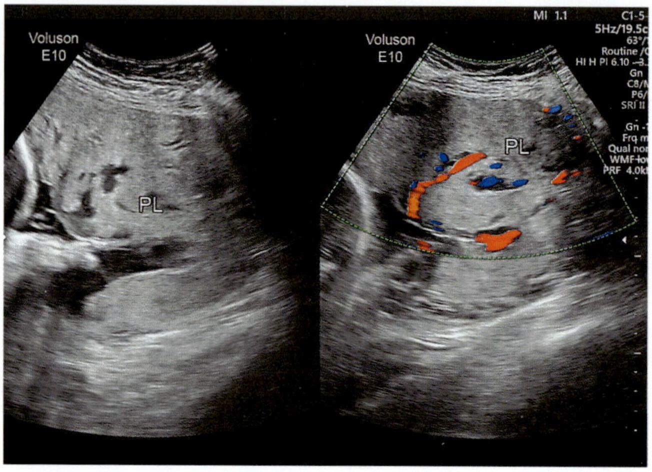

Fig. 16: Ultrasonography showing placenta previa.
(PL: placenta)
Courtesy: Professor Kamal Oswal, Head, Department of Radiodiagnosis, Vivekananda Institute of Medical Sciences, Kolkata, West Bengal, India.

the placenta previa and a high negative predictive value at any gestational age. Placenta previa is diagnosed when placenta covers the internal os or reaches the os. A second USG assessment is recommended at 32 weeks, if persists repeat transvaginal ultrasound (TVS) is recommended at 36 weeks gestation. Low-lying placenta is diagnosed when the placental margin is <2 cm from the cervical internal os, not covering it and repeated at 32 weeks, if persists again done at 36 weeks. Vasa previa is to be excluded if the low-lying placenta/placenta previa is resolved in subsequent sonography and tracing of umbilical cord insertion is done. Placenta accreta spectrum is always searched for in placenta previa.

Usefulness of cervical length measurement in USG—a short cervical length before 34 weeks increases preterm emergency delivery and there may be massive hemorrhage during sections.

Confirmation of placenta previa is done with the help of standard sonographic technique by which the site of placental implantation can be precisely found and seen at lower uterine segment.

A painless bleeding in second half of pregnancy should be considered as placenta previa until and unless proved otherwise.

Screening for Placenta Previa or Low-lying Placenta

Midpregnancy routine fetal anomaly scan should include localization of placenta to identify at risk for placenta previa or low-lying placenta. If there is placenta previa or low-lying placenta at anomaly scan follow-up by TVS is done at 32 weeks of gestation to diagnose persistent low-lying placenta and/or placenta previa. In case of persistent low-lying placenta/placenta previa at 32 weeks which remains asymptomatic TVS is recommended at 36 weeks to inform discussion about mode of delivery.

Role of Magnetic Resonance Imaging

Magnetic resonance imaging is excellent for diagnosis of placenta previa, but not for routine use, most useful for evaluation of placenta accreta spectrum.

Dangers of Placenta Previa

Maternal Dangers

Hemorrhage, shock, increased operative interference, PPH, retained placenta due to increased surface area and morbid adhesion, and sepsis.

NB: Placenta previa may be complicated with abruptio placentae in 10% cases.

Reasons of more chance of PPH in placenta previa: As placenta is implanted in lower uterine segment, there is less retractile to arrest the bleeding. Sometimes there may be morbid adhesion of placenta (placenta accreta, increta, and percreta). Larger surface area of placenta causes more bleeding. Due to preexisting anemia in APH slight PPH has profound effect on maternal health.

Though maternal deaths have been reduced from placenta previa, contribution of placenta previa in hemorrhagic death is still high.

Fetal Dangers in Antepartum Hemorrhage

There is possibility of low-birth-weight baby due to prematurity. FGR is unlikely. Asphyxia due to maternal hypotension, premature separation of placenta. Fetal malformation—there is more chance of fetal malformation in placenta previa.

Management of Placenta Previa

Role of Antenatal Care in Placenta Previa

Antenatal care is tailored. Placenta previa and low-lying placenta are screened during midtrimester anomaly scan. Routine antenatal care improves anemia, can diagnose the APH earlier and can prevent complications. Emphasis is given on prevention and treatment of anemia. Warning hemorrhage should always be investigated. Blood grouping and typing are done. It is marked as high-risk case—increased maternal and fetal surveillance are needed.

Management: All cases are taken admitted. Maternal condition, severity of blood loss, and fetal condition are assessed. Immediate infusion of intravenous (IV) fluid (crystalloids) with large bore needle, and blood requisition is done. Usually the first bleeding stops. A gentle speculum examination should be done 2–3 days after cessation of bleeding to visualize any local lesion.

All APH cases are considered as placenta previa until and otherwise proved.

Internal examination per vaginal (P/V) should never be done except in operation theater because it may cause torrential bleeding. Localization of the placenta is done by USG.

Conservative management or active management—decision is made depending on the bleeding status and fetal maturity. Mode of termination depends on the condition of the patient, type of placenta previa, and other associated obstetric condition.

Investigations are sent for blood for complete hemogram, bleeding time, clotting time, and clot retraction time.

Blood for grouping and cross matching are done. Sonography is done to detect placental site and for presence of any retroplacental clot.

Expectant Management in Placenta Previa

Macafee and Johnson (1945) advocated this expectant management in order to continue the pregnancy as far as possible to attain the fetal maturity without compromising the maternal condition and popularly known as Macafee and Johnson regime.

The indications of expectant treatment are duration of pregnancy is <37 weeks, there is no active vaginal bleeding, fetal condition is good, and maternal condition is not exsanguinated.

The components of Macafee and Johnson regime are bed rest, adequate nutrition, and hematinics, to watch for any vaginal bleeding, examination of vulval pads, physical and obstetrical examination of mother routinely, to monitor fetal condition clinically and by USG at 2–3 weeks interval. Gentle speculum examination with the help of Cusco's speculum is done 2–3 days after cessation of bleeding to exclude the presence of cervical polyp or any vaginal lesions.

Ideally expectant treatment in placenta previa should be given at hospital. In rare instances, when bleeding is spotting type, patient settled, fetal condition is good, where the residence is very nearby, and the patient and her relatives are well aware of the risk, the patient can be kept at home with provision of immediate transportation. Woman should be informed to attend hospital immediately, if there is any bleeding, spotting, contraction, pain, or even suprapubic ache. Mother with major placenta previa and having recurrent bleeding should be kept in hospital from 34 weeks. Home management is obviously economical. Every case should be individualized.

The contraindications of expectant treatment pregnancy are if the period of gestation is 37 weeks duration or more, patient is in labor, bleeding is not controlled/patient's condition is exsanguinated even if there is no bleeding at present, and fetus is dead or grossly congenitally anomalous.

Role of Steroid, Tocolytics, or Cerclage Operation

A single course of antenatal corticosteroid is recommended between 34+0 and 35+6 weeks of gestation in low-lying placenta or placenta previa and is best before 34+0 weeks of gestation where there is risk for preterm birth to accelerate lung maturity.

Tocolytics and cerclage operation have little role in placenta previa.

If tocolytic is used, not >48 hours. Ca-channel blocker nifedipine is best to avoid.

Time and Mode of Termination of Pregnancy in Placenta Previa

In uncomplicated placenta previa delivery is considered between 36^{+0} and 37^{+0} weeks of gestation. Late preterm delivery (34^{+0} to 36^{+0} weeks) is considered where there is history of vaginal bleeding or associated with risk factors for preterm delivery (RCOG 2018). In suspected morbidly adherent placenta delivery is recommended at 35–36 completed weeks.

Delivery is mostly done by cesarean. In well selected cases vaginal delivery may be attempted by ARM followed by oxytocin depending upon the type of placenta previa, amount of bleeding, condition of fetus, and other obstetric factors. The place of vaginal delivery is very limited.

Vaginal delivery can be allowed in low-lying placenta, margin 2 cm away from the cervical os where bleeding per vagina is minimal or nil, the mother's condition is good, no fetal distress, and no other obstetric factor is present. It is best determined by relation between the leading placental edge and fetal head position with the help of TVS.

"Double Setup" Examination

Digital cervical examination in the operation room to take decision about the mode of delivery for localization of placenta keeping all preparations for CS is called "*double setup*" examination. This digital examination, even if mild, may be a cause of torrential hemorrhage. However, the need of double setup examination is rare nowadays due to the wider availability of USG which helps in placental localization and makes easy to take the decision of route of delivery beforehand.

Digital vaginal examination is also very restricted in suspected placenta previa. It is only done when USG excludes the placenta previa and APH is associated with pain and uterine contraction.

Indications for Cesarean Delivery

Practically all cases of placenta previa is delivered by CS except a very few cases of low-lying placenta (minor degree) where vaginal delivery can be attempted.

The indications are—(1) all cases of major degree placenta previa, (2) in minor degree placenta previa where ARM fails to control the bleeding or there is fetal distress, (3) other obstetric factors are malpresentation, elderly primi, post-CS pregnancy with prior cesarean delivery, and contracted pelvis.

Optimization of Delivery of Women with Placenta Previa

Woman and relatives should be discussed regarding the delivery, indication of blood and blood products transfusion, and the need of hysterectomy are discussed. In anterior low-lying placenta and placenta previa there is high risk of massive hemorrhage and hysterectomy may be needed. Delivery is done in a setup with blood transfusion and critical care facility. Senior obstetrician and senior anesthetist should be present in planned cesarean delivery and be available at emergency.

Types of Cesarean Delivery in Placenta Previa

Both *lower segment or classical* type incision have advantages and disadvantages. Nowadays, most surgeons prefer to do lower segment cesarean section (LSCS) because they are well accustomed with this technique.

Advantages of LSCS in placenta previa are that surgeon is well accustomed with this technique, maternal sinuses on placental bed are well visible and easy to tackle, and if needed decision of hysterectomy can be taken. If there is placenta accreta it can be managed effectively. Disadvantages of LSCS are there may be profuse bleeding from the large dilated vessels situated over the anterior wall of lower uterine segment in anterior placenta previa. In LSCS the placenta is to be cut through resulting severe blood loss from fetus and fetus may be exsanguinated.

Techniques of Cesarean Delivery in Placenta Previa

Longitudinal abdominal skin incision is beneficial. The dilated veins on the anterior wall are ligated above and below and the incision is given in between.

If placenta is anterior—either of the two approaches is followed: (1) going through the placenta by incising it—requires speedy delivery of fetus as significant loss of fetal blood occurs resulting fetal anoxia or (2) fingers are entered through the edge of the placenta above or below whichever is nearer and passing through the membranes—this procedure may be associated with undue delay and there may be fetal blood loss from partially separated placenta.

Following delivery of baby umbilical cord is clamped immediately. Maternal or fetal outcomes are rarely compromised even incision is given through placenta. Oxytocin infusion is started.

Tackling of Placental Bed Hemorrhage

Due to the poorly contracted smooth muscle in lower uterine segment, there may be uncontrollable bleeding. Initial management is uterotonic followed by pressure by hot mop.

If not controlled, "*oversewing suture*" with 0-chromic catgut, "*Cho circular sutures*" around the bleeding area in 1 cm interval, compression sutures that traversed anterior, and posterior uterine wall like "*Cho multiple square sutures*" or "*cervical isthmic sutures*" etc. are applied (These are described in chapter of PPH, Chapter 19).

Tamponade with Bakri or Foley balloon can be very useful. Some advocate combined use of Bakri balloon and compression sutures. Tightly packing the lower uterine segment with gauze and removal of gauze after 12 hours transvaginally have also been reported with success. Other options are uterine and internal iliac artery ligation. Pelvic artery embolization is becoming popular where the facility is available. Subendometrial injection of vasopressin at the placental site bleeding has been reported.

In uterine atony—uterus is massaged, hot mops compression given, oxytocic is repeated. In rare cases of brisk hemorrhages, *stepwise uterine devascularization and even hysterectomy* is needed when conservative methods fail (see Chapter 19 of PPH). Hysterectomy may also be needed in morbid adhesions of placenta.

Advantages of classical cesarean section in placenta previa: Lower segment is avoided, so that in anterior placenta previa the injury of vessels and cutting through the placenta can be avoided.

Disadvantages of classical cesarean section: All the disadvantages of classical section are there. Surgeons, nowadays, are not well conversant with this technique. Placental bed and lower segment are not well visible, therefore difficult to tackle the bleeding and morbid adhesion, if any.

Special Problems of Placenta Previa in a Pregnancy with Prior Cesarean Section

- Previous CS itself is a risk factor (five times more common) for placenta previa as discussed earlier.
- Women with a history of previous cesarean who have either placenta previa or anterior placenta implanted over old CS scar are at increased risk of morbid adhesion (placenta accreta spectrum) and should be managed as a case of placenta accreta, with proper preparation for surgery (detailed in the Placenta Accreta Spectrum, Chapter 11).

- Ultrasound and MRI help to diagnose morbid adhesion of placenta.
- In a suspected placenta previa accreta skin incision is better to be vertical, uterine incision (vertical) should be given at a site distant from the placenta and baby is delivered without disturbing the placenta so that placenta can be managed conservatively or to do elective hysterectomy keeping placenta in situ and without disturbing it if accreta is confirmed.
- Going through the placenta after incising it in placenta previa accreta invites profuse bleeding and hysterectomy becomes mandatory if accreta is confirmed. An ultrasound scan before starting the surgery is essential to plot out the placenta (detailed in the Placenta Accreta Spectrum, Chapter 11).

Anesthesia in Antepartum Hemorrhage

Regional anesthesia is the recommended method, if there is no specific contraindication and there is less blood loss than general anesthesia. When maternal or fetal condition is compromised general anesthesia should be considered to facilitate maternal resuscitation.

Management of Labor in Vaginal Delivery in Placenta Previa

Continuous fetal heart monitoring should be done. If bleeding continues or increases liberal cesarean delivery is contemplated.

Active management of third stage of labor is done as there is more chance of PPH. Following delivery of placenta, the patient is closely observed to detect PPH at earliest.

CHAPTER 11

Placenta Accreta Spectrum

Learning Objectives

- Incidence
- Different Varieties
- Federation of Gynecology and Obstetrics Classification of Placenta Accreta Spectrum (2019)
- Complications
- Risk Factors and Etiology
- Pathophysiology
- Diagnosis
- Imaging in Placenta Accreta Spectrum
- Management
- Delivery and Cesarean Hysterectomy
- Alternate Methods of Management

INTRODUCTION

Placenta accreta spectrum (PAS) is associated with significant morbidity and mortality due to life-threatening hemorrhage and it is one of the leading causes of peripartum hysterectomy. Its remarkable rising frequency has made it one of the most dreadful problems in obstetrics.

It is a condition where the placenta is directly adhered to the uterine myometrium wall due to absence of the decidua basalis. PAS is also referred to as morbidly adherent placenta, which includes a range of pathologic adherence of the placenta, namely placenta accreta, increta, and percreta. It is also called placenta accreta syndrome and pernicious placenta previa with accreta and abnormally adherent placenta. "Accreta" comes from Latin ac- + crescere to grow from adhesion or become attached to. The term "placenta accrete" was first described by FC Irving (obstetrician) and A Hertig (pathologist) from Boston in 1937.

INCIDENCE

Hundred years back the incidence was 1 in 20,000 births, in 1980s it was 1 in 2,500 and in 2015 1 in 731 and more recently, it is 1 in 300 [American College of Obstetricians and Gynecologists (ACOG), 2018]. The reason is not very clear. Increase in cesarean section rate with increase of placenta previa with implantation of placenta over scar is a definite cause, but there may be other factors which need extensive research to reveal. Whether the surgical technique and suture materials used in cesarean delivery have any effect is still unclear.

DIFFERENT VARIETIES

By the depth of trophoblastic growth, the variants of PAS are:

- Placenta accreta—placental villi is attached to the myometrium—80%.
- Placenta increta—placental villi invades the myometrium—15%.
- Placenta percreta—placental villi penetrates through myometrium to reach the serous coat of uterus—5%.

However, in the referral center, majority (>50%) are percreta and the accreta and increta are of equal percentage near 25% each.

Morbid adhesion of placenta may be focal or total. Focal means only a single lobule (partly or fully) is abnormally adherent. It is called total placenta accreta when abnormal attachment involves all lobules.

FEDERATION OF GYNECOLOGY AND OBSTETRICS CLASSIFICATION OF PLACENTA ACCRETA SPECTRUM (2019)

Grade 1: Abnormally adherent placenta (placenta adherent or accreta) **(Fig. 1)**

Grade 2: Abnormally invasive placenta (increta) **(Fig. 2)**

Grade 3: Abnormally invasive placenta (percreta)

Grade 3a: Limited to the uterine serosa **(Figs. 3 and 4)**

Grade 3b: With urinary bladder invasion **(Fig. 5)**

Grade 3c: With invasion of other pelvic tissue/organ

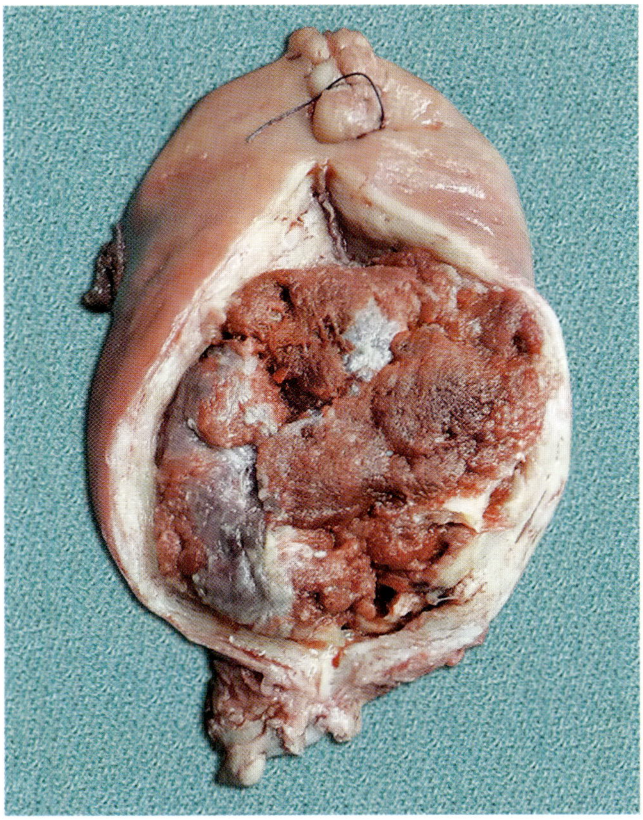

Fig. 1: Abnormally adherent placenta (placenta accreta)—placental villi attached to myometrium *(FIGO Grade 1)*.

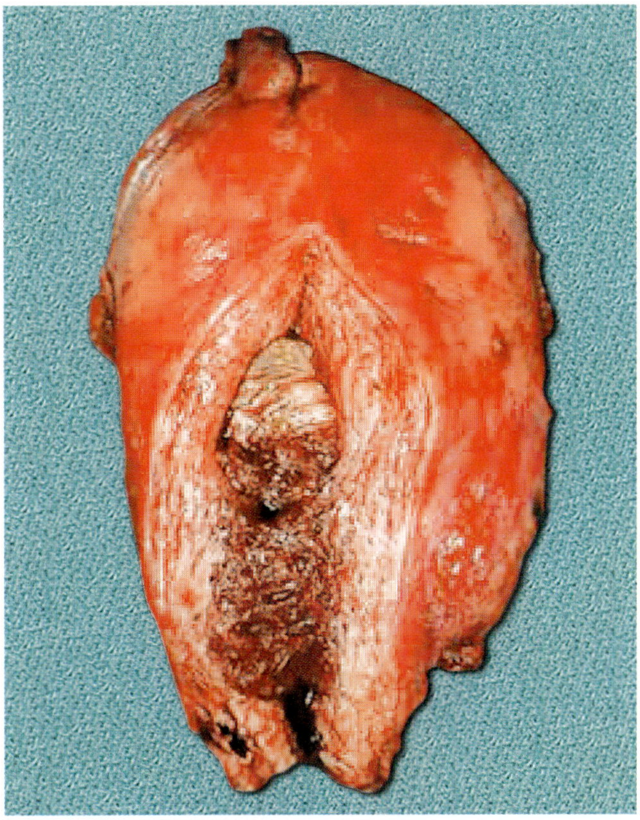

Fig. 2: Abnormally invasive placenta (increta)—part of myometrium invaded *(FIGO Grade 2)*.

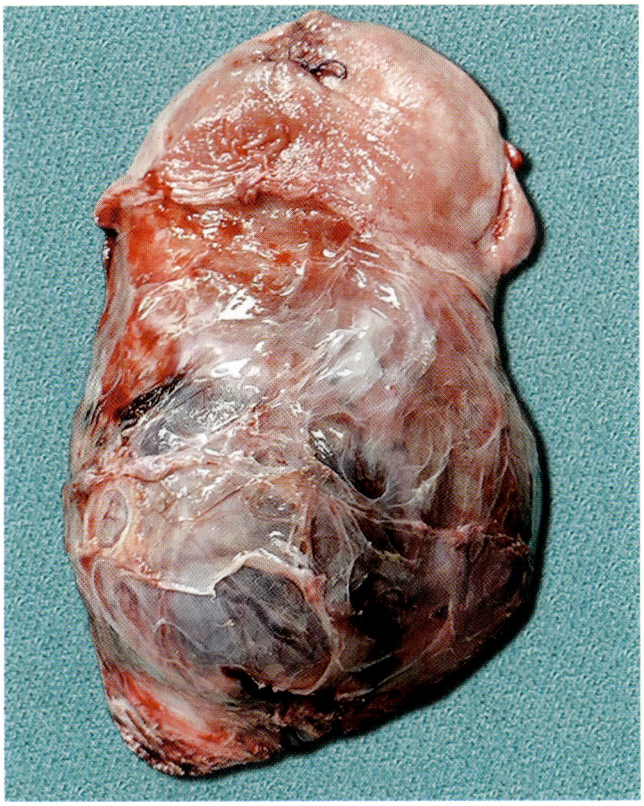

Fig. 3: Specimen of uterus following obstetric hysterectomy, only thin serosa is present (percreta) *(FIGO Grade 3a)*.

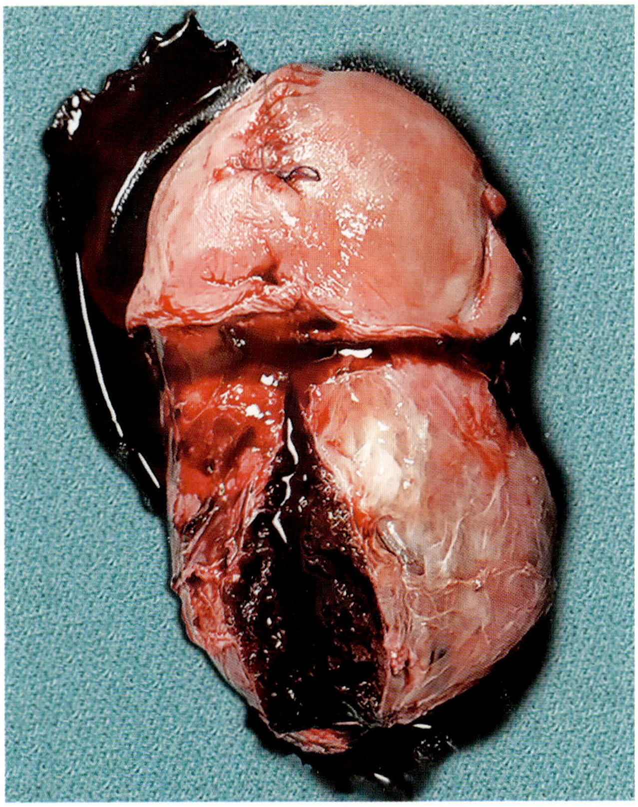

Fig. 4: Same specimen as in Figure 3 to cut open—incision given over serosa, there is no myometrium (percreta) *(FIGO Grade 3a)*.

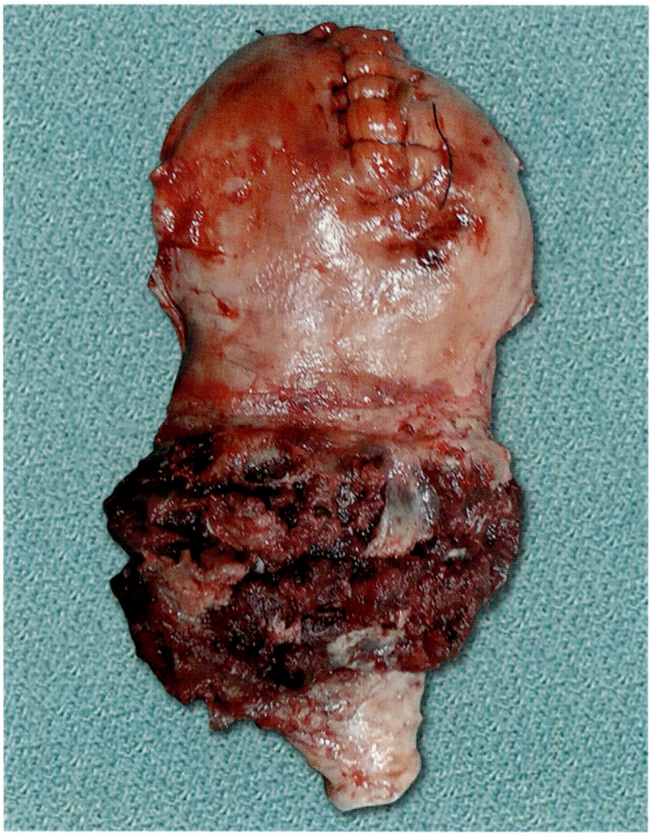

Fig. 5: Another specimen—no serosa and no myometrium, bladder involvement (percreta) (*FIGO Grade 3b*).
Courtesy: Professor RP Ganguly and Dr Anindya Das, RG Kar Medical College and Hospital, Kolkata, West Bengal, India.

COMPLICATIONS

Maternal mortality—7%

Morbidity—massive hemorrhage (3–5 L), disseminated intravascular coagulation (DIC), acute kidney injury (AKI), acute respiratory distress syndrome (ARDS), need for hysterectomy, postoperative bleeding needing repeat surgery, injury to ureter, bladder, bowel, etc., transfusion reaction, infection, and thromboembolism.

RISK FACTORS AND ETIOLOGY

The important risk factors for PAS are:

- Prior cesarean delivery is the most common risk factor—the risk rises as the number of prior cesarean sections increases. Associated placenta previa—*combination of placenta previa and history of prior cesarean delivery has higher chance of accreta*. PAS occurs in 3% of women with placenta previa without prior cesarean deliveries.
- History of accreta in a previous pregnancy/manual removal of placenta
- Prior uterine surgeries, e.g., myomectomy, endometrial resection
- Vigorous endometrial curettage and Asherman syndrome
- Endometritis
- Uterine anomalies
- In vitro fertilization (IVF) procedures/intrauterine device (IUD)
- Advanced maternal age and multiparity
- Abnormal results of some *placental biomarkers* increase the risk of PAS. Among those are maternal serum alpha-fetoprotein, pregnancy-associated plasma protein A, pro B-type natriuretic peptide, troponin, free β-human chorionic gonadotropin (hCG) [messenger ribonucleic acid (mRNA)], and human placental lactogen and total placental cell-free mRNA. But all these are poor predictor and not clinically useful.

PATHOPHYSIOLOGY

Prior uterine surgeries increase trophoblastic invasion. Defective formation of decidua—partial or total absence of the decidua basalis and imperfect development of the fibrinoid or Nitabuch layer causes abnormal placental adherence to the myometrium leading to abnormal infiltration of deep placental anchoring villi of the placenta into myometrium, sometimes involving bladder. Mere decidual defect is not solely responsible for PAS. "Constitutional endometrial defect" of endometrium is the reason for hyper-invasiveness of placenta. Immunologically mediated hyper-invasiveness has been explored. Some genes that code for adherence and remodeling are expressed.

Cesarean scar pregnancy (CSP) and placenta accreta syndrome share the same histopathology for which CSP and PAS are considered in a spectrum of the same disorder **(Fig. 6)**.

DIAGNOSIS

Antenatal Diagnosis

- Antenatal diagnosis of PAS is highly desirable for the planning of management.
- The presence of risk factors as above are taken into consideration.
- Antepartum hemorrhage (APH) may occur due to coexisting placenta previa. Placenta previa is associated in >80% cases. History of first- and second-trimester hemorrhage may be present.
- Imaging—sonography is primary modality for antenatal diagnosis (see below). Other is magnetic resonance imaging (MRI).

The *prior cesarean delivery and the presence of an anterior low-lying placenta* should be thought of higher risk of PAS.

Following vaginal delivery: Diagnosis is done following the failure to remove the retained placenta manually.

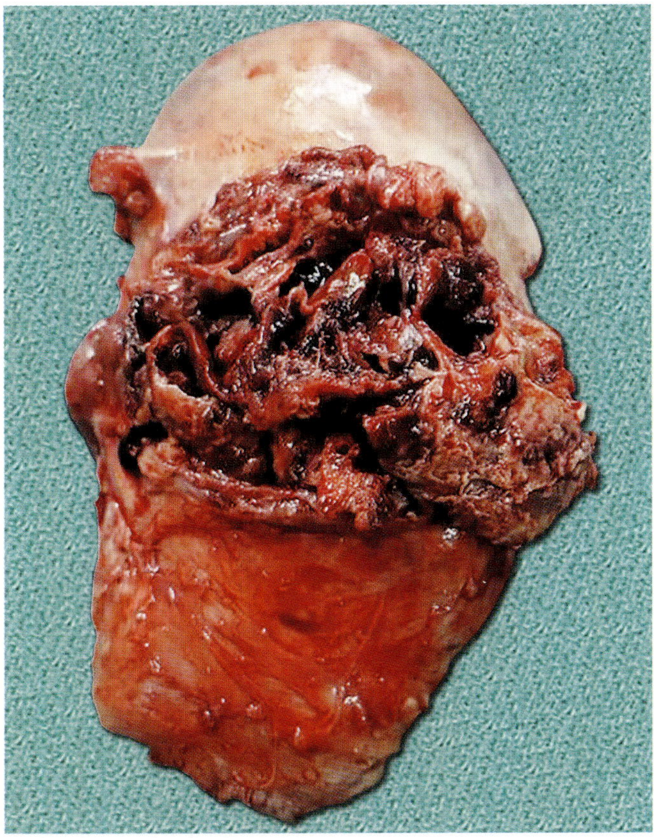

Fig. 6: Cesarean scar pregnancy 16 weeks post-cesarean section second gravida, medical termination of pregnancy attempted followed by profuse bleeding.
Courtesy: Dr Anirban Mondal, Associate Professor, Bankura Sammilani Medical College, West Bengal, India.

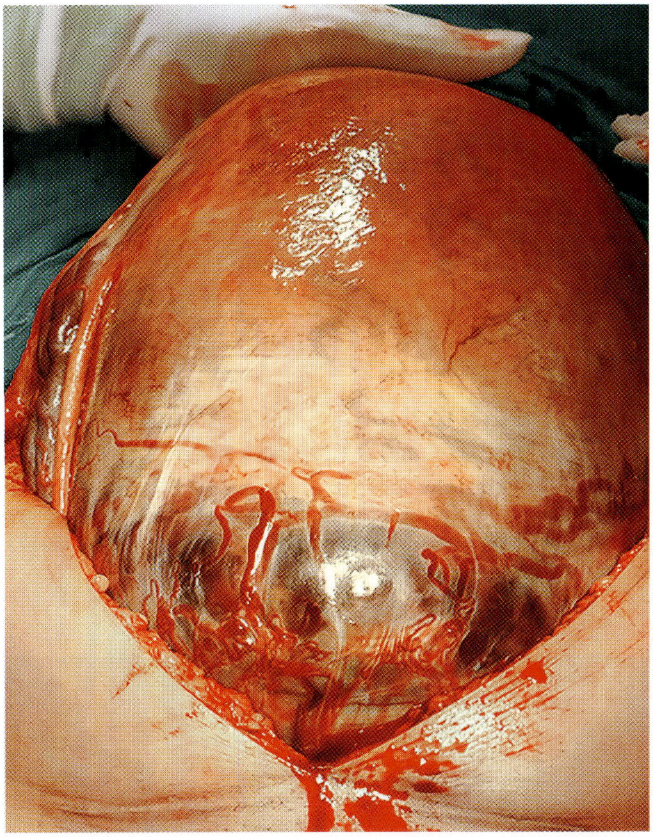

Fig. 7: Following laparotomy typical findings of prominent vessels on lower uterine segment in placenta accreta spectrum.

During cesarean section: The following laparotomy typical findings of prominent vessels on lower uterine segment **(Fig. 7)** are visualized. Inability to deliver the placenta during cesarean section due to absence of plane of cleavage is highly suspicious. Rarely, intraperitoneal hemorrhage is seen in case of placenta percreta (placental villi penetrates the serous coat; **Fig. 8**).

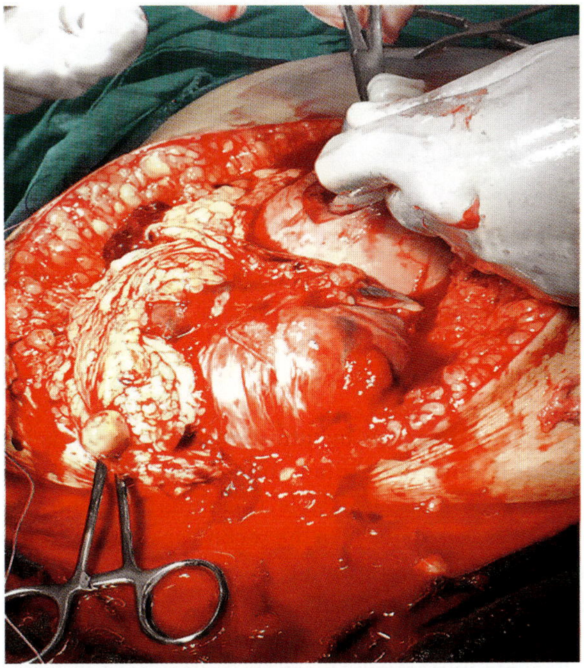

Fig. 8: Intraperitoneal hemorrhage in case of placenta percreta (placental villi penetrates the serous coat. Baby is delivered through fundal incision.
Courtesy: Professor Abhijit Rakhsit, RG Kar Medical College, Kolkata, West Bengal, India.

IMAGING IN PLACENTA ACCRETA SPECTRUM

Sonographic Features (Figs. 9 to 11)

- Loss of the normal hypoechoic zone between the placenta and myometrium
- Decreased (<1 mm) retroplacental myometrial thickness
- Abnormalities of the uterine serosa-bladder interface (placental bulging), and
- Extension of placenta into myometrium, serosa, or bladder

Color flow Doppler **(Fig. 11)** shows (1) multiple placental vascular lacunae and (2) turbulent lacunar blood flow which is the most common finding of PAS. Others are subplacental vascularity and uterovascular hypervascularity.

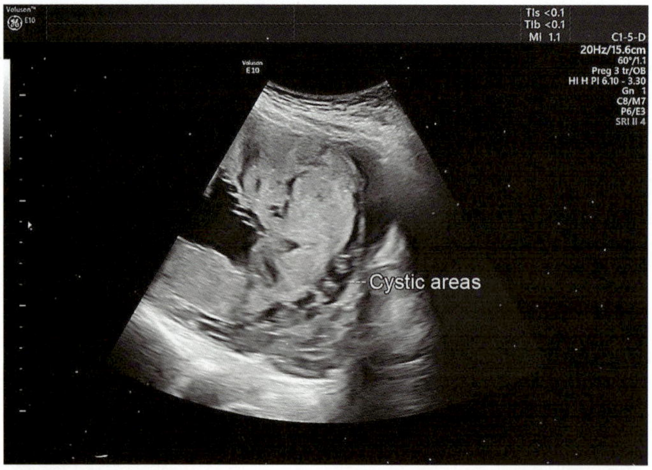

Fig. 9: Ultrasonography shows multiple placental vascular lacunae (cystic spaces), loss of the normal hypoechoic zone between the placenta and myometrium, and decreased (<1 mm) myometrial thickness.

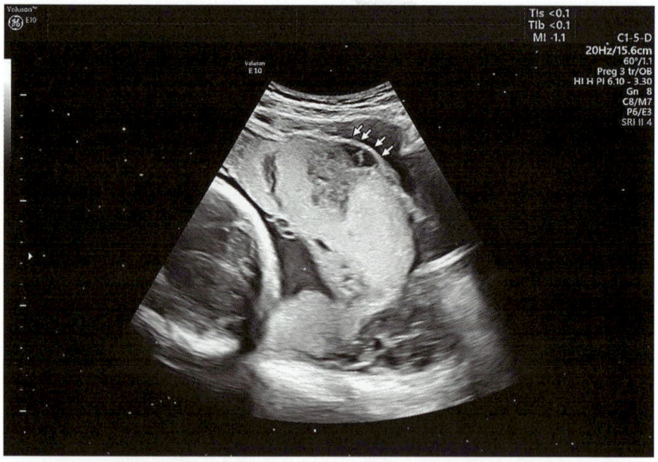

Fig. 10: Only serous coat is visible, in some places very thin myometrium is present.
Courtesy: Professor Kamal Oswal, Head, Department of Radiodiagnosis, Vivekananda Institute of Medical Sciences, Kolkata, West Bengal, India

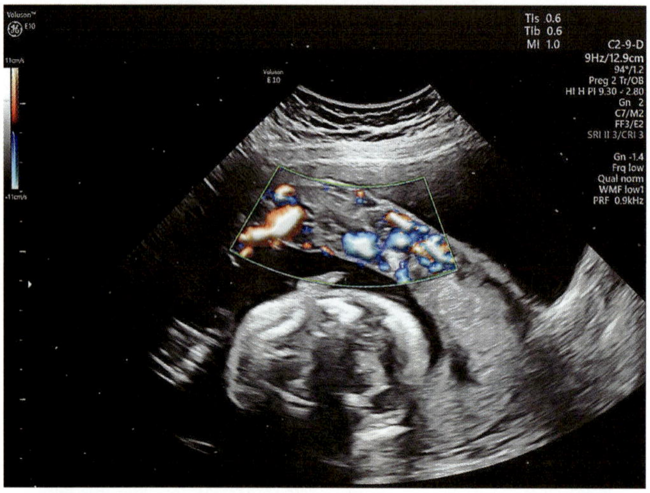

Fig. 11: Ultrasonography color Doppler shows turbulent lacunar blood flow in placenta accreta spectrum.
Courtesy: Professor Kamal Oswal, Head, Department of Radiodiagnosis, Vivekananda Institute of Medical Sciences, Kolkata, West Bengal, India.

Antenatal diagnosis by ultrasonography (USG) is highly accurate if done by skilled sonologist. USG features of placenta accreta may be visible as early as the first trimester but majority is diagnosed in the second and third trimesters. Transvaginal sonography (TVS) is not contraindicated. Presence of placenta previa is the common association seen in >80% cases of PAS.

Placenta in posterior location is diagnosed in late, and has more surgical complications.

Placenta accreta index (Yule et al, Am J Obstet Gynecol S105, 2020) has been proposed to predict the severity for need of hysterectomy. These include number of previous cesarean deliveries, location of placenta, bridging vessels, lacunae, and the shortest myometrial distance.

Screening by Ultrasonography

In a woman with a history of prior cesarean section (CS) having an anterior low-lying placenta or placenta previa during the routine fetal anomaly scan PAS is screened. There is no clear-cut guideline in number and optimal timing of ultrasound in PAS. In asymptomatic woman, it is reasonable to do at 18–20, 28–30, and 32–34 weeks, of gestation. This will allow for the assessment of placental location and invasion to optimize timing of delivery, and possible bladder invasion and possibility of preterm labor by measuring *cervical length*.

First-trimester USG finding of gestational sac found in the lower uterine segment with multiple irregular vascular spaces within the placental bed in first trimester is strongly associated with PAS.

Cesarean scar pregnancy diagnosed in the first trimester may develop subsequent PAS, if pregnancy is untreated.

Role of Magnetic Resonance Imaging in Diagnosis (Fig. 12)

Diagnostic accuracy of PAS by MRI and ultrasound is almost similar if done by skilled personnel. MRI is complemented to USG for diagnosis of difficult cases, posterior placenta previa, and to assess depth of invasion, lateral extension of myometrial invasion (ACOG 2018).

Histopathology (Fig. 13)

Histopathology following hysterectomy shows myometrial invasion of placental tissue and trophoblastic cells in nests and clusters.

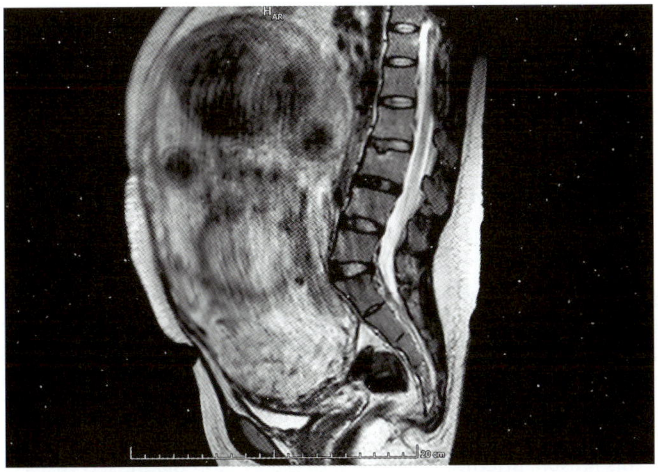

Fig. 12: Magnetic resonance imaging of 33 years old with prior cesarean delivery (CD) at 36 weeks' gestation with occasional spotting with complete placenta previa (type IV) and placenta accreta. The placenta is bulging in the previous CS scar which was completely thinned out and placenta had encroached but peritoneum was intact.

Courtesy: Dr Pesona Grace Lucksom, Professor, Department of Obstetrics and Gynecology, Sikkim Manipal Institute of Medical Sciences, Gangtok, Sikkim, India.

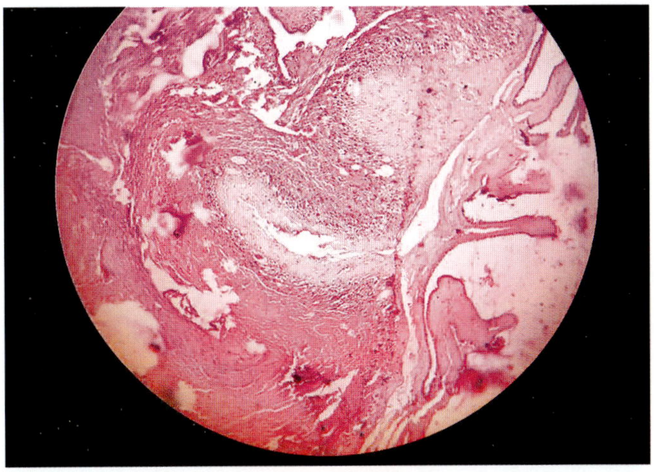

Fig. 13: Histopathology shows placental tissue, trophoblastic cells in nests, and clusters invading within myometrium. Features consistent with placenta increta invading more than half of myometrial thickness.

MANAGEMENT

Management of the Morbid Adherent Placenta (Placenta Accreta Spectrum)

- Cesarean hysterectomy
- Conservative or
- Expectant approaches are the options for management of the morbid adherent placenta.

However, cesarean hysterectomy is the treatment of choice in most of the cases. Conservative or expectant approaches are done in very special situation, in well-selected cases.

Approach in Management in Placenta Accreta Spectrum

Planned delivery should be the aim in a diagnosed case of PAS in a *tertiary care center (level III or IV)* equipped with adult intensive care unit (ICU), neonatal ICU, and immediate access to blood products. The surgical team should consist of experienced obstetric surgeon, oncosurgeon, senior anesthetist, and urological surgeon. It is better to have interventional radiologist if there is facility. Delivery is best scheduled for peak availability of all resource persons.

Timing of Delivery in Relation to Period of Gestation

A window of $34^{0/7}$– $35^{6/7}$ weeks of gestation is suggested as the preferred gestational age for scheduled cesarean delivery or hysterectomy (ACOG 2018). In other opinion (NICE 2018), planned delivery at 3^{5+0} to 3^{6+6} weeks of gestation is best to balance between fetal maturity and the risk of unscheduled delivery provided there is no risk factor for preterm delivery.

A cesarean delivery followed immediately by cesarean hysterectomy before the onset of labor improves maternal outcomes. Waiting after $36^{0/7}$ weeks of gestation is avoided because about one-half of women with PAS beyond 36 weeks need urgent delivery for bleeding at unscheduled time.

Earlier delivery is needed in presence of continuous bleeding, preeclampsia, maternal comorbidities, labor, prelabor rupture of membranes (PROM), or fetal compromise.

Corticosteroid is recommended in women with antenatally diagnosed accreta and anticipated delivery before $37^{0/7}$ weeks of gestation.

Preoperative steps which should be taken are: (1) Maximization of Hb level; (2) Counseling regarding severe hemorrhage and availability of blood and blood products and risks of urinary tract injury; (3) Consent for hysterectomy; (4) Preoperative placement of balloon-tipped catheters into the internal iliac arteries for inflation after delivery for occlusion of blood vessels or catheter for embolization; (5) Many prefer ureteric stenting (cystoscopic); (6) at least two large intravenous (IV) cannula should be placed.

Type of Surgery Planned in Established Case of Placenta Percreta or Increta

Cesarean hysterectomy with the placenta left in situ after delivery of the fetus is the most accepted approach in diagnosed case of PAS. Attempt of removal of placenta (extirpative technique—see later) is associated with significant risk of profuse hemorrhage **(Fig. 14)** and are strongly discouraged.

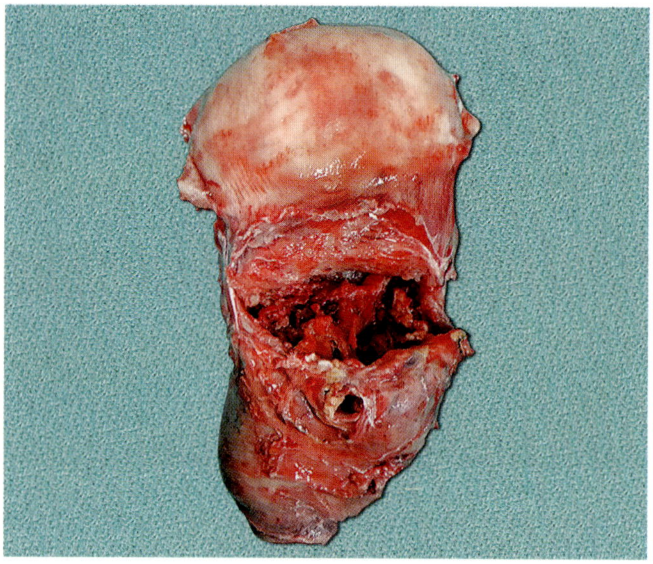

Fig. 14: Cesarean hysterectomy specimen with morbid adhesion of placenta which was removed partially in a second gravida with living issue one at 32 weeks of pregnancy presented with antepartum hemorrhage in a post-cesarean delivery pregnancy with recurrent bleeding. There was severe bleeding and hypotension during surgery and needed massive transfusion of blood and blood products to save. For this reason, attempt of removal of placenta in diagnosed cases of placenta accreta spectrum is strongly discouraged.
Courtesy: Dr Sandip Sarkar, Associate Professor, RG Kar Medical College and Hospital, Kolkata, West Bengal, India.

DELIVERY AND CESAREAN HYSTERECTOMY

Steps of Surgery (Figs. 15 to 25)

Vertical skin incision is preferred by many for better access **(Fig. 15)**. After opening the abdomen inspection of the uterus is done **(Figs. 16 and 17)** to discern the level of placental invasion and to mark the upper level of placental location, above which uterine incision is given. Vertical uterine incision is given and it may be higher, even *transfundal* **(Fig. 18)**. Baby is delivered **(Fig. 19)** first. Without attempting the delivery of the placenta assessment of extent of invasion is done. In obvious increta and percreta, hysterectomy is the best course and delivery of placenta is not attempted. Cord is clamped and cut after delivery of the baby and pushed inside **(Fig. 20)** after ligature. Uterotonic is withheld. Tranexamic acid (1 g slow IV) is given immediately prior or during CS delivery. Uterine wound is closed after pushing the cord. Hysterectomy (total) is performed preserving the ovaries, but fallopian tubes should be removed for reducing cancer ovary risk. Round ligament is divided as laterally as possible to permit access to pelvic side walls. *Internal artery ligation*, before proceeding to hysterectomy or other uterine devascularization, decreases blood loss, but its efficacy has not been full proven **(Fig. 21)**. Hysterectomy is proceeded **(Figs. 22 and 23)**. Separation of bladder may be very difficult sometimes in morbid adhesion of placenta due to invasion of bladder which needs very meticulous dissection **(Fig. 24)**. Occasionally, bladder may be injured or sometimes intentional cystotomy and partial bladder excision are done which is repaired in layers and postoperative bladder drainage is given for prolonged period. After completion of hysterectomy **(Fig. 25)** completion of hemostasis is secured **(Fig. 26)**. **Figure 27** shows specimen of uterus with morbidly adherent placenta following hysterectomy.

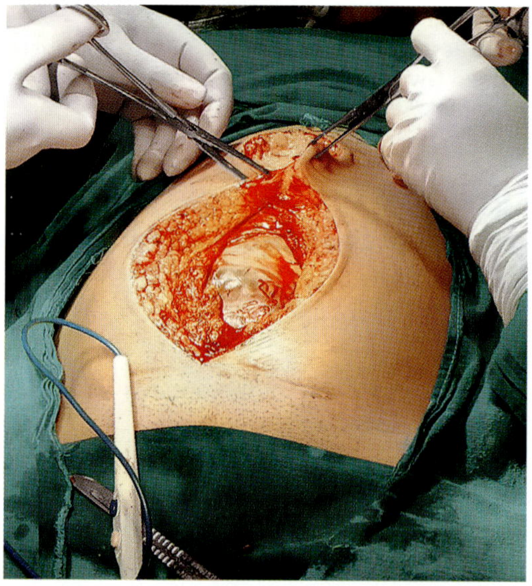

Fig. 15: Infraumbilical vertical skin incision.

Delayed Hysterectomy

Delayed hysterectomy with placenta in situ may be considered in case of extensive pelvic invasion.

Modified radical hysterectomy for PAS has also been described where more retroperitoneal dissection is done to open paravescical space and to do superior dissection to expose bifurcation of common iliac arteries and ureters and extensive dissection is done.

Additional Therapy with Surgery

Internal iliac artery embolization by *interventional radiology* in cases of persistent or uncontrolled hemorrhage may be useful.

Inflation of balloon-tipped intra-arterial catheters into the internal iliac arteries placed preoperatively is done after delivery for occlusion of blood vessels.

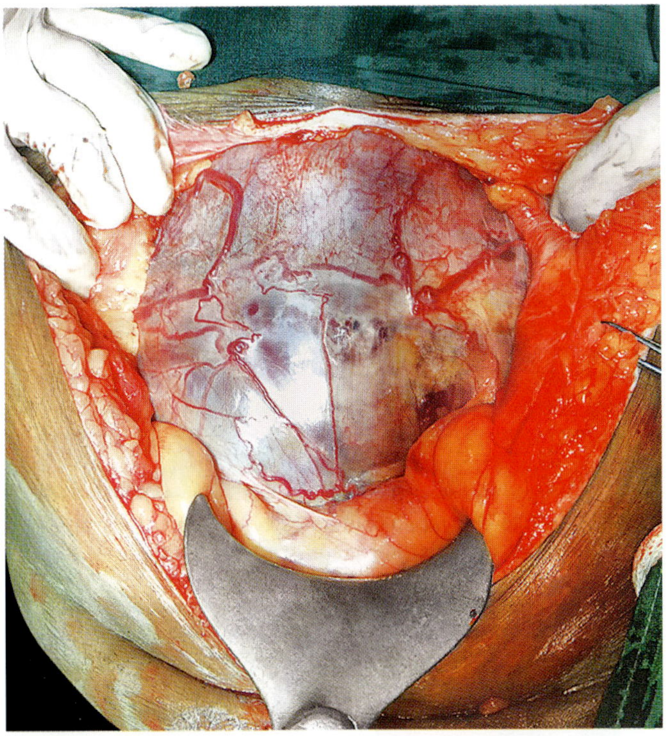

Fig. 16: On opening the abdomen prominent vasculature on lower uterine segment indicating placental invasion.

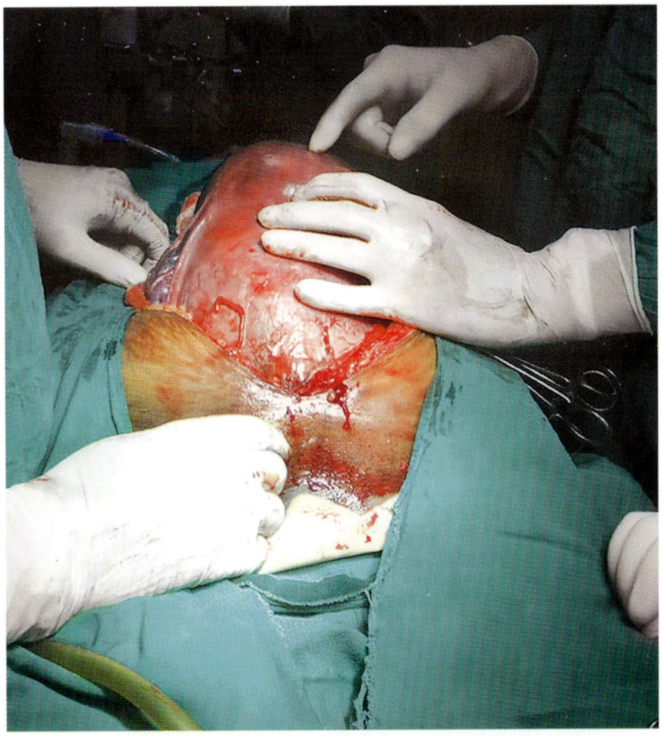

Fig. 17: Inspection of the uterus is done to discern the level of placental invasion and to mark the upper level of placental location, above which uterine incision is given.

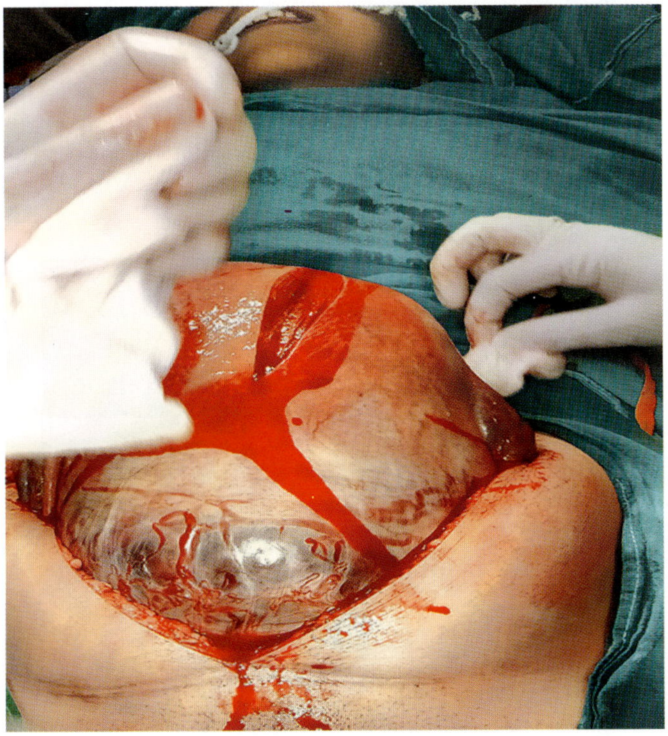

Fig. 18: Transfundal vertical incision above the level of the placenta.

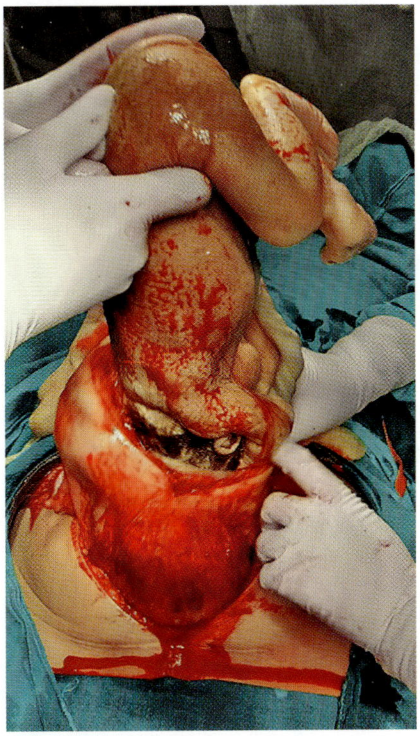

Fig. 19: Baby is delivered through fundus.

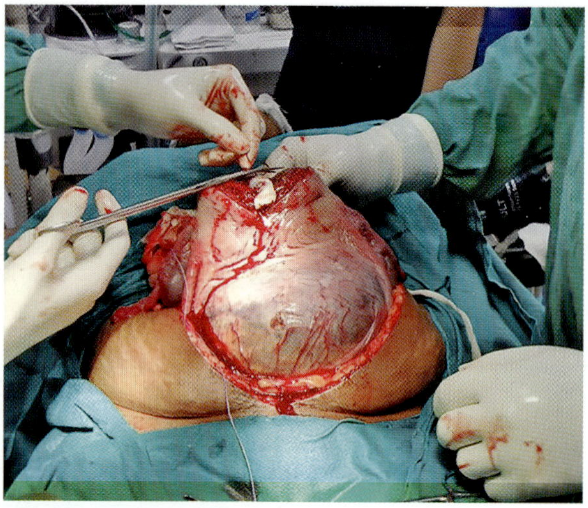

Fig. 20: Cord is clamped, cut, tied, reposed, and wound repaired.

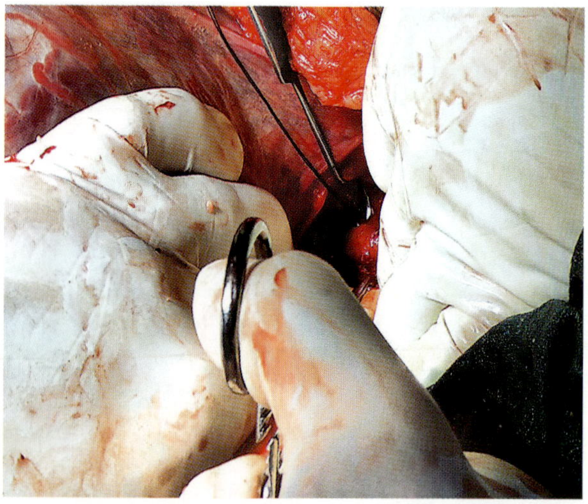

Fig. 21: Following repair of uterine wound internal iliac artery ligation is done using aneurism needle (both sides).

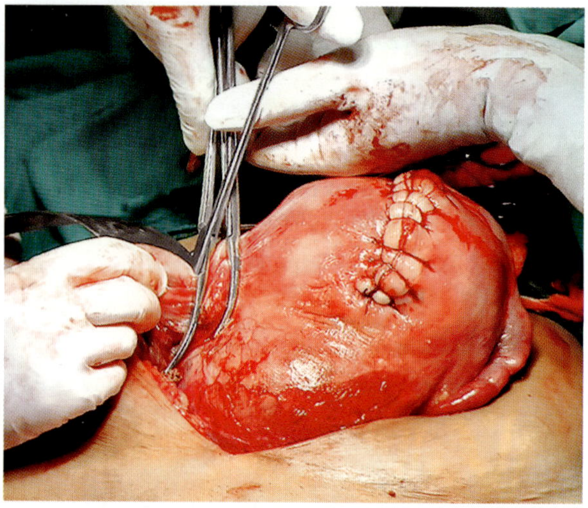

Fig. 22: Hysterectomy proceeded. Pedicle containing fallopian tube, ovarian ligament, and mesosalpinx is clamped, cut, and tied leaving behind ovary.

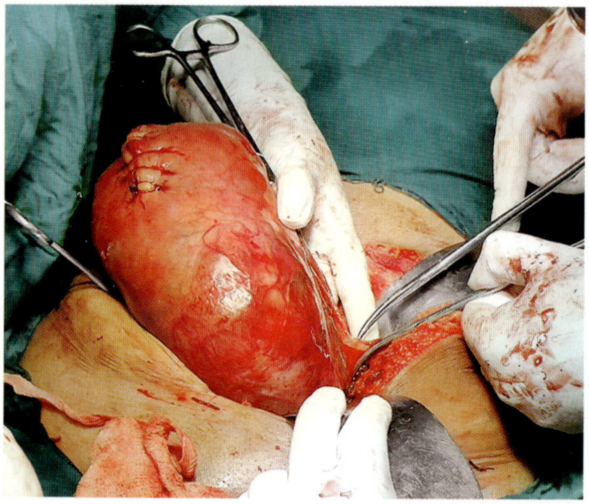

Fig. 23: Hysterectomy proceeded—clamping, cutting, and tying of pedicle opposite side.

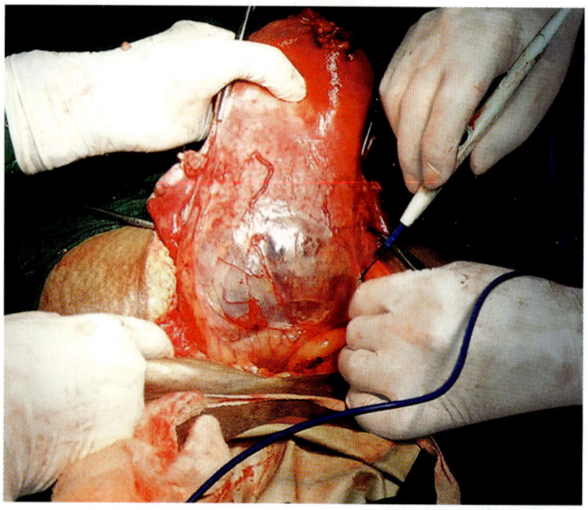

Fig. 24: After cutting uterovescical fold of peritoneum bladder is separated meticulously which is the most difficult part to avoid injury.

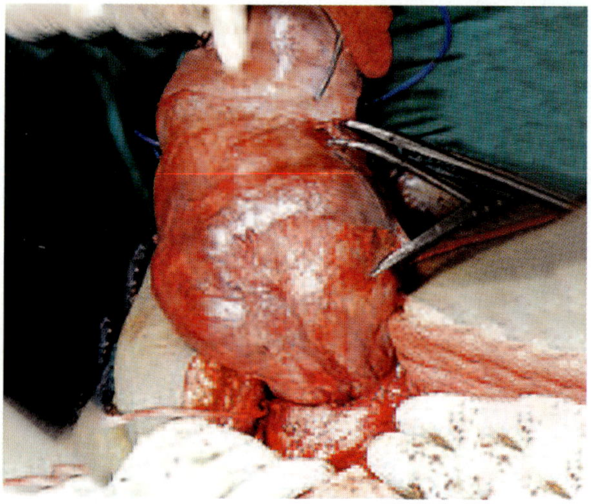

Fig. 25: Hysterectomy—last part near the vault of vagina.
Courtesy: Professor Debdutta Ghose and Dr Chandos Saha, RG Kar Medical College, Kolkata, West Bengal, India.

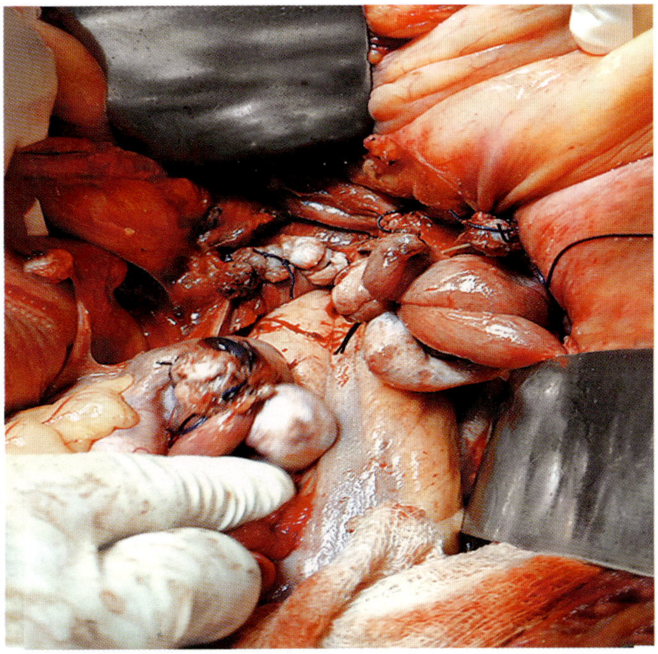

Fig. 26: Vaginal vault repaired following removal of uterus—complete hemostasis secured.

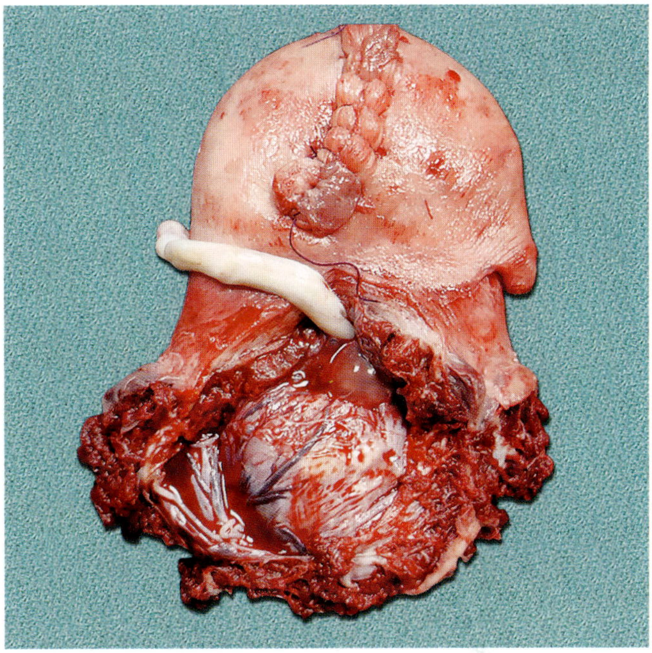

Fig. 27: Hysterectomy specimen to cut open from behind to show the adherent placenta to anterior wall.
Courtesy: Dr Sumon Poddar and Dr Dipro Saha, RG Kar Medical College, Kolkata, West Bengal, India.

Pelvic pressure packing, and aortic compression or clamping are other measures to control severe and intractable pelvic hemorrhage.

Blood and blood products—the use of a 1:1:1 to 1:2:4 strategy of packed red blood cells: fresh frozen plasma: platelets are reasonable to combat blood loss. Tranexamic acid is used as adjunctive therapy.

Postoperative thromboprophylaxis is given.

Other Novel Technique of Hysterectomy

There are many modification techniques described to minimize blood loss (early devascularization, or using stapling or vessel sealer), e.g., *posterior retrograde hysterectomy via pouch of Douglas (POD), modified radical hysterectomy*.

ALTERNATE METHODS OF MANAGEMENT

- Conservative
- Expectant approaches (leaving the placenta in situ) to preserve uterus with considerable risk with adequate counseling and informed consent are done rarely.

1. *Conservative management* is defined as forcible manual removal of placenta *(extirpative technique)* or uteroplacental tissue without removal of the uterus. In partial adhesion (focal) of placenta when depth is less, removal of placental tissue is done with hemostatic suture placement (e.g., oversewing suture) and balloon tamponade. Ligation of internal iliac arteries and uterine arteries may be required. Due to possibility of massive hemorrhage extirpative technique should be abandoned [Federation of Gynecology and Obstetrics (FIGO), 2018]. Salvation hysterectomy may be needed after attempt of conservative treatment **(Fig. 14)** with potential threatening of life.
2. *Expectant management* is defined as leaving the placenta either partially or totally in situ and is seldom done. When the placenta is left in situ, regular follow-up, ultrasound, MRI, and access to emergency care for complications, such as bleeding or infection should be available and there may be need for secondary hysterectomy. All possibilities, complications, and subsequent interventions should be informed to the patient and relatives. Serial serum β-hCG is not informative.

Methotrexate is given with an expectation for placental rapid involution and resorption, but it is not recommended now for unproven benefit rather having significant adverse effects (maternal hematologic and nephrologic toxicities). Methotrexate acts on rapidly dividing cells and at third-trimester division of placental cells is limited. Further, methotrexate is contraindicated in breastfeeding because of neonatal morbidity.

A Rare Case of Placenta Percreta with Conservative Management

In very rare instance, there may be placenta percreta perforating through the serosa in upper uterine segment without history of cesarean delivery. Description of such an extremely rare case with conservative management is illustrated in **Figures 28A to C**.

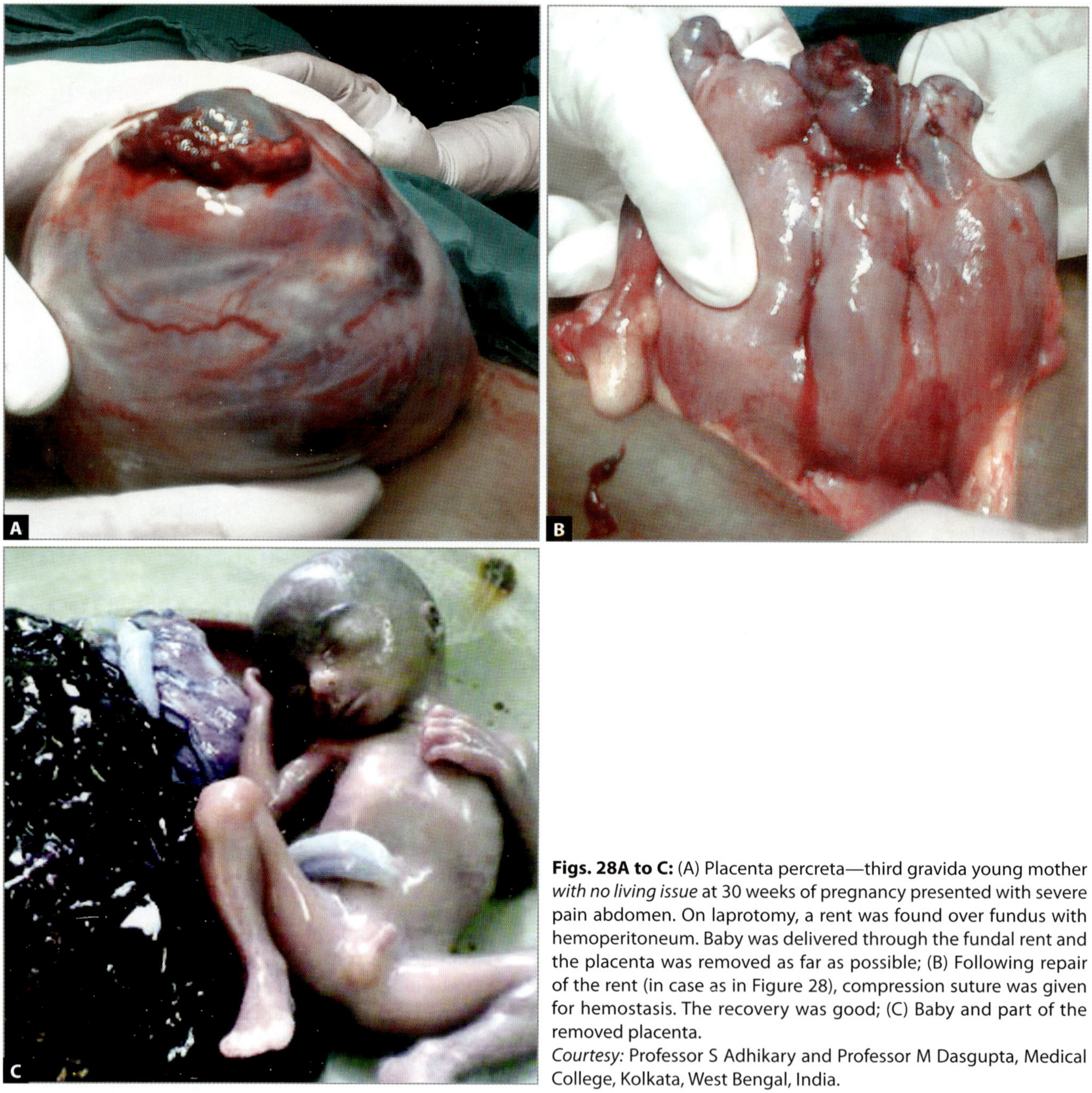

Figs. 28A to C: (A) Placenta percreta—third gravida young mother *with no living issue* at 30 weeks of pregnancy presented with severe pain abdomen. On laprotomy, a rent was found over fundus with hemoperitoneum. Baby was delivered through the fundal rent and the placenta was removed as far as possible; (B) Following repair of the rent (in case as in Figure 28), compression suture was given for hemostasis. The recovery was good; (C) Baby and part of the removed placenta.
Courtesy: Professor S Adhikary and Professor M Dasgupta, Medical College, Kolkata, West Bengal, India.

Unexpected and Unplanned Discovery of Placenta Accreta Spectrum Peroperatively

Occasionally, PAS is discovered during attempt of cesarean delivery. On opening the abdomen, it is immediately apparent that placenta accreta is present by typical look of lower uterine segment with prominent vessels **(Fig. 16)**. If mother and fetus are stable *the cesarean section is delayed until the appropriate staff and resource persons and adequate blood products are available.*

This may require abdominal incision closure and *urgent transfer of the patient to a higher center.* If morbid adhesion is inadvertently discovered with the uterus already open after delivery of baby, uterine closure is done rapidly and hysterectomy is proceeded. Other measures taken are pelvic pressure packing, tranexamic acid infusion, and blood transfusion.

Anesthesia

The surgical procedure can be done safely with regional anesthesia but it may need to convert to general anesthesia, if needed.

CHAPTER 12

Induction and Augmentation of Labor

Learning Objectives

- Definitions
- Indications
- Contraindications
- Determining Factors for Success of Induction
- Methods of Induction of Labor
- Failed Induction
- Risks and Complications

DEFINITIONS

Induction of Labor

Induction of labor means artificial onset of uterine contractions beyond the age of fetal viability by any means, either medical, surgical, or mechanical expecting vaginal delivery. In closed and uneffaced cervix, induction of labor commences with cervical ripening.

Augmentation of Labor

It is the hastening of the process of labor which has already started, by using oxytocics, amniotomy, or both.

Hence, induction is done before the onset of labor and augmentation is given after the labor has started.

INDICATIONS

The purpose of induction of labor is to accomplish vaginal delivery instead of continuation of pregnancy for the benefit of the baby or mother or both.

Fetal reasons are diabetes mellitus, Rh-incompatibility, postmaturity, intrauterine growth restriction, and fetus with major congenital anomaly (hydrocephalus, anencephaly, achondroplasia, etc.)

Maternal reasons are intrauterine fetal demise (IUFD), renal disease such as nephrotic syndrome, liver disease, and autoimmune disorders.

Both fetal and maternal reasons are pregnancy-induced hypertension—preeclampsia, eclampsia, placental abruption, and premature rupture of membranes.

Among these, common indications of induction of labor are postmaturity, pregnancy-induced hypertension (PIH), premature rupture of membranes, accidental hemorrhage, diabetes mellitus, and IUFD.

Elective Induction

Elective induction is a type of induction where everything is normal and the induction is not essential. It is done for the convenience of the obstetrician and the patient. However, elective induction at term is not recommended [American College of Obstetricians and Gynecologists (ACOG) 2019] and this practice should not be encouraged as the induction procedure is not without complication and inherent risks are explained with informed consent.

CONTRAINDICATIONS

Not every pregnant mother is suitable for induction of labor. The contraindications are contracted pelvis, malpresentation like transverse lie/cord prolapse, major degree placenta previa, active genital herpes, previous history of classical cesarean section, history of myomectomy with opening of cavity, cervical cancer, and nonreassuring fetal heart rate pattern [category III fetal heart sound (FHS)].

Two factors must be checked before induction: (1) accurate gestation age (where preterm delivery is not the indication of induction) and (2) fetal lung maturity.

DETERMINING FACTORS FOR SUCCESS OF INDUCTION

- Gestational age—more near the date, more the chance of success

- Parity—chance of success of induction is more in multipara than nulliparous woman
- Younger age, body mass index (BMI) <30 kg/m^2, birth weight <3,500 g favor induction
- Cervical "ripeness" or "favorability"
- Bishop score (see below)—high score favors induction. Bishop score is the most important predictive factor.
- Procedures adopted for induction

Bishop Score (Table 1)

Bishop score (Bishop EH 1964) is a preinduction cervical assessment by which the success of induction of labor can be anticipated. It is, in fact, the assessment of ripeness of the cervix.

TABLE 1: Bishop score.

	Score			
Cervical state	***0***	***1***	***2***	***3***
Dilatation (cm)	Closed	1–2	3–4	5 +
Effacement	0–30	40–50	60–70	≥80
Consistency	Firm	Medium	Soft	–
Position	Posterior	Middle	Anterior	–
Station of head	– 3	– 2	– 1	0

Total score is 13.

A Bishop score of ≤6 or less is unfavorable for induction of labor and a score of >8 indicates a high chance of successful induction. 3 cm—0 score, 2 cm—score 1, 1 cm—2 score, and 0 cm—3 score.

In *modified Bishop scoring system*, the length (in cm) of cervix is used instead of effacement.

Simplified Bishop Score

Simplified Bishop score consists of three of the original five parameters, namely cervical dilation, station, and effacement, which have been shown to have similar or better positive- or negative-predictive value in comparison to the conventional five scoring system.

Role of transvaginal sonography to predict induction: Measurement of cervical length by transvaginal sonography (TVS) is an alternative method. However, a large data from a meta-analysis shows low sensitivity and specificity with limited predictive value.

METHODS OF INDUCTION OF LABOR

- Medical
- *Surgical:* Artificial rupture of membranes (ARM; amniotomy). Amniotomy is preferred in labor augmentation to induction.
- *Mechanical:* Stripping of membranes, extra-amniotic saline infusion (EASI), transcervical balloon, and hygroscopic cervical dilators.

Agents for Medical Induction

The following pharmacological agents are used for medical induction:

- Oxytocin
- *Prostaglandins*:
  - PGE2 (Dinoprostone) gel/tape/suppository
  - PGE1 (Misoprostol) tablet
  - PGF2α (Dinoprost)
  - Antiprogesterone—mifepristone (RU 486)
  - Relaxin
  - *Nitric oxide donor—isosorbide mononitrate and glycerine trinitrate:* They are less effective than prostaglandin and associated with significant nausea, vomiting, and headaches.

Oxytocin

Oxytocin is given through intravenous infusion. Usually, two or five units are mixed with 500 mL Ringer solution. The drip rate is calculated according to the milliunits (mU) needed per minute, starting with 4 mU/min and gradually escalating for every 20 minutes to increase up to 16 mU/min.

Calculation of milliunits from the drop of fluid/minute: When 1 unit (1,000 mU) oxytocin is mixed with 500 mL Ringer solution, 15 drops contain 2 mU as *15 drops are equivalent to 1 mL of fluid* in a standard I/V set. When 2 units are mixed with 500 mL Ringer solution, 15 drops contain 4 mU, 30 drops contain 8 mU, and 60 drops contain 16 mU. When 4 units are mixed with 500 mL of Ringer solution, 15 drops contain 8 mU, 30 drops contain 16 mU, and 60 drops contain 32 mU.

During the infusion, the patient's pulse, blood pressure, and urine output are monitored periodically. Contraction of the uterus—frequency per 10 minutes, intensity (by dipping the fingers over uterus), and duration—is observed. Fetal heart sound is monitored every 15 minutes. After the onset of labor, progress is assessed by dilatation of the cervix, station and rotation of fetal head. Counting the infusion drops per minute is adjusted.

The maximum dose of oxytocin differs in patients. The average maximum effective dose is 36 mU/min. However, it can be increased to 72 mU/min. With increase of dose of oxytocin renal free water clearance drops markedly. Infusion of an appreciable amount of fluid along with oxytocin water intoxication may occur resulting in coma, convulsion, and even death. When a high dose of oxytocin is needed, it is justified to increase the concentration instead of diluted oxytocin with much amount of fluid. Crystalloids, such as normal saline or Ringer lactate, should be used.

In hyperstimulation of uterus evidenced by frequent uterine contraction and persistence of uterine contraction for more than 1 minute, absence of relaxation phase in between contractions and in appearance of fetal distress (evidenced by abnormal fetal heart sound and meconium-stained liquor), oxytocin drip is stopped. Currently, "uterine tachysystole" (>5 contractions in 10 minutes) is the preferred term to any other terminology.

Prostaglandins Commonly Used for Induction

- Dinoprostone (PGE2 500 μg)—Cerviprime gel. Vaginal suppository (20 mg) Vaginal insert/tape (Propess/Cervidil) containing 10 mg dinoprostone **(Fig. 1)**
- PGE1 (Misoprostol) tablet—25 or 50 μg

Repetition of dose

Dinoprostone (PGE2) gel: The prefilled syringe is inserted intracervically and gel is released just below the internal os. Following insertion of Cerviprime gel, the patient's condition, uterine activity, and FHS are monitored. The patient is not allowed to move for at least 30 minutes. If after 6 hours, no uterine contraction starts or Bishop score is <7, the dose is repeated, and a maximum of three doses in 24 hours can be repeated. In the meantime, Bishop score is expected to be good (say >6), when artificial rupture of membranes (ARM) is done and oxytocin drip is given immediately or after few hours. Vaginal suppository (20 mg) is not indicated for cervical ripening; rather, it is used for termination in fetal death in between 12 and 28 weeks' pregnancy.

Dinoprostol vaginal insert/tape with its advantages: Dinoproston vaginal tape (Propess, Cervidil-10 mg vaginal pessary/insert) is a thin, flat, semitransparent polymeric wafer which is rectangular in shape contained within a knitted polyester sac. It is provided with a long tail for easy removal from the vagina. It is used as a single dose administered high into the posterior vaginal fornix transversely using a small amount of water. After the vaginal delivery system has been inserted, the tape may be cut with scissors so that there is sufficient tape length outside the vagina to allow removal. It is removed after 12 hours or with onset of labor and at least 30 minutes before oxytocin administration. The patient remains recumbent for at least 2 hours after insertion. The rate of release of drug is 0.3 mg/h. It cannot be kept for more than 24 hours. It is important to monitor uterine contractions and fetal condition at frequent regular intervals. The advantage of vaginal delivery system/insert in cervical ripening over gel is that it can be removed quickly and easily if there is fetal distress, uterine hyperstimulation, hypertonic uterine contraction, systemic side effects such as nausea, vomiting, hypotension, or tachycardia, and spontaneous rupture of membranes.

Induction to delivery interval with dinoprostone is maximum 24 hours as shown in most meta-analyses.

Misoprostol in induction of labor: PGE1 (Misoprostol) tablet—Misoprostol (25 μg) tablet is given either orally or vaginally. The patient's condition, uterine activity, and FHS are monitored. The dose is repeated in 4–6 hours' interval.

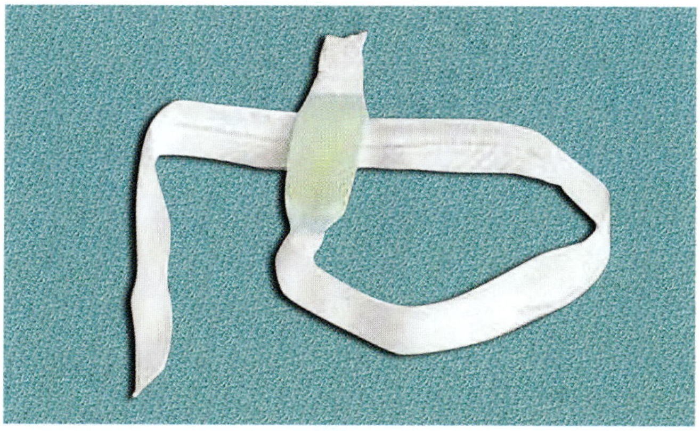

Fig. 1: Prostaglandin vaginal insert (tape)—Propess/Cervidil.

Mechanical Methods

Different varieties of mechanical methods are as follows:

- Transcervical Foley balloon catheter with or without EASI or double balloon
- Hygroscopic cervical dilators (Dilapan-S) correspond to laminaria tent used for medical termination of pregnancy (MTP)
- Sweeping of membranes (stripping)

Procedures of Extra-amniotic Saline Infusion (Fig. 2)

A Foley catheter is introduced through the cervical canal and balloons are inflated. About 200 mL of warm saline water is introduced into the extra-amniotic space. When the labor starts, oxytocin is infused. EASI acts by liberation of prostaglandin, cervix becomes favorable, and onset of labor occurs. EASI is much less hypertonus than prostaglandins.

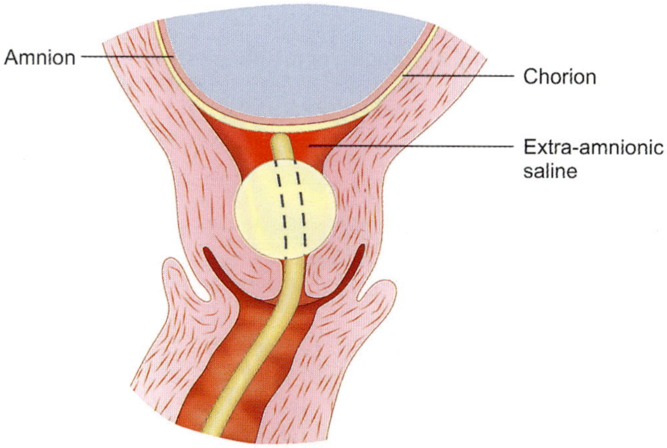

Fig. 2: Saline infusion in the extra-amniotic space with the help of Foley catheter that is placed through the cervix. The 30 mL balloon is inflated with saline and pulled snugly against the internal os, and the catheter is taped to the thigh. Room temperature normal saline is infused through the catheter port of the Foley at 30 or 40 mL/h by the intravenous infusion pump.

In transcervical Foley catheter and PGE2 gel for induction at term cesarean delivery rate does not differ as shown by PROBAAT-P and M trials.

Sweeping (Stripping) of Membranes (Fig. 3)

It is a method by which the membranes are stripped off with the help of fingers introduced through the cervical canal in between the membranes and lower uterine segment of the uterus throughout the circumference **(Fig. 3)**. Separation of membranes results in liberation of prostaglandins which is responsible for onset of labor.

Hygroscopic Osmotic Cervical Dilators

Laminaria tent, laminaria japonicum, or Dilapan-S, which is used for MTP, is also effective and safe for labor induction. Chance of infection is a concern. Laminaria tent is Chinese seaweeds. When it is introduced in the cervical canal and kept in situ for 12 hours, it swells up by its hygroscopic nature about four times its diameter and makes the cervix soft and dilatable. It should be inserted properly so that the tip of the laminaria tent is just placed at the level of internal os **(Figs. 4 and 5)**.

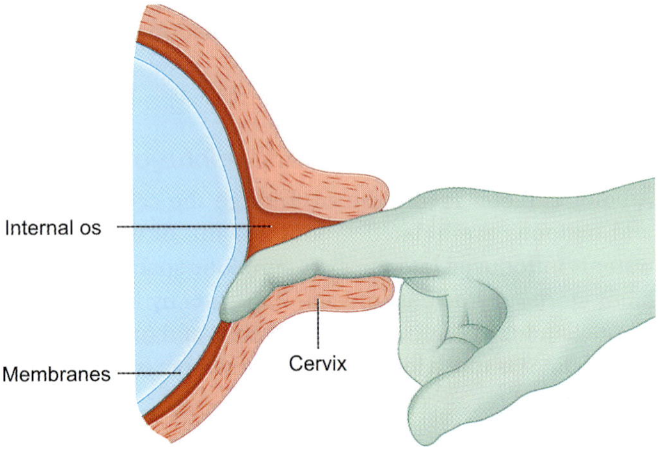

Fig. 3: Stripping of membranes.

Favorable Cervix and Unfavorable Cervix

When Bishop score is 6 or less, it is called unfavorable cervix; when Bishop score >6, it is called favorable cervix. In Bishop score >8, there is a high chance of successful induction. Ripe cervix is soft, thin, effaced, or becoming effaced and one finger dilatable. Unripe cervix is one which is hard, long, closed, and not effaced.

Ripening of Cervix

Ripening is a process by which the cervix becomes soft and thin. Alteration of collagen and hyaluronic acid ratio occurs in ripening by the action of hormones. It occurs prior to onset of labor. In case of unripe cervix, ripening is made by using ripening agents. Methods which are applied for induction of labor can be used for ripening of cervix.

Induction, cervical ripening in prior cesarean delivery, pregnancy, and risk of uterine scar rupture: There is a three-fold increase of scar rupture with oxytocin and more with prostaglandin when the patient is in labor. For vaginal birth after cesarean (VBAC) and trial of labor after cesarean (TOLAC), misoprostol should be avoided and PGE2 should be used cautiously. The mechanical method is a suitable option for these women. The use of prostaglandins for preinduction cervical ripening or for labor induction is not recommended by ACOG (2019).

Agents used for preinduction cervical ripening: The agents used locally for induction of labor are used for cervical ripening. These are:

- Dinoprostone—gel, vaginal tape—followed by amniotomy
- *Misoprostol tablet:* 25–50 µg vaginal, oral, and buccal is used widely for preinduction cervical ripening as "off label" drug safely
- Foley catheter

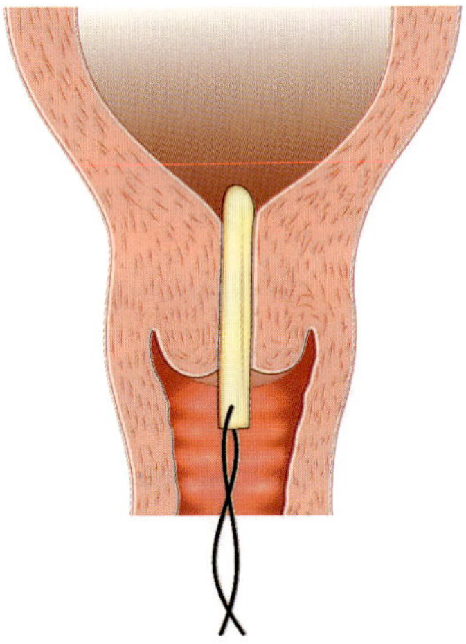

Fig. 4: Correct application of laminaria tent. The upper end of the laminaria tent is placed up to the internal os.

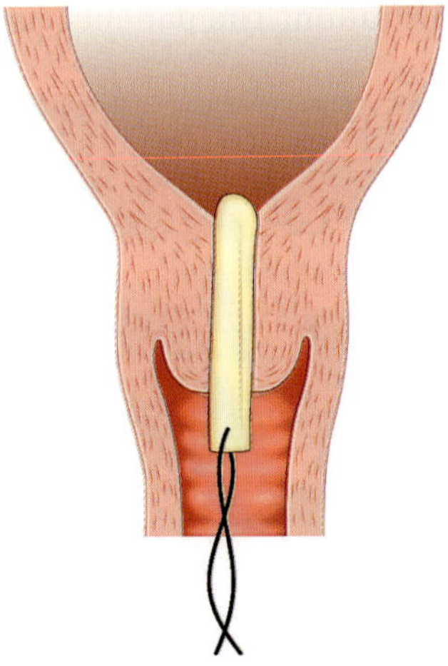

Fig. 5: Laminaria tent is swollen after several hours.

FAILED INDUCTION

If after an attempt of sufficient induction, the onset of labor does not occur (has not entered the active phase of labor) it is called "failed induction." Before declaration of failed induction, it must be sure that sufficient attempt was made for cervical ripening and adequate dose of oxytocin with reasonable period of time (minimum 12–24 hours) has been administered. However, till now the exact time limit has not been set to call failed induction, the next step depends on the primary indication. If it is done for fetal or maternal reason, cesarean section is performed liberally. If it is attempted for other less indicated reasons, the conservative approach may be applied.

RISKS AND COMPLICATIONS

- The most important concern of induction of labor is to increase the cesarean delivery rate by two- to three-fold, more in nullipara. However, recent data shows comparable, even lower, rates of cesarean delivery in induction of labor in comparison to spontaneous labor [ARRIVE Trial (A Randomized Trial of Induction versus Expectant Management), 2020]
- Prolonged labor
- Postpartum hemorrhage (PPH) and uterine atony for which there is an increased chance of peripartum hysterectomy.
- Uterine rupture
- Prematurity—nonmedically indicated delivery prior to 39 weeks should be avoided.
- Infection—maternal (chorioamnionitis) and fetal
- Uterine tachysystole (more than five contractions in a 10-minute period) resulting in fetal distress
- Nausea, vomiting, and diarrhea for oral prostaglandin
- Water toxication due to oxytocin
- Cord prolapse in ARM

Surgical Induction (Figs. 6 and 7)

Surgical induction is the artificial rupture of membranes, or also called amniotomy. It is performed using Kocher forceps or Hollister amniotomy hook.

Indications of Surgical Induction

Induction and augmentation of labor, placental abruption, pregnancy-induced hypertension (PIH), diabetes mellitus, and chronic hydramnios are indications of surgical induction. Combined induction is done in all cases of surgical induction. In combined technique, usually the medical method is done first followed by surgical induction. However, the advantage of ARM is that the color of the liquor can be seen and if it is thick meconium stained, induction is abandoned in favor of cesarean delivery.

Artificial low rupture of membranes: The important indications of artificial low rupture of membranes are surgical induction of labor and augmentation of labor.

Contraindications of artificial low rupture of membranes IUFD:

- Cord presentation, vasa previa
- Where presenting part is high up (chance of cord prolapse)
- Polyhydramnios (fear of accidental hemorrhage and cord prolapse)

Steps of Surgical Induction (ARM) (Figs. 6 and 7)

The patient is placed in thigh flexed, leg flexed, and abducted on the OT table. No anesthesia is needed. FHS is ausculted. Evacuation of the bladder is done or the patient is asked to pass urine herself.

Per vaginal examination is done. Fundus of uterus is fixed by assistant. Left index and middle fingers are passed inside vagina **(Figs. 6 and 7)**. The closed Kocher artery forceps **(Fig. 8)** is passed through the cervical canal under the guidance of left index and middle fingers and membranes are touched. Membranes are ruptured by sharp thrusting of the tip of forceps. If not successful, membranes are caught by forceps and torn by pulling. Care should be taken not to grasp the maternal tissue. Color of the liquor is noted. Vaginal examination is done to exclude prolapse of the cord or any bleeding. FHS is again ausculted.

If the liquor is found thick, meconium-stained fetal distress is likely. Resuscitative measures are taken with left lateral position, oxygen administration, and 5% Dextrose infusion. Decision is taken for termination of pregnancy by cesarean delivery.

Sometimes, blood may come out following ARM. This is due to injury of the placenta which is low down or there may be presence of vasa previa, placental abruption, or injury to maternal or fetal soft tissue.

The liquor may not come out due to the presence of less liquor or due to engagement of the head. The presenting part is pushed up to disengage and liquor is allowed to drain. This step is needed to see the color of liquor.

Labor usually takes 12–24 hours to start after ARM.

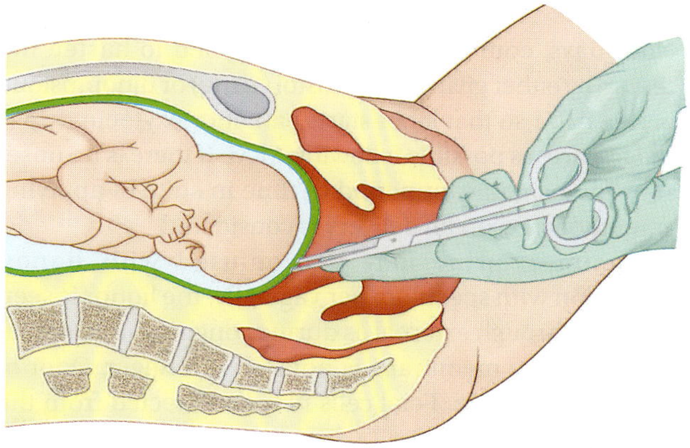

Fig. 6: Low rupture of membranes with Kocher forceps.

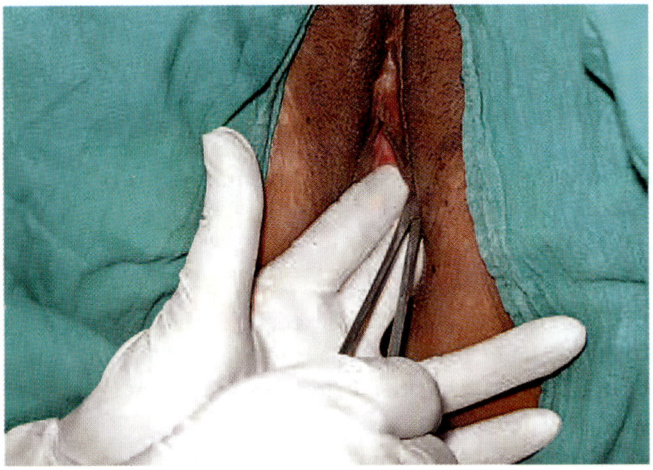

Fig. 7: Surgical method—low rupture of membranes with Kocher forceps.

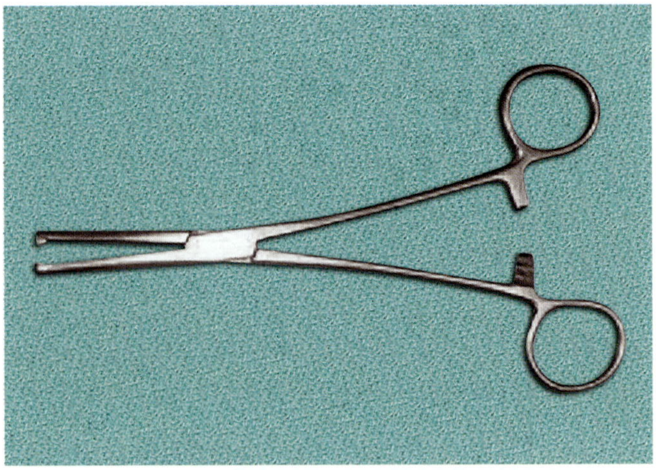

Fig. 8: Kocher artery forceps (straight).

Flowchart 1: Protocol of induction of labor.

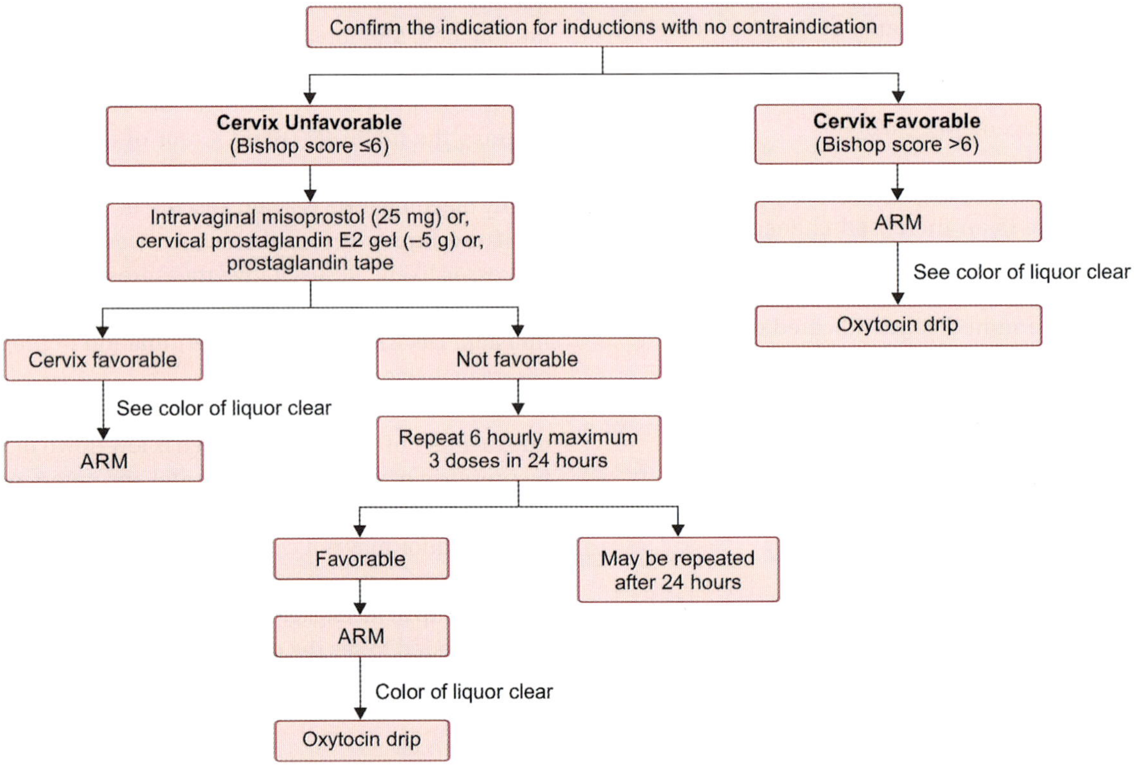

Nowadays, combined method is applied to hasten the procedure by either giving misoprostol (25 μg) or dinoprostone gel before ARM so that labor starts earlier or oxytocin drip is started as early as possible following ARM. If there is no onset of labor for a significant period of time in spite of applying other methods, cesarean delivery is considered.

Sometimes, urine may be confused with liquor. By inspection with speculum per vaginally, the liquor is seen to come out through external os during coughing. By internal examination, the membrane is not felt with finger. Odor of urine is characteristic. Fetal cells may be detected from the fluid if it is amniotic fluid.

Protocol of induction of labor is given in **Flowchart 1**.

Dangers of ARM are bleeding, cord prolapse, and injury of maternal and fetal tissues.

High rupture of membranes: High rupture of membranes using Drew-Smythe catheter, a Y-shaped metallic catheter with two curvatures, and a stellate inside is an obsolete method. In this method, the membranes are ruptured above the presenting part and liquor is drained. It was practiced to drain the fluid in hydramnios to prevent cord prolapse and to prevent placental abruption. Injury of placenta, uterine walls, and fetal parts may occur because it is a blind procedure and there is chance of infection.

CHAPTER 13

Obstructed Labor: Symphysiotomy, Duhrssen's Incision, Impacted Head, and Vaginal Septum

Learning Objectives

- Causes of Obstructed Labor
- Sequel of Obstructed Labor
- Diagnosis a Case of Obstructed Labor
- Prevention of Obstructed Labor
- Definitive Management of Obstructed Labor
- Cervical Dystocia
- Duhrssen's Incision
- Symphysiotomy
- Hydrocephalus
- Impacted Head
- Vaginal Septum

DEFINITION

Obstructed labor is the type of labor where there is no progress of labor due to insuperable mechanical obstruction in spite of good uterine contraction. Incidence of obstructed labor is 1–2% in referral hospital. However, this incidence is decreased recently due to improved labor care and increased institutional delivery.

CAUSES OF OBSTRUCTED LABOR

The causes may be due to faults in (A) passage, (B) passenger, and (C) power:

- *Faults in the passage*: Contracted pelvis and cephalopelvic disproportion (CPD), pelvic soft tissue tumor like uterine fibroid in lower uterine segment or in the cervix and ovarian tumor, and cervical dystocia
- *Faults in the passenger*: Large baby (macrosomia); malpresentation—occipito-posterior, brow, face and transverse lie, and shoulder dystocia; and congenital anomaly of fetus—hydrocephalus, fetal ascites and tumor, and conjoined twin
- *Faults in the power*: Constriction ring

SEQUEL OF OBSTRUCTED LABOR

Maternal Effects

Mother becomes exhausted and dehydrated, and features of metabolic acidosis develop, maternal sepsis develops, and there is increase in intensity, frequency, and duration of uterine contractions making the uterus tonically contracted with less and less relaxation phase.

As there is mechanical obstruction, the upper uterine segment contracts and retracts and the lower uterine segment becomes dilated and thinner, and as a result there will be formation of a pathological retraction ring known as *Bandl's ring*. With progress, Bandl's ring becomes oblique and gradually ascends upward and as a result the upper uterine segment becomes thicker and smaller and lower uterine segment becomes larger and thinner (For details see Author's *Bedside Clinics in Obstetrics*, 5th edition).

In case of multigravida, with dilatation and thinning of the lower segment, the lower segment ruptures if immediate intervention is not done.

In case of primigravida, labor becomes standstill resulting secondary uterine inertia with features of dehydration and exhaustion and development of sepsis.

Chance of PPH is more, mostly due to atonicity. Formation of vesicovaginal fistula—during obstructed labor, the bladder, bladder neck, and the upper part of urethra are compressed by fetal head against the symphysis pubis and later the tissue becomes devitalized (avascular necrosis), and sloughed to develop genitourinary fistula. Maternal death may occur due to *ruptured uterus, septicemia,* and *PPH*. Obstructed labor contributes 8% of all maternal deaths in the world.

Fetal Effects

Fetal asphyxia, intracranial hemorrhage, intranatal fetal death, and neonatal septicemia and its consequences.

DIAGNOSIS A CASE OF OBSTRUCTED LABOR

History: There is history of prolonged labor.

Physical examination: Mother is exhausted, there are features of dehydration—dry tongue, shrunken eyes, and less and concentrated urinary output. Pulse rate is increased and temperature is raised.

Abdominal examination: Uterus becomes tonically contracted, hard, and tender. There is formation of *Bandl's ring or pathological retraction ring* which is felt at the junction of upper uterine segment and lower uterine segment. Fetal parts are palpable with difficulty. Urinary bladder becomes thick and is palpable abdominally. Fetal heart sound (FHS) may or may not be audible. It is irregular and there is presence of bradycardia.

Vaginal examination: Vagina becomes dry and hot, there may be offensive discharge per vagina, usually cervical os is fully dilated, presenting part is impacted in the pelvis with development of large caput and excessive molding in case of cephalic presentation. There may be hand prolapse in shoulder presentation with impaction of shoulder.

Difference between the constriction ring and pathological retraction ring (Bandl's ring) is given in **Table 1**.

> *Discovery of pathological retraction ring or Bandl's ring:*
> It was Ludwig Bandl (1842–1892) who discovered Bandl's ring. As a student, Ludwig Bandl discovered Bandl's ring in 1870 while performing an autopsy on a dead body of a gravid woman who committed suicide during labor. Bandl also first pointed out that rupture is always confined to the lower segment of the uterus. Ludwig Bandl worked in Vienna and Prague.

PREVENTION OF OBSTRUCTED LABOR

Cephalopelvic disproportion should be diagnosed in late antenatal period or in early labor.

All malpresentations and malpositions should be diagnosed in time and managed in tertiary care center so that early intervention can be done before development of obstructed labor. Use of partography in all labor cases prevents obstructed labor.

DEFINITIVE MANAGEMENT OF OBSTRUCTED LABOR

General management: Correction of dehydration by intravenous Ringer lactate solution which may be up to 3 L and catheterization is done. Broad-spectrum antibiotic is administered. Oxytocin drip is omitted. Vaginal swab is sent for culture sensitivity.

Obstetric management: Ruptured uterus is excluded always. If baby is alive, immediate *cesarean section* is done. If the baby is dead with no ruptured uterus or no sign of impending ruptured uterus, *destructive operation* is performed. However, if the obstetrician is not well conversant with the procedure of destructive operation, cesarean delivery is an alternative safer procedure in spite of dead baby. Continuous bladder drainage is given for 10 days after delivery to prevent vesicovaginal fistula.

CERVICAL DYSTOCIA

Cervical dystocia refers to a condition when in spite of good uterine contraction, cervix fails to dilate and the labor becomes prolonged.

Cervical dystocia may be primary or secondary to scar formation following previous obstetric tear or gynecological operation such as amputation or conization.

Diagnosis

The cervix becomes firm; anterior lip becomes edematous **(Figs. 1 and 2)**, and fails to dilate. In second stage, annular detachment of cervix may occur.

Management

Cesarean section may be needed in most of the cases. In some of the cases where cervix becomes thin and

TABLE 1: Difference between the constriction ring and pathological retraction ring (Bandl's ring).

Constriction ring	*Bandl's ring (pathological retraction ring)*
1. Due to the localized contraction of uterine myometrium	1. Formed at the junction due to different nature of functions of upper active segment and lower passive segment
2. May form anywhere in the uterus, but usually over the neck of the fetus	2. Formed at the junction of upper active segment and lower passive segment which moves upward gradually
3. Cause of obstructed labor	3. Effect of obstructed labor
4. May occur in any stage of labor	4. Formed usually in the second stage of labor
5. Ring is neither visible nor felt. The feeling of uterus is normal. Fetal parts are felt.	5. Ring is visible and felt from outside. Uterus becomes tense and tender, and fetal parts are not easily felt.
6. Maternal and fetal distress appear late	6. Patient is in distressed condition. Fetal distress or even fetal death may occur.
7. Uterine rupture unlikely	7. Rupture of uterus may occur in multigravida.
8. Delivery after making the ring relaxed with relaxing agent or deep anesthesia or incising the ring during cesarean section	8. Usually delivered by cesarean section or destructive operation after excluding rupture

presenting part descends, pushing up of cervix with fingers during contraction or application of ventouse may facilitate vaginal delivery.

Duhrssen's incision of cervix at 2 and 10 o' clock positions is an alternative and effective procedure where cervical dilatation is not more than half but cervix is very thin.

DUHRSSEN'S INCISION

The incision over undilated cervix facilitating the delivery of fetal head is known for more than century. It is not popular for its complication and serious life-threatening hemorrhage. For this reason, its application is limited to arrest of aftercoming head of a preterm neonate. It is desirable that cervix is completely effaced.

Procedure ***(Fig. 3)****:* Vaginal wall is retracted with the help of retractor. One or two fingers is placed inside the cervix to guard the fetal head and cervix is cut with the help of scissor at 2 o'clock position and another at 10 o'clock position if required. Then delivery is accomplished. Following delivery extension to upward is excluded. The incision is repaired interlocking absorbable stitches like repair of cervical tear **(Fig. 4)**.

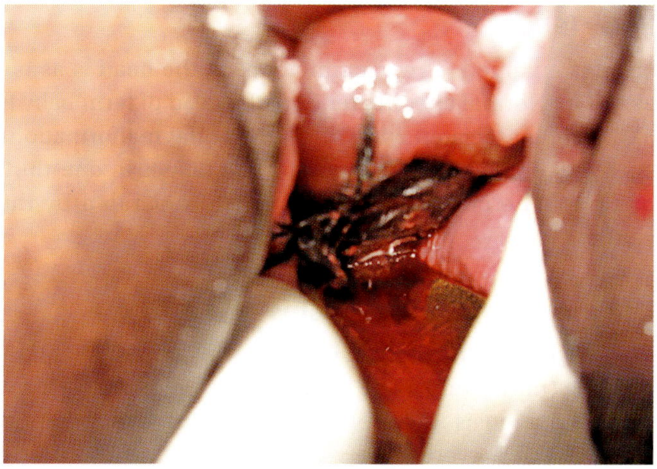

Fig. 1: Cervical dystocia—edematous cervical lip.

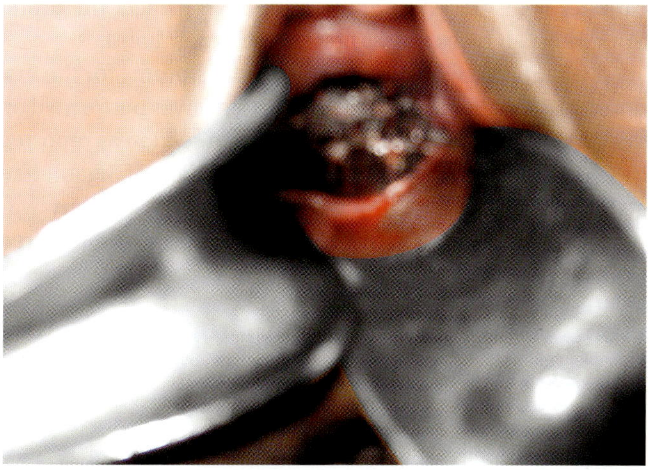

Fig. 2: Secondary cervical dystocia.
Courtesy: Professor Debdutta Ghosh, Department of Gynecology and Obstetrics, RG Kar Medical College, Kolkata, West Bengal, India.

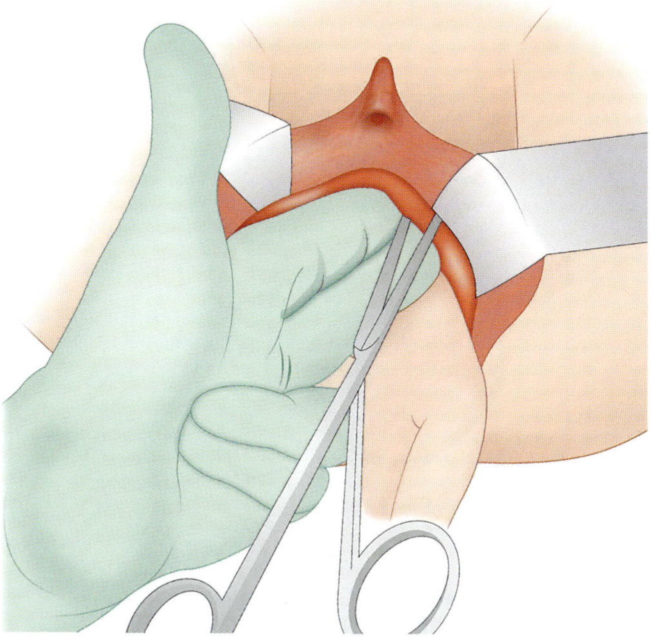

Fig. 3: Duhrssen's incision.

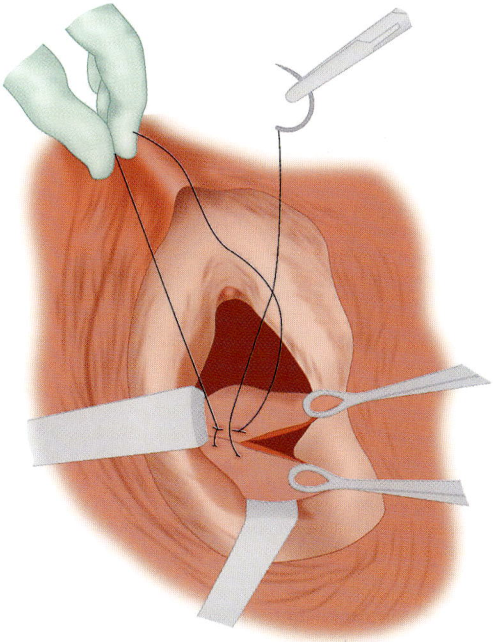

Fig. 4: Duhrssen's incision—it is repaired like cervical tear.

SYMPHYSIOTOMY (FIGS. 5 AND 6)

Symphysiotomy is a procedure by which the symphysis pubic joint is cut to widen pelvis and to facilitate delivery.

Where there is chance of survival of the fetus, symphysiotomy is an alternative procedure to cesarean delivery in obstructed labor due to outlet contraction with vertex presentation. This procedure is practiced in some developing countries. It is particularly useful in *shoulder dystocia* cases.

In this method, symphyseal cartilage and few of its ligamentous support is cut to widen the symphysial joint up to 2.5 cm under local analgesia. Index finger of the left hand is kept behind the urethra and the previously introduced catheter is displaced from the midline to protect the ureter from injury. It takes not >5 minutes in expert hand.

It was Sigault who performed symphysiotomy for the first time in 1777 in living woman. Before that it was performed on dead alternative to postmortem cesarean section as reported by Claude-De La Corvee in 1655. The patient of Sigault had given birth to four still born before symphysiotomy was performed to deliver a living baby. However, she suffered from a urinary fistula in rest of her life.

Congenital Anomalies of Fetus Which may Cause Obstructed Labor (Dystocia) (Figs. 7 to 10)

- Hydrocephalus **(Fig. 7)**
- Fetal ascites **(Fig. 8)**
- Neck swelling—cystic hygroma
- Conjoined twin **(Fig. 9)**
- Any swelling of thorax like lymphangioma **(Fig. 10)**

HYDROCEPHALUS

Hydrocephalus is a type of congenital malformation which is due to the accumulation of excessive amount of cerebrospinal fluid (CSF) in the ventricle resulting enlargement of the fetal skull. The amount may range from 0.5 to 1.5 L. Incidence of hydrocephalus is 1 in 2,000 births. Recurrence rate of hydrocephalus delivery is 5%.

Physical Description of a Hydrocephalus Baby (Fig. 7)

Head is enlarged. The circumference of the head is as big as 76 cm. Normal circumference of the head of term baby is 32–38 cm. Associated with other congenital malformations such as spina bifida, meningocele, and talipes in one-third of cases. The cranial bones are widely separated by the sutures.

Diagnosis of Hydrocephalus

The diagnosis can be made by clinical examination and by imaging (ultrasound). The mild varieties frequently escape clinical diagnosis and are diagnosed by ultrasonography. However, the severe variety can be diagnosed by clinical examination.

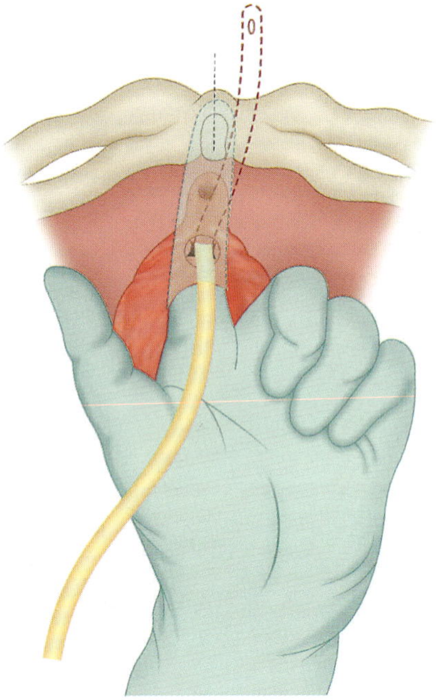

Fig. 5: Symphysiotomy—finger is introduced behind the pubic symphysis to prevent injury of urethra.

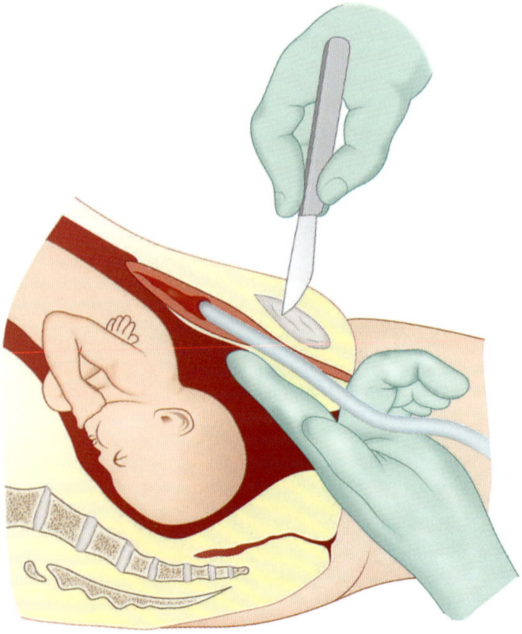

Fig. 6: Symphysiotomy—pubic symphysis is severed with scalpel.

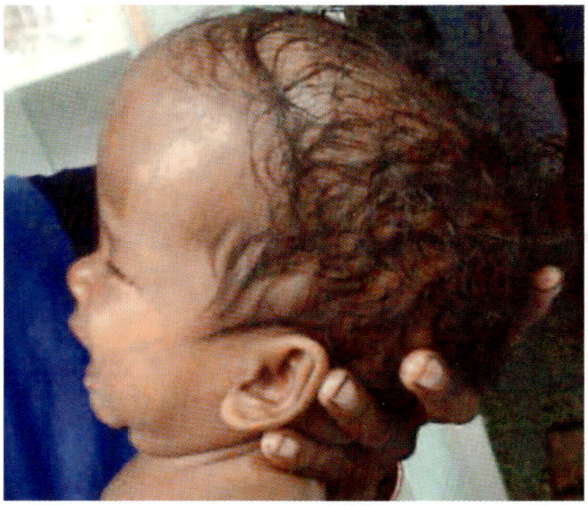

Fig. 7: Hydrocephalus.
Courtesy: Dr Sudipto Bandyopadhyay, NCU, Purulia, West Bengal, India.

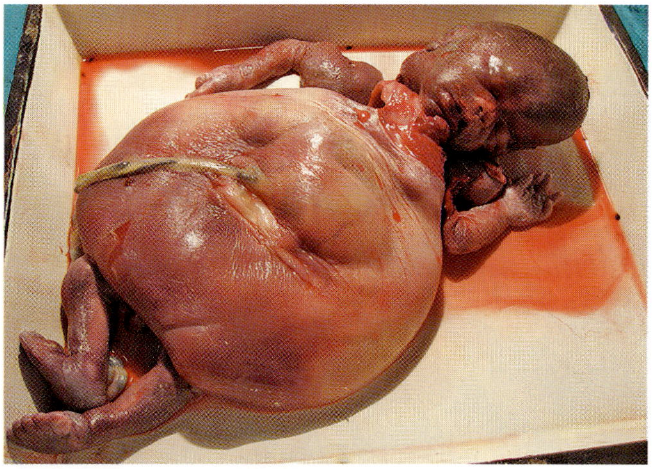

Fig. 8: Fetal ascites.
Courtesy: Dr Debjani Deb, Associate Professor, Bankura Sammilani Medical College and Hospital, Bankura, West Bengal, India.

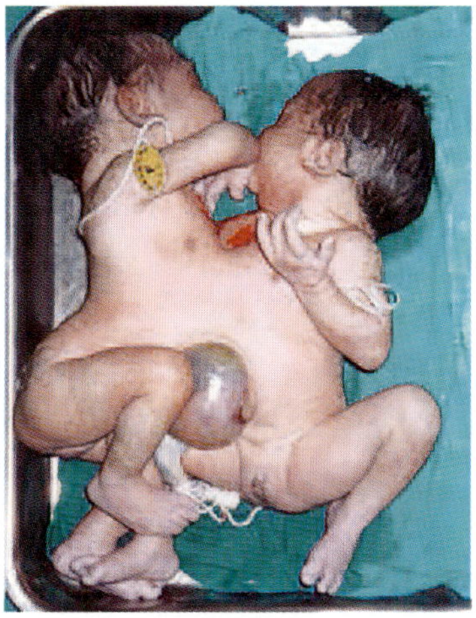

Fig. 9: Conjoined twin.

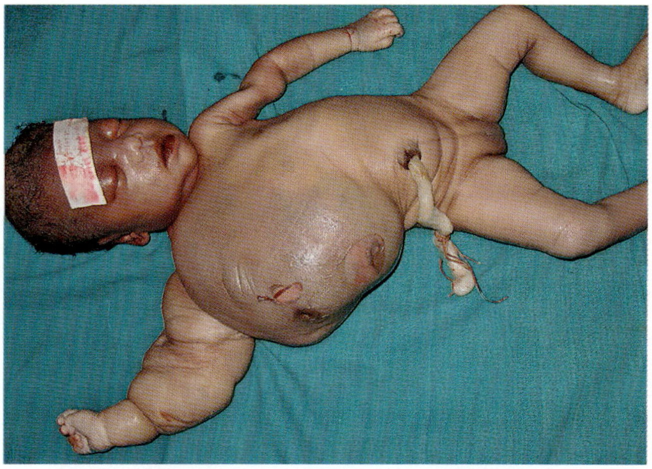

Fig. 10: Fetal thoracic lymphangioma.

During antenatal period, per abdominal examination shows broad globular firm head which is palpable above the symphysis. The head is softer than normal head and feels like a ping-pong ball. The head cannot be pushed down inside the pelvic cavity. Fetal heart sound is situated above the umbilicus. The most common presentation is vertex but in one-third cases, presentation is breech.

Per vaginal examination shows (if patient is in labor) widening of the sutures and fontanels, and the head is in high up position. There may be crackling sound on depressing the skull bones. During breech delivery head is obstructed following delivery of trunk **(Figs. 11 and 12)**.

X-ray shows large globular cranial shadow and comparatively the face shadow is small. Skull bones are thinner with gaping of the sutures. In breech presentation, normal head may be misdiagnosed as hydrocephalus in X-ray as it lies close to X-ray tube.

In sonography **(Fig. 13)**, head circumference is increased; there is dilatation of the lateral ventricle (ventriculomegaly). Choroid plexus is separated from the walls of the ventricle looking "*dangling choroids*" appearance. There is thinning of cerebral cortex. Brain tissue becomes paper-like thin. USG can diagnose as early as 16 weeks of pregnancy.

Different causes of ventriculomegaly are chromosomal abnormalities, genetic disorder, spina bifida, and infections such as toxoplasmosis and cytomegalovirus.

Dangers of Hydrocephalus

Maternal: Dystocia is inevitable. Chance of obstructed labor with ruptured uterus if not diagnosed in time.

Fetal: Except in mild variety, fetal prognosis is very poor. Babies are stillborn or die in neonatal period. Early delivery followed by shunting operation is an alternative option, but the chance of normalcy is less.

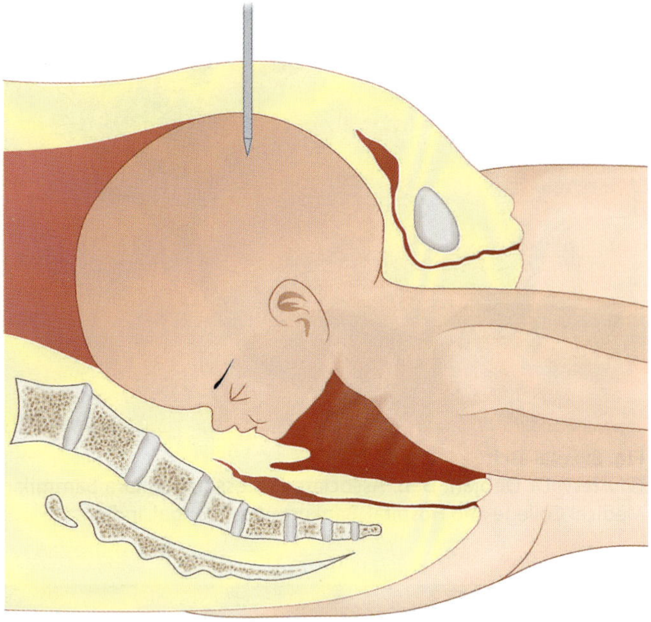

Fig. 11: Cranial compression through abdominal approach in aftercoming head of the breech.

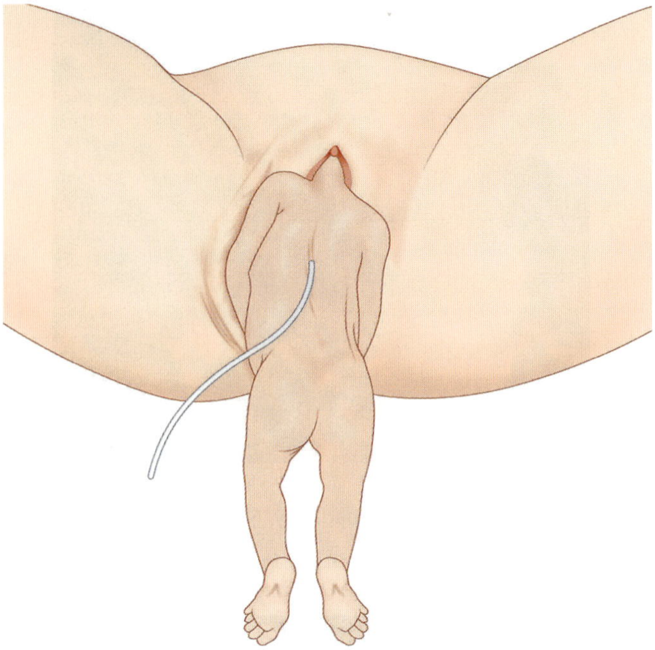

Fig. 12: Cerebrospinal fluid (CSF) can be withdrawn through spine when aftercoming head of the breech is too high in hydrocephalus.

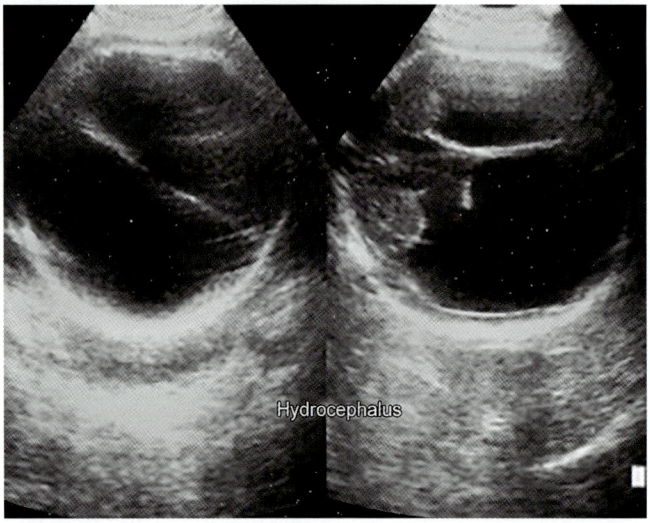

Fig. 13: USG showing hydrocephalus.
Courtesy: Professor Madan Karmakar, Department of Radiodiagnosis, Institute of Postgraduate Medical Education and Research, Kolkata, West Bengal, India.

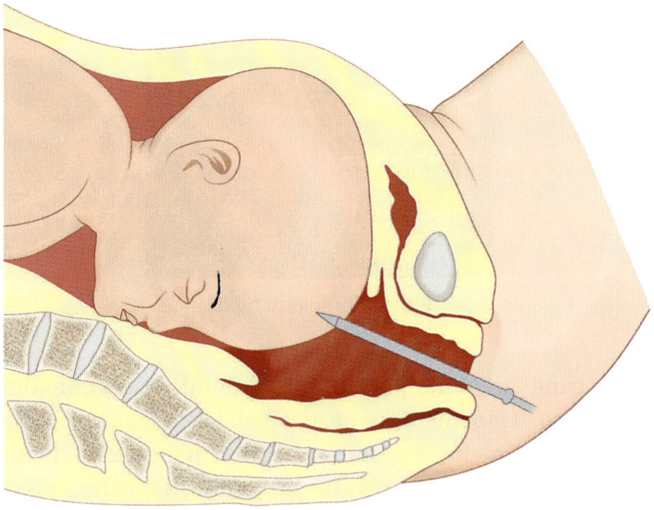

Fig. 14: Cephalocentesis (craniocentesis) through vaginal approach with wide bore needle.

Management of a Case of Pregnancy with Hydrocephalus

As hydrocephalus is not diagnosed in first half of pregnancy but in later half of pregnancy (which does usually occur), the pregnancy is continued till it is inducible, usually after 36 weeks. *Cephalocentesis* or also called *craniocentesis* is the mainstay of management. The technique varies depending on the fetal presentation.

Induction is done with low amniotomy. After onset of labor when os becomes 3–4 cm, *cranial decompression (cephalocentesis)* is performed transvaginally in vertex presentation with the help of perforator or sharp-pointed scissors by which the CSF is drained and head gets collapsed. Long wide bore needle (8 inch, 17-gauge needle) is used **(Fig. 14)**. Spontaneous delivery is awaited. *Hydrocephalus is the only indication of craniotomy in living baby.*

Alternatively, after evacuation of the bladder, decompression **(Fig. 11)** through the *abdominal approach* using wide bore stout needle (preferably by ultrasound guidance) can be done.

When the presentation is breech, fetus is delivered up to the neck and then head is perforated and decompressed through the *suboccipital* region. If aftercoming head is too high, it can be approached through the cervical spinal canal **(Fig. 12)**.

Following placental delivery, exploration of the birth canal is done to exclude ruptured uterus. During cesarean delivery, it is better to drain CSF by needle before incising the uterus in diagnosed cases. This will avoid the extension of low transverse or vertical incision.

Is there any indication of medical termination of pregnancy (MTP) in hydrocephalus?

Hydrocephalus is rarely diagnosed before first half of pregnancy, if not associated with other congenital anomaly.

According to recent Indian MTP Act (2021), MTP can be considered from 20 weeks up to 24 weeks with opinion of two registered practitioners. After 24 weeks, the opinion of medical board is needed [Detailed in the Chapter 3 (MTP Act)].

IMPACTED HEAD

When the head is impacted in the pelvic cavity, it is unlikely that vaginal delivery is possible. If the baby is viable only option is cesarean delivery. Cesarean delivery at this stage is also challenging.

There are various disadvantages of cesarean delivery in the second stage. Cesarean delivery is technically difficult with the head sometimes deeply impacted in the maternal pelvis. There is risk of injury to both mother and fetus. There may be tears in relation to the uterine incision, hemorrhage, blood transfusion, bladder trauma, and requirement for intensive care.

There are various techniques of delivery of impacted head during cesarean delivery. These are: (1) push method, (2) pull method, (3) forceps—single blade (Vectis)/double blade, and (4) Patwardhan's technique and fetal pillow. These are detailed in the Chapter 16 of Cesarean Delivery.

VAGINAL SEPTUM (FIGS. 15 TO 18)

Congenital septa may be transverse or longitudinal.

Transverse septum may be complete or may be perforated. In complete transverse, septum infertility is the consequence. In perforated septum, obstructed labor supervenes. Congenital perforated septum or acquired perforated strictures are sometimes misdiagnosed as undilated cervix. In advance labor after full dilatation of cervix, the presenting part bulges over the septum downward. If the opening is large head may negotiate or passes after slight stretching with fingers. Sometimes, crucial incision is needed for completion of delivery. Urethra and rectum are to be cared of during incision. In very thick septum, cesarean delivery is done.

Longitudinal septum divides the vagina into right and left part and may be associated with uterine anomaly. It may be partial either in upper part (common) or lower part of the vagina, or may be complete throughout the vagina. During labor complete longitudinal septum usually does not cause obstruction as fetus passes in one side of the dilated vagina easily. In case of incomplete longitudinal septum, obstruction may supervene sometimes, for which resection should be done during antenatal period in case of diagnosed cases. Not uncommonly occur that a patient may present in advanced labor in partial longitudinal septum in lower part of the vagina. In most of the cases, septum becomes attenuated by the pressure of descending fetal head. Sometimes, dystocia may occur. Then, the septum is kept away by putting fingers between

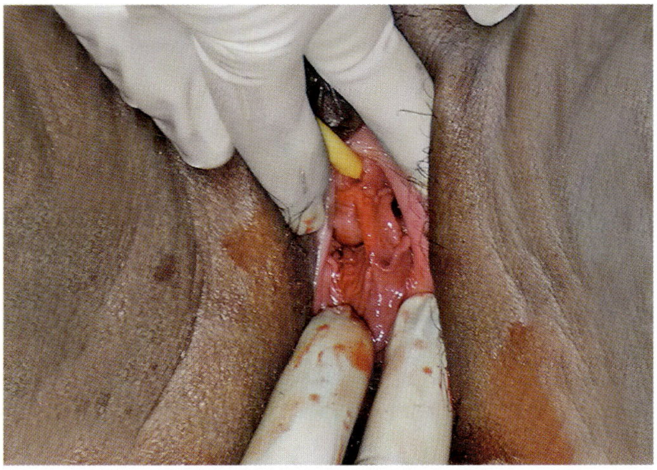

Fig. 15: Longitudinal septum of the vagina shown immediately after cesarean delivery in didelphic uterus.

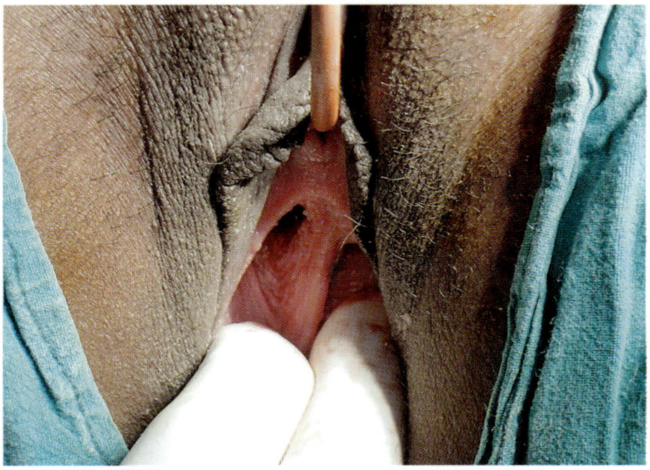

Fig. 16: Longitudinal septum diagnosed during antenatal period.

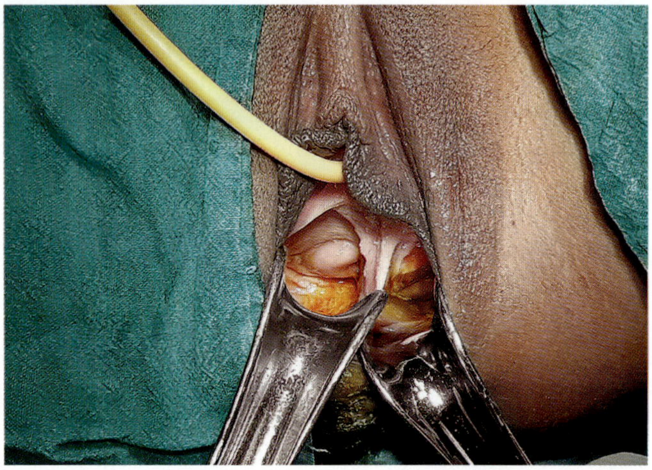

Fig. 17: Vaginal longitudinal septum with uterine didelphys to show two cervix by two speculum in a patient who came with infertility.

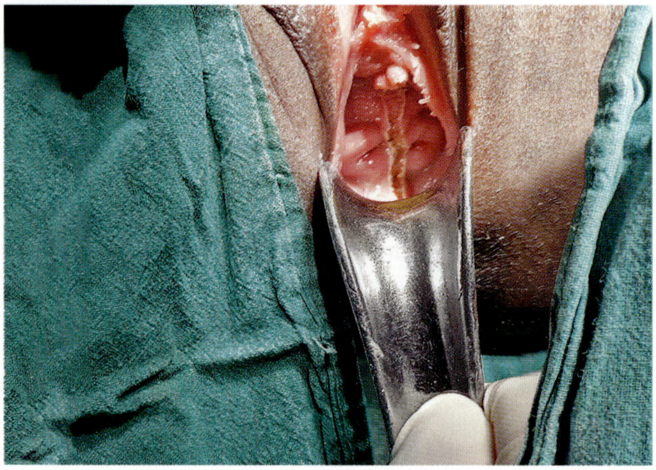

Fig. 18: Two cervix after resection of vaginal septum.

the septum and the fetal head and septum is transacted with scissors under good analgesia. During superior dissection, urethra is to be cared to prevent injury. In thick septum, transection is done between clamps. Cut ends are ligated with absorbable simple stitches or with transfixing stitches.

CHAPTER 14

Shoulder Dystocia

Learning Objectives

- Incidence
- Mechanism
- Risk Factors
- Prediction
- Prevention
- Hazards
- Diagnosis of a Case of Shoulder Dystocia
- Management of a Case of Shoulder Dystocia

INTRODUCTION

Shoulder dystocia is one of the dreadful and emergency conditions in obstetrics with significant maternal morbidity and neonatal morbidity and mortality. It has been described in medical literature for more than two centuries.

DEFINITION

Following delivery of the head in case of longitudinal lie, there is difficulty in delivery of the shoulder. This condition is called shoulder dystocia.

The interval between the delivery of head and shoulder exceeding 1 minute is arbitrarily called shoulder dystocia. The normal mean time from head to body delivery is 24 seconds.

Shoulder dystocia is an emergency condition as the umbilical cord is compressed inside the birth canal. It needs immediate intervention to free the shoulder to save the baby.

Cases other than shoulder dystocia where there is difficulty of completion of vaginal delivery are locked twins, conjoined twins, constriction ring, and short umbilical cord.

INCIDENCE

The incidence of shoulder dystocia is <1% and currently the incidence is increasing.

MECHANISM

In normal labor, during delivery of shoulder, bisacromial diameter enters into one oblique diameter in the pelvis and then rotates to occupy the anteroposterior diameter of the pelvis. In shoulder dystocia, bisacromial diameter primarily occupies the anteroposterior diameter of the inlet instead of oblique diameter and tends to enter through the anteroposterior diameter.

Usually, the anterior shoulder (unilateral) is impacted over the symphysis pubis and the posterior shoulder enters into the pelvis. Rarely, both shoulders (bilateral) may impact above the pelvic brim.

RISK FACTORS

The risk factors of shoulder dystocia are:

- Fetal macrosomia
- Maternal obesity
- Maternal diabetes
- Platypelloid and contracted pelvis
- Postdated pregnancy
- History of shoulder dystocia in previous pregnancy
- Epidural anesthesia
- Augmentation of labor with oxytocin
- Arrest disorder of first stage
- Prolonged second stage
- Instrumental vaginal delivery (midforceps)

PREDICTION

Prediction is not possible in majority of the cases due to the absence of risk factors. The risk factors as stated are taken into account. Prolonged first stage and second stage may be associated with shoulder dystocia.

PREVENTION

As prediction can rarely be done, prevention is very difficult. Elective cesarean delivery in cases of estimated baby weight of 5,000 g in a nondiabetic mother or 4,500 g in a diabetic mother is considered safe. Early labor has been studied but it is not recommended before 39 weeks [American College of Obstetricians and Gynecologists (ACOG) 2019]. Recurrent shoulder dystocia may occur in 5–15% cases. Cesarean delivery is not necessarily indicated in all women with a previous history of shoulder dystocia. Parameters such as gestational age, fetal weight, maternal glucose level, and degree of neonatal injury in previous birth are considered for decision-making (ACOG 2019). The pros and cons of the mode of delivery are discussed with the woman who has encountered shoulder dystocia in previous pregnancy.

HAZARDS

- *Fetal hazards are more than mother:* Transient Erb or Duchenne brachial plexus injury is the most common and occurs in 10–15% cases. Fractures of the humerus and clavicle are other possibilities. Fetal asphyxia is common. Hypoxic ischemic encephalopathy (HIE) is common. Fetal or neonatal death may occur.
- *Maternal hazards:* Postpartum hemorrhage occurs mostly from uterine atonicity and also maternal genital tract injuries due to manipulative and operative interferences.

  Recurrent shoulder dystocia occurs in 4–10% cases.

DIAGNOSIS OF A CASE OF SHOULDER DYSTOCIA

Chin is tucked over the perineum following delivery of the head **(Fig. 1)**. There is failure of complete spontaneous restitution (*Turtle sign*).

MANAGEMENT OF A CASE OF SHOULDER DYSTOCIA

Call for help—assistant, anesthetist, and pediatrician are involved. The aim is to deliver the baby as quick as possible to avoid prolonged cord compression and to minimize head-to-body delivery time. On the other hand, it must be taken into consideration that too much and inappropriate manipulation may cause fetal and maternal injury.

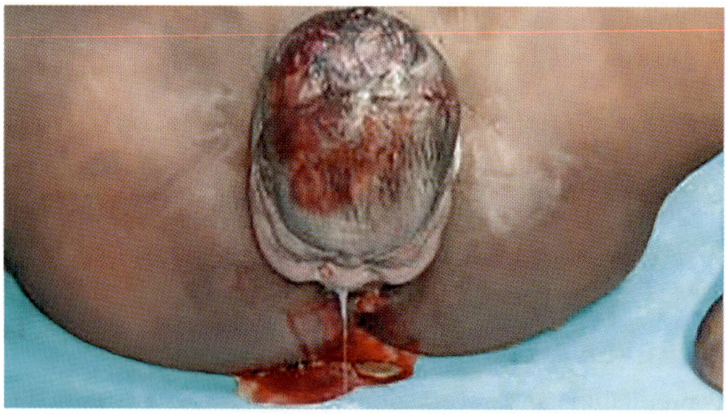

Fig. 1: Chin is tucked over the perineum.

Catheterization is done to evacuate the urinary bladder. A large mediolateral episiotomy is given if it is already not given earlier. A gentle traction with maternal expulsion force and suprapubic pressure by assistant may deliver the shoulder in some cases. *However, any fundal pressure and undue traction of head and neck are avoided.* If this procedure fails, the subsequent procedures are as follows:

- *McRobert's maneuver* ***(Figs. 2 and 3):*** The legs are abducted and sharply flexed upon the abdomen. It needs two assistants. The legs are removed from the stirrup, the thighs are sharply flexed upto the abdomen keeping the knees flexed assistant also gives simultaneous suprapubic pressure. This procedure straightens the sacrum relative to the lumbar vertebrae, rotates the symphysis pubis toward the maternal head, and decreases the angle of pelvic inclination and free the impacted anterior shoulder. This is the first step and an effective method. This maneuver is based on the mobility of sacroiliac joint.
- *Wood's corkscrew maneuver (1943)* ***(Fig. 4):*** Posterior shoulder is rotated in a corkscrew manner by 180° to make it anterior and is delivered under the symphysis pubis. This method is done under general anesthesia by inserting two fingers in the posterior wall of the vagina and like Lovset's maneuver in breech presentation.
- *Posterior arm extraction method:* Delivery of the posterior shoulder may be done by sweeping the posterior arm across the chest and thereafter delivering by gentle traction. Shoulder is then rotated in one oblique diameter and then delivered.
- *Rubin's method (1964):*
  - *First maneuver:* Applying force to the maternal abdomen, fetal shoulders are rocked from side to side.
  - *Second maneuver:* If the above method fails, the accessible fetal shoulder is pushed by pelvic hand

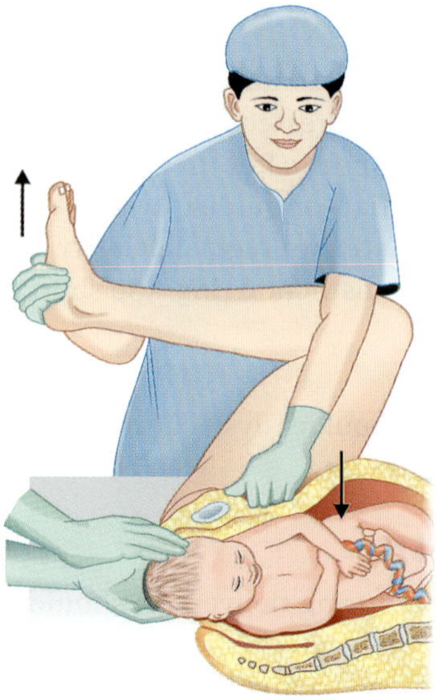

Fig. 2: McRobert's maneuver.

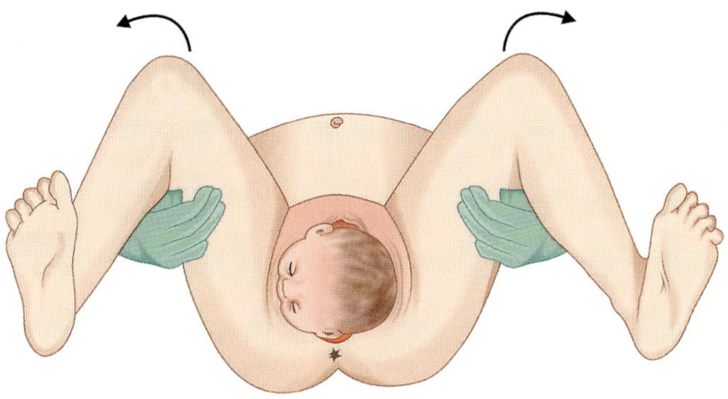

Fig. 3: McRobert's maneuver. The legs are abducted and sharply flexed upon the abdomen.

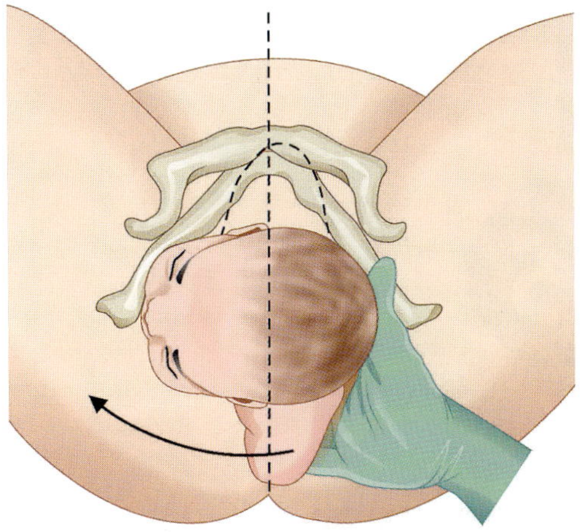

Fig. 4: Wood's corkscrew maneuver.

toward the anterior chest wall of the fetus that results in abduction of both shoulders, thus reducing the shoulder-to-shoulder diameter which will free the impacted shoulder.

- *Deliberate fracture of the anterior clavicle:* It is done by thumb to press the anterior clavicle toward and against the pubic rami and impaction of shoulder is freed. However, it is very difficult to do clavicle fracture in practice.
- *All-fours maneuver:* In this method, the woman is positioned on her hands and knees. This posture helps rotation of maternal pelvis and release of anterior shoulder is expected.
- *Posterior axilla sling traction (PAST):* In this method, a urinary catheter or suction catheter is passed through the posterior axilla as a sling and by outward traction the posterior arm is delivered. Humeral fracture and Erb palsy are potential complications.

Cleidotomy of one or both clavicles with scissors reduces the girth of the shoulder. This is done only in a dead fetus or living anencephalic baby.

- *Zavanelli maneuver of cephalic replacement:* The head is pushed into the vagina under anesthesia after making the head occipitoanterior or occipitoposterior and the baby is delivered abdominally by cesarean section. Terbutaline (0.25 mg SC) is used to relax the uterus. Uterine rupture may occur occasionally. Fetal injuries are common mostly due to prior manipulation. Moreover, the baby may die in the meantime.

Symphysiotomy is an alternative method practiced by an experienced obstetrician. In this method, symphyseal cartilage and few of its ligamentous support are cut to widen the symphysial joint up to 2.5 cm under local analgesia. The index finger of the left hand is kept behind the urethra and the previously introduced catheter is displaced from the midline to protect the ureter from injury. It takes not more than 5 minutes in expert hand. It should be attempted only after standard maneuver due to maternal morbidity. However, the decision should be taken quickly for the sake of health of neonate.

According to ACOG (2002), none of the methods is superior to other. However, McRobert's maneuver is considered as a reasonable initial approach.

Shoulder dystocia drill: The drill is a set of maneuvers performed sequentially to complete vaginal delivery in shoulder dystocia.

The sequences are:

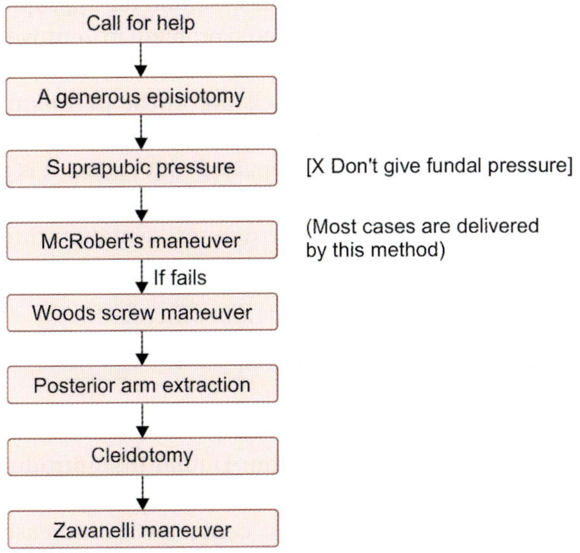

A "shoulder dystocia drill" should be practiced among all faculties, residents, anesthetists, and nurse practitioners. It is unpredictable but not uncommon and an emergency. Most cases of shoulder dystocia are relieved successfully by sequential applications of maneuvers.

CHAPTER 15

Episiotomy and Obstetric Anal Sphincter Injuries

Learning Objectives

- Episiotomy
- Types, Procedure, Repair, Complications
- Anatomy of Anal Canal and Anal Sphincter
- Anal Incontinence
- OASIS
- Episiotomy Wound Dehiscence

INTRODUCTION

Perineal tear in vaginal child birth is common and lesser degree may occur up to 50–75% cases and vaginal introitus is most commonly involved. Third- and fourth-degree lacerations involve the anal sphincter and called obstetric anal sphincter injuries (OASIS) and the incidence of OASIS is 5% or less. Other than short-term morbidities of blood loss, pain in puerperium, infection, and wound disruption, OASIS is associated with serious anal incontinence in long run. Hence, proper knowledge is essential for appropriate management of this underestimated problem to improve the quality of life.

Episiotomy is a planned incision on the perineum to increase the vulval outlet during last part of second stage of labor. This surgical incision is repaired with suture. It is also called "perineotomy". The idea of episiotomy was to prevent the vaginal and surrounding structures laceration during vaginal birth to ease the delivery of the baby and to reduce the delivery time.

EPISIOTOMY

History of Episiotomy

A midwife Sir Fielding Ould from Dublin first introduced episiotomy in 1741. It took more than 100 years to make it practice. In the first half of last century with increase in hospital delivery the rate of episiotomy increased substantially throughout the world. In 1920 De Lee introduced prophylactic forceps with routine use of episiotomy in all nulliparous women with an idea to protect both mother and baby.

Advantages Claimed in Routine Episiotomy

Maternal Benefits

- It avoids perineal laceration, and hematoma.
- By planned incision—easy to repair and heals well than laceration.
- Second stage of labor can be shortened.
- It improves sexual function, reduces risk of rectal and urinary incontinence, and prevents genital prolapse by minimizing trauma to the pelvic floor and by preserving the muscle relaxation of the pelvic floor and perineum.

Fetal Benefits

By preventing a prolonged second stage fetal asphyxia, cranial injury, cerebral hemorrhage, and mental retardation can be prevented. Episiotomy minimizes trauma to fetal head, especially in premature baby, and makes easy delivery of aftercoming head of breech.

In spite of the fact that episiotomy was one of the most commonly performed surgical procedures globally, it is practiced without strong scientific evidence of its usefulness and risk factors are not studied well.

Alleged Risks of Routine Episiotomy

- Unavoidable extension of episiotomy incision involving anal sphincter and rectum resulting third- and fourth-degree tears (OASIS).
- Routine bleeding sometimes excessive and hematoma formation

- Improper anatomical repair resulting asymmetry and skin tag.
- Unsatisfactory anatomic results such as skin tags, asymmetry, introital narrowing, anal fistula, rectal fistula, and prolapse of vagina.
- Edema and pain
- Wound sepsis and disruption
- Dyspareunia
- Overall more cost in routine episiotomy

Recent View on Episiotomy—Restrictive versus Routine?

Routine episiotomy is not recommended now. "Restrictive episiotomy" is preferred to "routine episiotomy" as it has a number of benefits over routine. American College of Obstetricians and Gynecologists (ACOG) (2020) recommends selective use of episiotomy rather than routine episiotomy. Other than immediate benefit the evidence of long-term major benefit following episiotomy is lacking. Episiotomy has few problems such as anatomical deformity, pain, dyspareunia, and blood loss. It neither decreases perineal damage nor reduces future vaginal prolapse or urinary incontinence. Rather in routine episiotomy, there is increase of third- and fourth-degree tears and subsequent dysfunction of anal sphincter muscle. However, there may be increased risk of anterior perineal injury involving anterior vaginal wall, labia, clitoris, or urethra following restrictive episiotomy, but there is little morbidity in anterior perineal trauma. World Health Organization (WHO) recommends to restrict episiotomy rate to 10% for normal deliveries.

Indications for the Restrictive Use of Episiotomy

Indications for the restrictive use of episiotomy are not always clear. However, the following are considered:

- Nullipara in selected cases
- Multigravida with rigid perineum
- Abnormal presentations and positions like occipitoposterior (OP), face, and breech.
- Instrumental vaginal delivery—forceps operation
- To cut short the second stage of labor in some maternal conditions like heart disease and eclampsia.
- Some fetal conditions like prematurity to minimize trauma to the fetal head.
- Predicted macrosomia
- Presumption of imminent tear
- Previous history of perineal operations such as pelvic floor repair, CPT repair.

Episiotomy in Assisted Vaginal Delivery (Ventouse and Forceps)

Risk of perineal laceration is more in the cases where assisted vaginal delivery (AVD) is indicated. Forceps delivery is a known risk factor of second- and third-degree tear, episiotomy does not always confer protection rather episiotomy itself may cause OASIS. Restrictive rule is followed here until clinically indicated for episiotomy and if given, mediolateral is preferred for protection of anal sphincter. There is less OASIS if forceps is applied in occipitoanterior position than in OP position. In vacuum extraction, OASIS is more in nulliparous than multiparous. Lateral episiotomy is associated with less OASIS in ventouse application whereas midline episiotomy increases it.

Different Degrees of Obstetric or Perineal Laceration (Figs. 1 to 4)

During childbirth some *perineal laceration* may occur spontaneously, or the midwife or obstetrician may give *episiotomy* to increase vaginal outlet to help the childbirth.

The updated international system classifies obstetric laceration into four types [Royal College of Obstetricians and Gynaecologists (RCOG) 2015]:

1. *First degree:* When injury occurs involving perineal skin, fourchette, and/or vaginal mucosa only **(Fig. 1)**.
2. *Second degree:* Tear extends to the fascia, muscles of the perineal body, and but not the anal sphincter **(Fig. 2)**.
3. *Third degree:* Injury to the perineum extending involving anal sphincter complex [external anal sphincter (EAS) and internal anal sphincter (IAS)] **(Fig. 3)**. Third degree is subdivided into 3a, 3b, and 3c.
   - *3a:* <50% of EAS complex
   - *3b:* >50% thickness involved.
   - *3c:* Both EAS and IAS torn, but anorectal mucosa intact
4. *Fourth-degree tear:* Perineal injury involving anal sphincter complex (EAS and IAS) and anorectal mucosa to expose the lumen of rectum **(Fig. 4)**.

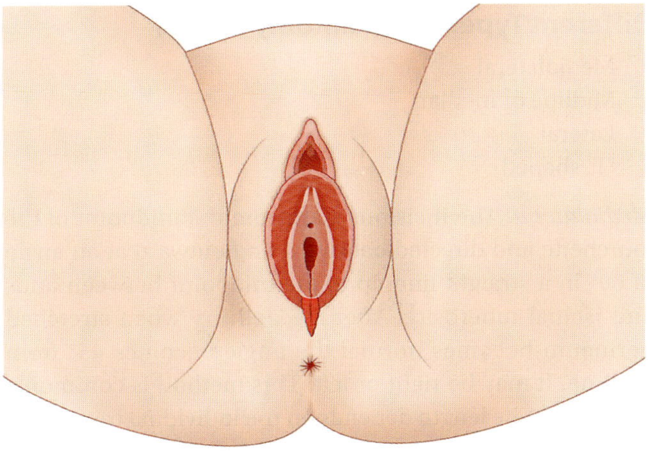

Fig. 1: *First-degree perineal tear:* Only vaginal and perineal skin involved.

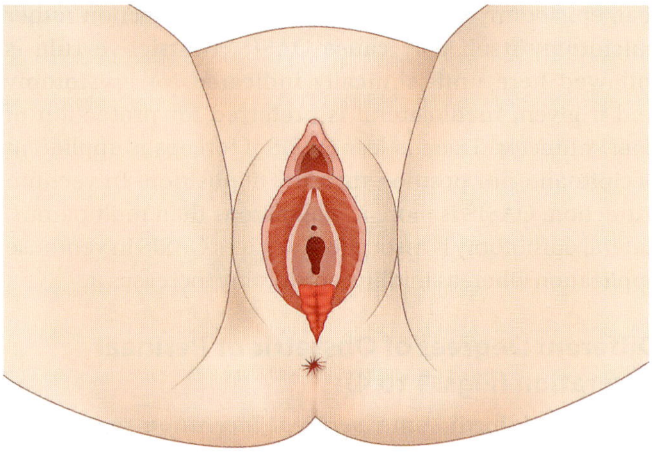

Fig. 2: *Second-degree perineal tear:* Perineal muscle involved.

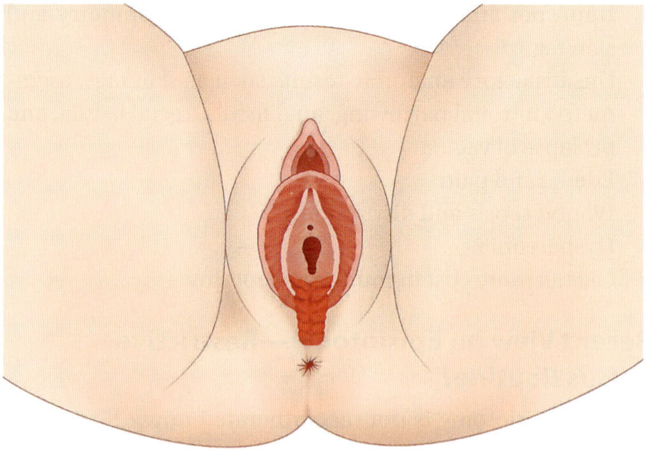

Fig. 3: *Third-degree perineal tear:* Anal sphincters involved.

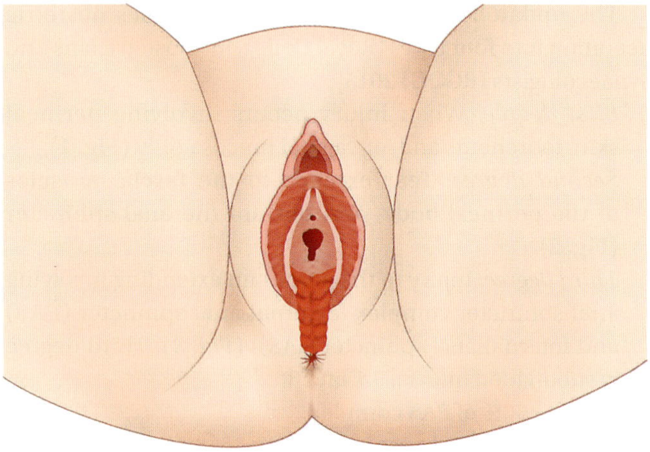

Fig. 4: *Fourth-degree perineal tear:* Rectal mucosa involved.

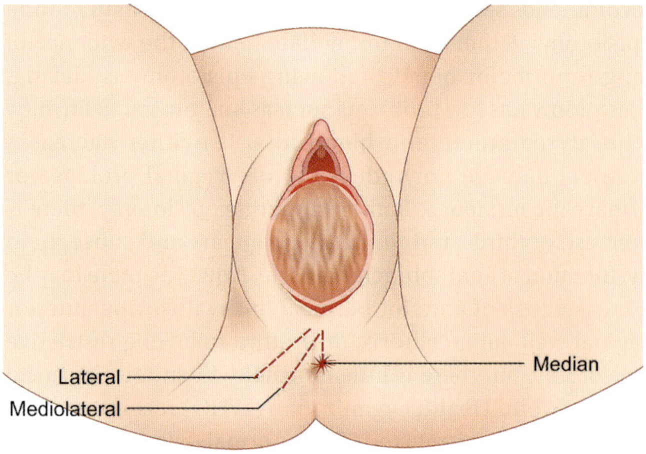

Fig. 5: Different types of episiotomy.

Obstetric anal sphincter injuries (OASIS) are comprised only third- and fourth-degree laceration. OASIS are the most severe form of perineal laceration and involves anal sphincter. It is discussed in details in this chapter.

Different Types of Episiotomy (Fig. 5)

- Mediolateral
- Midline or median
- Lateral
- "J" shaped

Mediolateral: The incisions start from the midpoint of the fourchette and directed backward and outward at an angle of 60° in a straight line up to the midpoint between anus and ischial tuberosity. After the delivery when stretched perineum becomes normal the angle becomes 45° from midline. It may be right or left. This method is commonly employed. The length depends on the individual case.

Advantage is that incision can be extended without involvement of rectum. Disadvantages are blood loss is more, apposition is not so good-like midline, more postoperative discomfort, more chance of wound gaping, and more incidence of dyspareunia.

Midline or median: It starts from the midpoint of fourchette and extends posteriorly for about 2.5 cm in the midline. Advantages are less bleeding, excellent anatomical apposition, repair is easy, union is good, and postoperative discomfort is less. However, if extension occurs, rectum will be involved resulting OASIS.

Lateral: Starting from 1–2 cm lateral from midline of fourchette directed laterally, more laterally than mediolateral toward ischial tuberosity left or right. The only advantage is that the introitus can be made wider. The disadvantages are excessive hemorrhage, poor healing, and injury of Bartholin's gland and its duct restricts its uses.

"J" shaped: It commences from the center of fourchette and is extended in a curved fashion in downward and outward direction. It is not so popular due to its technical difficulty, excessive bleeding, malapposition, and poor healing with occurrence of more dyspareunia.

Midline (median) and mediolateral episiotomies involve structures those found with second-degree laceration, and their repairs are similar.

Anatomical structures incised in episiotomy **(Fig. 6)** are vaginal mucosa, superficial and deep transverse perineal muscles, bulbospongiosus and few fibers of levator ani muscle with their fascia, subcutaneous tissue, and perineal skin. Blood vessels are anterior branches of internal pudendal vessels and branches of nerves. In lateral episiotomy, more fatty tissues are damaged, more muscle bulk are cut, and larger blood vessels are injured (labial branch of external pudendal artery).

Procedures of Episiotomy

Timing of episiotomy is important. Episiotomy is given when the head does not recede in between contractions, perineum becomes bulged, thin, and threatens to be ruptured **(Fig. 7)**. It synchronizes with just before crowning.

The instruments and gadgets required in episiotomy and its repair are: (1) swab-holding forceps, (2) syringe, (3) needle holder, (4) artery forceps, (5) scissors, (6) dissecting forceps, (7) lignocaine solution, (8) Sims speculum, (9) providone iodine solution, (10) Vicryl, and (11) catgut.

Episiotomy scissor and its repair set are displayed in **Figures 8 and 9**, respectively.

Sequential Steps

- Position—supine, thighs flexed and knees flexed, patient is on labor table.
- Antiseptic swabbing and draping
- Bladder catheterization
- Per vaginal examination
- Anesthesia—perineal infiltration with 10 mL 1% Xylocaine or pudendal block with perineal infiltration **(Fig. 10)**.
- Two fingers of left hand are placed between the presenting part and the posterior vaginal wall, and the perineum is

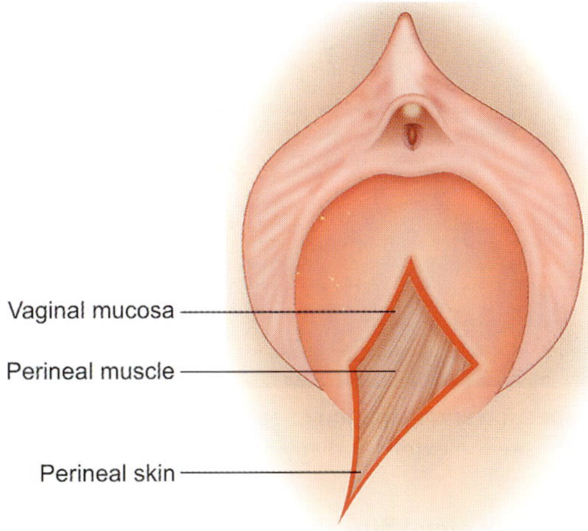

Fig. 6: Structures incised in episiotomy.

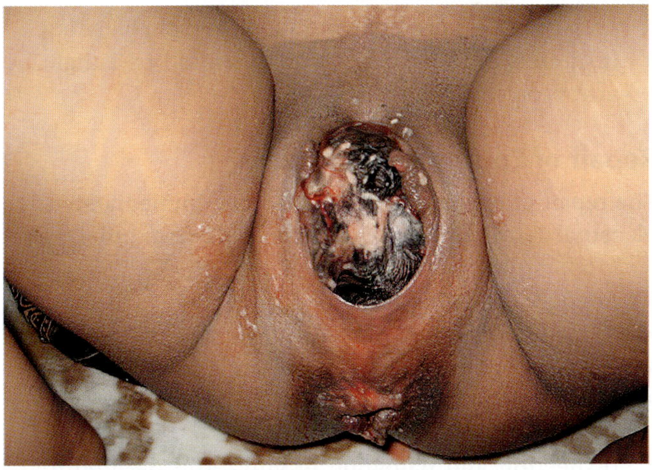

Fig. 7: Timing of performing episiotomy.

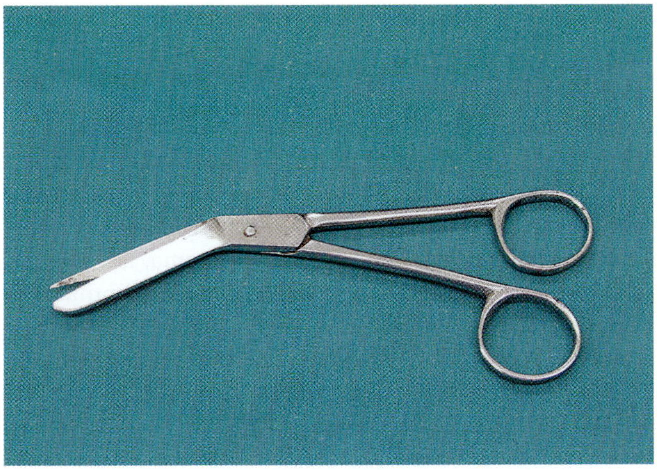

Fig. 8: Episiotomy scissor.

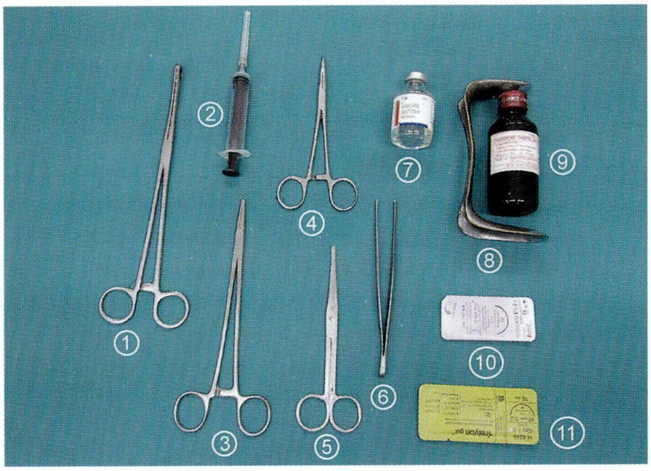

Fig. 9: Episiotomy and its repair set. (1) Swab-holding forceps; (2) Syringe; (3) Needle holder; (4) Artery forceps; (5) Scissors; (6) Dissecting forceps; (7) Lignocaine solution; (8) Sims speculum; (9) Providone iodine solution; (10) Vicryl; (11) Catgut.

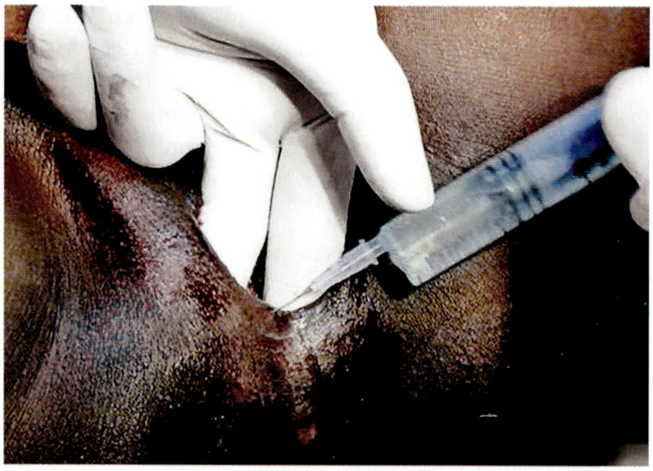

Fig. 10: Perineal infiltration of lignocaine.

cut with the scissors (blunt blade inside vagina) starting from midpoint of fourchette and extending downward and backward on right or left side **(Fig. 11)**.

- The fetus and afterbirths are delivered. A sanitary pad is pressed in the episiotomy wound to prevent bleeding.
- If there is any spurting vessel, it should be caught by artery forceps.

Repair of Episiotomy Wound

The repair of episiotomy wound is done immediately after placental delivery excluding any cervical tear or other tear.

- Mother is in lithotomy position.
- Adequate light source
- Catheterization
- Cleaning of the wound with antiseptic solutions
- Local infiltration of 1% Xylocaine (already given) **(Fig. 10)** or pudendal block
- Inspection and palpation of vulva and perineum are done to see the extent, any other laceration **(Fig. 12)**. Following instrumental delivery cervix is also examined for any bleeding and tear.

Repair is done in *three layers* in the following manner:

- Vaginal mucosa is repaired first **(Figs. 13A and B)**—the first stitch is placed beyond the apex of cut wound. Subsequently, the cut margins are repaired with continuous interlocking stitches up to the introitus.
- Then, perineal muscles are apposed **(Figs. 14A and B)**—by interrupted stitches. Care is taken to include all muscles, to obliterate dead space and to secure hemostasis to prevent vulval hematoma.
- Finally perineal skin and subcutaneous tissues **(Figs. 15A and B)** are repaired by interrupted mattress stitches.
- Any pack kept in vagina before repair is removed.
- Per rectal examination is done to see whether rectal mucosa has been included in stitches or there is any vulval hematoma.

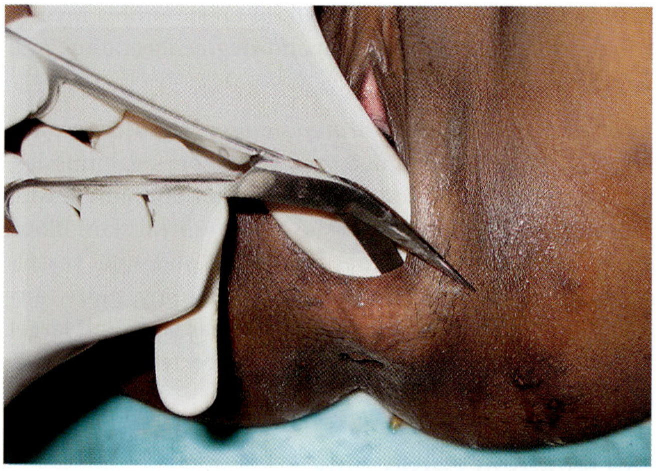

Fig. 11: Left mediolateral episiotomy.

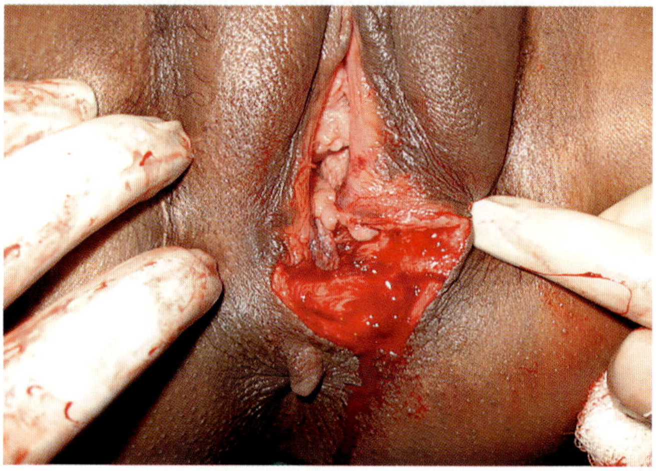

Fig. 12: Inspection and palpation of episiotomy wound are done to see the extent and any other laceration.

- If there is any rectal bite, the stitch is to be removed.

Midline episiotomy is shown diagrammatically in **Figures 16 to 19**. After repair wound is finally inspected for any bleeding or breakage of skin **(Fig. 20)**.

Complications of Episiotomy

Immediate complications are extension of the wound, CPT (OASIS), rectovaginal fistula (RVF), severe hemorrhage, vulval hematoma **(Fig. 21)**, retention of urine, infection, nonhealing, wound dehiscence, excessive pain (causes are vulval hematoma, paravaginal hematoma, ischiorectal hematoma, and perineal cellulitis). Vulval hematoma following repair is not uncommon and is ungently managed **(Fig. 22)**. Delayed complications are painful scar, RVF **(Fig. 23)**, and dyspareunia.

Care for Episiotomy Wound

Patient is advised to keep the wound dry. Wound is dressed with antiseptic ointment or solution at least twice daily, particularly after urination and defecation. Analgesics

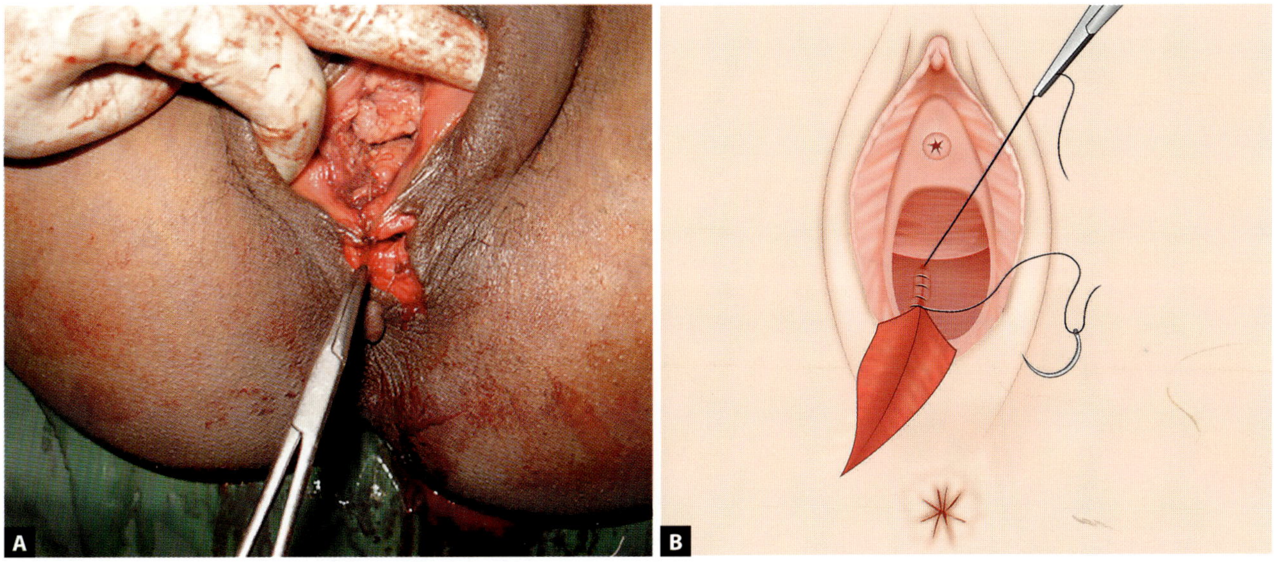

Figs. 13A and B: Mediolateral episiotomy. Vaginal mucosa is repaired first.

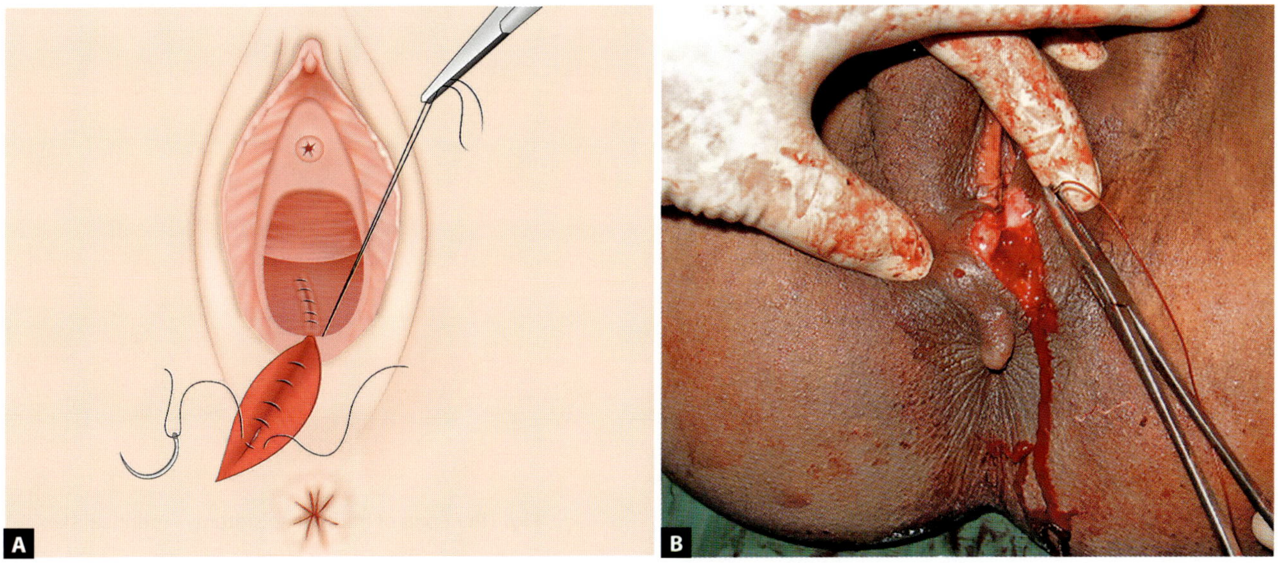

Figs. 14A and B: Perineal muscles are apposed.

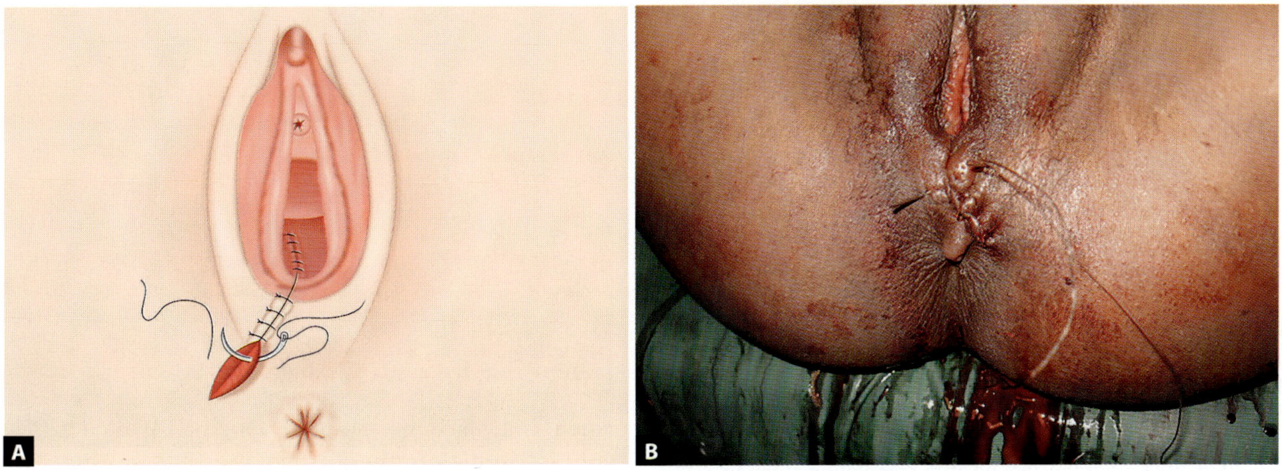

Figs. 15A and B: Perineal skin and subcutaneous tissues.

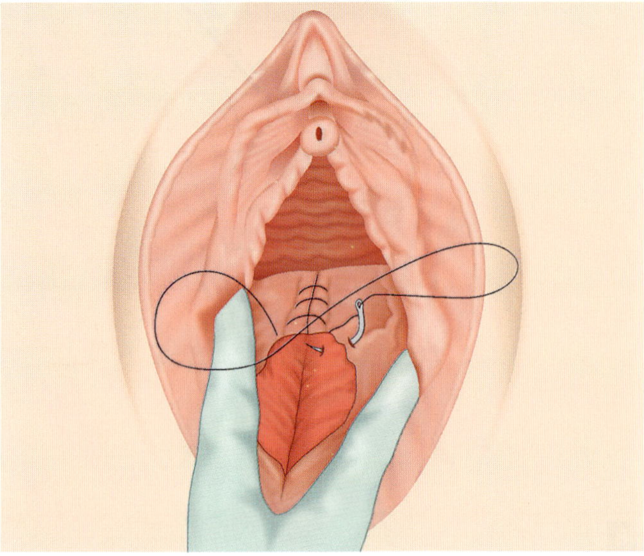

Fig. 16: Repair of midline episiotomy—vaginal mucosa.

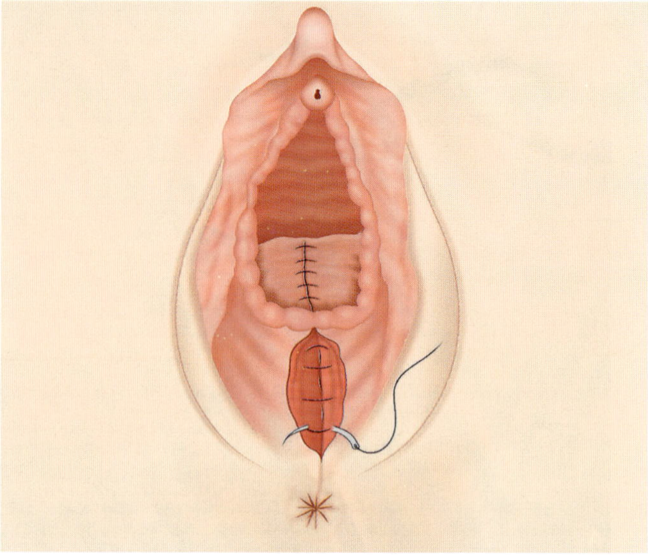

Fig. 17: Repair of midline episiotomy—perineal muscle.

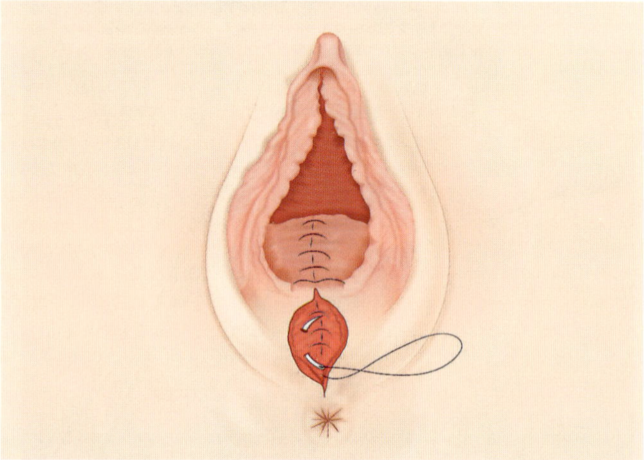

Fig. 18: Repair of midline episiotomy—perineal muscle.

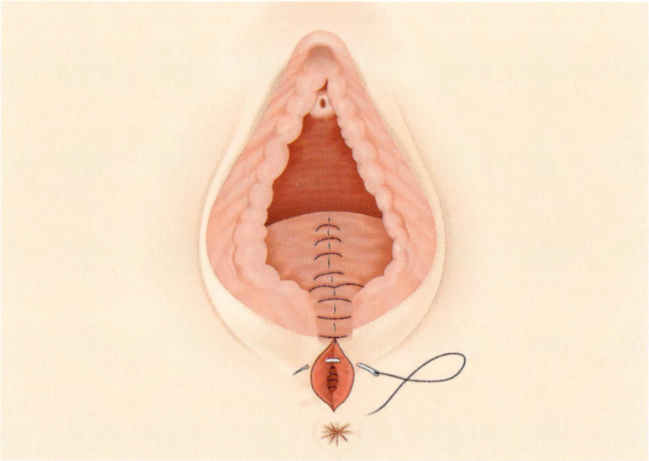

Fig. 19: Repair of midline episiotomy—perineal skin.

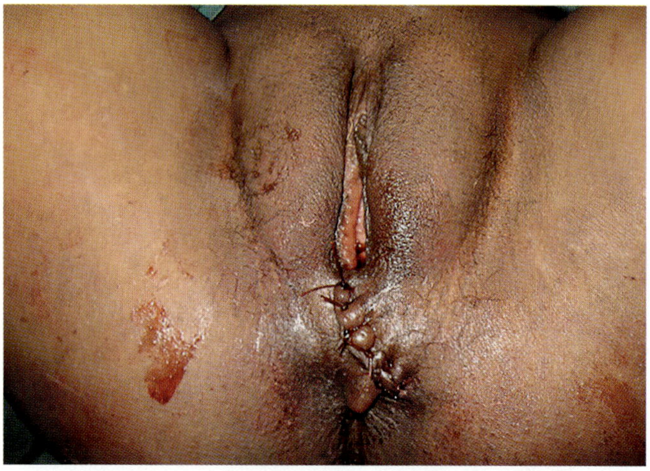

Fig. 20: Episiotomy wound after completion of repair.

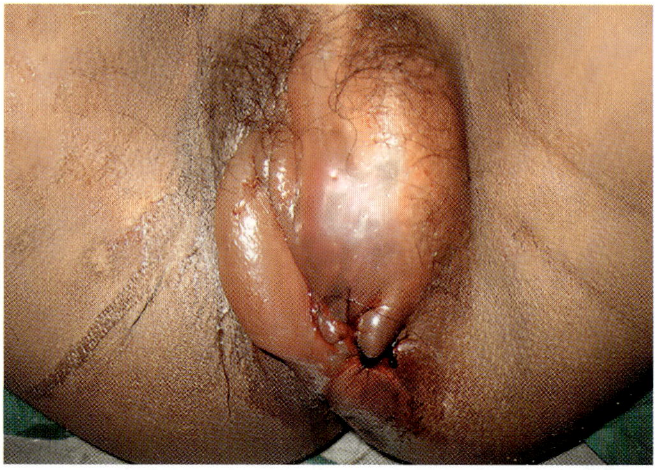

Fig. 21: Vulval hematoma developed following repair of episiotomy.

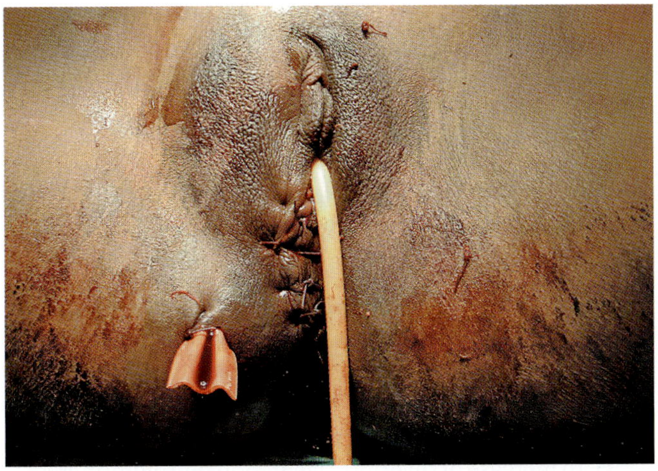

Fig. 22: Rubber drain has been given following repair of vulval hematoma.

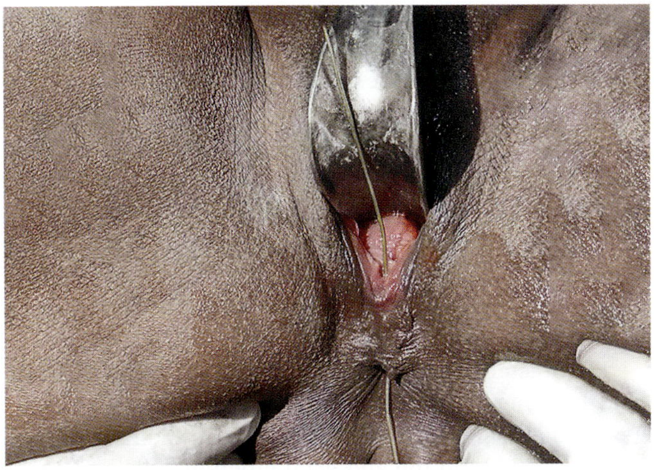

Fig. 23: Small rectovaginal fistula following vaginal delivery with episiotomy. Patient complained of loose stool occasional per vagina. A probe is passed through the fistula to demonstrate the fistulous tract.

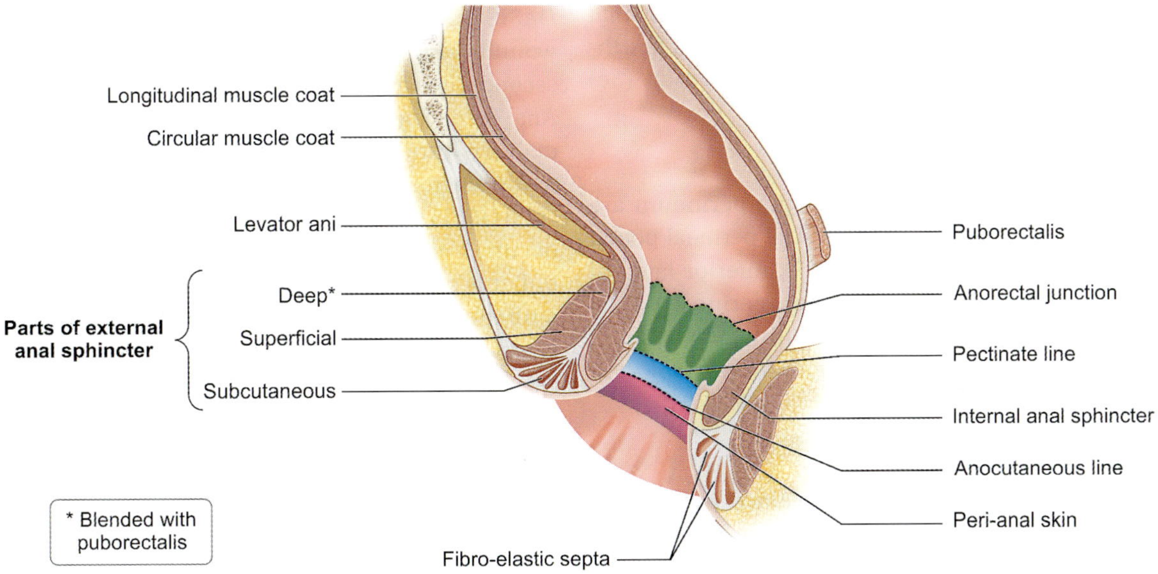

Fig. 24: Anatomy of anal canal and anal sphincter.

and antibiotics are usually not prescribed routinely. As episiotomy wound is stitched with absorbable suture, removal of stitch is not needed.

ANATOMY OF ANAL CANAL AND ANAL SPHINCTER (FIG. 24)

The length of anal canal is 4–5 cm and it starts as continuation of rectum at the level of levator ani attachment. From inside outward it has mucosa, IAS, intersphincteric space outside which lies the EAS in lower part and puborectalis in upper part. IAS is the continuation of smooth circular muscle fiber of rectum. Intersphincteric space contains the extension of the rectal longitudinal smooth muscle layer. The mucosa contains the columnar epithelium in cephalad and simple stratified squamous epithelium caudally, in between lies the dentate or pectinate line. Anal cushions are the three submucous arteriovenous plexuses which are highly vascular and helps for complete closure and continence of the anal canal to some extent.

Hemorrhoids are the venous engorgement in the cushion and may result from pregnancy, excess straining and hard stool as a result of degeneration and loss of support by connective tissue. External hemorrhoids which lie below the pectinate line may be painful and may be seen as mass. Above the pectinate line there may be internal hemorrhoids which may bleed or prolapse but unlikely painful.

Anus has two sphincters, namely IASs and EAS. IAS and EAS along with puborectalis muscle form the anal sphincter complex.

Outside IAS lies the EAS in its lower part and puborectalis in upper portion. The length of IAS is 3–4 cm and at its distal part there is overlapping with EAS.

Internal anal sphincter maintains the anal canal resting pressure and responsible for fecal incontinence significantly. It becomes relaxed before defecation.

External anal sphincter is a circular muscle ring throughout the circumference of IAS on its lower part. It is attached anteriorly with perineal body and posteriorly with coccyx by anococcygeal ligament. It has three parts, namely subcutaneous, superficial, and deep. For anal continence it has great role. In addition, to keep the resting continence it prevents incontinence in urgency by squeezing pressure.

Puborectalis which is one of the three muscles of levator ani (the other two are pubococcygeus and iliococcygeous) lies medially and extends from pubic bone on either side and comes behind the anorectal junction acting as a sling maintaining the continence.

Hence, the continence of anal canal is maintained by EAS (major role), IAS, puborectalis, and anal cushion.

As the sphincters are close to the vagina, it is likely that they are torn during vaginal delivery. IAS is injured in fourth-degree tear and advanced third-degree laceration (3c) resulting anal incontinence.

Structure of Perineum

Structures from superficial to deep in the perineum are skin, fascia of Colles, contents of superficial perineal pouch (superficial transverse perinei and EAS), inferior layer of urogenital diaphragm, contents of deep perineal pouch (transverse perinei profundus and sphincter vaginae), superior layer of urogenital diaphragm, levator ani, and pelvic cellular tissue.

ANAL INCONTINENCE

Anal incontinence is defined as the complaint of involuntary loss of flatus and/or liquid or solid feces affecting quality of life.

Mechanism of Continence of Flatus and/or Feces and Mechanism of Disruption (Pathophysiology of Anal Incontinence)

The perineal body lies between the vagina and the rectum. It is mostly formed by the bulbocavernosus and transverse perineal muscles and other muscles are puborectalis and the EAS. The anal sphincter complex (EAS and IAS) lies below the perineal body and extends for a distance of 3–4 cm.

The EAS is composed of skeletal muscle. The IAS, which overlaps and lies above the EAS, is composed of smooth muscle which is continuous with the smooth muscle of the colon.

In urgency, EAS and puborectalis maintain the continence. Puborectalis muscle provides continence of hard stool whereas external and internal sphincters are responsible for maintenance of flatus and liquid stool. The IAS provides most of the resting tone of anus and is essential for maintenance of continence.

Anal cushions help for complete closure and continence of the anal canal to some extent. Laceration of these sphincters is associated with anal incontinence.

OASIS

OASIS means obstetric anal sphincter injuries including both third- and fourth-degree perineal tears.

Impact of OASIS

Obstetric anal sphincter injuries are associated with social, psychological, and clinical impact. Pain, dyspareunia, fecal urgency, anal incontinence, and difficulty of passage of stool are the symptoms.

With increase of severity of laceration morbidity increases. Third- and fourth-degree lacerations are associated with short- and long-term adverse effects and primary risk factors for anal incontinence. There are more bleeding and pain in OASIS in comparison to simple laceration. Infection and wound disruption are more common in OASIS. First- and second-degree tears are mostly healed with less consequences. Anal incontinence increases double in OASIS than vaginal delivery without OASIS. Anal incontinence occurs more in fourth-degree than in third-degree lacerations.

If OASIS is not repaired immediately or wound disruption occurs it may result old CPT occurs with incontinence of flatus and feces **(Fig. 25)**. The details are described in author's *Bedside Clinics in Gynecology*, 2nd edition 2023, published by Jaypee Brothers Medical Publishers.

Diagnosis and Identification of OASIS

Clinical examination—inspection and palpation with good analgesics, exposure, good light after cleaning the blood from perineum, posterior vaginal wall, and surroundings of anal canal and rectum **(Fig. 26A)**.

Endoanal ultrasound—*occult OASIS* is better diagnosed by ultrasonography. Intrapartum endoanal ultrasound

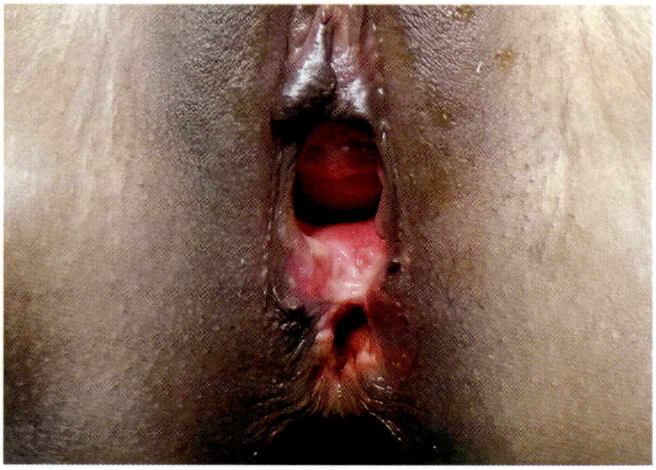

Fig. 25: Old complete perineal tear (involving anal mucosa).

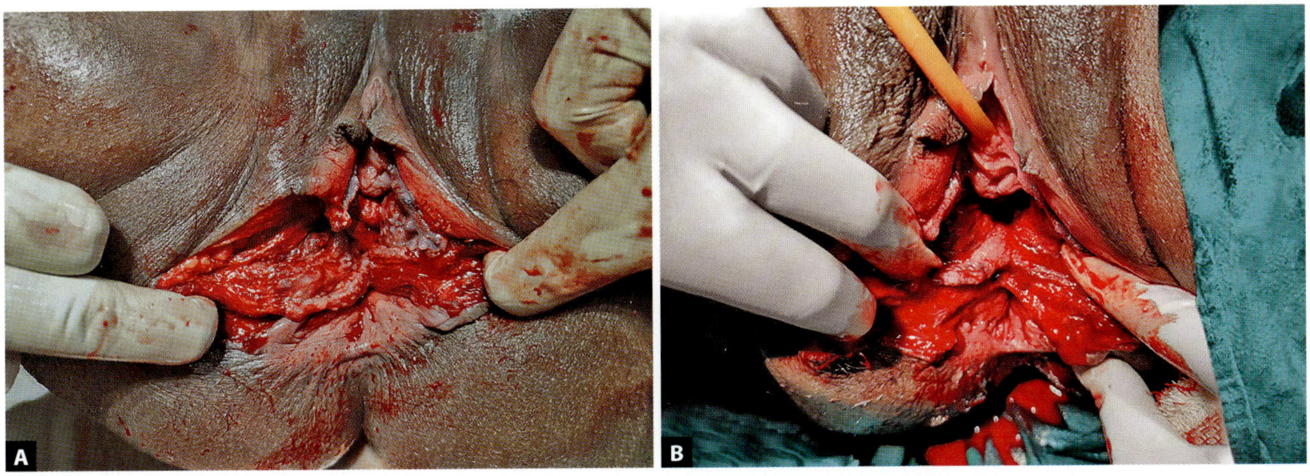

Figs. 26A and B: (A) Fourth-degree perineal tear following forceps delivery. Primi at 39 weeks exceeded second one and half hours and developed fetal bradycardia and meconium-stained liquor. A 3.055 kg baby was delivered by low forceps, there was a tight loop of cord around the neck. Baby cried immediately after birth; (B) Laceration is thoroughly examined to see the extent of injury in the case as described in Figure 26A.

during labor is used to diagnose clinically occult tear but is not routinely recommended by ACOG (2020).

Risk Factors of OASIS

Various risk factors are nulliparity, elderly mother, prolonged second stage, midline (median) episiotomy, prolonged second stage, precipitate labor, and persistent OP position. Operative delivery and large baby >4 kg increase the risk of OASIS. OASIS is more common in Asian race or Indian race.

Causes of OASIS

- Mismanaged second stage
- Operative vaginal delivery (OVD)—more on forceps than ventouse
- Malpresentation—OP, aftercoming head of breech
- Precipitate labor
- Delivery of large baby
- Shoulder dystocia
- Extension of median episiotomy wound

Prevention of OASIS in Vaginal Delivery and Operative Vaginal Delivery

Removal of blades before the delivery of head, asking mother to prevent bearing down during forceps removal and head delivery and simultaneous application of pressure over perineum by an assistant also prevent the advanced perineal tears (OASIS).

Surgical Repair of OASIS

Before repair perineum is thoroughly examined, including rectal examination, to assess the severity and extent of the laceration **(Fig. 26B)**. Failure of detection of OASIS and its repair may cause inadequate repair that may result wound complications and anal incontinence. It should always be done in operation theater.

Prerequisites

- Good anesthesia either general anesthesia or spinal
- Wide exposure, good light, and instruments for retraction
- Experienced operator and assistants
- Cleaning of blood and blood clots

Sequential Steps (Figs. 27 to 34)

- Repair of rectal mucosa in fourth-degree tear—continuous nonlocking with rapidly absorbable monofilament suture 2-0 to 4-0 gauge **(Figs. 27A and B)**
- Repair of IAS—continuous nonlocking suture 3-0 to 4-0 gauge, monofilament suture
- Repair of EAS—end-to-end repair or overlapping repair **(Figs. 28 to 30)**
- Repair of vaginal mucosa and deeper tissues—single continuous locking sutures—delayed absorbable (Polyglactin 910 Vicryl 2-0 or 3-0 gauge suture) **(Figs. 31A and B)**
- Repair of perineal muscles—superficial transverse perineal and bulbospongiosus—continuous nonlocking suture **(Fig. 32)**
- Repair of perineal skin—done by interrupted absorbable sutures **(Figs. 33 and 34)**. Subcuticular stitch is a good option.

End-to-end EAS repair is done in 3a and 3b OASIS **(Fig. 35A)**—four fascial stitches are applied first surrounding the sphincter posterior, inferior, anterior, and superior. Also a single figure of eight stitches is placed to appose the torn ends of EAS muscles. Delayed absorbable (Vicryl 2-0 or 3-0 gauge) suture is used.

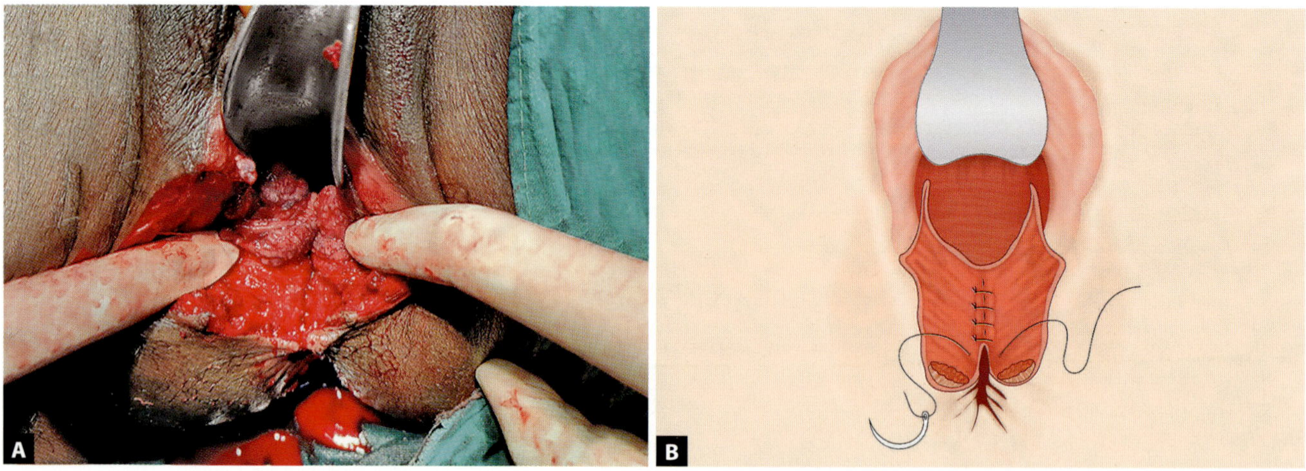

Figs. 27A and B: (A) Repair of anorectal mucosa; (B) Repair of anorectal mucosa (diagrammatic).

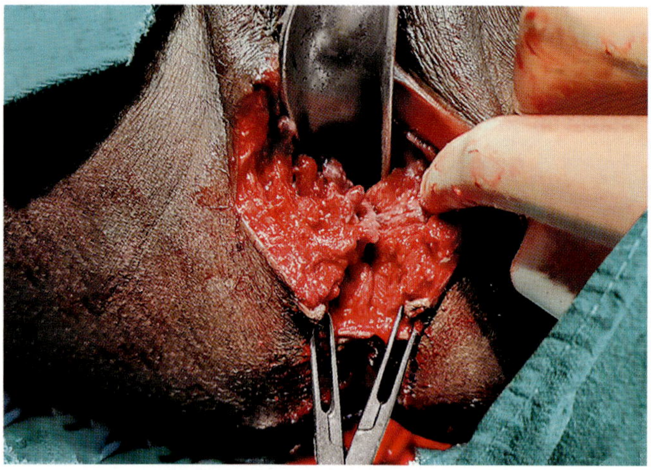

Fig. 28: Torn ends of external sphincters are identified and held with Allis forceps on two sides.

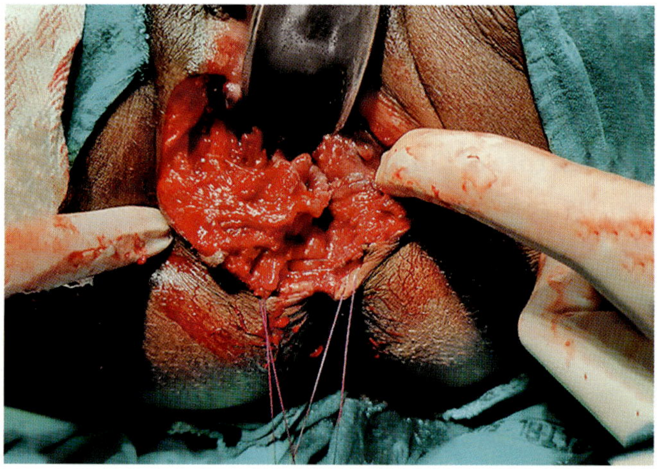

Fig. 29: Sphincters are on the process of repairing.

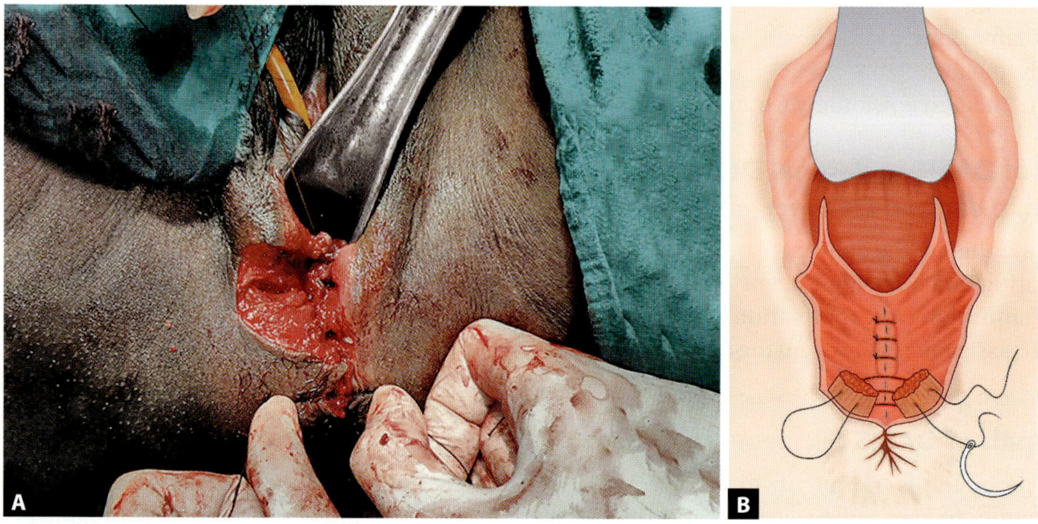

Figs. 30A and B: (A) Sphincters apposed and tied with each other; (B) Apposition of torn anal sphincter ends (diagrammatic).

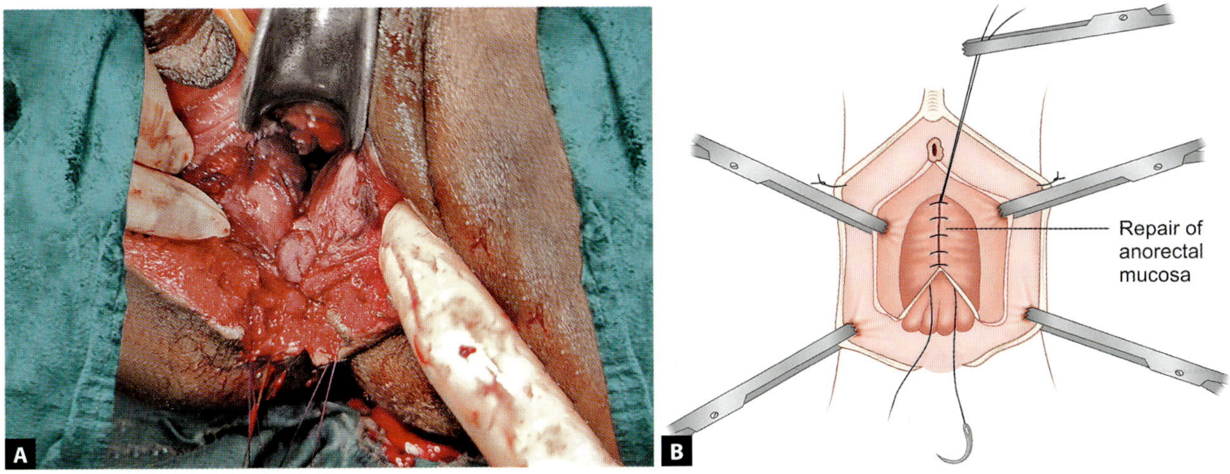

Figs. 31A and B: (A) Apex of the cut end of vaginal mucosa is identified and repaired with continuous stitches; (B) Completion of repair of vaginal mucosa.

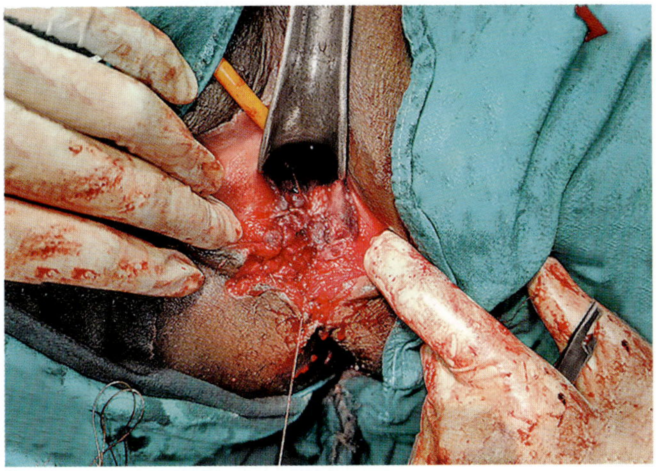

Fig. 32: Repair of perineal muscles.

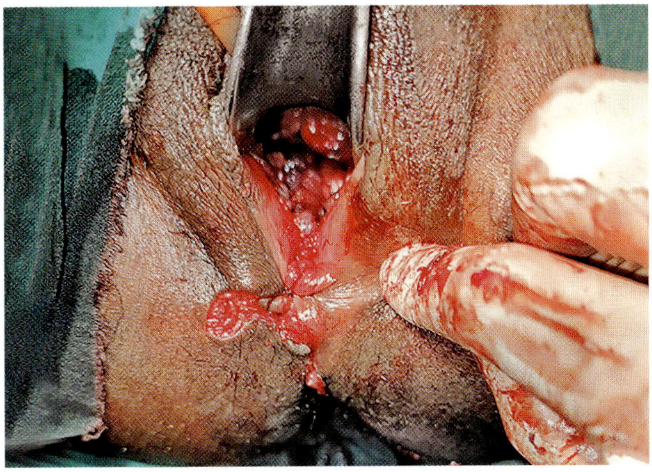

Fig. 33: Repair of perineal skin.

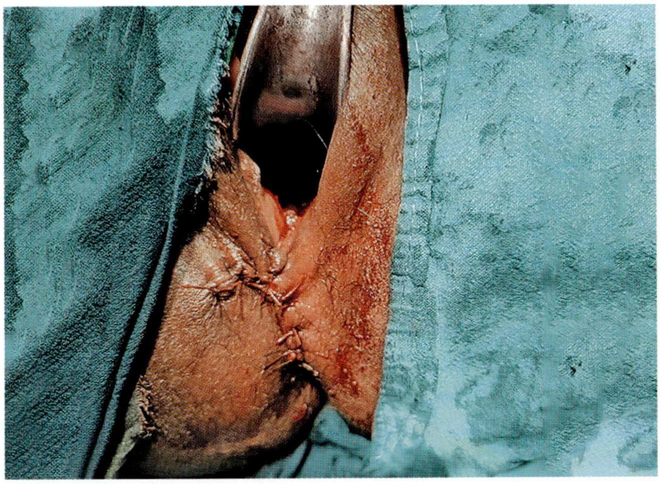

Fig. 34: Completion of repair of perineal skin.
Courtesy: Dr Anumita Chandra and Dr Nikita Achal, RG Kar Medical College, Kolkata, West Bengal, India for all original figures from 26 to 34.

Overlapping repair of EAS is done in full thickness torn **(Fig. 35B)**. Torn ends are identified first, then dissected for 1.5 cm each length free of fascia, overlapped, 4–6 mattress stitches are given (*vest-over-pants technique*). Here also delayed absorbable (Vicryl 2-0 or 3-0 gauge) suture is used.

Postoperative Care after Repair of OASIS

For prevention of infection, single dose of antibiotic is administered peroperatively, second-generation cephalosporine is effective. Perineal care by using hand shower or warm water to clean the wound and anus is suggested two to three times daily and after micturition and defecation. Warm sitz bath is useful. Ice application locally may reduce swelling and pain to some extent. Postoperative oral laxative like lactulose is suggested to prevent hard stool. However, very liquid stool may pass through repaired layer and hard stool can break the stitches. Enema is avoided. For pain relief very good analgesic, usually nonsteroidal anti-inflammatory

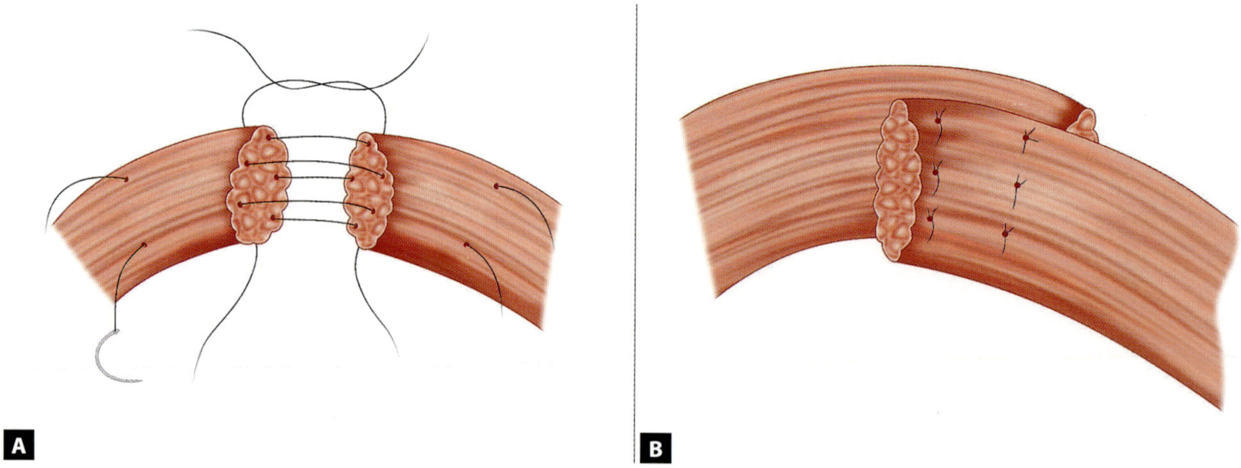

Figs. 35A and B: (A) Repair of external ani sphincter—end to end; (B) Repair of external ani sphincter—overlapping.

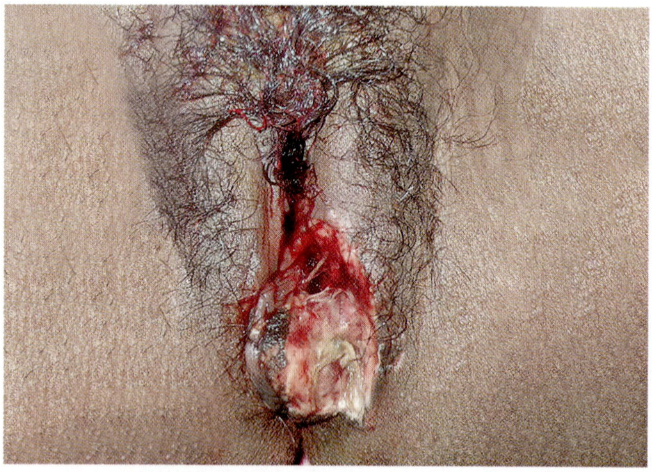

Fig. 36: Episiotomy wound dehiscence with infection.
Courtesy: Dr Anirban Mondal, Associate Professor, Bankura Sammilani Medical College, Bankura, West Bengal, India.

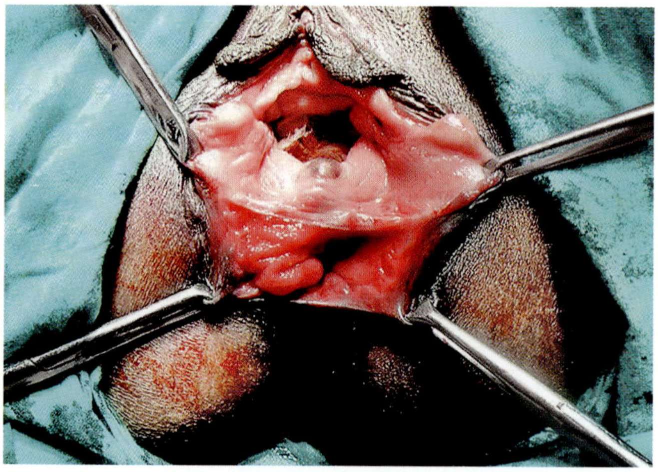

Fig. 37: Old complete perineal tear.

drug (NSAID), or in severe cases codeine containing analgesic is prescribed. In persistent pain, hematoma and cellulitis are to be ruled out.

Follow-up

Woman is followed up within 8–12 weeks to assess the healing of wound and if there is complication like anal incontinence. >75% women become asymptomatic. Mothers with persistent symptoms are examined carefully. For assessment of anal sphincter defects *endoanal ultrasonography* and/or manometry may be helpful. Intercourse is avoided before 3–6 months in laceration, not before follow-up.

Mode of Delivery Following Obstetric Anal Sphincter Injuries

The risk of repeat OASIS is high (five-fold) following vaginal delivery and woman should be counseled before vaginal delivery for future risks. Many prefer to do elective cesarean delivery with history of OASIS to prevent future anal incontinence.

EPISIOTOMY WOUND DEHISCENCE

Though rare in developed country, wound dehiscence **(Fig. 36)** is not uncommon in developing country. The incidence ranges from 1 to 5%. The common association of wound dehiscence is wound infection. Commonly the patient presents with pain pus discharge and sometimes fever.

Management consists of broad spectrum antibiotic, orally in mild infection, parenteral in severe infection, and analgesics. The most important part is complete opening of wound, drainage of pus, wound debridement with removal of sutures, and irrigation which is usually done in operation theater with anesthesia following which daily dressing is done.

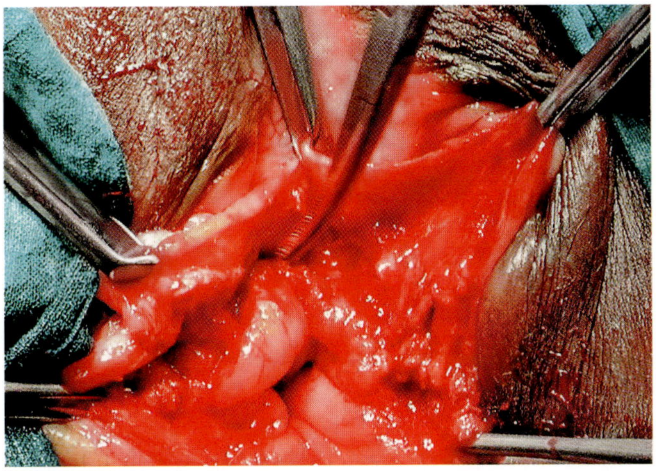

Fig. 38: Dissection done for repair of old complete perineal tear.

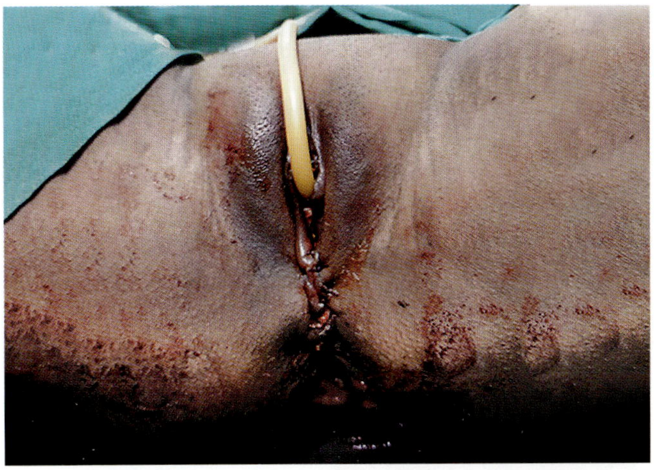

Fig. 39: After repair of old complete perineal tear.

Traditionally, the repair was made delayed for at least 3 months giving time for complete resolution of wound with free of infection and chance of breakage is less. In recent days, the concept of early repair has come that will correct sexual and bowel function early. As soon as the granulation tissue is formed secondary repair is performed which takes about 1 week. The success of primary repair is >90% in terms of healing and continence of flatus and faces.

In case of OASIS, the sphincter torn ends which are usually retracted are freed of fibrous tissue, mobilized, and apposed **(Figs. 37 to 39)**. The wound is repaired like primary repair. In secondary repair overlapping stitch is preferred to end-to-end method.

CHAPTER 16

Cesarean Delivery

Learning Objectives

- History
- Definition
- Indications
- Types
- Reasons of Stronger (Sound) Scar in LSCS than Classical One
- Preoperative Procedures and Care
- Perioperative Care
- Steps of Lower-segment Cesarean Delivery
- Variation in Technical Aspects of Cesarean Delivery and Current Recommendation
- CAESAR Study
- Indications of Forceps Application during Cesarean Delivery
- Technique of Classical Cesarean Delivery (Upper Uterine)
- Postoperative care
- Complications
- Cesarean Delivery in Special Situations
- Incidences

INTRODUCTION

Cesarean delivery (CD) or cesarean section (CS) which is, in fact, the delivery of the baby through abdominal route is the most common surgery in modern obstetrics. During last few decades, the incidence has sharply risen due to various reasons, which is also a real concern. In the era of small family norm in majority cases, the outcome is good, but it is not without complications rather it is potential for many adverse, sometimes serious outcomes such as placenta accreta spectrum (PAS) in next pregnancy. Knowledge and study on this subject are essential for every obstetrician.

HISTORY

Though CD in modern medicine is documented in mid-70th century, the idea of delivery of living baby is known from ancient time in myths and history. Brahma is said to emerge from the umbilicus of his mother in 5636 BCE. Buddha is described to be delivered from the right flank of his mother Maya. In Greek–Roman mythology, there are descriptions of birth from unusual sites of important personalities, gods, heroes, and super human.

The most controversial early story of successful operative deliveries was the tale of Jacob Nufer, a sowgelder. It was 1500 AD when Jacob Nufer performed the cesarean operation on his wife. After 7 days in labor and failure attempts by thirteen midwives, her husband Jacob Nufer did the operation desperately after taking permission from the local authority. The mother lived and gave birth normally to five children subsequently. The cesarean baby lived till 77 years. The Jacob Nufer story was first related after >80 years of the supposed event by Caspar Bauhin (1581), which was originally written by Francois Rousset, physician to the Duke of Savoy. The Nufer story was again described later in mid-18th century by the reviewer and John Burton. This entire story is under suspicion and difficult to believe especially for the subsequent events.

Whatever may be, before the modern CD came into practice and reported, physicians like Francis Rousset would believe in 16th century that cesarean operation is not only feasible but also could save the lives of both mother and baby.

Francois Mauriceau, a French obstetrician, is the first to report CD on living women in 1668. At that time, the maternal mortality was extremely high and till the end of 19th century, it was about 85–100%. And the main reason was the uterine wound was kept unrepaired. Bleeding and severe infection due to unrepaired uterus result in severe morbidity and mortality. Eduardo Poro from Italy first performed subtotal hysterectomy following delivery of the baby in 1876 and mother survived. In his technique after the delivery of baby, fundus of uterus was amputated and the cervical stump marsupialized to anterior abdominal wall. With the Poro's technique, maternal mortality decreased significantly.

It was Saenger from Germany who sutured uterine wall to preserve uterus first in 1882. He used to deliver the baby through a vertical incision above the level of lower uterine segment. After removing the placenta, wound was repaired by two layers—first deep layer with silver wire and second layer with fine silk. Kreher performed transverse lower-segment operation first in 1881. Fritz Frank described first the operation with extraperitoneal low-transverse uterine incision in 1907. He emphasized that there are less blood loss and less chance of infection in this method. Kronig advocated transperitoneal approach with vertical incision in 1912. Beck in 1919 and De Lee in 1922 popularized lower-segment operation by vertical incision. It was Munro Kerr who popularized semilunar transverse lower-segment incision for CD in 1926. Till then, many modifications have occurred in suture techniques and also the number of layers repaired, etc., but Munro Kerr's operative technique is still widely accepted. In last few decades, less tissue reactive suture materials have been available, serosal and parietal peritoneum omitted, running suture instead of interrupted sutures and blunt dissection instead of traditional sharp entry have been introduced. Overall, the use of prophylactic antibiotic, availability of blood transfusions, and improved anesthesia technique dramatically reduced morbidity and mortality and CD has now become a safer surgery.

Origin of the Term "Cesarean"

There is lot of controversies on the origin of the term "cesarean". One view is that the term originated from a Roman Law-Lex Caesarea (7015 BC). The law stated that a dying woman should be delivered abdominally to get a live baby. This law was applicable also in the era of Julius Caesar. Another view is that the term cesarean delivery was derived after the name of Caesar. This view is discarded by the fact that Aurelia, mother of Julius Caesar, lived to hear of her son's invasion of Britain. Third possible origin includes the Latin word "Caedare", which means to cut and the term "caesones" that was applied to infants born by postmortem operations.

Till 1598, the procedure was known as cesarean operation after which the term "operation" was replaced by "section". At present, the term "delivery" has become popular instead of "section".

DEFINITION

Cesarean section is an operative procedure where a birth of fetus occurs through incisions in the abdominal wall (laparotomy) and the uterine wall (hysterotomy). CD is an alternative nomenclature of CS and more meaningful so far as birth is concerned. Removal of baby from abdominal cavity following uterine rupture or in secondary abdominal pregnancy is not CD.

INDICATIONS

The common indications are cephalopelvic disproportion (CPD), post-CD, fetal distress, placenta previa, malpresentation and malposition, and abnormal uterine action.

The absolute indications are central placenta previa, severe CPD or contracted pelvis, carcinoma cervix—advanced stage, mass in the pelvis—cervical fibroid, broad ligament fibroid or impacted ovarian mass, and vaginal stenosis, septum, and acquired vaginal atresia.

Recurrent indications of CD are severe CPD or contracted pelvis, vaginal stenosis, septum, acquired vaginal atresia, and malformation of the uterus.

Indications in Details

- *Power*: Uterine dystocia not corrected by medical method, and constriction ring.
- Passage—bony—contracted pelvis, CPD, soft tissue—cervical fibroid, broad ligament fibroid, ovarian tumor, carcinoma cervix, vaginal obstruction, previous history of vesicovaginal fistula (VVF) repair, malformation of the uterus.
- *Passenger (fetal reason)*—big baby, malpresentations such as breech, brow, mentoposterior face, malposition—occipitoposterior, twin pregnancy when first twin is nonvertex. *Fetal complications*: Growth restricted fetus, cord prolapse, fetal distress, Rh incomparability, and previous history of repeated fetal death.
- *Maternal reasons*: Placenta previa (type II posterior, type III, and IV), some cases of abruptio placentae, severe preeclampsia and eclampsia, diabetes, post-CS pregnancy, in some heart diseases (coarctation of aorta, Marfan's syndrome)
- *Others*: Elderly primi, bad obstetric history (BOH), failed forceps, failed induction, and cesarean delivery on maternal request (CDMR).

Cesarean delivery on maternal request: Reasons of maternal request are fear of pain, reduction of fetal injury, convenience, and protection of pelvic floor. Fetal birth injury, hypoxic-ischemic encephalopathy, and infection are slightly less in CD. There is conflict on this issue in one side the maternal desire, and on the other side the obstetrician's own decision. There is still no consensus recommendation. CDMR in woman desiring multiple children is better discouraged to avoid the future consequences of multiple cesarean birth. CMDR should not be done before 39 weeks (ACOG, 2020).

TYPES

According to the site of incision on uterus—Cesarean delivery is classified as lower segment and upper segment.

According to time of operation it may be elective or emergency.

Elective CD is a planned CD where prior planning is done in respect to timing, place, and surgical team before allowing the mother going to labor. The term "scheduled CS" can be used for elective CD to differentiate it from nonlabor emergency CD.

Emergency CD is a type of CD, which is performed in acute obstetric emergency irrespective of whether mother is in labor or not. Emergency may be due to fetal or maternal cause or both. This is an important component of emergency obstetric care (EmOC) to reduce maternal mortality.

Different Types of Uterine Incision for Cesarean Delivery

- Transverse lower uterine segment incision, which is commonly done
- Vertical incision entirely on lower segment
- Classical CD incision, which in fact starts as low vertical incision and extended to upper uterine segment (body of uterus)
- Fundal or even posterior incision in placenta accrete spectrum.

Lower-segment Cesarean Delivery

In lower-segment cesarean delivery, uterus is entered through the lower uterine segment where loose peritoneum is attached. This is commonly transverse and may be vertical as well. The term is either LUCS (lower uterine cesarean section) or LSCS. In LSCS, transverse incision is preferred because it is wide enough for delivery of the fetus. In some conditions, where lower segment is not formed, like in cases of transverse lie and delivery of small baby with breech presentation, low vertical incision is given.

Vertical incision may be entirely on lower segment. In classical section, incision starts as low vertical incision and extends to body.

Advantages of lower segment CD over classical CD are bleeding is less, repair is good, peritonization is good, postoperative peritonitis, adhesion formation (bowel or omentum), and intestinal obstruction are less. Besides, postoperative recovery is good, wound healing is good, scar becomes sound (strong), and chance of rupture is less (1% or less).

Classical Cesarean Delivery

Classical CD is not practiced nowadays but can be done only in few instances, e.g., where lower segment is not accessible like multiple or large fibroid, gross adhesions, and severe contracted pelvis. This method is also useful in transverse lie with a large fetus, especially when membranes are ruptured and shoulder is impacted, in cases of very small fetus, especially in breech, where lower segment is not thinned out, excessive maternal obesity, carcinoma cervix, following repair of high VVF, sometimes Type III and IV placenta previa (not absolute) and in postmortem CD.

There are few advantages of classical CD over lower-segment CD. The area can be approached easily and incision is given when lower uterine segment is not approachable. In some cases, such as in placenta previa, delivery of fetus is easier and safer.

The disadvantages of classical CD over lower-segment CD are many. Hemorrhage is more, apposition of layers is not good, peritonization is not good, postoperatively, more chance of peritonitis and more chance of adhesion formation. Postoperative recovery is not as good as LSCS and morbidity is high. Wound healing is not good due to imperfect apposition, hematoma formation, due to uterine contraction and relaxation and the presence of tension in muscles and there is more chance of gutter formation inside. It is seen that scar becomes weaker and chance of rupture is more (5–10%).

REASONS OF STRONGER (SOUND) SCAR IN LSCS THAN CLASSICAL ONE

Anatomical apposition with perfect hemostasis occurs in LSCS scar, whereas in classical section, thick margins are apposed unevenly with pockets of hematoma formation followed by abscess where there may be formation of gutter inside. Healing is good in LSCS as the lower segment does not contract or retract, which mostly occurs in upper segment. In the next pregnancy, stretching is less on the LSCS scar in contrast to the classical scar where stretching occurs in perpendicular direction to the scar as the wound is longitudinal. In the next pregnancy, implanted placenta usually occurs in upper segment, which makes the upper uterine scar weak. All these factors explain why less risk of rupture in LSCS scar.

PREOPERATIVE PROCEDURES AND CARE

Informed consent and counseling: Woman should be discussed freely about the indication, procedures, alternatives, goals, limitations, potential operative risks involved, need for blood transfusion, and effect on future pregnancy. In case of pregnancy with previous CS, trial of labor (TOLAC) is discussed. Other intervention such as tubal sterilization or intrauterine contraceptive device (IUCD) insertion during CD, if planned, prior consent should be taken. Patient's autonomy should always be respected. Refusal of required intervention should be documented and future consequences should be informed in written.

PERIOPERATIVE CARE

- Patient should be evaluated by operative and anesthetic team. All investigation reports are examined including recent hematocrit and blood grouping typing.

- Nothing per mouth at least for 4–6 hours is desirable. In the current ERAS (enhanced recovery after surgery) protocol, patient should stop intake of solid food for 6 hours before surgery. Bowel preparation is not necessary. Some amount of clear liquid may be allowed up to 2 hours in otherwise uncomplicated cases.
- Regional anesthesia is the choice of anesthesia. Liquid antacid (nonparticulate) is administered to neutralize gastric acid that may prevent gastric aspiration. Injection ranitidine 150 mg intramuscular (IM) or intravenous (IV) is given before operation. Antiemetic (injection Reglan) is given IV. For emergency procedure, Ryle's tube suction is done and, in that case, regional anesthesia is preferred.
- Intravenous channel is made. Volume preloading with crystalloid or colloid is done in regional anesthesia to reduce the risk of hypotension.
- Preparation of abdominal skin is done by shaving and scrubbing with antiseptic solution. Hair removal is not mandatory until and unless it is on surgical site. Clipping and chemical epilation is better than shaving.
- An indwelling catheter is usually given to make the bladder empty during surgery and also to measure output in per- and postoperative period.
- To auscult the fetal heart sound (FHS) at OT table is mandatory.
- In pregnancy, as venous thromboembolism is increased, thromboprophylaxis is to be kept under consideration. ACOG (2020) recommends pneumatic compression stockings before CD.
- Pregnant woman having specific comorbidity such as diabetes needs specific care.

Antibiotic Prophylaxis

For infection prevention, single dose of prophylactic antibiotic is administered, preferably within 60 minutes of planned CD or in emergency cases as early as possible. A single dose of antibiotic of β-lactam group cephalosporin such as Cefazolin 1 g or extended penicillin is good choice. In case of excess blood loss (>1,500 mL) or increased operative time (>3 hours), additional dose should be given. In obese patient, 2 g dose or 3 g dose is recommended (CDCP). In *Staphylococcus aureus*-resistant cases, vancomycin single dose (15 g/kg) is given in addition.

Anesthesia

Regional anesthesia is safer and results in less maternal and neonatal morbidity than general anesthesia (GA). Spinal, epidural, or GA will be decided by the anesthetist after consultation with the patient.

STEPS OF LOWER-SEGMENT CESAREAN DELIVERY

Common instruments, which are used in CD, are given in **Figures 1 to 14**. These are female rubber catheter **(Fig. 1)**, Foley catheter **(Fig. 2)**, swab-holding forceps **(Fig. 3)**, scalpel with blade **(Fig. 4)**, scissors **(Fig. 5)**, artery forceps **(Fig. 6)**, Kocher artery forceps **(Fig. 7)**, Allis tissue forceps **(Fig. 8)**, Doyen's retractor **(Fig. 9)**, Green Armytage forceps (not used nowadays, instead Allis tissue forceps used) **(Fig. 10)**, needle holder **(Fig. 11)**, sterile mucus sucker **(Fig. 12)**, chromic catgut with needle **(Fig. 13)**, and delayed absorbable suture (polyglactin 910) with needle **(Fig. 14)**.

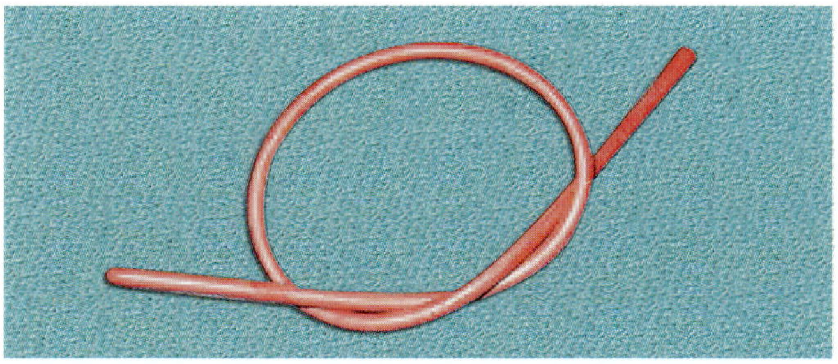

Fig. 1: Female rubber catheter.

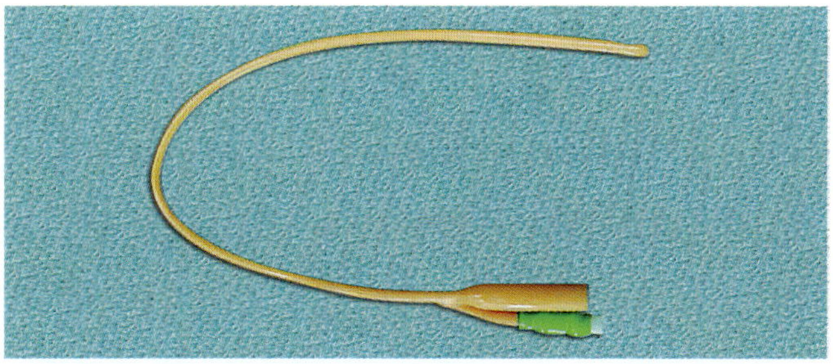

Fig. 2: Foley catheter.

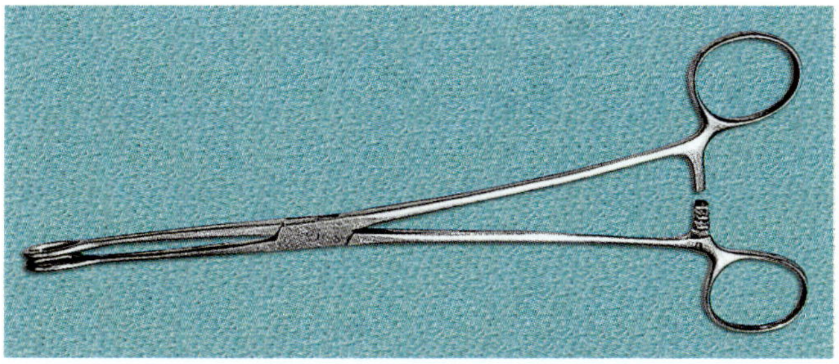

Fig. 3: Swab-holding forceps.

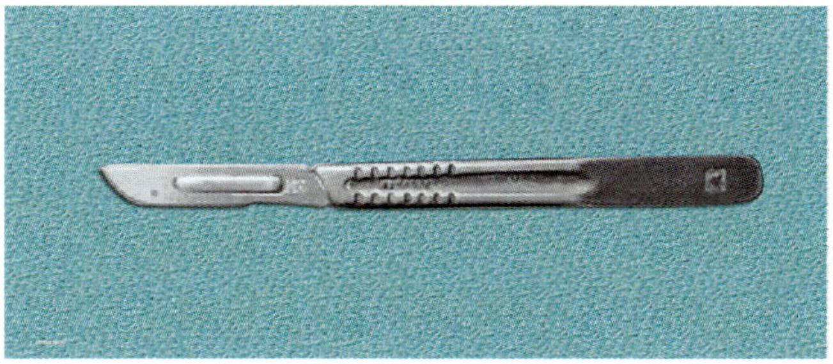

Fig. 4: Scalpel with blade.

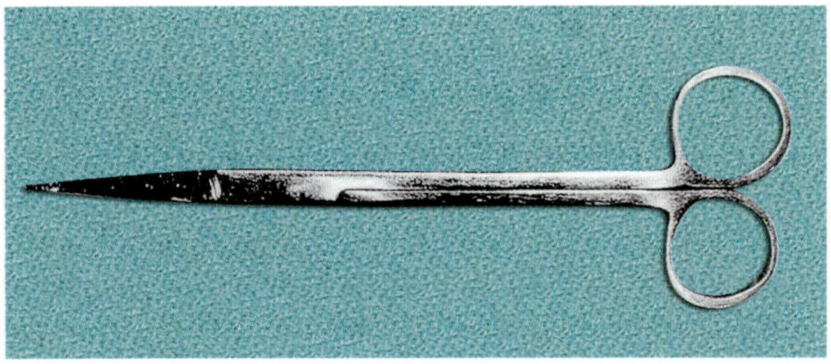

Fig. 5: Scissors.

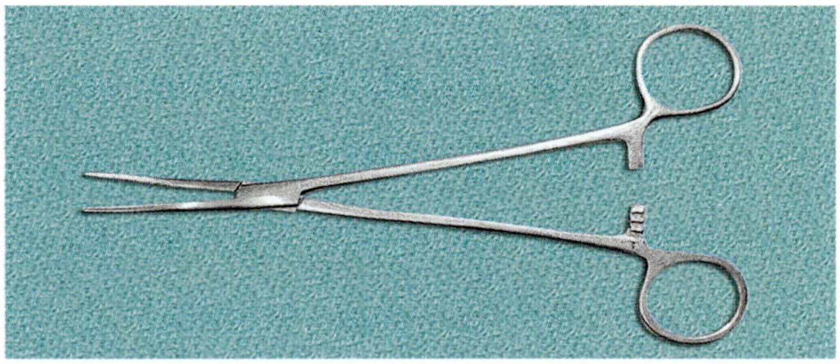

Fig. 6: Artery forceps

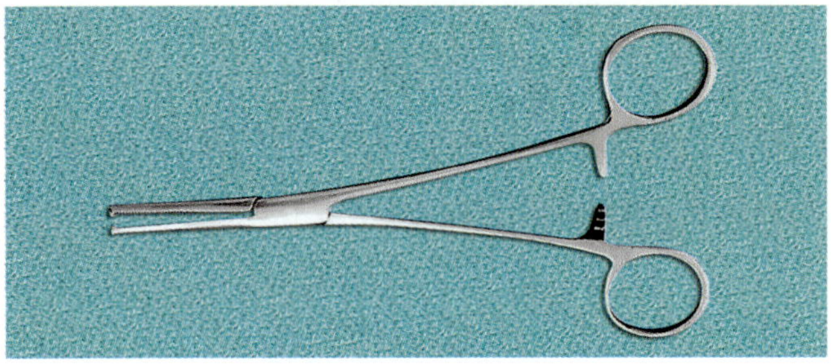

Fig. 7: Kocher artery forceps.

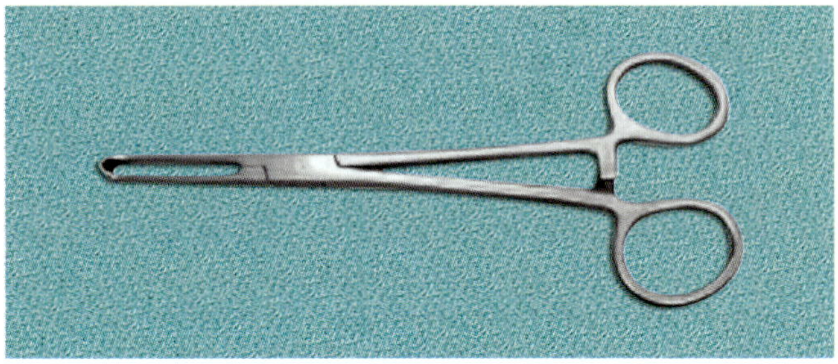

Fig. 8: Allis tissue forceps

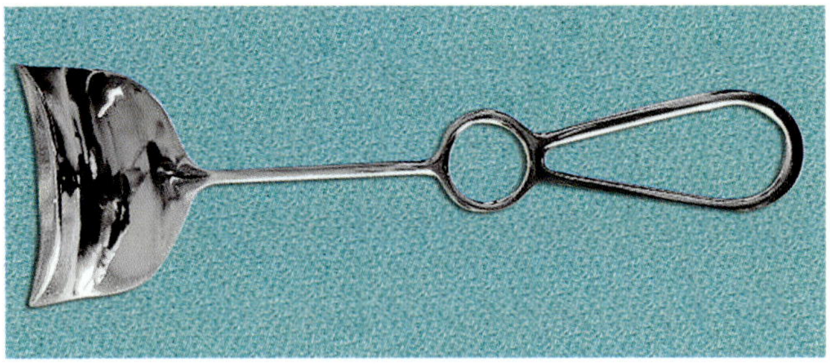

Fig. 9: Doyen's retractor.

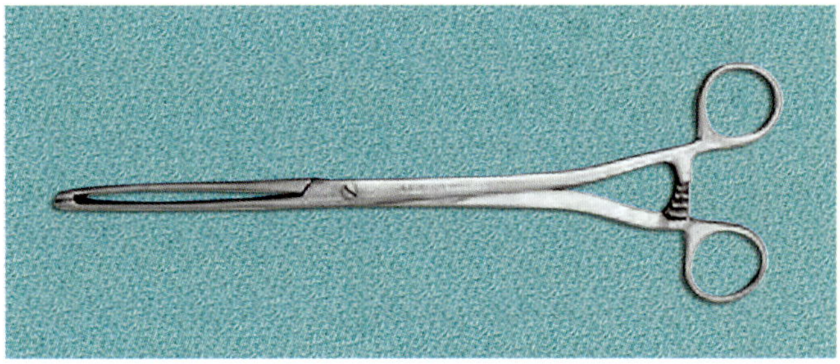

Fig. 10: Green Armytage forceps (not used nowadays, instead Allis tissue forceps used).

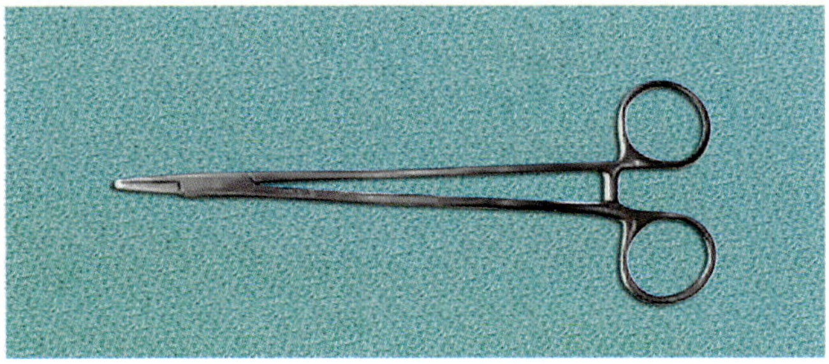

Fig. 11: Needle holder.

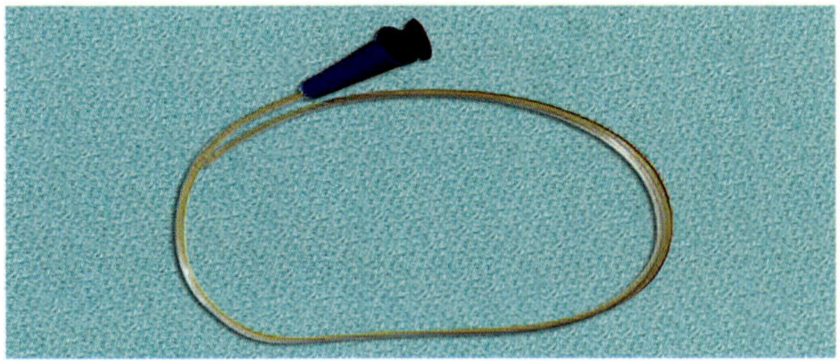

Fig. 12: Sterile mucus sucker.

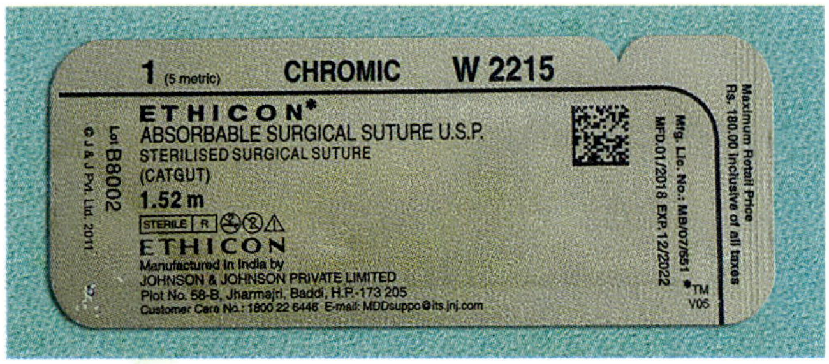

Fig. 13: Chromic catgut with needle.

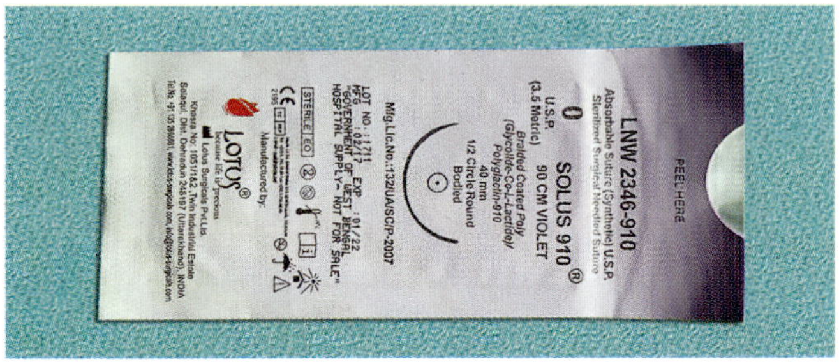

Fig. 14: Delayed absorbable suture (polyglactin 910) with needle.

Details of the Procedure of Lower-segment Cesarean Delivery (Figs. 15 to 53)

Details of steps are shown in the Figures from ***Figs. 15 to 53****.*

Patient is made supine position (15° tilt to left side may be done to avoid supine hypotension syndrome **Fig. 15**). FHS is again auscultated when patient is on OT table. Anesthesia is given, usually regional. Catheterization is done with rubber catheter for evacuation of bladder. Antiseptic dressing of the abdominal skin is done before operation with chlorhexidine-alcohol or povidone-iodine solutions. Chlorhexidine-alcohol is said to be superior. Then after the skin made dry draping is done.

Opening the Abdomen

Skin incision: Usually, Pfannenstiel incision **(Fig. 16)** is given. This is a suprapubic low transverse "smile" like incision 3 cm above the symphysis pubis at the level of pubic hairline, slightly curved, 12-15 cm in length (see below). Alternatively, midline vertical incision can be given (see later). For morbid obese woman, periumbilical midline incision is preferred.

Subcutaneous tissue **(Fig. 17)** layer is sharply dissected to reach rectus sheath. Superior epigastric vessels may be encountered much lateral to midline which is either diathermy coagulated or ligated with plain catgut (3-0).

Recuts sheath is cut transversely with sharp incision **(Figs. 18 to 20)**. Anterior rectus sheath is composed of two layers—external oblique aponeurosis and fused aponeurosis of internal oblique and transverse abdominis muscles. Inferior epigastric vessels, which lie lateral to rectus abdominis, are not usually injured and, if injured, need ligation or coagulation. By holding the cut margins of rectus sheath at midline, both below and above flaps are separated from rectus abdominis below up to symphysis pubis and above to the extent as needed **(Fig. 21)**. The vessels coursing between muscle and sheath are secured by coagulation or stitches and complete hemostasis done.

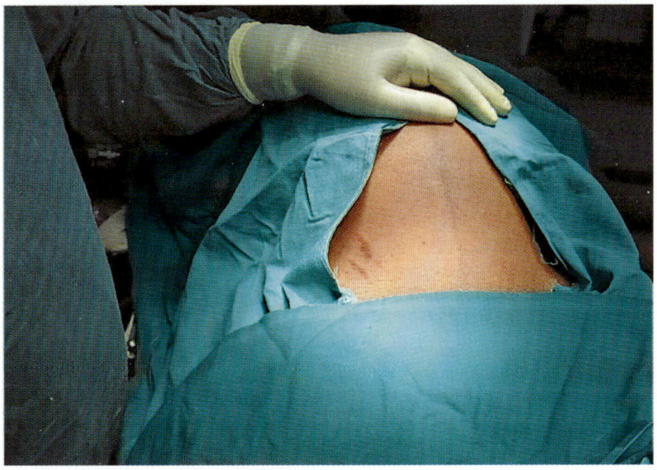

Fig. 15: Mother is on operation theater (OT) table and made supine position, antiseptic dressing and draping done.

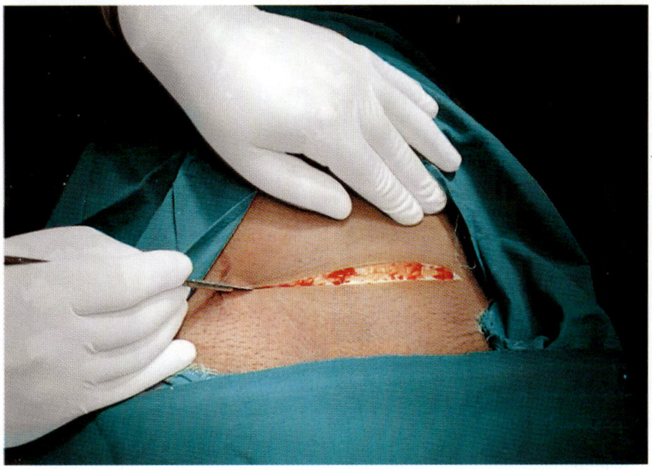

Fig. 16: Transverse (Pfannenstiel) skin incision is given.

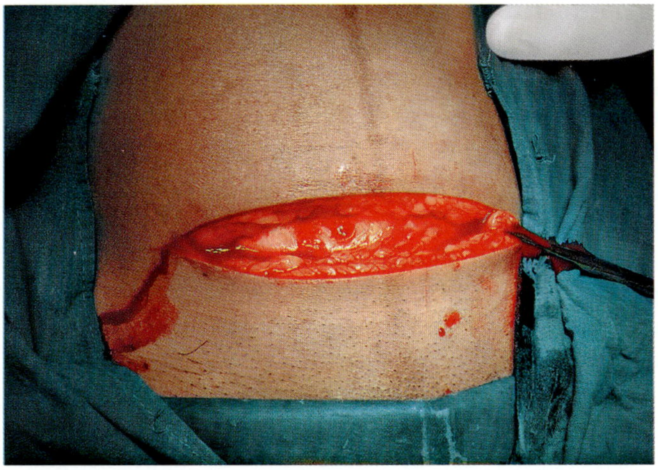

Fig. 17: Subcutaneous tissue layer is sharply dissected to reach rectus sheath.

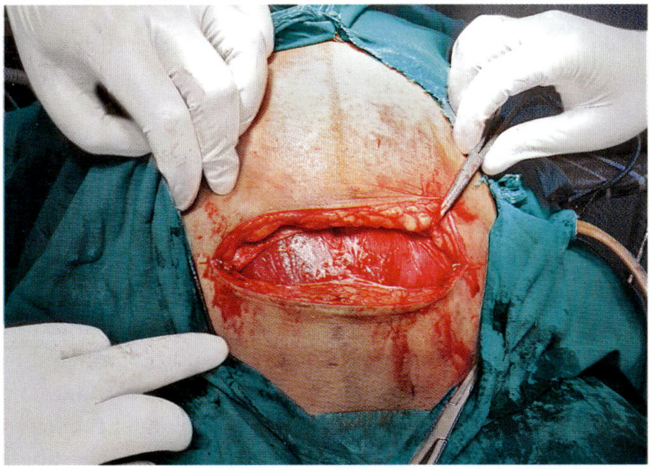

Fig. 18: Recuts sheath is cut transversely with sharp incision.

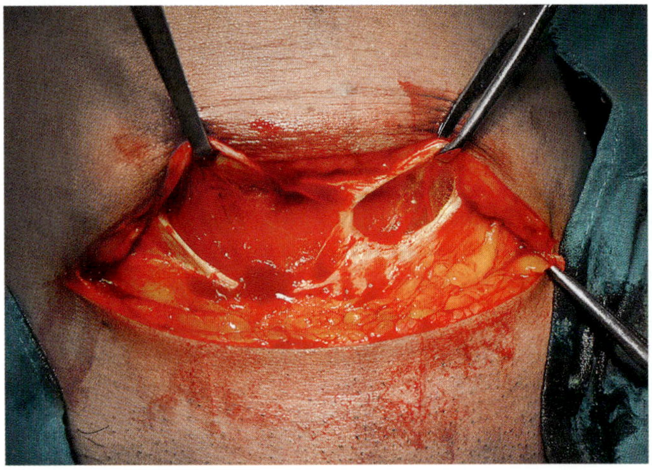

Fig. 19: Rectus sheath is made separated from rectus abdominis muscle.

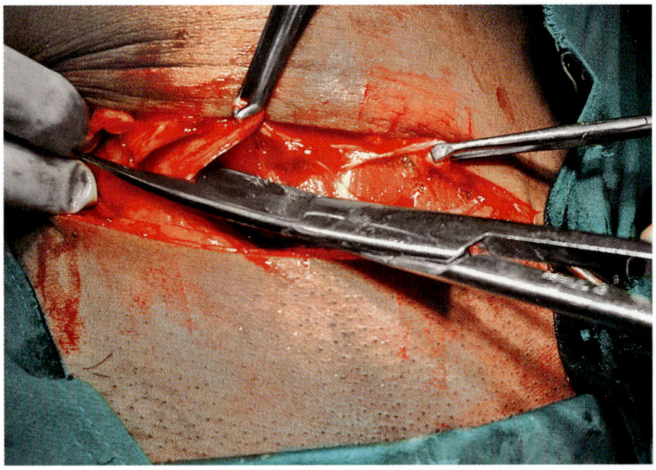

Fig. 20: Dissection of rectus sheath is extended laterally.

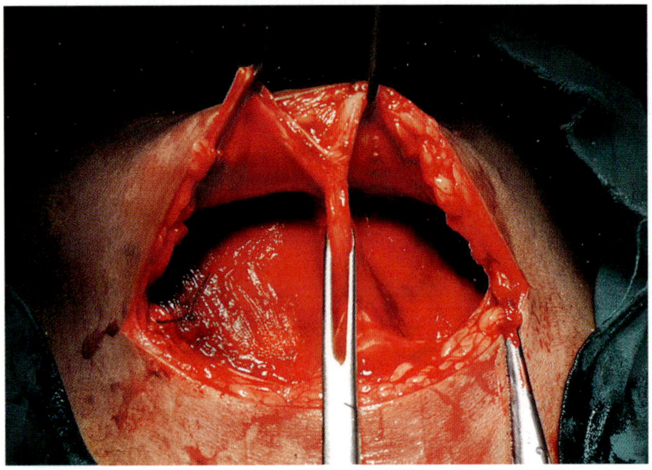

Fig. 21: By holding the cut margins of rectus sheath at midline, both below and above flaps are separated from rectus abdominis and from linea alba.

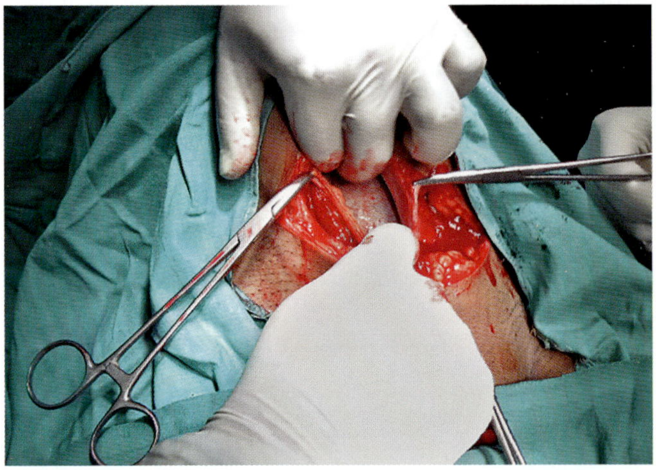

Fig. 22: Peritoneum cavity is entered after cutting the peritoneum and extraperitoneal fossa.

Careful hemostasis is very crucial to prevent hematoma and infection prevention.

Rectus muscles and pyramidalis are retracted laterally starting from above (there is no posterior layer of rectus sheath in lower abdomen).

Opening of peritoneal cavity: Transversalis fascia with preperitoneal fat is dissected to reach peritoneum, which is opened (**Fig. 22**) very carefully by lifting with two artery forceps and not to do any inadvertent injury of omentum, bowel, and bladder, and thus abdominal cavity is entered. Holding the peritoneum in upper part prevents injury of bladder. Before opening it, the peritoneum is palpated to exclude the inclusion of omentum, bowel, and bladder. The incision is then extended below up to the bladder reflection and superiorly above the arcuate line where transverse fibers of posterior layer of rectus sheath may need to be cut. It is to be remembered that bladder is elevated and edematous in obstructed labor. One must be careful also about the presence of any of intra-abdominal adhesion in case of previous abdominal surgery.

After Opening the Abdomen

Doyen's retractor is introduced to retract the lower cut margin of abdominal wound (**Fig. 23**). Packing with moist sponge is done (not mandatory). Fundus is palpated and position of round ligaments is identified to see whether uterus is rotated, if so, it is corrected manually so that incision becomes central.

Lower uterine segment is identified by the presence of loose peritoneum (uterovesical fold of peritoneum) in lower part of the uterus and above the upper margin of bladder.

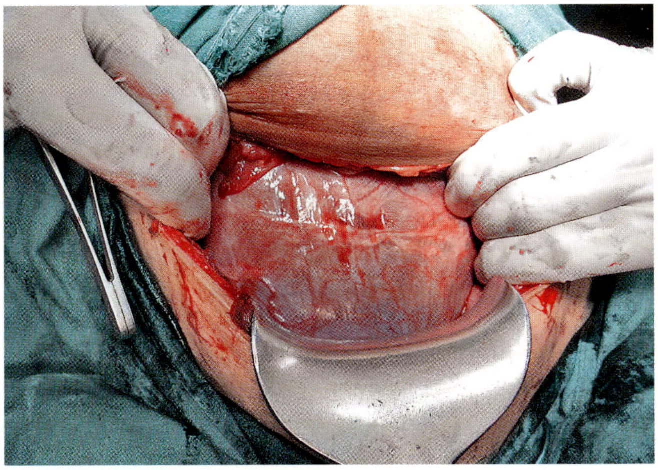

Fig. 23: Doyen's retractor is introduced to retract the lower cut margin of abdominal wound and to see the lower uterine segment.

Incision over Uterus

Commonly low transverse incision is given until and unless other type of incision is indicated. Loose peritoneum is grasped **(Figs. 24 and 25)** and incised transversely within a scalpel or scissors after separating from myometrium for about 2 cm wide. Beneath the peritoneum scissors are introduced between peritoneum and myometrium and peritoneum is incised extending laterally and slightly upward for about 10 cm **(Figs. 26 and 27)**. Bladder is gently separated (not too much) by blunt or sharp dissection. In pregnancy with prior CS, blunt dissection is avoided. In adhesion, sharp dissection is done. This bladder flap development is not done by all as avoiding this skin incision to delivery time is shortened. It is still a routine procedure, but should not be dissected too laterally which may cause

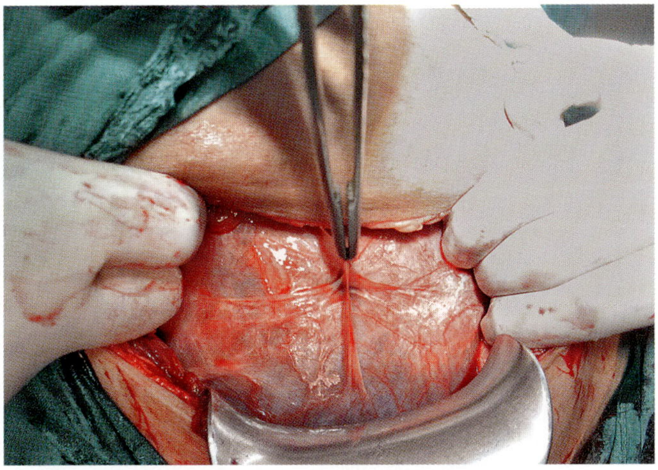

Fig. 24: Lower segment is identified by attachment of loose peritoneum and reflexion of uterovesical fold of peritoneum.

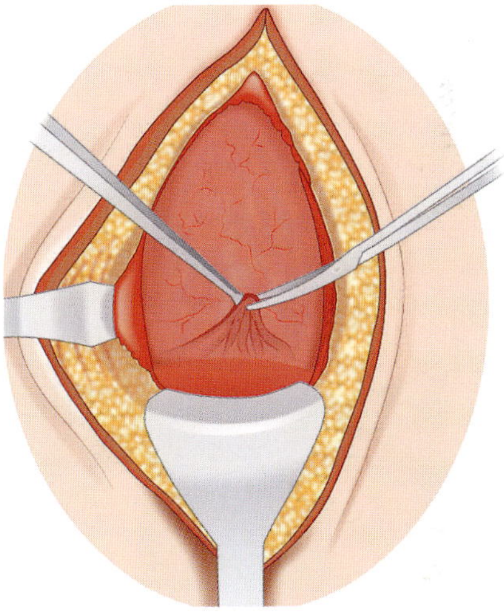

Fig. 25: Identification of the lower uterine segment by presence of loose peritoneum.

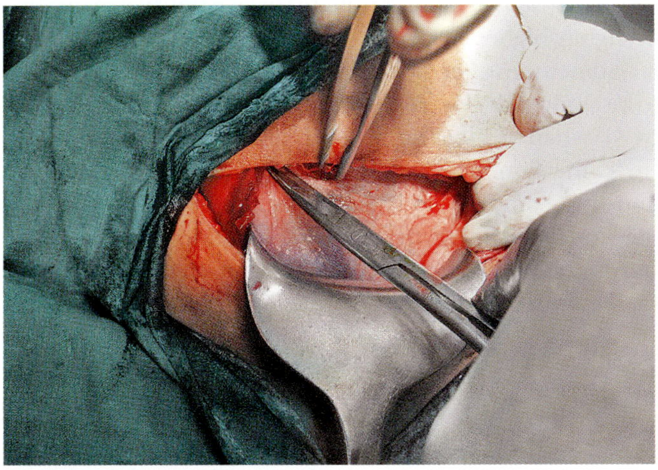

Fig. 26: Beneath the peritoneum scissors are introduced between peritoneum and myometrium and peritoneum is incised extending laterally and slightly upward for about 10 cm.

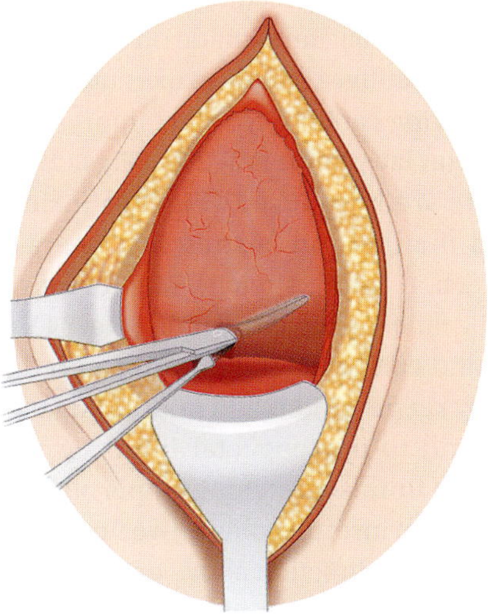

Fig. 27: Loose uterovesical peritoneum is cut with scissors.

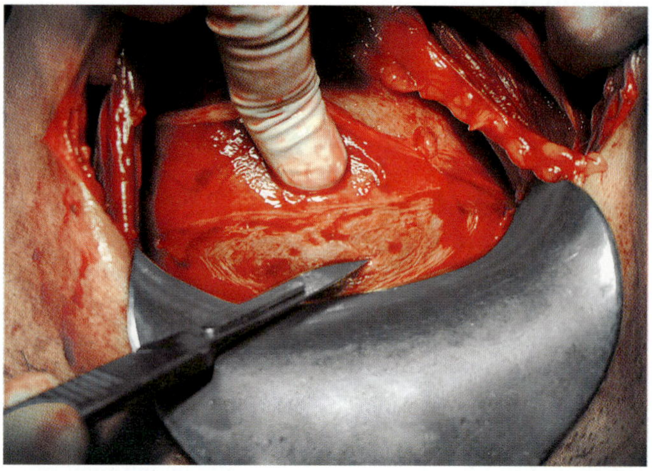

Fig. 28: Lower segment is transversely cut with scalpel after bladder is gently separated (not too much) by blunt or sharp dissection.

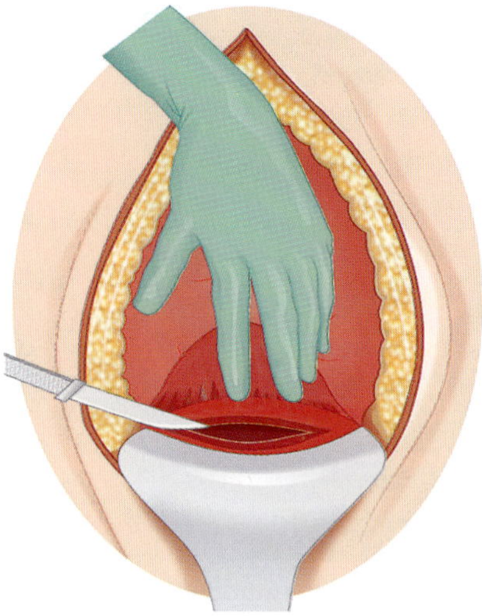

Fig. 29: Incision over the uterine myometrium with scalpel.

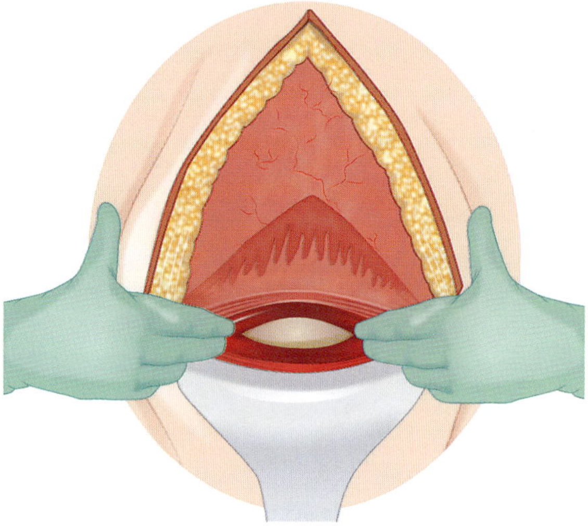

Fig. 30: Uterine wound is extended laterally.

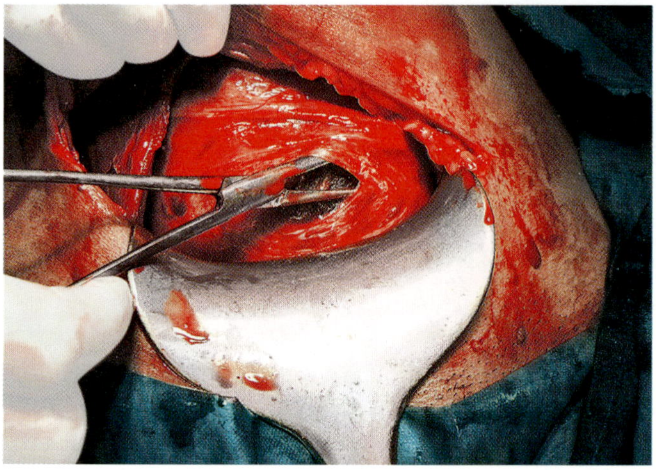

Fig. 31: Uterine cavity is opened with tip of the artery forceps and fetal head is visible after rupturing the membranes.

vessel injury and severe bleeding. With the help of a scalpel, a small transverse incision is made on the uterine wall in the midline with repetitive shallow strokes until the membranes are seen by taking care not to inflict injury to the fetal parts (chance of fetal laceration is 1–2%) **(Figs. 28 and 29)**. Two index fingers are introduced **(Fig. 30)** inside the uterine wound and the incision is stretched laterally and slight upward direction (blunt stretch). Membranes are ruptured and amniotic fluid is allowed to drain **(Fig. 31)**. Alternatively, uterine wound can be extended with sharp dissection also by scissors by keeping index and middle finger inside behind the lateral end to prevent fetal injury. Another method of blunt dissection is stretching upper margin and lower margin of incision inserting one or two fingers in the midline, pulling in opposite direction above and below. This method is claimed to be safer. Blunt method is associated with less operative time, less chance of extension, and lesser blood loss. In advanced labor, it is better to give transverse incision at slightly higher level.

Sometimes after giving low transverse incision if it seems to be inadequate for baby delivery uterine wound is extended by "J"-shaped incision, a "U" incision or by inverted "T". In "J" incision, one corner of incision is extended upward and it becomes U incision, if made bilateral. "J"-shaped incision is preferred to inverted "T". But in all these cases, intraoperative blood loss is more and chance of rupture increases in trial of labor (TOLAC) in future pregnancies.

Delivery of the Head

The amniotic fluid and blood are suctioned by the assistant to clean the area. Surgeon's right hand is slipped into the uterine cavity between symphysis pubis and fetal head **(Figs. 32 and 33)**. Doyen's retractor is removed by the assistant. As the occiput comes into the incision, head is

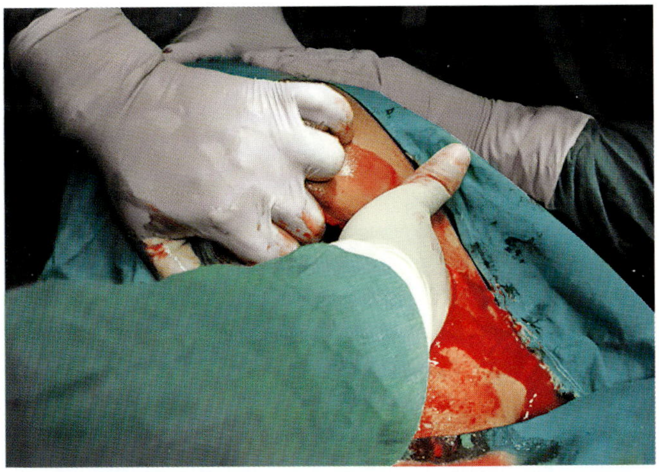

Fig. 32: Surgeon's right hand is slipped into the uterine cavity between symphysis pubis and fetal head. Doyen's retractor is removed by the assistant.

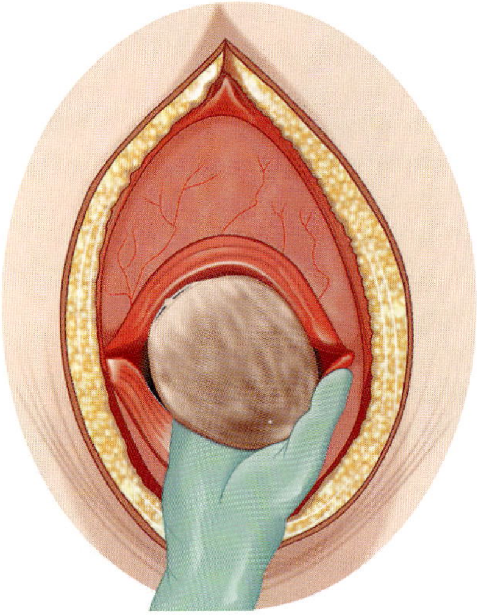

Fig. 33: Right hand is introduced in uterine cavity after rupturing the membranes.

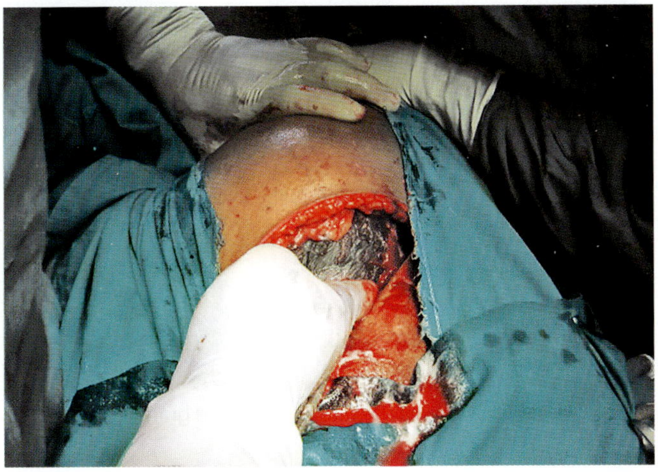

Fig. 34: The surgeon will always avoid flexing of the wrist and lower margin of the uterine wound is used as fulcrum.

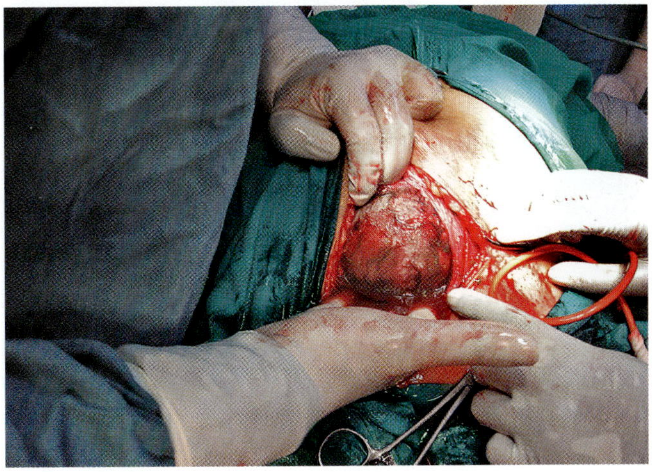

Fig. 35: Head comes out through uterine wound.

lifted slightly over the fingers and palm. Head is delivered through the wound aided by modest fundal pressure by assistant. The surgeon will always avoid flexing of the wrist and lower margin of the uterine wound is used as fulcrum **(Figs. 34 to 37)**. This step will prevent the extension of angles laterally and below to vagina that might cause injury to uterine artery and hematoma formation. Head is delivered over the plam gently any cord round the neck is searched for and, if so, it is slipped overhead.

Routine suction of baby is not recommended now **(Fig. 38)**. The shoulders are delivered using gentle traction and fundal pressure. The rest part of the baby is delivered slowly. Baby is shifted to mother's chest (skin-to-skin contact). Skin-to-skin contact between newborn and mother is also recommended by ACOG (2020). Umbilical cord is cut in-between clamps and now delayed cord clamping is recommended.

Administration of Oxytocics

Immediately after the delivery of the baby, oxytocin infusion is started by adding 20 units in 1 liter of crystalloid at a rate of 10 mL per minute. Bolus IV injection of oxytocin (10 units) can be given, but avoided for fear of hypotension. The dose can be altered as per need. Dose is tapered when uterus becomes well contracted. Alternatively, carbetocin, a synthetic oxytocin analog, 100 µg in IV bolus single dose over 1 minute or IM is used. Carbetocin has a property quick onset action of oxytocin and long-acting effect of ergometrine. It is suitable but expensive. However, oxytocin is recommended as first-line drug by WHO (2018) and International Federation of Gynecology and Obstetrics (FIGO) (2022) in active management of the third stage of labour (AMTSL). In addition, injection tranexamic acid 1 g IV slowly is given. Administration of tranexamic acid 10–20 minutes before skin

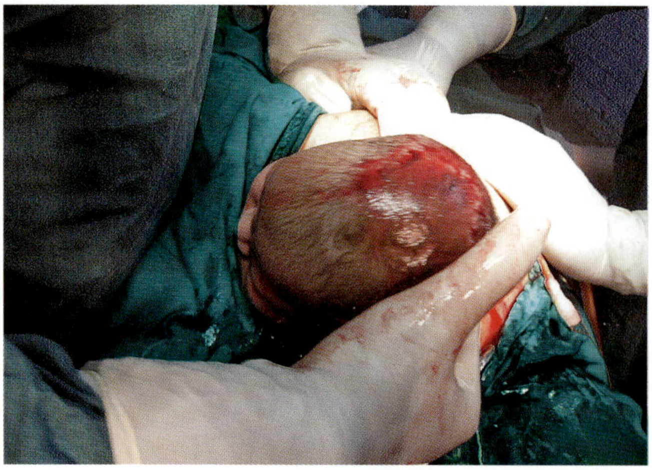

Fig. 36: Head is delivered over the palm gently.

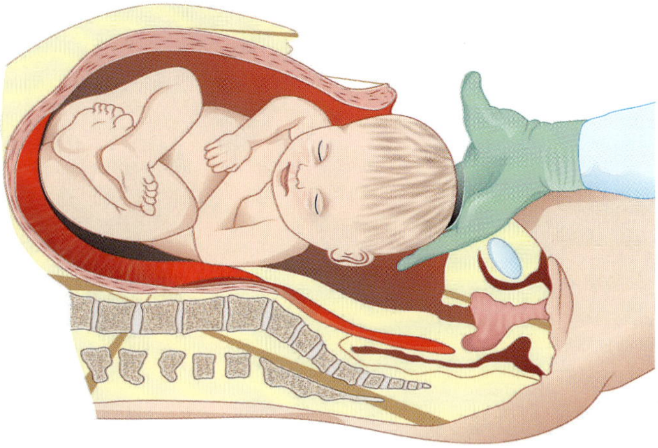

Fig. 37: Head is delivered over the palm gently.

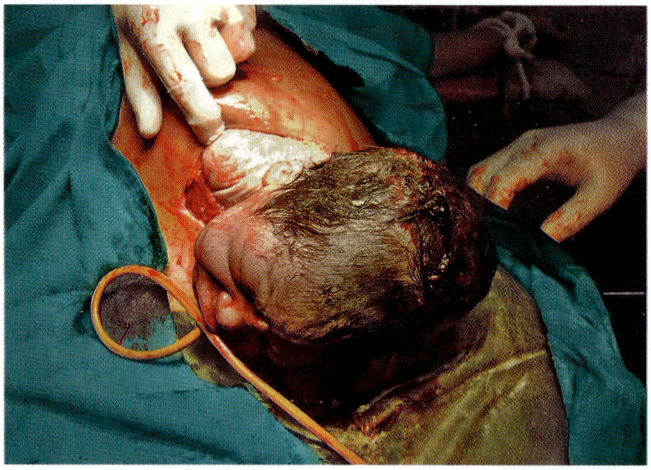

Fig. 38: After the delivery of the head mouth cavity is sucked. Routines sucking is not encouraged now if the baby is not compromised.

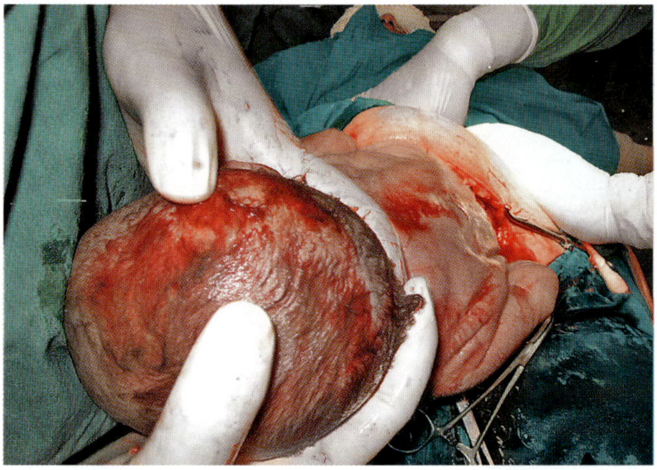

Fig. 39: Trunk of the baby is delivered gradually.

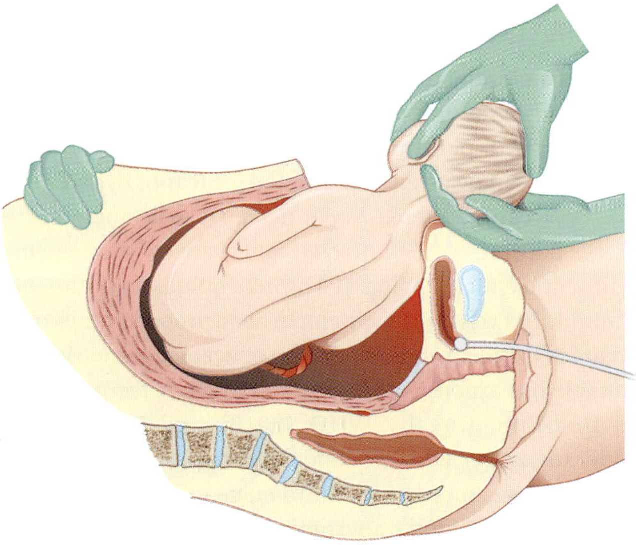

Fig. 40: Anterior shoulder is delivered.

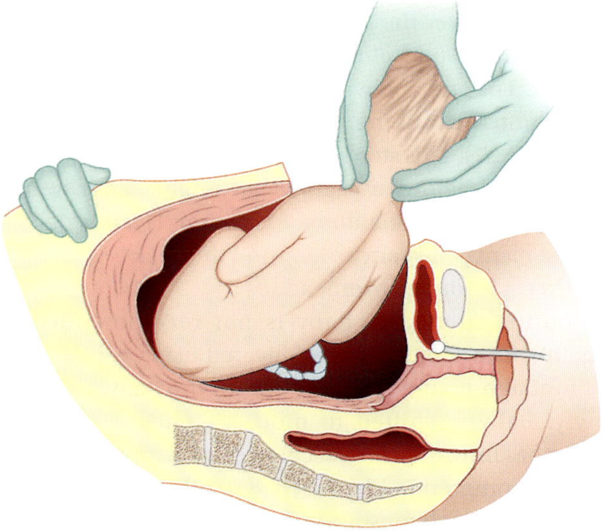

Fig. 41: Posterior shoulder is delivered.

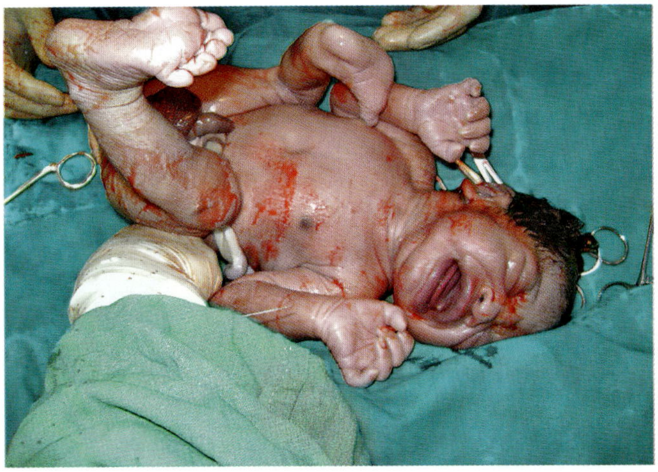

Fig. 42: Baby after complete birth and delayed cord clamping done.

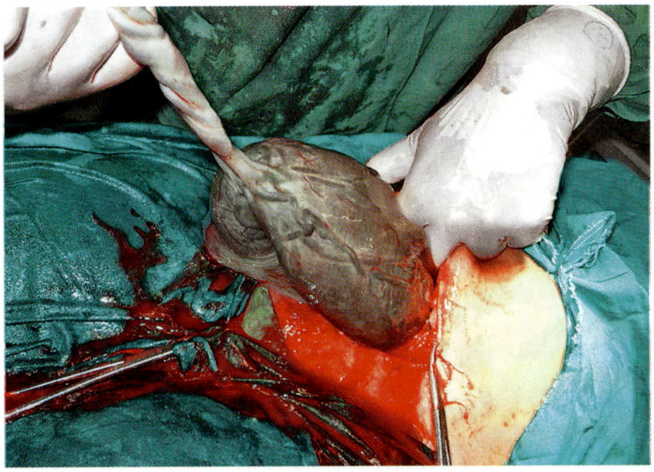

Fig. 43: The placenta and membranes are delivered by controlled cord traction.

incision reduces the risk of postpartum hemorrhage (PPH). Other oxytocics used for PPH prevention are misoprostol, methyl ergometrine, combination of methyl ergometrine, and oxytocin. Each has advantages and disadvantages. Trunk is delivered gradually **(Fig. 39)**. Anterior **(Fig. 40)** and posterior **(Fig. 41)** shoulders are delivered. Following delivery of baby **(Fig. 42)** delayed cord clamping is done.

Removal of Placenta and Membranes

Placenta and membranes are removed through traction of the cord gently by the right hand while pushing the uterus toward umbilicus with the left hand (controlled cord traction as recommended by WHO) **(Figs. 43 and 44)**. Routine manual removal of placenta is discarded as it is associated with risk of infection and more blood loss. Examination of placenta and membranes is done for any missing bits. Uterine cavity is inspected and is either suctioned or wiped out with a gauze pack to remove any left out small bit of placenta, membranes, vernix, clots, and any debris. Any membranes are removed by sponge-holding forceps. Wiping the cavity with laparotomy sponge (mop) is also practiced. Previous practice of dilatation of closed cervix by double-gloved fingers or artery forceps through the CS wound is discouraged.

The margins on the uterine wound are held by Allis tissue forceps or Green Armytage forceps. Four forceps are required, two for two angles, one for upper flap, and the other one for lower flap **(Figs. 45 and 46)**. Postpartum intrauterine contraceptive device (PPIUCD), if planned, is inserted before closure.

Repair of Uterine Wounds

Uterine wound is repaired in the following layers, presently one or two layers.

First layer includes deeper muscles of uterus excluding decidua with running-lock suture stitches using 0 or number 1 chromic catgut or polyglactin 910 (Vicryl) suture with round body needle starting from one angle to the end of another angle **(Figs. 47 and 48)**. The sutures at the both extreme sides should be placed just beyond the angles. No difference of adverse pregnancy outcome in terms of uterine rupture is found on suture type by CORONIS Collaborative 2016 group study.

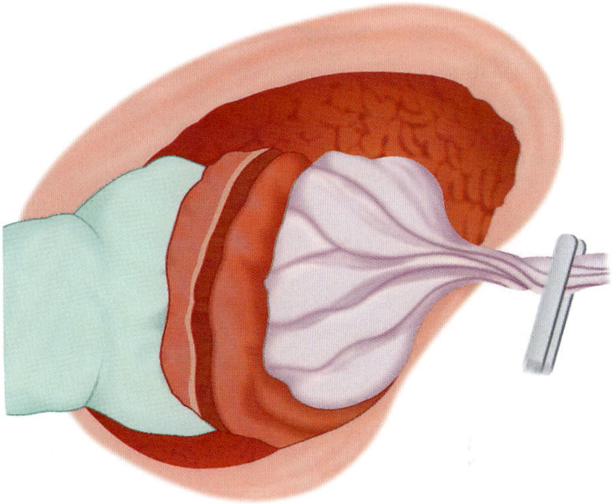

Fig. 44: Placenta and membranes are delivered.

Second layer **(Fig. 49)** includes superficial muscles and fascia with continuous stitches using same suture material as first layer, and inverting the first layer. Third layer *of visceral peritoneum*, which was given previously, is now omitted **(Fig. 50)**. Omission of repair of visceral peritoneum results in no postoperative complications as suggested by multiple randomized trials.

Closure of uterine wound by *single layer* instead of two (first and second layers) is of no difference so far as short-term outcome is concerned. However, second layer is given as a means to secure hemostasis and to improve integrity

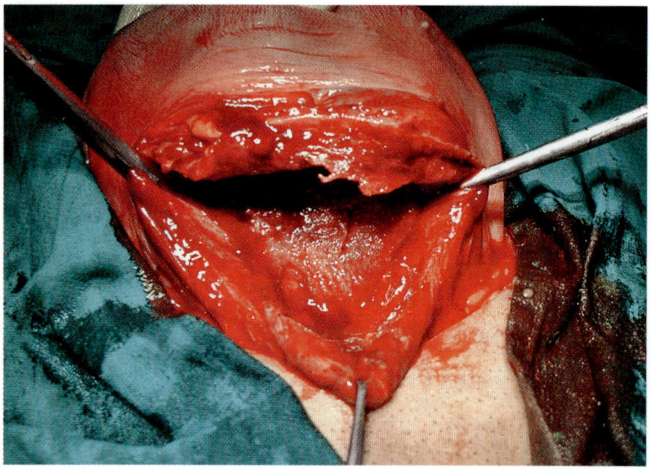

Fig. 45: Upper and lower margins and two angles of the uterine wound are visible.

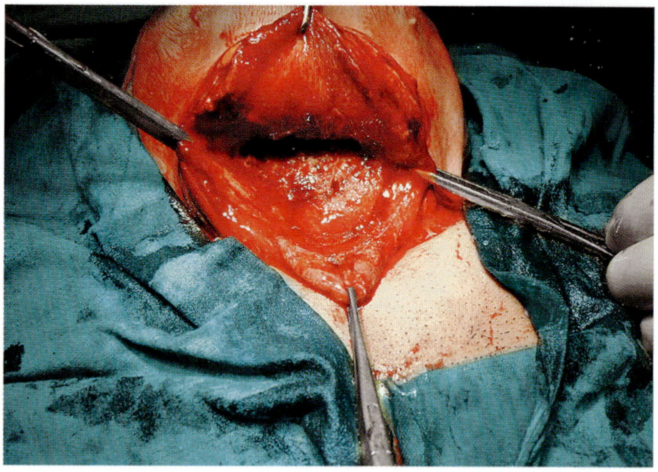

Fig. 46: The margins on the uterine wound are held by four Allis tissue forceps or Green Armytage forceps, two for two angles, one for upper flap, and the other one for lower flap.

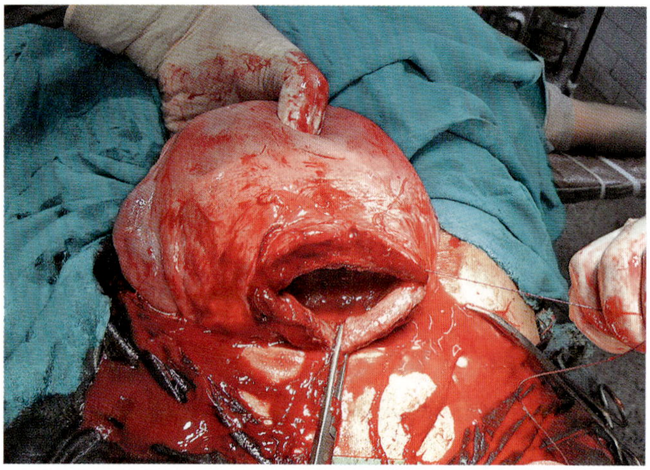

Fig. 47: Uterine wound is repaired by starting from one angle.

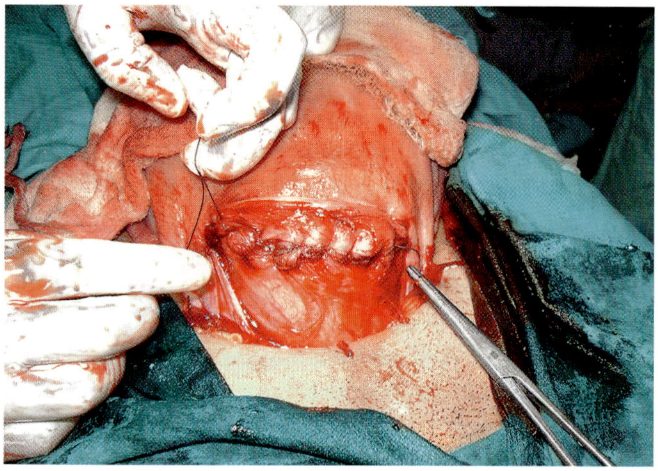

Fig. 48: Repair of first layer is done with continuous interlocking suture using 0 or number 1 chromic catgut or polyglactin 910 (Vicryl) suture with round body needle starting from one angle to the end of another angle.

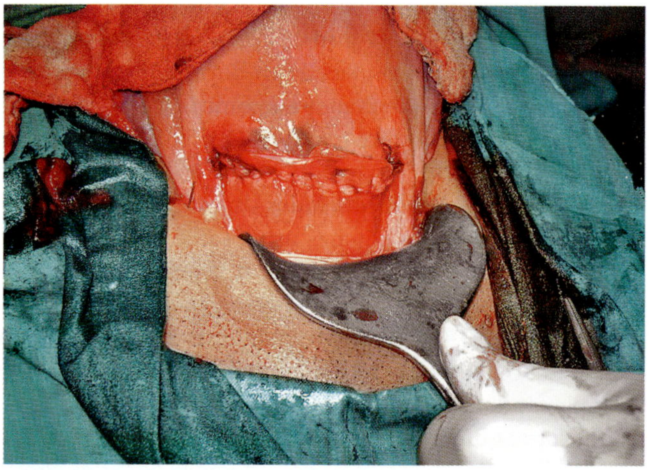

Fig. 49: Second layer includes superficial muscles and fascia with continuous stitches using same suture material as first layer, and inverting the first layer. Third layer *of visceral peritoneum*, which was given previously, is now omitted.

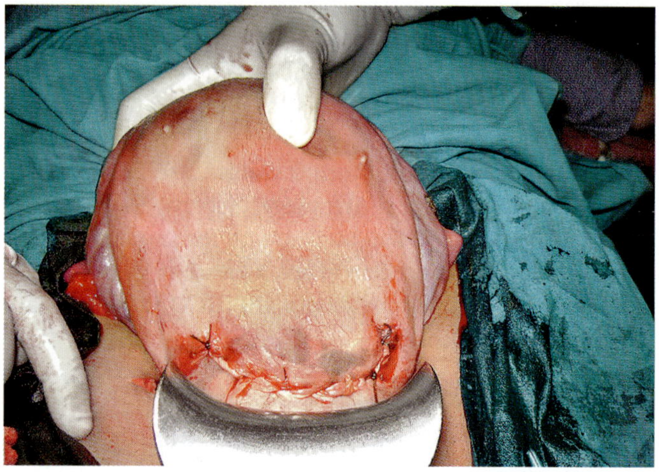

Fig. 50: Third layer of visceral peritoneum has been shown here, but now it is omitted.

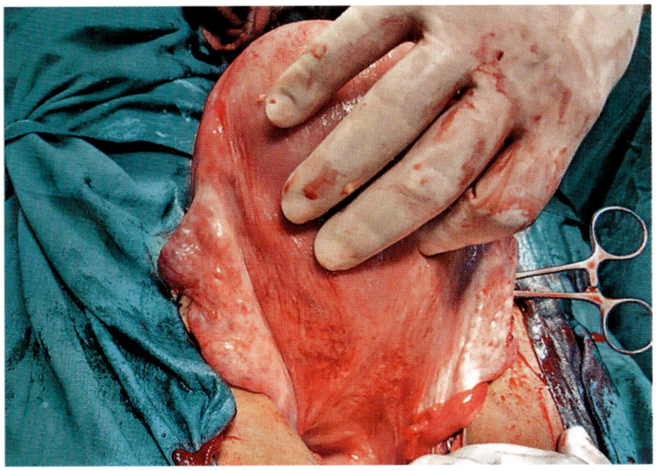

Fig. 51: Posterior wall of uterus including broad ligament and uterine wound are inspected to be sure about complete hemostasis or to exclude any hematoma formation.

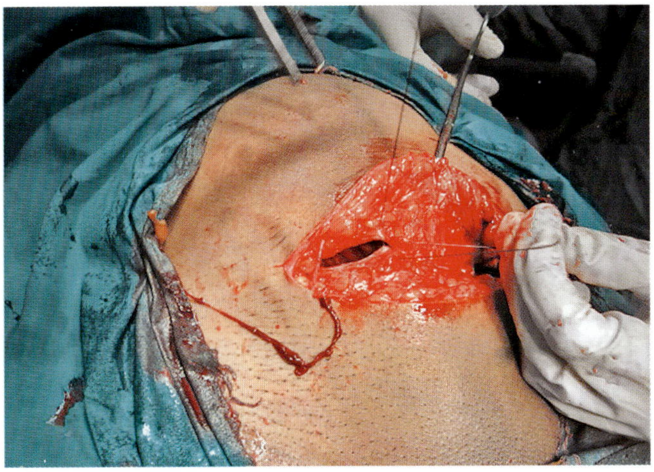

Fig. 52: Rectus sheath is repaired with delayed absorbable continuous and nonlocking suture.

of scar and reasonable to apply in those planning future pregnancies (see below).

Exteriorization of uterus: Many surgeons prefer to repair the uterine wound after eventrating (exteriorization) the uterus. In that case, reintroduction of Doyen's retractor is not needed at this time. Doyen's retractors and packs are removed.

Peritoneal cavity is cleaned suctioning blood and amniotic fluid. Routine irrigation is not done. Posterior wall of uterus including broad ligament and uterine wound is inspected to be sure about complete hemostasis or to exclude any hematoma formation **(Fig. 51)**. Permanent sterilization in the form of tubal ligation, if preplanned, is performed. Counting of instruments, needles, and packs is done.

Closure of Abdomen

The layers are peritoneum, rectus muscle, rectus sheath, and skin. Peritoneum closure is not recommended due to lack of benefit by the recent studies. Rectus muscles may be apposed with one or two figure of eight sutures with 0 or number 1 catgut stitches but not mandatory. Rectus sheath is repaired **(Fig. 52)** with delayed absorbable continuous and non-locking suture. If subcutaneous tissue is >2 cm, it is closed separately with continuous or interrupted stitches with plain catgut or delayed absorbable suture. Skin is sutured with continuous subcuticular stitch using 3-0 or 4-0 delayed absorbable suture or interrupted nonabsorbable suture **(Fig. 53)**, which needs removal on 5th or 6th day. Alternatively, skin can be closed by glue or with staples. Staples are associated with more skin separation. There is no evidence of good result with negative pressure wound dressing in obese women.

Vagina is cleaned and swabbed, and examined whether there is undue bleeding per vagina.

The average blood loss in LSCS is about 500–1,000 mL in otherwise uncomplicated cases. It should not exceed 1,000 mL.

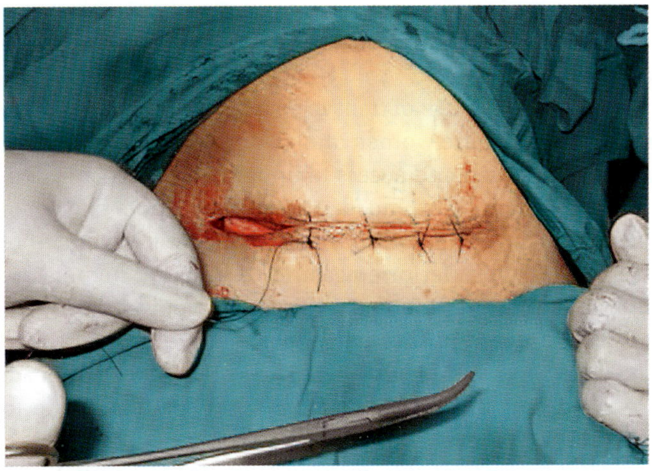

Fig. 53: Skin is sutured with interrupted nonabsorbable suture which needs removal or with continuous subcuticular stitch using 3-0 or 4-0 delayed absorbable suture.

Instrument, Needle and Sponge Count in Cesarean Delivery or Any Open Cavity Operation

Count should be taken for four times—first during the unpacking and set up of instruments and sponges, second before starting of the surgical procedure, third when closure begins, and final count is done during final skin closure.

VARIATION IN TECHNICAL ASPECTS OF CESAREAN DELIVERY AND CURRENT RECOMMENDATION

Types of Skin Incision

A transverse incision is preferred where it is feasible for its advantages. However, emergency entry is quicker in vertical incision during primary and repeat CD **(Fig. 54)**. With high infection risk, patient's midline incision is favored as in transverse incision chance of collection of

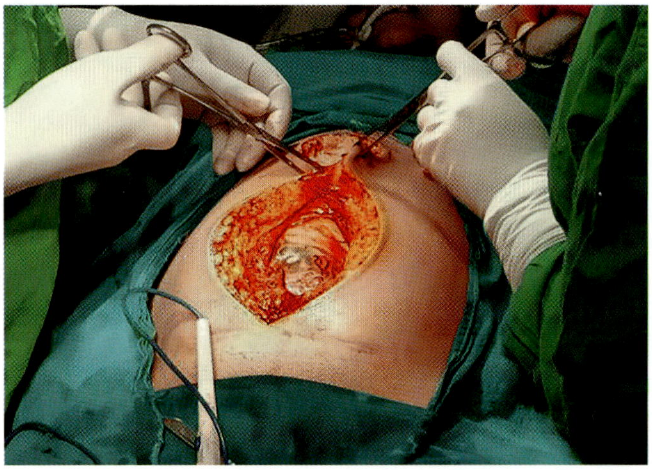

Fig. 54: Midline vertical skin incision.

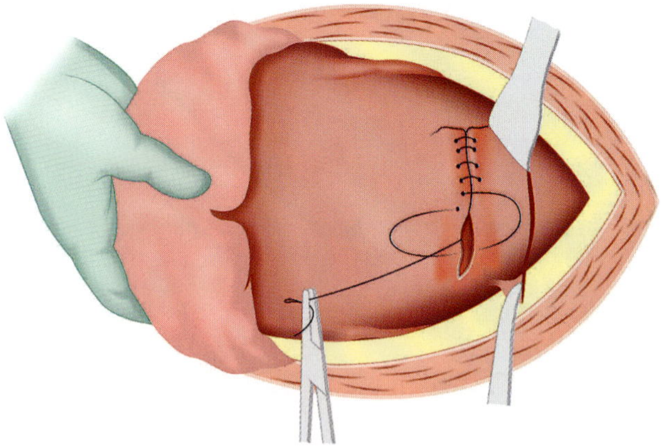

Fig. 55: Uterine wounds are repaired with continuous interlock stitches (single layer) is not recommended.

purulent fluid is more in layers of parietes. The advantages of transverse incision of skin are cosmetic, chance of wound dehiscence is less, and probability of incisional hernia is also less.

The disadvantage of transverse incision is less exposure, especially in obese women and also where wide operating space is required and access to upper abdomen is needed. Incision cannot be extended. Anatomically, more chance of blood loss and hematoma formation due to involvement of superficial and inferior epigastric vessels and higher rate of neural injury of ilioinguinal and iliohypogastric nerves are encountered in transverse incision. More time is also needed. There is difficulty in delivery of nonengaged head. Repeat CD is more time consuming and difficult due to scarring in Pfannenstiel incision.

Midline vertical skin incision **(Fig. 54)** is about 12–15 cm length extended below up to 2–3 cm above the superior border of symphysis pubis. Subcutaneous layer is cut by scalpel or diathermy to expose the rectus sheath. Linea alba is opened starting first in upper part very gently by lifting to avoid injury to intra-abdominal structures. Rectus muscle and pyramidalis are separated in midline. Peritoneum is opened carefully similar to transverse incision.

Advantages and Disadvantages of Exteriorization of Uterus

Advantages: Relaxed, atonic uterus can be identified quickly and uterine massage can be given well. Incision and bleeding points are visualized well and repaired more easily. Adnexal exposure is good; hence, tubectomy is easier if it is needed.

Disadvantages are discomfort and vomiting. However, there are no increased febrile morbidity and no increased blood loss.

Current recommendation (NICE guideline): Intraperitoneal repair of the uterus should be undertaken in CD. Exteriorization of the uterus is not recommended because it is associated with more pain and does not improve operative outcomes such as hemorrhage and infection. The CORONIS Collaborative Group (2013) trial found no difference in terms of endometritis and transfusion on randomly assigned nearly 5,000 parturients.

Number of Layers of Uterine Incision to be Repaired

There has been much tendency recently repairing uterine wound in two layers, even in one layer without much adverse outcome. In a meta-analysis (2017), a single-layer closure **(Fig. 55)** showed thinner myometrium in comparison to repair by double layer on, but no difference in scar defect or rupture is proved. As per NICE guideline, the effectiveness and safety of single layer closure of the uterine incision are uncertain. Except within a research context, the uterine incision should be sutured with two layers. Neither the visceral nor the parietal peritoneum should be sutured at CS because this reduces operating time.

Joel–Cohen and Misgav–Ladach Method of Cesarean Delivery

In Misgav–Ladach Hospital at Jerusalem, several works have been done to standardize the technique of CD. The principal features include:

- Joel–Cohen's method of opening the abdomen
- Single-layer suturing of uterus
- Nonclosure of visceral and parietal layers of peritoneum. There is more blunt dissection than sharp.

In Joel–Cohen technique **(Fig. 56)**, a transverse straight 10-cm skin incision is given 3 cm below the line that joins the anterior superior iliac spines, slightly above the level of Pfannenstiel incision. Subcutaneous tissue layer is cut 2–3 cm wide in the midline by sharp dissection up to the

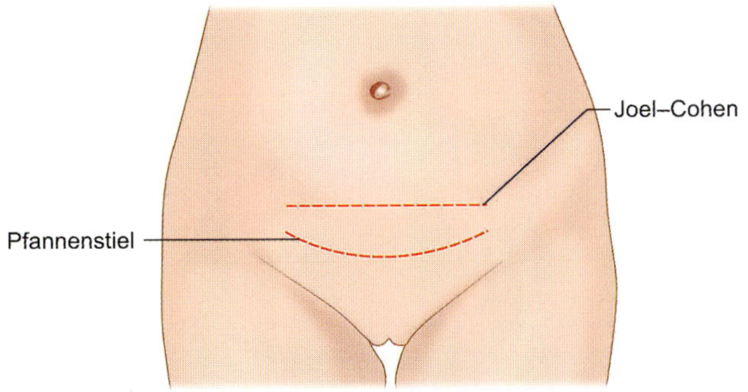

Fig. 56: Joel–Cohen incision and Pfannenstiel incision.

rectus fascia. Now, a small transverse incision is given in rectus fascia. A curved scissors is entered laterally to cut the rectus fascia beneath the subcutaneous fat, which is still intact. This is done on both sides.

On the lateral margins of rectus fascial incision, a finger is hooked on either side and stretched horizontally. As the rectus abdominis muscles are visible, the index finger of each hand one above and one below is inserted between the rectus abdominis bellies. Two index fingers are moved simultaneously one above and one below to separate the rectus abdominis further. Peritoneum is opened by sharp dissection and extended sharply above downwards. In Misgav-Ladach technique, dissection is done with the index fingers simultaneously in opposition direction to open the peritoneum bluntly. The layers of the abdomen are manually stretched laterally on both sides simultaneously to make the abdominal opening wide.

Uterovesical fold of peritoneum is incised and bladder is pushed below bluntly to expose the lower uterine segment. Uterine myometrium is incised transversely in midline to open and laterally extended with one finger both sides. Baby and placenta are delivered in similar way. Uterine wound is closed with interrupted sutures.

In Misgav-Ladach technique, uterine wound is repaired by continuous locking stitches in single layer.

Joel-Cohen incision is associated with shorter operating time, less blood loss, and reduced postoperative febrile morbidity.

Pfannenstiel incision **(Fig. 56)** is a low transverse "smile" like incision 3 cm above the symphysis pubis at the level of pubic hairline, slightly curved (12–15 cm in length) (*see* also Chapter 1). The Pfannenstiel incision and Joel-Cohen incisions are both acceptable choices.

Opening of Uterus: Blunt versus Sharp

When there is a well-formed lower uterine segment, blunt rather than sharp extension of the uterine incision should be used because it reduces blood loss and incidence of postpartum hemorrhage and the need for transfusion at CS are less.

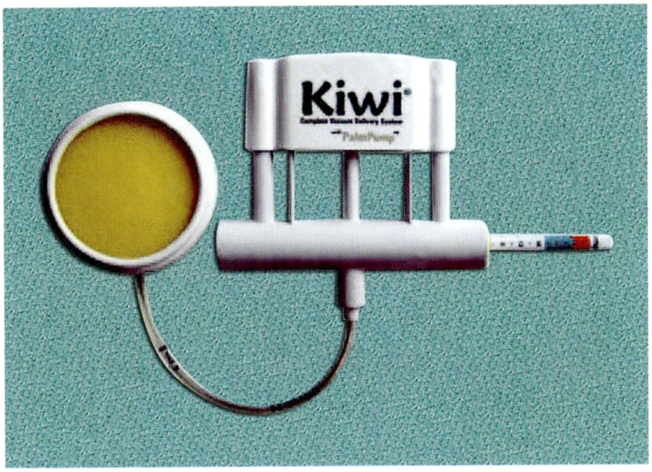

Fig. 57: Vacuum delivery system with palm pump.

CAESAR STUDY

CAESAR study report (2010) shows that there are no differences in any of the short-term morbidity outcomes between:

- Single- versus double-layer closure of the uterine incision
- Closure versus nonclosure of the pelvic peritoneum
- Liberal versus restricted use of a subrectus sheath drain although there is a difference in the duration of surgery in single- versus double-layer closure of the uterine incision. CAESAR study is the largest randomized trial of CS surgical techniques.

INDICATIONS OF FORCEPS APPLICATION DURING CESAREAN DELIVERY

- In floating head
- In case of deeply engaged head
- In aftercoming head of the breech

Recently, ventouse (*palm pump*) is also used to deliver fetal head **(Fig. 57)**. Application of forceps is done either by both blades or by single blade using as Vectis. Both blades **(Figs. 58 and 59)** are applied together as vaginal delivery (commonly). Classical forceps such as Simpson, Elliot, and Das's forceps are used. Wrigley is not a bad choice. Rarely, single blade can be used as Vectis.

TECHNIQUE OF CLASSICAL CESAREAN DELIVERY (UPPER UTERINE)

The vertical incision **(Fig. 60)** is given with a scalpel in upper segment of the uterus as low as possible depending on the availability of the lower uterine segment. If bladder dissection could not be done due to adhesions, fibroid or placenta percreta incision is given above the level of bladder. Incision is extended upward with scissors long enough to permit the delivery of the fetus (excessive hemorrhage occurs

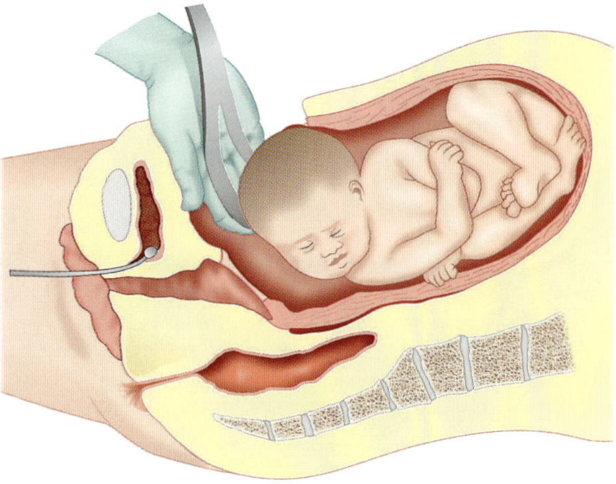

Fig. 58: Delivery of head by forceps in cesarean section (both blade).

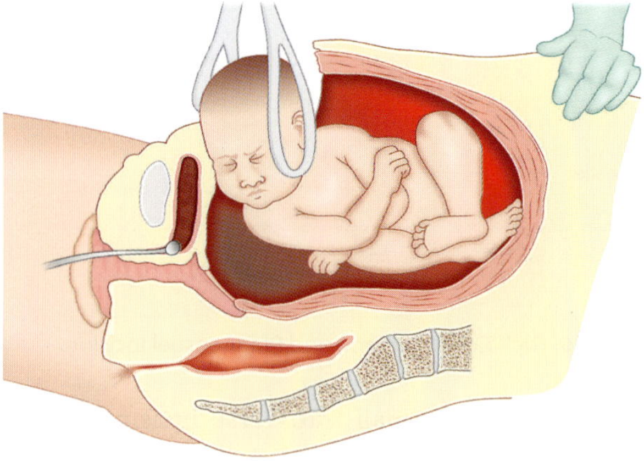

Fig. 59: Delivery of head by forceps in cesarean section (first blade).

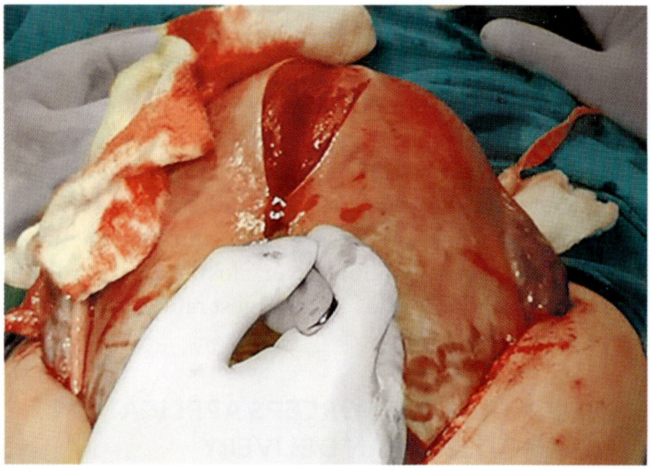

Fig. 60: Classical upper uterine segment incision.

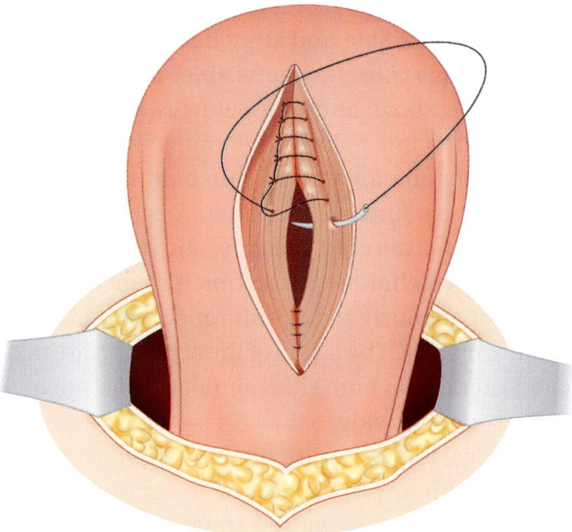

Fig. 61: Deeper part of myometrium are repaired with continuous interlocking suture by 1–0 chromic catgut in classical upper uterine segment cesarean.

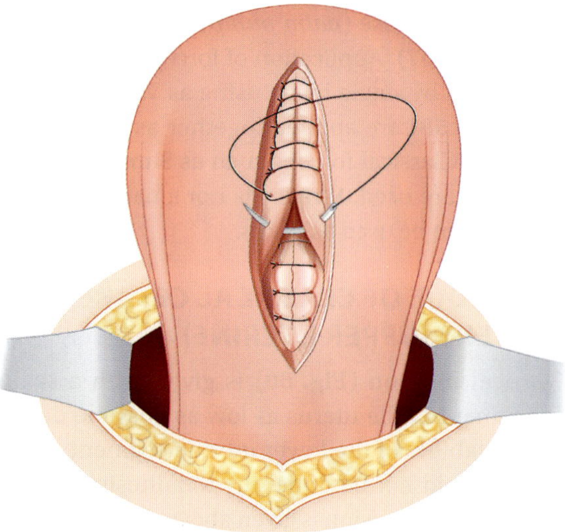

Fig. 62: The superficial part of myometrium is closed with similar suture with continuous interlocking suture in classical upper uterine segment cesarean.

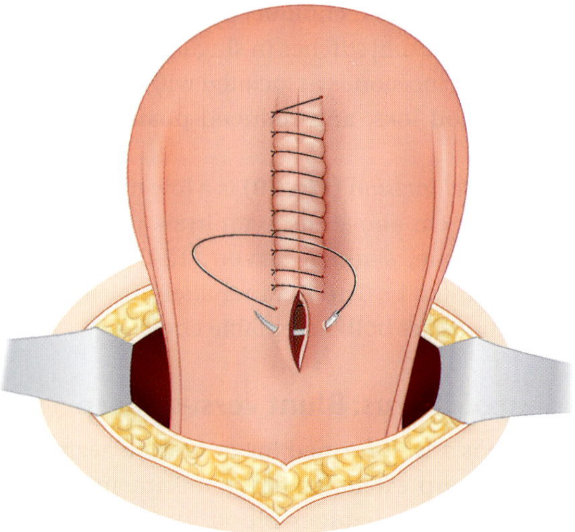

Fig. 63: The outer half is closed with continuous suture in classical upper uterine segment cesarean.

at this stage). Baby followed by placenta and membranes is delivered as quickly as possible. Repair of uterine wound is done quickly **(Figs. 61 to 63)**. Deeper half and superficial part of myometrium is repaired by continuous interlocking suture with 1-0 chromic catgut. The outer layer (serosal layer) is approximated with 2-0 chromic catgut with either continuous or figure-of-eight sutures. The assistant should compress the uterus from each side medially during tying the sutures.

POSTOPERATIVE CARE

Care of a Patient of Cesarean Delivery during Postoperative Period

- *Observation (at recovery area):* The patient is monitored in respect of consciousness, pulse, BP, vaginal bleeding, and contractility of uterus (by palpation) every half hour, even 15 minutes interval for 2 hours, then hourly at least for 6 hours (observed on a one-to-one basis).
- Patient is shifted to postpartum ward when vital signs are stable, vaginal bleeding minimal and urine output adequate. Clinical assessment of patient is done four hourly. It includes pulse, respiration, saturation, pallor, uterine tone, surgical site bleeding, vaginal bleeding, and urine output. In any case, if urine output becomes <30 mL/h, the cause must be evaluated. Pallor, tachycardia, hypotension, and oliguria are suspicious of internal hemorrhage in absence of revealed PPH. Hematocrit is estimated next morning or earlier if more than average blood loss or clinically indicated.
- Intravenous fluid with Ringer lactate and /or 5% dextrose normal saline (DNS) of amount 2–2.5 L is transfused in 24 hours. 10 units of oxytocin is mixed with one unit of 540 mL fluid,. Not more than 3 units containing oxytocin are not needed. Blood transfusion is usually not needed in uncomplicated patient. Input and output are recorded and balance is maintained.
- *Analgesics and sedatives:* Injection pethidine 100 mg IM is given and repeated as needed. Alternatively, morphine or neuraxial analgesia in intrathecal or epidural route can be continued for 24 hours. Nonsteroidal anti-inflammatory drugs should also be offered. Transversus abdominis plane (TAP) block or patient-controlled analgesia (PCA) are the recent options.
- *Bladder evacuation:* Continuous bladder drainage by Foley catheter is for accurate assessment of urine output and to remove after 6–12 hours. Immediate postoperative removal of catheter is recommended by ERAS Society (2019) but it is not consensus. Patient is encouraged to pass urine herself as early as possible.
- *Antibiotics:* Single dose of prophylactic broad-spectrum antibiotics as described above is given. Antibiotic is continued for 2–3 days in susceptible cases.
- *Breastfeeding:* Baby is put on breastfeeding in earliest possible time (usually within few hours). Early skin-to-skin contact between the woman and her baby should be encouraged.
- Oral fluid is started after 12 hours. However, recent strategy is to start liquids, even solid foods early in uncomplicated cases even within hours of surgery (Macones, 2019) in women who are recovering well after CS. Conventionally, IPS is observed and solid oral food is usually allowed from 2nd day.
- Laxative may be given on 3rd day, if patient does not pass stool by this time.
- *Ambulation:* Patient is allowed to go out of bed as early as possible. Risk of venous thromboembolism event (VTE) is decreased in early ambulation. Walking is encouraged early. Moving to toilet is promoted initially with the assistance, then walking without support as early as possible. Deep breathing and coughing are encouraged. An abdominal binder is not routinely prescribed, except in woman with lax abdomen.
- Abdominal stitches are removed on 5th or 6th day if nonabsorbable suture is used and then discharged. Patient is discharged earlier (within 3–4 days) if subcuticular nonabsorbable suture is given. Staples, if used, are removed on 4th postoperative day if wound looks healthy. Early ambulation and early discharge are encouraged nowadays by applying absorbable subcuticular stitches. However, before earlier discharge, woman and newborn are properly examined as postpartum eclampsia and neonatal jaundice may develop within 5–6 days.
- During discharge, mother is advised such as vaginal birth, e.g., nutrition, exercise, hygiene, breastfeeding, breast hygiene, routine iron therapy, and contraceptive.
- After 1st week, mother will start activity of caring of bay herself and own care. She will be aware of taking care of the cesarean scar wound and to report for any problem.
- Near half of the couple, resume normal sexual activity after 6 weeks. Average time to join normal office work is about 3 months.
- Follow-up postnatal check-up is mandatory within 6 weeks.

COMPLICATIONS

Peroperative Complications

- *Hemorrhage*—atonic (primary PPH) and traumatic tear of the uterine vessels
- *Injury*—bladder, ureter, intestine and omentum, and extension of uterine wound
- Difficulty in delivery of fetus and difficulty in delivery of placenta—in placenta accrete increta and percreta
- Aspiration pneumonitis; anesthetic complications.

Postoperative Complications

Immediate:
- Shock and hypotension
- Hemorrhage—PPH
- Rectus sheath hematoma (*see* Chapter 17)
- Broad ligament hematoma (*see* Chapter 21)
- Sepsis—peritonitis, pelvic infection, and genital tract infection
- Abdominal distention
- Intestinal obstruction
- Thromboembolic phenomenon—pulmonary embolism
- Problems related to skin wound—dehiscence, collection of blood, serous fluid and pus, and burst abdomen.

Delayed:
- Chronic pelvic pain
- Incisional hernia
- Intestinal obstruction
- Pelvic adhesions
- Increased chance of placenta previa in future pregnancies
- Subsequent pregnancy complications—uterine scar rupture, placenta previa, PAS, placental abruption, preterm birth, fetal growth restriction (FGR), stillbirth, and difficulty in CD due to intra-abdominal adhesion. Repeat cesarean birth in next pregnancy is another concern.

Fetal risk: Physical injury—scalp laceration, transient tachypnea, and fetal asphyxia due to delayed delivery

Maternal mortality in cesarean delivery: Average maternal mortality in developed country is 2–4/1 lakh. It is 10 times than that of vaginal birth; in developing country, it is 10–20 per one lakh CD.

Causes of maternal death in cesarean delivery are: (1) Hemorrhage, (2) infection, (3) anesthetic complications, and (4) pulmonary embolism.

Perinatal mortality in cesarean delivery: Perinatal mortality is 6–11%. The causes are asphyxia, septicemia, prematurity, low-birth weight baby, and respiratory distress syndrome (RDS).

For rectus sheath hematoma following cesarean delivery see Chapter 17.

Abdominal Distention in Postoperative Period following Cesarean Delivery: Causes and Stepwise Management

The important pathological causes are peritonitis, fluid electrolyte imbalance, unnoticed intestinal injury, intestinal obstruction, abdominopelvic hemorrhage (especially broad ligament hematoma), and foreign body.

Management: Management depends on the type of distention, progress of distention, and condition of the mother. Some form of paralytic ileus is common in all laparotomy cases. In CD, it is quiet less and normally passes off.

In soft distension, which persists after 2nd day, suction, IV saline infusion, sedation, and omission of oral fluid are done; usually, it is relieved on next day in most of the cases.

If the abdomen is rigid, IPS less or not audible and distension increases with nausea, vomiting, colicky pain, and no passage of flatus and feces—the above treatment is continued for few more days. Straight X ray abdomen is done to exclude bowel obstruction. Complete hemogram, blood picture, electrolytes, and vaginal swab for CS are sent. Antibiotics are changed accordingly. Fluid and electrolytes are maintained. Blood transfusion is given if indicated. Ultrasonography (USG) whole abdomen and computed tomography (CT) scan abdomen are helpful to reach diagnosis. Further management depends on the probable diagnosis.

Almost in every case, abdominal distention should not be left beyond 6 days and laparotomy should be considered. Earlier the laparotomy, better is the prognosis.

Ogilvie syndrome: It is one rare cause of postoperative abdominal distension. It is a dynamic colonic ileus causing pseudo-obstruction and is found in 1 in 1,500 pregnancies, mostly postpartum commonly after CD. It is manifested by huge distension of abdomen with involvement of cecum and right hemicolon and may cause perforation. Management consists of decompression by neostigmine (2 mg) infusion or colonoscopic decompression or laparotomy for perforation.

CESAREAN DELIVERY IN SPECIAL SITUATIONS

Cesarean Delivery in Placenta Previa

Practically, all cases of placenta previa are delivered by CD except a very few cases of low-lying placenta (minor degree) where vaginal delivery can be attempted.

Cesarean delivery in placenta previa is challenging due to various reasons—(1) health of the woman may be compromised due to hemorrhage, (2) incision on lower uterine segment in presence of placenta in lower uterine segment anteriorly and delivery of baby may cause severe hemorrhage endangering both mother and baby, (3) chance of placental bed hemorrhage in noncontractile lower uterine segment, and (4) possibility of morbid adhesion of placenta, especially in pregnancy with prior CD.

Indications, types of CD, uterine incision, difficulty during baby delivery, and tackling of placental bed hemorrhages during surgery and managing problems of placenta previa in a pregnancy with prior CS are discussed in Chapter 10 (Placental Disorder and Hemorrhages) and Chapter 11 (Placenta Accreta Spectrum).

Indications of CD and precautions to be taken in abruptio placentae are described in Chapter 10 (Placental Disorder and Hemorrhages).

Cesarean Delivery in Placenta Accreta Spectrum

As there is sharp increase in the incidence of PAS, every obstetrician must be acquainted with dealing such case. CS in PAS is highly challenging. In diagnosed cases, planned CS is done and usually followed by hysterectomy. Midline vertical skin incision is preferred. Uterine incision is given on fundal above the level of placenta. The details of steps are elaborated in the chapter of Chapter 11 (Placenta accreta spectrum).

Cesarean Delivery in Prolonged Second Stage

Both maternal and neonatal morbidity are increased in CD in second stage. There may be double the risk of intraoperative trauma in CS at full dilatation compared with CD during the first stage of labor. The increase of neonatal morbidity is probably more due to the prolongation of the labor, which leads to hypoxia than the procedure of delivery.

In prolonged second stage, if there are features of obstructed labor and head is high up, CS is safely performed.

When the head is engaged in prolonged second stage, the management is very crucial either by safe instrumental delivery or by CD. Instrumental vaginal birth should be considered for prolonged second stage if the "safety criteria" have been fulfilled. This is safe to carry out as a "trial" in theater with easy recourse to CD, if the attempt is unsuccessful.

Cesarean delivery in second stage, especially in deeply engaged head, is also a substantially riskier procedure associated with both maternal and neonatal complications. There is potential for injury to both mother and fetus. There may be tears in relation to the uterine incision, intraoperative bleeding, postpartum hemorrhage, blood transfusion, bladder trauma, postoperative sepsis, pyrexia, increase of length of hospital stay, and requirement for intensive care. To minimize the maternal and neonatal morbidity, several techniques have been developed undertaken during CD in deeply engaged head.

Tackling Deeply Engaged Head in Cesarean Delivery

- *Push technique*: Attempt is made to introduce the fingers below the presenting part and the fetal head is lifted. If not possible, the assistant is asked to push the fetal head per vaginally **(Fig. 64A and B)**.
- *Forceps delivery*: Single blade can be used as vectis or with the applications of double blade forceps, delivery is done through the uterine wound.
- *Pull technique*: Reverse breech extraction is done—first delivery of the podalic end is done followed by that of head. In this method, wound extension and uterine vessel injury become less.
- *Patwardhan's technique* **(*Fig. 65*)**: Delivery of one shoulder first, followed by delivery of other, so that back comes anterior (to make occipitoanterior) followed by delivery of trunk keeping the two hands of the surgeon behind the ventral aspect of fetus and the buttocks along with legs are delivered and finally the fetal head. Delivery of the inside hand technique is to insert your index and middle finger above the shoulder, bring the fingers in front of the chest, then laterally behind the ventral aspect of upper arm and by pushing outward to the lateral end of uterine wound the hand is delivered. After delivery of both hands, the trunk and lower limbs are delivered as described.
- *Fetal pillow* **(Fig. 66)**: Fetal pillow (FP) is a silicone balloon which is used vaginally for upward displacement of fetal head to make the delivery of head easier during

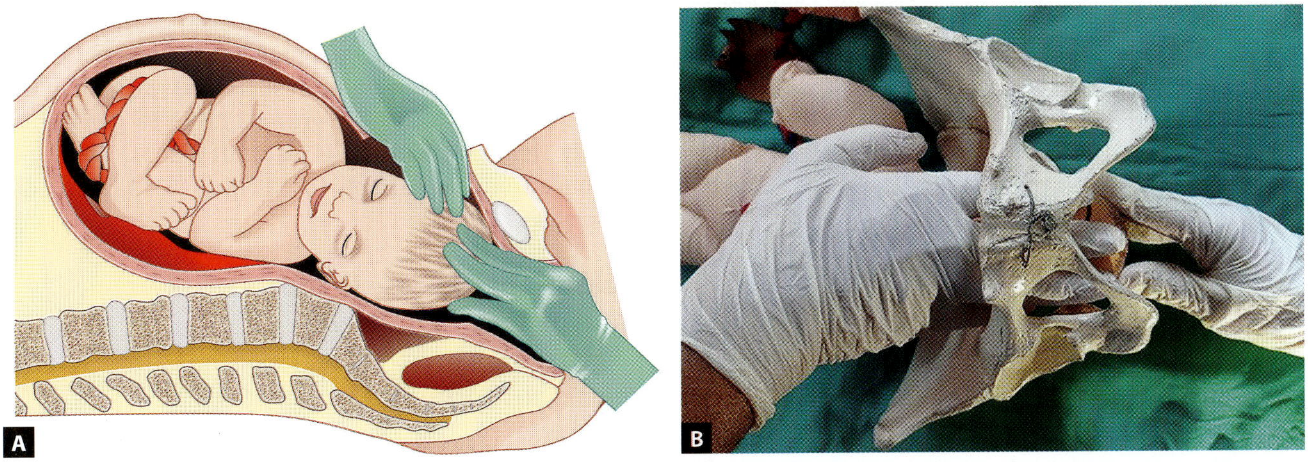

Fig. 64A and B: (A) Push technique to deliver the impacted head in cesarean section; (B) Push technique to deliver the impacted head in caesarean section with model.

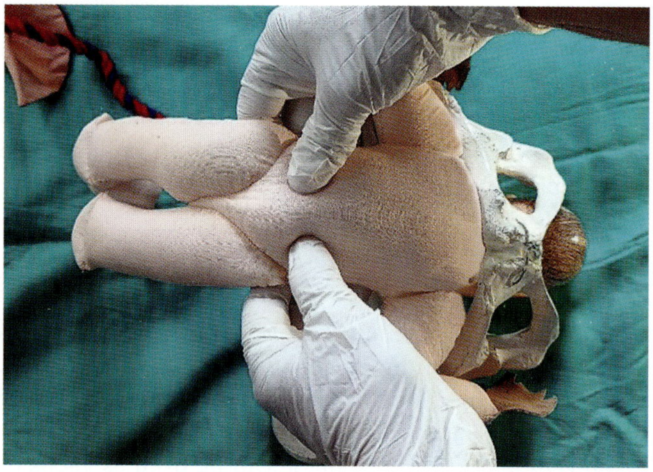

Fig. 65: Patwardhan's technique.

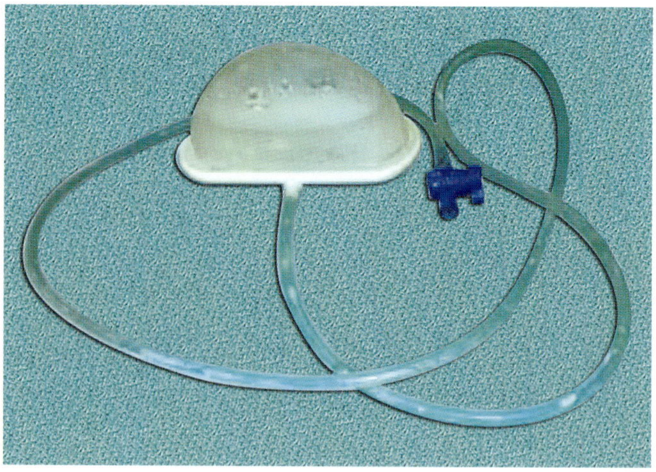

Fig. 66: Fetal pillow.

CD in deeply engaged head in second stage of labor. It is inserted vaginally prior to performing a CS at full dilation. After insertion, the balloon is inflated with 180 mL of sterile saline and produces a large bubble of fluid in the pelvic cavity and results in a 3–4 cm upward displacement of fetal head. Uterine incision is given slightly higher on a wider and thicker part of the lower segment and head is delivered easily with minimum manipulation. After the delivery, device is deflated by opening the two-way tap and is removed by gentle pulling at the tubing. It is claimed to reduce significant reduction in the maternal and perinatal morbidity compared to the conventional technique for head delivery particularly in cases of obstructed labor.

Tackling Floating Head during Cesarean Delivery

- Amniotic fluid is drained as much as possible and then delivery of head becomes easier.
- Forceps may be used to deliver the fetal head as described. Alternatively, ventouse device and Palm pam are used.
- Internal podalic version and breech extraction are done, but these should be done before allowing drainage of amniotic fluid.

Cesarean Delivery in Transverse Lie

Problem is that lower uterine segment is not thinned out and remains thick and small. Uterine wound is extended by "J"-shaped incision **(Fig. 67)**, a "U" incision or by inverted "T". In "J" incision, one corner of incision is extended upward and it becomes "U" incision if made bilateral. "J"-shaped incision is preferred to inverted "T". Intraoperative blood loss is more and chance of rupture increases in trial of labor in future pregnancies. Some prefers vertical incision in transverse lie.

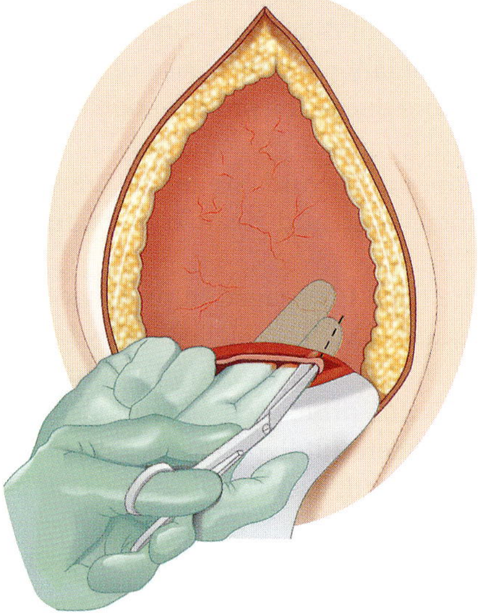

Fig. 67: "J"-shaped incision.

INCIDENCES

In England, it was 9% in 1980 and 21% in 2001. In USA, the rate was 32.9% in 2009. Paraguay has the highest CD rate (41.4%) and Israel has the lowest (15.4%). CD rate in India is 21.5% (urban 32.3% and rural 17.6%) as per National Family Health Survey (NFHS-5) (2019–2021) data. It has increased in comparison to NFHS-4 (2015–2016) data, which was 17.2%.

Reasons of Increase in the Rate of Cesarean Delivery

Injudicious decision of primary CD

- Due to increased number of pregnancies with prior CD
- Injudicious decision of induction of labor, which ultimately increases the CD in nulliparous

- Liberal CD due to malpresentation/malposition such as breech and occipitoposterior
- Decreased number of instrumental vaginal delivery such as forceps and ventouse
- Due to increase in the age of marriage and increase in the number of elderly primigravida—more CD.
- Identifications of high-risk women and elective CD
- Identification of the high-risk baby
- Wider use of electronic fetal monitoring is associated with an increased CD
- Small family norm and improved anesthesia—increase in CD rate
- Fear of litigation in fetal death/asphyxia
- Patient's demand for CD
- Fear of pain during birth in normal delivery
- Very safe procedure in many parts of the world
- Convenience to schedule the time of birth, suitable for family and healthcare provider
- Choosing the day and time of birth for cultural reason
- Perceived by many as less traumatic to baby
- Less pelvic floor damage with less stress urinary incontinence in CD as perceived by many.

Strategies to Reduce Cesarean Delivery Rate

- Decision of primary CD should be taken very judiciously and should be restricted to genuine indicated cases. Primary means first cesarean irrespective of previous vaginal births. >50% are primary CD and >50% of primary CD is due to nonprogress of labor and nonassuring CTG.
- Selected postcesarean pregnancy should be attempted for vaginal birth (VBAC). Rate of trial of labor after cesarean delivery (TOLAC) is low in many of the places; the success rate of vaginal birth after CD (VBAC) is high and may be as high as 80%.
- Judicious selection of cases for induction of labor—proper selection of cases will restrict pre-labor LUCS proved by many study and country (USA).
- Malpresentation such as breech should be managed through external cephalic version (ECV) or assistant vaginal breech delivery.
- Careful labor monitoring using partograph and active management of labor
- Decision of CD should not be based on CTG diagnosis of fetal distress alone, but should be confirmed by scalp blood pH.
- Decision of CD should always be taken by consultant obstetrician. This will reduce CD rate.
- Amnioinfusion, especially in advanced labor, though not universally recommended
- To encourage destructive operation in fetal death instead of doing CD
- Universal implementation of Robson's criteria as WHO guideline (2017).

Robson's Criteria

Rising rate of CD is now an important issue in obstetrics and a major public health concern globally. In last few decades, there has been dramatic increase of CD rate as high as 30% or even more to unprecedented levels in some places with parallel concern about its consequences. WHO considered CD rate to be limited within 15% in 1985. There are various reasons for increase of CD rate as above. There is consensus that CD rate to be checked and to be reduced. Michael Robson in 2001 had developed standard criteria and classification that would help healthcare facilities to optimize CD use. WHO (2015) proposed the use of the Robson classification system as a global standard for assessing, monitoring, and comparing CD rates both within healthcare facilities over time and between facilities.

Robson criteria are also called *Ten Group Classification System (TGCS)*.

This system classifies CD in ten categories based on six basic obstetric characteristics (variables), which help comparison of CD rates with minimum confounding factors.

The six basic obstetric characteristics are:

1. Parity (nulliparous, multiparous)
2. With or without previous CD
3. Onset of labor (spontaneous/induced or pre-labor CD)
4. Number of fetuses (singleton or multiple)
5. Gestational age (preterm: <37 weeks or term ≥37 weeks)
6. Presentation/lie of fetus (cephalic, breech presentation, or transverse lie).

Based on these six variables, *10 groups are classified* as follows:

1. *Group 1:* Nulliparous, singleton, cephalic, ≥37 weeks, spontaneous labor
2. *Group 2:* Nulliparous, singleton, cephalic, ≥37 weeks, either had labor induced or CD before labor
3. *Group 3*: Multiparous, singleton, cephalic, ≥37 weeks, without a previous uterine scar, spontaneous labor
4. *Group 4:* Multiparous, singleton, cephalic, ≥37 weeks, without a previous uterine scar, either had labor-induced or by CD before labor
5. *Group 5:* Multiparous, singleton, cephalic, ≥37 weeks with at least one previous uterine scar
6. *Group 6:* Nulliparous with single breech pregnancy
7. *Group 7:* Multiparous, single breech pregnancy
8. *Group 8:* Multiple pregnancies (twins or higher orders multiples) including women with previous uterine scar
9. *Group 9:* Singleton, transverse, or oblique lie including women with previous uterine scar
10. *Group 10:* Singleton, cephalic, <37 weeks.

Every pregnant woman admitted for delivery is classified in one of the ten groups based on the six basic obstetric characteristics.

The results can be compared between the hospitals, countries, and regions. With this system, the groups of women which contribute most and least to overall CD rates will be identified and analyzed, thus can help to formulate strategies to reduce the CD rate. It will also be able to assess the quality of care and of clinical management practices by analyzing outcomes by groups of women.

The criteria do not consider whether CD rate is high or low but it will assess whether it is appropriate or not, considering relevant information.

In some studies, using Robson criteria, highest contribution of CD is found to be the group 5 (previous CD, term, singleton, and cephalic) and for primary CD, groups 1 and 2 (induction and CD before labor) are the major contributors.

Appropriate selection of cases for primary CD and VBAC in repeat CD cases can reduce significant number of cases of CD. The Robson *"10 groups" system* is clinically relevant, simple, robust, and reproducible. This system is adopted recently in many countries such as UK, Scandinavia, and Canada. WHO (November 2017) has published guidelines for its use, implementation, and interpretation.

CONCLUSION

Cesarean delivery is the most common major surgery performed in obstetrics. Introduction of CD has revolutionized the fetomaternal outcome in modern obstetrics. Improved operative technique, safe anesthesia, and availability of antibiotics have made it safer. But, it is not out of danger; sometimes, complications may be serious in nature. Besides the immediate complications, the long-term morbidities associated with CD include repeat cesarean birth, and complications in next pregnancy such as rupture uterus and the risks of placental abnormalities such as placenta previa and PAS. Rising rate of CD is now an important issue in obstetrics and a major public health concern globally. Optimizing the rate and maximizing the safety are the future strategy.

CHAPTER

17

Rectus Sheath Hematoma Following Cesarean Delivery

Learning Objectives

- Anatomical Considerations
- Causes of Rectus Sheath Hematoma in Lower Uterine Cesarean Delivery
- Diagnosis
- Classification
- Differential Diagnosis
- Management
- Prevention
- Prognosis

INTRODUCTION

Rectus sheath hematoma (RSH) is a collection of blood beneath the rectus sheath from the blood vessels coursing through it or injury to the muscle itself. RSH following cesarean section (CS) is not infrequently encountered in clinical practice; it is mostly of mild variety. But late diagnosis may result in severe morbidity and even may be fatal in undetected cases of severe RSH; the overall mortality rate is reported to be 4%.

Rectus sheath hematoma is the most common of three causes of relaparotomy following CS; the other two are postpartum hemorrhage (PPH) and intraperitoneal hemorrhage.

ANATOMICAL CONSIDERATIONS

In rectus sheath, hematoma blood is collected beneath the rectus sheath from the injury of the blood vessels coursing through it **(Fig. 1)**. Knowledge of anatomy of anterior abdominal wall will help to prevent and manage this common morbid problem in obstetrics. Anatomy of anterior wall is described in Chapter 1, **(Figs. 46 to 48)**.

The anterior abdominal wall consists of skin, superficial fascia, deep fascia and then laterally external oblique, internal oblique, and transversus abdominis muscle and their aponeurosis medially to fuse rectus sheath, anterior rectus sheath, and posterior rectus sheath in between which lie rectus abdominis and below pyramidalis. In the lower abdomen below the arcuate line, there is no rectus sheath posteriorly and weak transversalis fascia and peritoneum support the rectus.

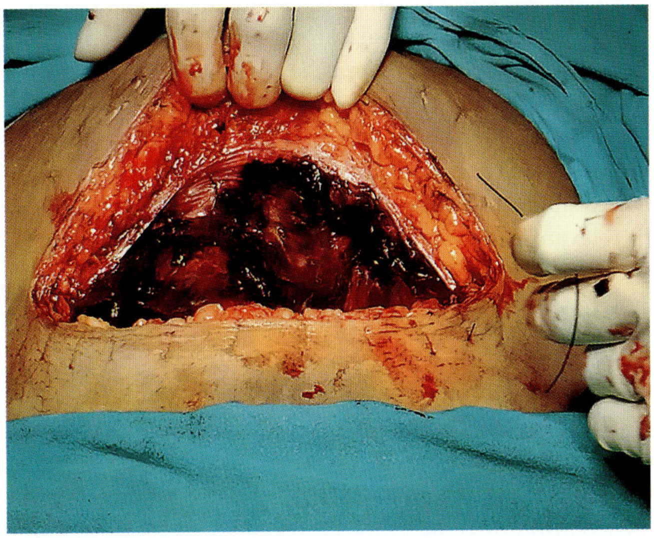

Fig. 1: Rectus sheath hematoma (RSH). A 28 years G2 P0 + 1 at 37 weeks' gestation undergone emergency lower uterine cesarean section (LUCS) due to severe preeclampsia (PE). She was on prophylactic magnesium sulfate ($MgSO_4$) and antihypertensive. RSH was diagnosed almost after 36 hours, when the patient developed severe pallor, tachycardia, hypotension, and oliguria. USG showed heterogeneous collection on the anterior wall. With simultaneous resuscitation, surgery was done, approximately 2–3 L of blood clot was removed within the rectus sheath (Fig. 3), no active bleeding point was noted, peritoneum was sutured, and drain was given. The patient received four units of packed red blood cells (PRBC), three units of fresh frozen plasma (FFP), and two units of platelets post-operatively. She recovered uneventfully.
Courtesy: Dr Sumon Poddar, Department of Gynecology and Obstetrics, RG Kar Medical College, Kolkata, West Bengal, India.

Vessels of concern in RSH are *superior epigastric artery, inferior epigastric artery* (IEA), and *perforator arteries*. Injury of *superior epigastric artery* (thoracic artery) which is a branch of the subclavian artery and which lies beneath the rectus muscle and in front of the posterior rectus sheath results in small hematoma and is not important from the obstetric point of view. *IEA*, a branch of the external iliac artery, which runs upward behind the rectus muscle is loosely supported by weak transversalis fascia and peritoneum as the rectus sheath is deficient below the arcuate line. This vessel commonly comes in the incision area of cesarean delivery and is more prone to be injured which may result in formation of large hematoma. *Perforator arteries* which have origin in bifurcations of the IEAs perforate the rectus abdominis muscle, traversing to the superficial tissues of the abdomen, and are most commonly injured while lifting the anterior rectus sheath from the rectus abdominis muscle. More details of anatomy of anterior abdominal wallare described in Chapter 1.

CAUSES OF RECTUS SHEATH HEMATOMA IN LOWER UTERINE CESAREAN DELIVERY

The important factors related to RSH following CS are inadequate hemostasis, needle laceration, slipped ligature, sawing effect of abdominal wall sutures, vigorous retraction, excessive separation of muscle, excessive undermining of muscles, and closure of abdomen in the hypotensive stage.

There are some nonsurgical causes of RSH such as acute paroxysmal coughing and asthmatic attacks which may not be relevant here.

DIAGNOSIS

Clinical

In the postoperative period, the patient develops more abdominal pain, abdominal swelling, orthostatic symptoms, and syncope.

Patient develops pallor, tachycardia, low BP, and oliguria. Tachycardia develops first followed by hypotension and diminished urinary output. Persistent tachycardia in the immediate postoperative period following cesarean delivery must be evaluated to detect early detection of RSH and intraperitoneal hemorrhage.

There may be tender abdominal mass which becomes prominent on leg-rising test. Tenderness remains the same or increases with head raising (*Carnett's sign*). Ecchymotic spots may be visible around stitch line or periumbilical areas (*Cullen's sign*).

On vaginal examination, no PPH is seen and the cervix may be drawn up and difficult to feel. In nonclosure of parietal peritoneum, blood goes directly into the peritoneal cavity resulting in hemoperitoneum and parietal swelling may not be so much evident in clinical examination and imaging.

Laboratory Tests

All the investigations which are done in a hemorrhagic patient are performed. These include complete blood count coagulation profile, liver function tests, and renal function tests. There may be low hemoglobin and altered coagulation profile and raised creatinine level.

Imaging

Ultrasonography shows homogeneous and sonolucent, but heterogeneous area in the presence of clot. Hemoperitoneum may be detected by imaging in nonclosure of parietal peritoneum as blood goes directly into the peritoneal cavity.

CT scan shows hyperdense mass and chronic hematoma may be iso/hypodense. The size, location, origin, extent, and nature of hematoma *are detected by CT scan*. The CT scan is reported to have a sensitivity and specificity reaching about 100%. RSH is classified on the basis of CT scan. The *role of MRI* is limited.

CLASSIFICATION

On the basis of CT scan, RSH may be classified into three types:

1. *Type I RSH*: Hematoma is small and confined within the rectus muscle and unilateral. There is no hemodynamic instability.
2. *Type II RSH*: Hematoma is also confined within the rectus muscle but can cross the midline and dissect the transversalis fascial plane. There is minimal or no hemodynamic instability.
3. *Type III RSH*: Hematoma is large, usually lies below the arcuate line, enters the prevesicular space of Retzius, and often presents with evidence of hemoperitoneum. It may require immediate surgical intervention.

DIFFERENTIAL DIAGNOSIS

Any other intra-abdominal bleeding from the uterine wound and broad ligament hematoma are the differential diagnoses. **Figure 2** shows bladder base hematoma following cesarean delivery.

MANAGEMENT

Resuscitation with IV fluid, packed red blood cell (PRBC) or other blood products, and antibiotics are administered according to severity. Aggressive therapies with intravenous fluid, PRBCs, or other blood products should be transfused when clinically indicated. The use of PRBC:fresh-frozen plasma:platelets in the ratio of 1:1:1 to 1:2:4 is reasonable to administer.

Surgical Management (Figs. 3 to 10)

- Surgical exploration is done in type III large hematomas, gradually increasing and in the case of presence of infection.
- It includes removal of stitches of skin and rectus sheath followed by inspection for bleeding vessels **(Fig. 3)**, evacuation of the hematoma, removal of blood clots **(Fig. 4)**, and irrigation with normal saline
- Any bleeding point is secured either by stitches **(Fig. 5)** or by using diathermy **(Fig. 6)**. Peritoneal cavity including uterine wound **(Fig. 7)** is explored. Rectus muscles are checked for complete hemostasis **(Fig. 8)**. Finally, repair of the rectus sheath **(Fig. 9)** and closure of the abdominal wall **(Fig. 10)** are done after putting one closed suction drain in the hematoma space and another in the peritoneal cavity.

Postoperative monitoring of vital parameters, urinary output, output through drain, and laboratory values is very important. The patient may need treatment in high dependency unit (HDU) or intensive therapy unit (ITU).

Alternative management includes transcatheter embolization with thrombin, gelfoam, or coil if available.

Conservative Management

Conservative management is indicated in small non-progressive hematomas (types I and II) where patients are stable hemodynamically and symptoms are mild and the

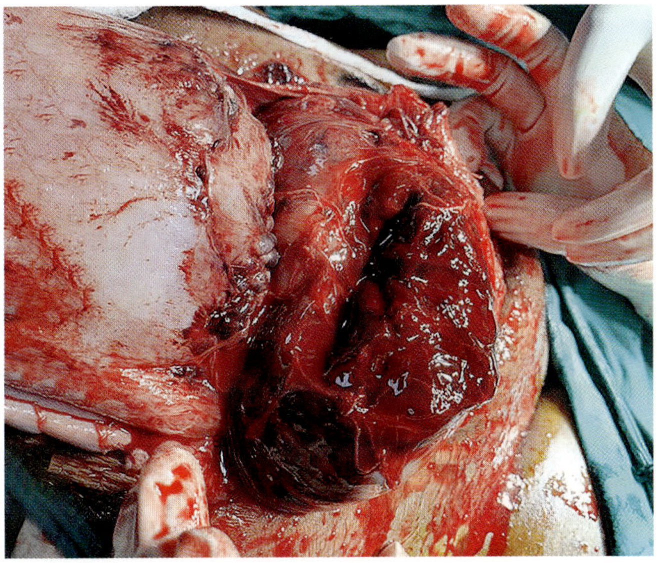

Fig. 2: Huge bladder base hematoma with broad ligament hematoma following lower uterine cesarean section (LUCS). Second para with prior cesarean section attended with shock 8 hours after cesarean section. Indication of cesarean section was prior cesarean section. She had a suprapubic mass separated from contracted uterus with the cervix drawn up. Immediate laparotomy was done with simultaneous resuscitation. There was large bladder base hematoma extending to broad ligament and retroperitoneal space on both sides. Obstetric hysterectomy with bilateral internal iliac ligation was contemplated. There was no injury on bladder wall.
Courtesy: Dr Shilpi Sharma and Dr Chiranjit Ghose, Department of Gynecology and Obstetrics, RG Kar Medical College, Kolkata, West Bengal, India.

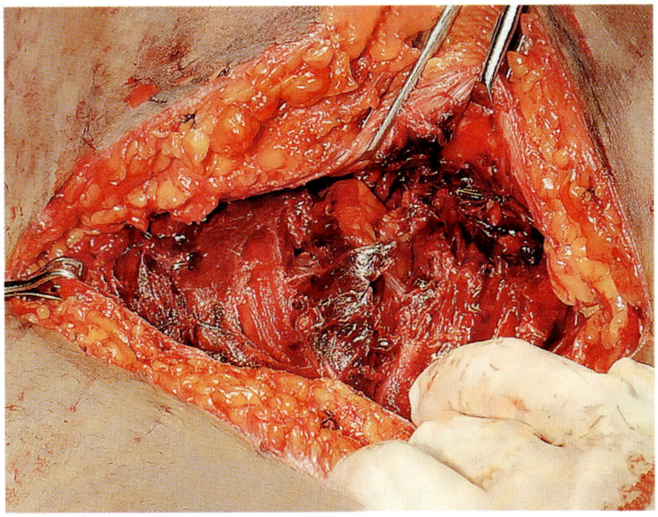

Fig. 3: Inspected for bleeding vessels.

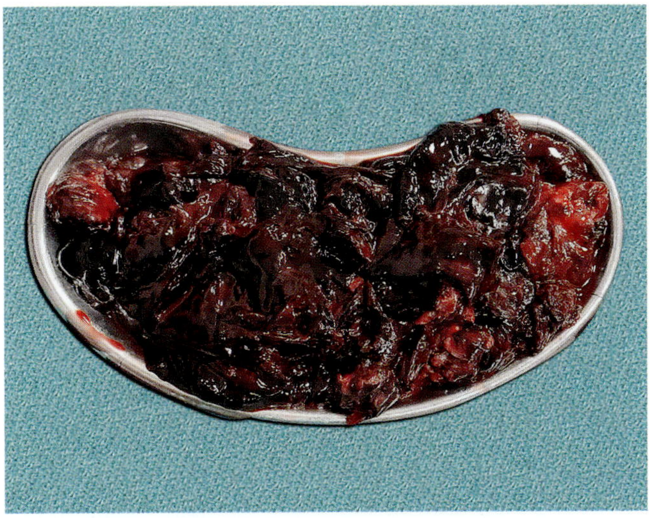

Fig. 4: Blood clots are removed as in the case in Figure 1.

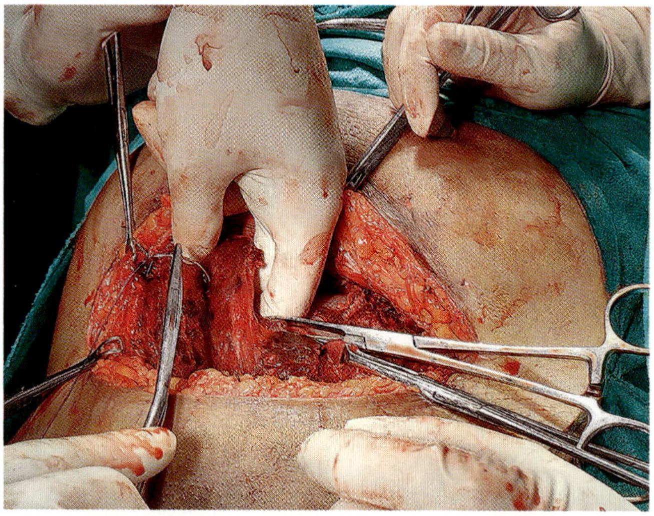

Fig. 5: Bleeding vessels are secured with stitches.

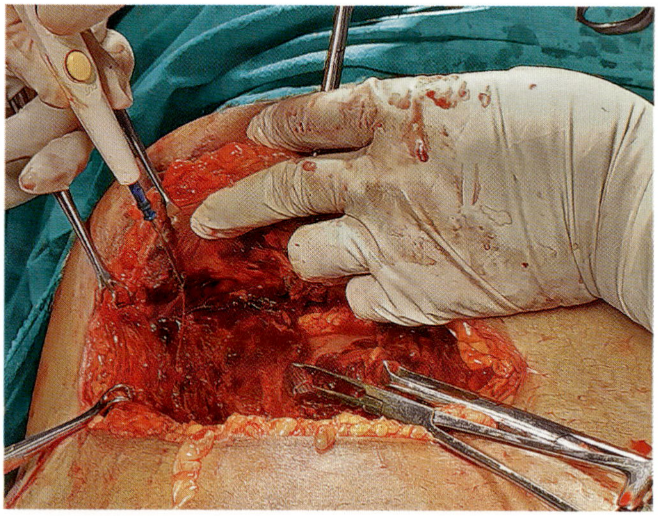

Fig. 6: Bleeding vessels are secured with diathermy.

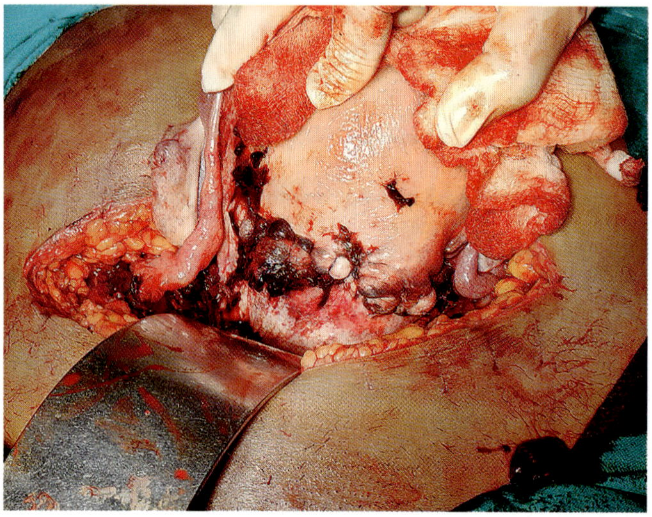

Fig. 7: Peritoneal cavity and uterine wound explored to search for any other source of bleeding.

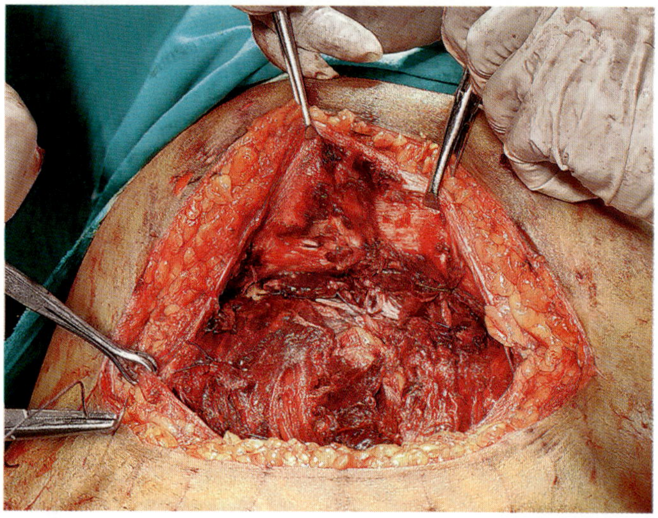

Fig. 8: Rectus muscles are checked for complete hemostasis.

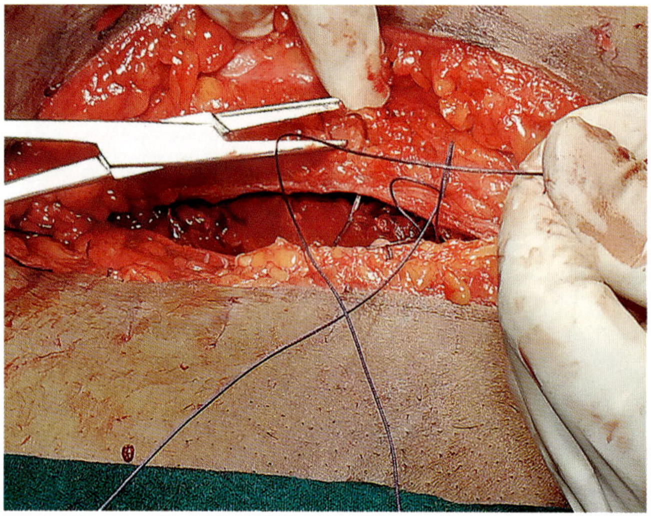

Fig. 9: Rectus sheath is repaired.

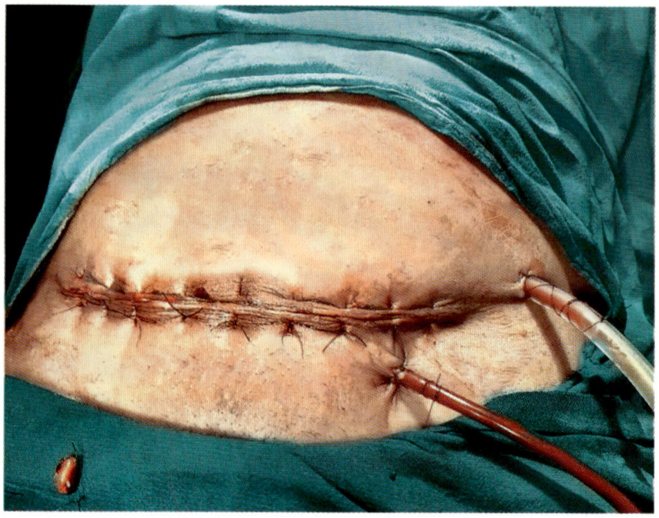

Fig. 10: Abdominal wall is closed after putting a closed suction drain in the hematoma space and another in peritoneal cavity.

diagnosis is certain. It consists of rest, analgesics, antibiotics, hematoma compression, and close monitoring.

PREVENTION

Separation of anterior rectus sheath should be done very cautiously and perforators should be secured properly. Direct injury to inferior epigastric vessels should be avoided. In nonclosure of parietal peritoneum, one must be very cautious to secure bleeding from margins. Before closing the abdomen, BP should be observed and hemostasis must be secured because bleeding points are often missed due to relative hypotension which is not uncommon in spinal anesthesia. Proper postoperative monitoring of the patient's vitals (BP, pulse, pallor, urine output) is essential to detect early detection of RSH. Anticoagulants in the postoperative period should be used judiciously.

PROGNOSIS

In early detection, prognosis is very good. Delayed diagnosis may result in severe morbidity and mortality. Mortality may be as high as 4%.

CONCLUSION

Any acute postoperative pain in the abdomen with fall in hematocrit, tachycardia, hypotension and oliguria and free fluid in abdomen must be suspicious of RSH. High index of suspicion, timely diagnosis, and prompt intervention can save the life, even in massive RSH.

CHAPTER

18

Operative Vaginal Delivery: Forceps, Ventouse, and Odon

Learning Objectives

- Obstetric Forceps
- Vacuum Extraction/Ventouse
- Odon
- Device

INTRODUCTION

Operative vaginal deliveries (OVDs) are performed by applying direct traction on the fetal skull with forceps or applying traction to the fetal scalp by means of a ventouse (vacuum extractor) to ease the vaginal delivery for the needs of mother and/or baby. For second stage operative delivery, critical balance is necessary between cesarean section and OVD. Over the past few decades, the rate of instrumental vaginal delivery has declined globally accounting increase of cesarean section rate in second stage which is of great concern. Training and practice of OVD are urgent to reduce the increased rate of cesarean section.

OBSTETRIC FORCEPS

History

The invention and evolution of forceps is a fascinating story which is rich in history. OVD has been described in Hindu medicine as far back as the 6th century BC. Instrumental delivery can be found in writings of Hippocrates between 500 BC and 500 AD. Intervention using surgical instruments for destructive operations even kitchen utensils would serve purely as an attempt to avoid maternal death. Forceps-assisted delivery to save both mother and baby was established by and developed over several centuries. It is said that obstetric forceps were invented by one of the Peter I and Peter II of Chamberlen family, probably by Peter I at the end of 15th century (around 1600 AD). Both the eldest and the youngest sons in Chamberlen family were named as Peter (Peter I and Peter II). This family was Huguenot refugee and came to England in 1569. This was kept secret in the Chamberlen family for 100 years or more. Peter I attended Anne of Denmark, Queen consort of James and other notable women of the society for confinements. Four generations of Chamberlen reigned in full swing with forceps till the death of Hugh Chamberlen the younger (junior) (Born 1664, died 1728).

Jean Palfyn is the first to publish forceps in 1720. He was anatomist and surgeon from city of Ghent. It was spoon-shaped instrument with wooden handle, two separate parallel handles bound together with tapes, not suitable for slipping overhead. Chapman first announced publicly the use of forceps by Chamberlen (1733).

In 1818, a number of Chamberlen's instruments were discovered in a well-concealed chest in Woodham Mortimer Hall, Essex. Obstetric forceps have been used near four and half centuries. Chamberlen forceps have been modified in several ways. Near 600 types of forceps model have been described.

The original Chamberlen forceps had only *cephalic curve*. It was André Levret from Paris who introduced the *pelvic curve* in 1747. William Smellie (1697–1763) of England also introduced a pelvic curve during the same time. Smellie simplified the lock and introduced an *English lock* (1752) and he was the first to recommend forceps in aftercoming head of breech. Handle curve with perineal curve was introduced by Aveling, James Hobson in 1868. Stéphane Tarnier (1828–1897), a French man, developed the *axis traction mechanism* in 1877. Bill from America developed axis traction to be fitted with the finger guard of many forceps. Later Alexander Russell Simpson, nephew of James Young Simpson (1880) and Robert Milne Murray, Edinburg (1891) designed simplified axis traction devices. Kielland from Norway introduced *rotational forceps* in 1916. Layman G Barton from New York developed another rotational forceps (Barton's forceps) in 1925 for Deep transverse arrest (DTA) where Kielland forceps are not useful. Edmund Brown Piper (1891–1935) from America developed (1929)

Piper forceps for suitable for delivery of aftercoming of head of breech with reverse pelvic curve and larger length. Much later (1967), long Piper forceps were modified by Leonard Laufer to make it shorter length and changing to pivot lock from English lock, suitable in cesarean section for delivering aftercoming head of breech. Sir Kedarnath Das from India (1923) devised lighter long forceps both with and without axis traction suitable for Indian women. American obstetrician Ralph Luikart modified blades (Luikart forceps) with *pseudofenestration* in 1937. Short forceps developed by Arthur Wrigley in 1935 (Wrigley's short forceps) is the modern version of Smellie's short forceps. Divergent outlet forceps were developed by Leonard Laufe (1968) to reduce fetal head compression. Héctor Salinas Benavides from Mexico designed a forceps *(Salinas forceps)* in 1965 with a property of excellent tractor and rotator. Two nonfenestrated parallel branches with a slight pelvic curvature join at the back by a frame with a system spring that dampens the traction force. Later, it was modified with straight branches. *VP Paily*, from Kerala, India, has developed few models of forceps especially for small baby.

History surrounding modification of forceps model and its use is very interesting. William Hunter (1718–1783), a fellow obstetrician of Smellie was appointed as physician to Queen Charlotte in 1762. Although, he was familiar but rarely used to apply forceps carrying with him a pair of rusty forceps to emphasize their infrequent use and to stress on natural birth. Thomas Denman (1733–1815) also developed forceps but imposed Denman conservatism (Hunterian-Denman legacy of conservatism) to control rampant use of forceps. Varieties of forceps with minimum trauma to baby and mother were developed by David Davis (1777–1841). In 1819, David Davis was appointed as obstetrician of Duchess of Kent following Charlotte's tragedy (1813, triple obstetric tragedy, see later).

In evolution and practice of forceps, many other stalwarts are involved and it is not possible to mention all about them. The name of James Young Simpson (1811–1870) is worth mentioning. He developed varieties of obstetric forceps including short forceps. His classical all-purpose model with fenestrated blade (Simpson forceps, 1848) is widely used and he is also known first to use chloroform anesthesia.

The popular solid blade forceps are Tucker-McLane. Many short forceps were devised in mid-19th century and thereafter, some of those are Oldham (1855) and Mattei (1853) short forceps. Neville-Barnes (1817–1907) forceps are well known in Britain.

Changes of Features of Forceps Over the Centuries

1. More than 600 varieties of forceps are described.
2. Alteration of materials, sizes, and shape
3. Structure of blade, disposition of branches, and lock
4. Introduction of pelvic curvature, perineal curvature, and handle curvature
5. Introduction of axis traction mechanism
6. Materials—wooden, ivory, leather, and metals
7. Change of carbon steel to stainless steel to make lighter and more strength
8. Disappearance of wooden and ivory for heat sterilization.

Landmark Changes of the Instruments

1. The original Chamberlen forceps had only cephalic curve.
2. Pelvic curvature was introduced by André Levret, 1747.
3. English lock was developed by William Smellie, 1752.
4. Perineal curve was introduced by RW Jhonson, 1769.
5. Handle curve was designed by Aveling, 1868.
6. Axis traction was first introduced by Tarnier, 1877.
7. Rotational forceps was developed by Kielland, 1916.

Varieties of Commonly used Forceps

- The obstetric forceps may be long, short, curved, and straight. It may be with axis traction, without axis traction, and rotational or nonrotational. There are some forceps with some special features.
- Long-curved obstetric forceps—examples are Das forceps, Simpson's forceps, and Elliot forceps (fenestrated blade), Luikart forceps (pseudofenestrated blade), and Tucker-McLane forceps (solid blade).
- Short-curved obstetric forceps—Wrigley's forceps, modified Simpson's short forceps
- Straight long obstetric forceps—Kielland forceps
- Rotational forceps—Kielland forceps, Burton forceps
- Axis traction mechanism—Tarnier, Das forceps, Milne Murray, and Bill axis traction device. The purpose of axis traction device is to pull along the axis of birth canal. A teaching model, Bill axis traction after fitting with the finger guard which is present in most of the forceps traction is given. It has an arrow and indicator line, if the arrow is found to point directly to the line pull, is likely to the least resistance along the axis of birth canal.
- Piper forceps—forceps for aftercoming head of breech.

Though, there are some common forceps, uses of type of forceps vary from country to country, preference is given to the instruments which are developed and available in the respective country.

Description of a Long-Curved Obstetric Forceps—Das Forceps (Fig. 1)

The basic features are like other all-purpose classical forceps, e.g., Simpson, Elliot, Bail-Williamson, Luikart, Tucker-Mclane, etc. with minor variations which are mentioned in description of respective forceps.

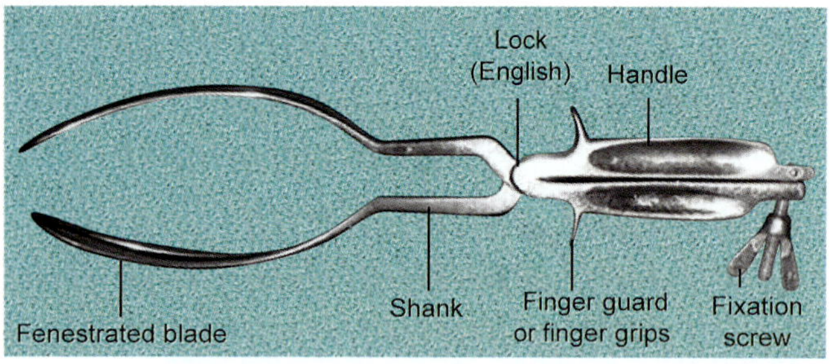

Fig. 1: *Das forceps:* Long curved, fenestrated blades, parallel shanks, and English lock with fixation screw.

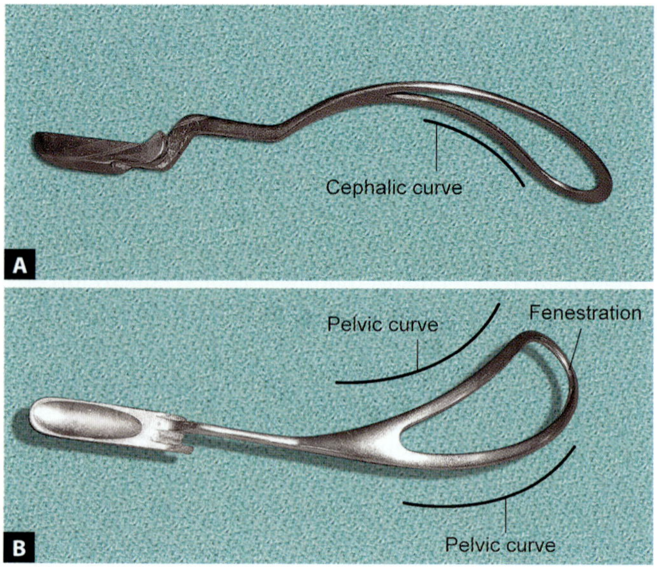

Figs. 2A and B: (A) Cephalic curve of short curve obstetric forceps (same as in long-curved obstetric forceps); (B) Pelvic curve of short-curved obstetric forceps (same as in long-curved obstetric forceps).

Das obstetric forceps consist of two halves, each half called a branch. Long-curved obstetric forceps is about 37 cm (15 inches) long (Das forceps). Each branch consists of (1) blade (fenestrated), (2) shank, (3) lock, (4) handle with finger guard or finger grip, (5) fixation screw (optional), and (6) axis traction device (optional). *Blade:* Each blade is named as right or left according to the relation to maternal pelvis, i.e., the side on which it is applied. Each blade has a toe, heal, and two curves (i) cephalic curve and (ii) pelvic curve. At the proximal part of the fenestration of the blades of long curved obstetric forceps, a slot may be present to accommodate the knob of axis traction rod.

Blades

Forceps blade may be (a) fenestrated (gap in the single blade)—Simpsons, Elliot, and Das; (b) pseudofenestrated—Luikart; and (c) solid—Tucker-McLane.

In solid blades both sides are smooth and a have disadvantage of slipping overhead, especially in molded head. Fenestration makes the instrument lighter and provides a good grip over the fetal head reducing head slipping and favors less compression. However, there may be forceps mark over face in this type even correctly applied, and friction of blade with the vaginal wall is disadvantage. Pseudofenestration has both advantages, outer smooth, not damaging vaginal wall and inner pseudofenestration for good grip of fetal head, chance of slipping is less. Application and removal are easier and safer than fenestrated blade.

Curve of Forceps (Figs. 2A and B)

Cephalic curve ***(Fig. 2A)****:* It is a curve on the flat surface which fits with the fetal head during application. The standard radius of curvature is 11.25 cm (41/2 inches). The distance between the tips is 2.5 cm (1 inch) and the widest gap in between the two articulated blades is 9 cm (33/8 inch) in Das forceps. The presence of gap in between the tips helps to avoid the grasping of neck and excess compression of head of the fetal head. The widest gap (9 cm) in between the blades provides a firm grip over the fetal head (biparietal diameter is 9.4 cm or 33/4 inches) without undue compression. All types of forceps have cephalic curve including Chamberlen forceps.

Pelvic curve ***(Fig. 2B)****:* This curve is on the edge of the blade to fit the curve of the sacrum (anatomical pelvic axis—curve of Carus). In pelvic application (see below), the pelvic curve is concave anteriorly and convex posteriorly. The presence of convexity is due to fitting with the concavity of the sacrum and the curve corresponds with the anatomical axis of pelvis. When the forceps are kept on horizontal surface keeping the tips upward pelvic curve is well observed. The radius of pelvic curve is 17.5 cm (7 inches). Pelvic curve was introduced by Levret from Paris in 1747.

Shank

It is a metal bar connecting the blade with the handle. It is usually 6.25 cm (2½ inches) of length in classical long forceps, may be altered. Shanks may be parallel (Das) or overlapping (Luikart, Tucker-Mclane). It gives the length of the instrument and so facilitates the locking and makes the traction easier. The shank is of minimal length in short obstetric forceps.

Lock

Lock is a part of forceps for articulation of two branches and, almost compulsory. Different types of locks are varieties of lock **(Fig. 3)**: (a) English lock **(Fig. 4)**, which consists of a socket system fitting each blade one another at the end of shank. This lock is most common. Smellie introduced the English lock (1752), (b) sliding lock—along the shank, (c) French lock—bolts or button at the joining of the shanks, (d) German lock—wing nut and screw at handle, and (e) pivot lock is present at the ends of the handles, as found in Laufe divergent forceps. Combination of French lock (button

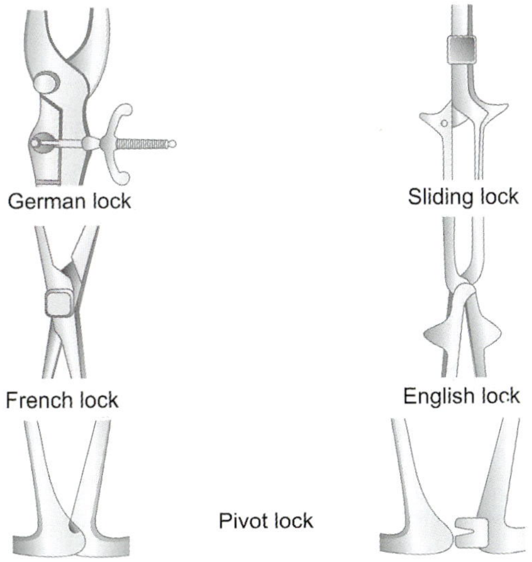

Fig. 3: Varieties of lock.

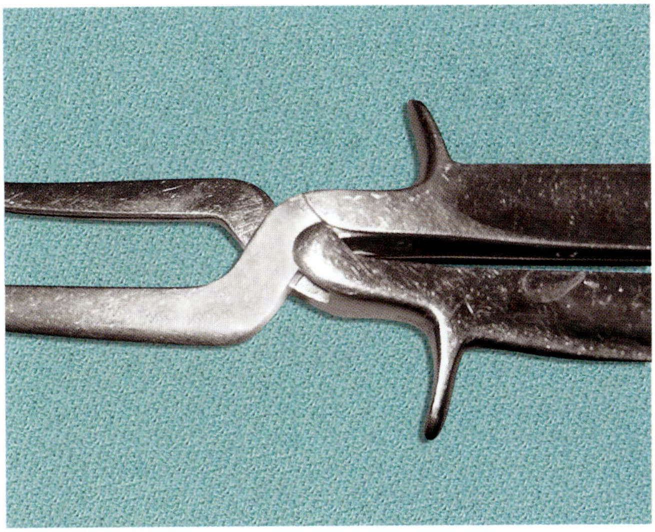

Fig. 4: English lock in long-curved obstetric forceps.

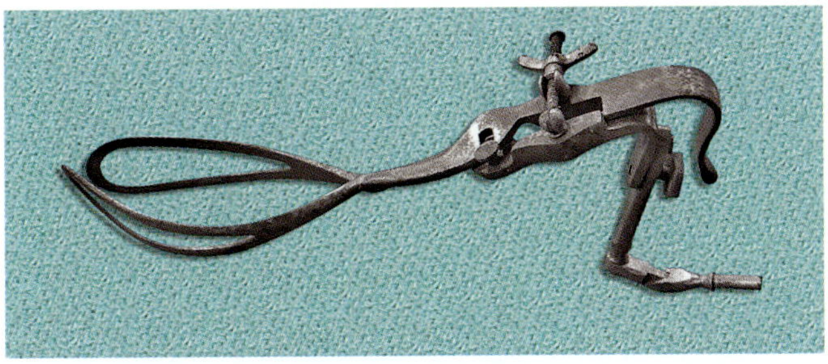

Fig. 5: Dewey's axis traction forceps (1900) with German lock.
Courtesy: RG Kar Medical College Forceps Gallery.

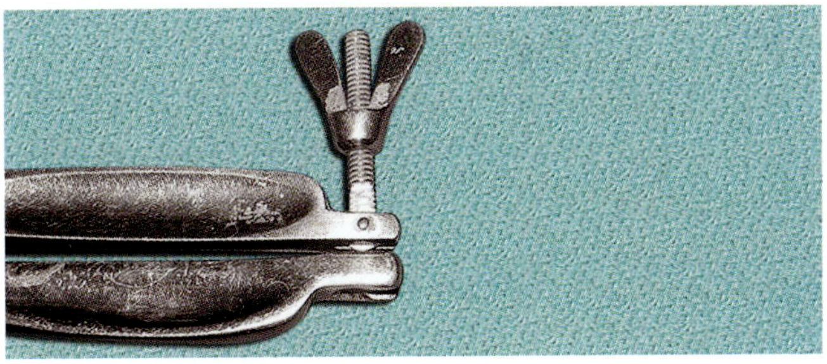

Fig. 6: Fixation screw attached with handle.

or bolt at joining of the shanks) and German lock (wing nut and screw at handles) are found in Dewey forceps **(Fig. 5)**.

Handle

The handle of each half is the most proximal part and made of long thick metal rods. The measurement of handle is 12.5 cm (5 inches). A finger guard or finger grip is usually present at the distal ends of the handle which helps in placing the fingers to give a pull or for fitting the Bill axis traction device.

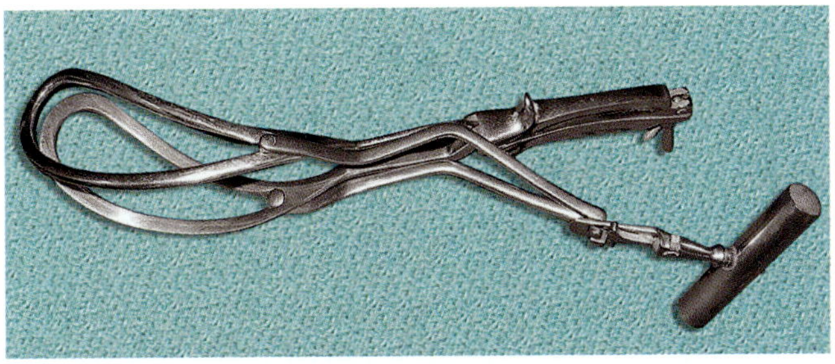

Fig. 7: Axis traction rod fitted with long-curved obstetric forceps (Das).

Fixation Screw

The fixation screw **(Fig. 6)** helps to keep the blades in position and is placed at the end or at the base of the handles. It does not cause any undue compression over the head but keeps the blades in proper fitting. The fixation screw is usually present on the left blade. Fixation screw is not compulsory component. It is present in Das forceps.

Axis Traction Device (Fig. 7)

Axis traction mechanism: This is the mechanism by which axis traction device is applied in midforceps operation. Axis traction device was developed by Tarnier in 1877. It helps to apply traction in the correct axis of the pelvis **(Figs. 8A and B)**. Less force is needed to deliver the fetal head.

Figure 9 shows axis traction device for Das forceps. Different parts of axis traction device are two axis traction rods (right and left)—each rod consists of a knob, a bar, and a groove and there is a traction handle **(Figs. 10A to C)**.

There are other varieties of like axis traction and Milne Murray (1891) and Bill axis traction. Tarnier original axis traction consists of hinged rods on the blades. Bill axis traction device is detachable and has a T-shaped handle and is designed to fit handle of many forceps including Simpson, Luikart, and Elliot.

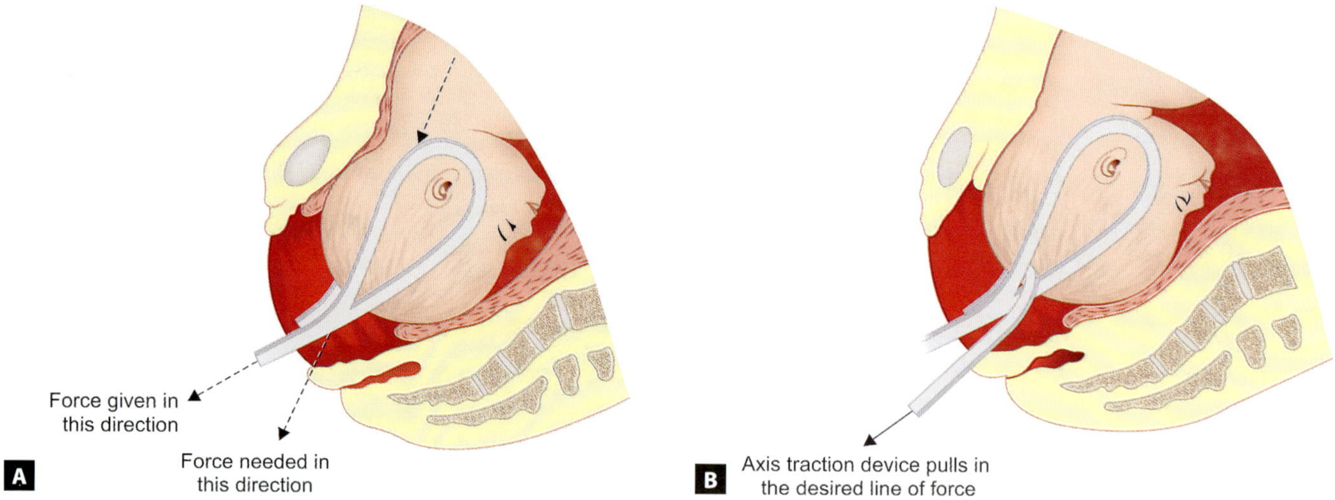

Figs. 8A and B: (A) Direction of forces desired and direction of forces give; (B) Advantages of axis traction.

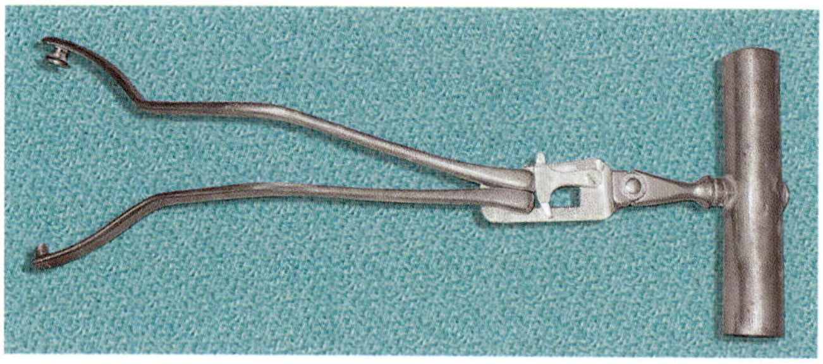

Fig. 9: Axis traction device.

Milne Murray and Das's model consist of two detachable axis traction rods (right and left). In Das's variety, each rod consists of a knob, a bar, and a groove with a single traction handle. Knob is for fitting with the groove of corresponding blade.

Identification of side (right or left) of the axis traction rods: The knob will be directed inward. The concavity lying anteriorly fits the convexity of perineum, and the groove attached to the bar points to the side of maternal pelvis to which the traction rod belongs. Left rod is attached with left blade and right rod with right blade before application of forceps.

Different Parts of Short-curved Obstetric Forceps (Wrigley's Forceps—Arthur Wrigley, 1935) (Fig. 11)

Shank is very small, Handle is small, cephalic curve is marked, pelvic curve is slight, instrument is lighter, and weight is about one-third of long curved forceps. There is no provision for axis traction.

Different Functions of Obstetric Forceps

Traction: While delivering forceps can exert traction on fetal head. Traction of 18 kg and 13 kg are needed in primigravida and multigravida respectively for midforceps operation.

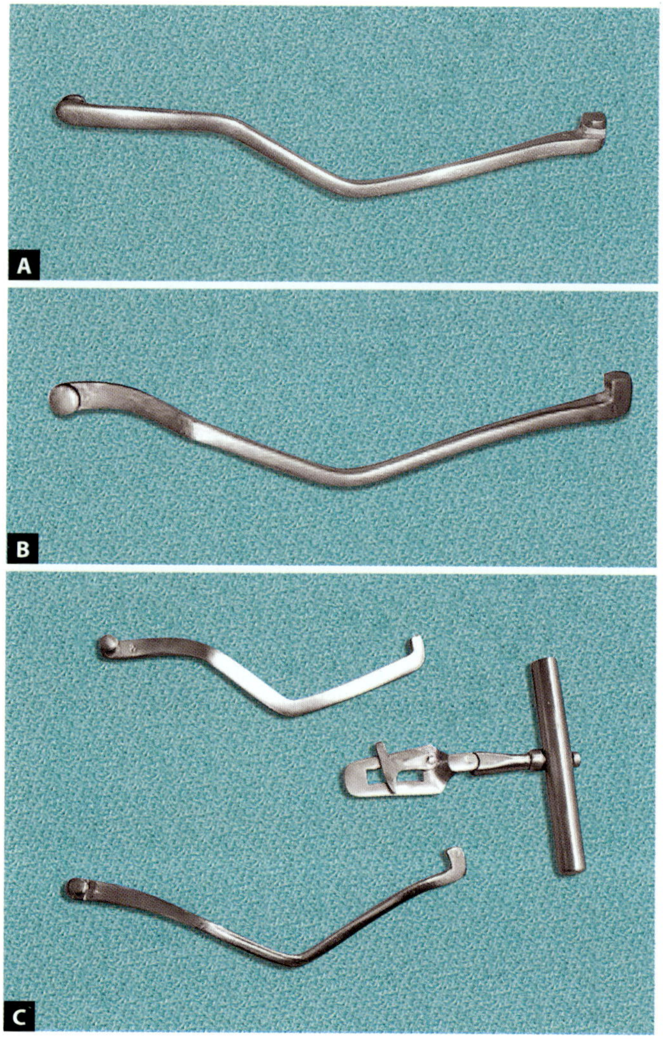

Figs. 10A to C: (A) Right axis traction rod; (B) Left axis traction rod; (C) Parts of axis traction device.

Protection: If properly applied it acts as a protective cage, especially in premature baby.

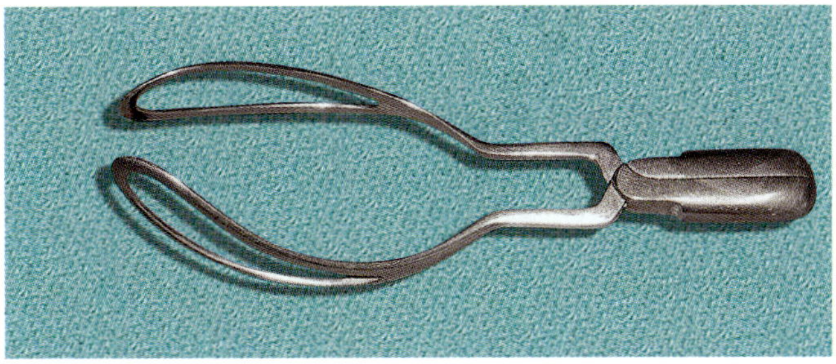

Fig. 11: Short-curved obstetric forceps (Wrigley's forceps).

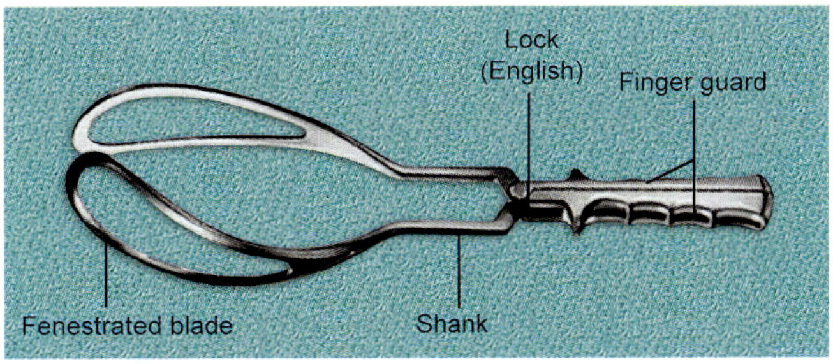

Fig. 12: Simpson's obstetric forceps—long curved, fenestrated blades, parallel shanks, and English lock.

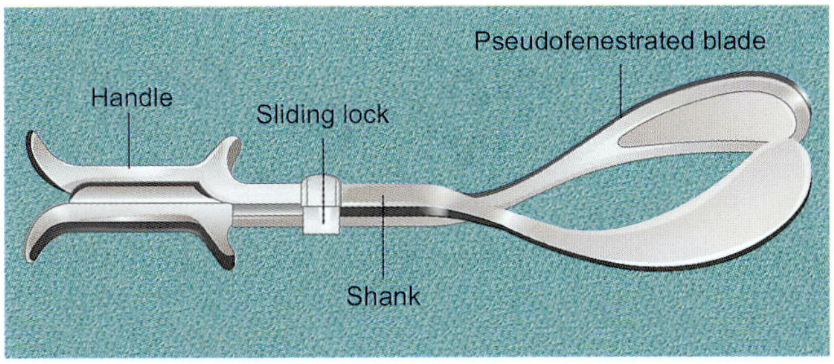

Fig. 13: Luikart obstetric forceps—long curved, overlapping shanks, pseudofenestrated blades, and tongue grooved handles.

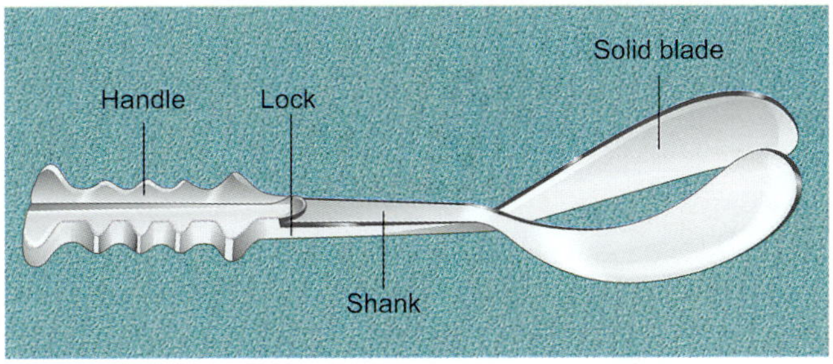

Fig. 14: Tucker–McLane forceps—long curved, solid blade, overlapping shank, and English lock.

Compression: This compression provides good grip of the fetal head without any harmful effect which is exerted on the base of the skull.

Rotation: Rotation can be done with the help of Kielland forceps (not used so commonly).

It is used as vectis to assist in delivery of fetal head in cesarean section (single blade). In cesarean section—head can be delivered with the help of obstetric forceps in case of floating head and deeply engaged head (see Chapter 16 Cesarean Delivery). A single blade can also be used as vectis in deeply engaged head.

Some Common Forceps

Wrigley's forceps ***(Fig. 11):*** Short-curved obstetric forceps, short shank, fenestrated, English lock, ideal for outlet forceps delivery.

Das forceps ***(Fig. 1):*** Long curved, fenestrated blades, parallel shanks, and English lock with fixation screw in handle of left branch, provision of axis traction.

Simpson's obstetric forceps ***(Fig. 12):*** Long curved, fenestrated blades, parallel shanks, and English lock. It can also be applied during cesarean delivery. Simpson developed various types of forceps, common is long-curved obstetric forceps. Other is short forceps. James Young Simpson (1811–1870) from Edinburg was the first one to introduce chloroform anesthesia in obstetrics also (1847).

Luikart forceps ***(Fig. 13):*** Long curved, pseudofenestrated blades, overlapping shanks, sliding lock, and tongue grooved handles with a bar on left branch. Corrects asynclitism and many advantages.

Elliot forceps: Long curved, overlapping shanks, English lock, and wheel (screw in handle of right branch).

Tucker-McLane forceps ***(Fig. 14):*** Long curved, solid blade, overlapping shank, and English lock.

Dewey forceps ***(Fig. 5):*** Long curved, fenestrated blades, combined (French and German) locks, axis traction.

Piper forceps ***(Fig. 15):*** This is a long forceps, fenestrated, English lock, with minimal or no pelvic curve with tapered blades but with marked perineal curve **(Fig. 15)**. This is suitable for delivering aftercoming head of breech developed (1929) by Edmund Brown Piper (1891-1935).

Kielland forceps ***(Fig. 16):*** More or less straight forceps long rotational obstetric forceps, fenestrated blade, longer than classical long-curved obstetric forceps—40 cm (16 inches). Radius of pelvic curve and cephalic curve are more. There is a reverse pelvic curve also. Knob on each blade indicates the side toward which occiput lies. There is a sliding lock for correction of asynclitism of fetal head. Blades are named as anterior and posterior, not right and left.

Barton forceps ***(Fig. 17):*** Barton forceps are long rotational forceps with detachable anterior blade with special function of correction of asynclitism, fenestrated with sliding lock. It is one type of rotational forceps used in deep transverse arrest in a flat pelvis where Kielland forceps is contraindicated. Barton forceps is more effective than Kielland forceps at "0"

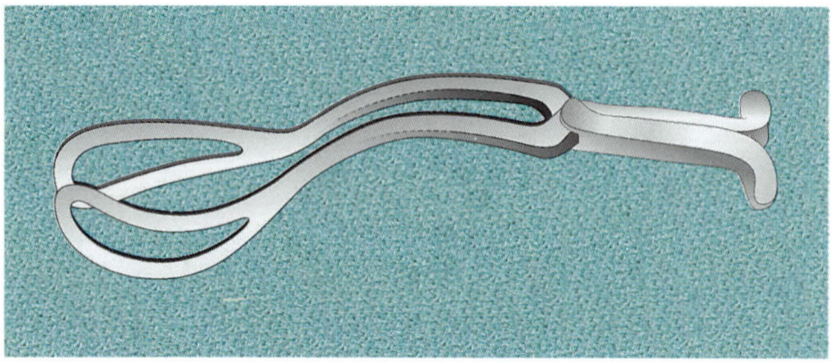

Fig. 15: Piper forceps.

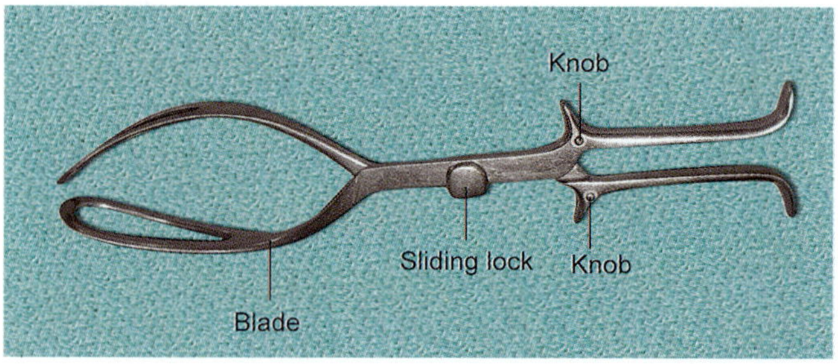

Fig. 16: Kielland forceps.

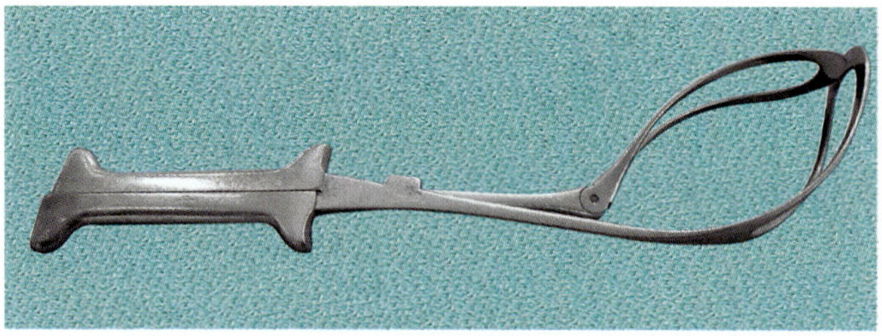

Fig. 17: Barton forceps.

station transverse arrest. It can also be used easily during cesarean section even by the beginners in floating head during cesarean section. It is better than any other forceps or ventouse for delivering floating head. It was developed by LG Barton from New York in 1925.

***VP Paily's forceps* (*Fig.18*)**: VP Paily from Kerala, India designed some special variety of forceps. Features are reduction of biparietal distance and reduction in pelvic curve, especially designed for small baby.

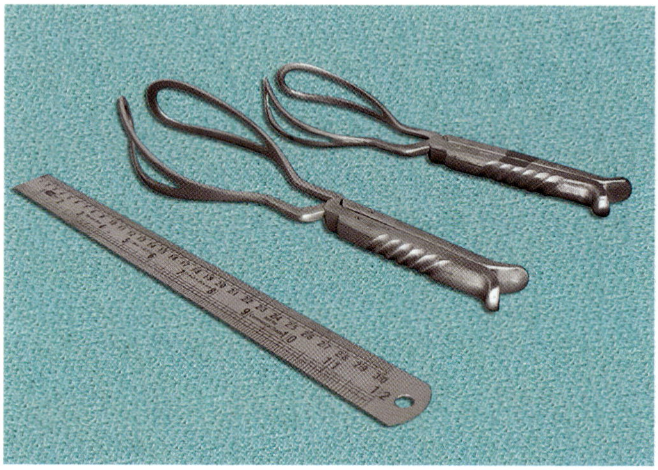

Fig. 18: *VP Paily's forceps:* Features are reduction of biparietal distance and reduction in pelvic curve. Especially designed for small baby.

Cephalic Application and Pelvic Application

Cephalic application (***Fig. 19***): The forceps blades are applied on the side of the head by which the biparietal diameter lies in widest gap between the two blades. The head is compressed by 0.4 cm (3/8 inches). This compression is not harmful for fetal head. The occipitomental diameter of the fetal head comes in correspondence to the long axis of the blades. This application is safe for the baby without any injury to the baby.

Pelvic application (***Fig. 20***): In this type of application, the blades are introduced by the side of the pelvis ignoring the position occupied by the fetal head. If there is no complete rotation of the fetal head, one blade may lie over the mastoid and the other on the malar region of the fetus causing undue compression over the fetal head beyond the margin of safety (**Fig. 21**). Hence, this type of application should always be avoided.

When there is complete rotation of the head (direct occipitoanterior), the cephalic and pelvic applications correspond and it is the ideal method of application. When there is incomplete rotation, rotation of the head manually or with forceps is done to bring the sagittal suture anteroposterior (AP) and forceps are applied. That said, cephalic application is done first and then rotated occipitoanterior to make direct occipitoanterior before traction is applied.

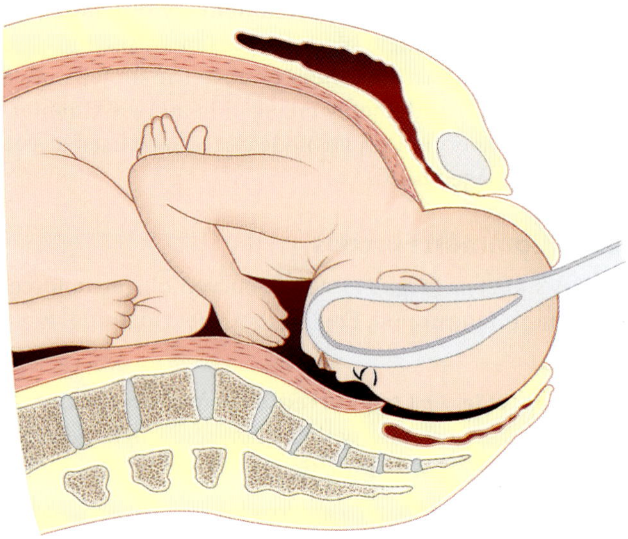

Fig. 19: Cephalic application.

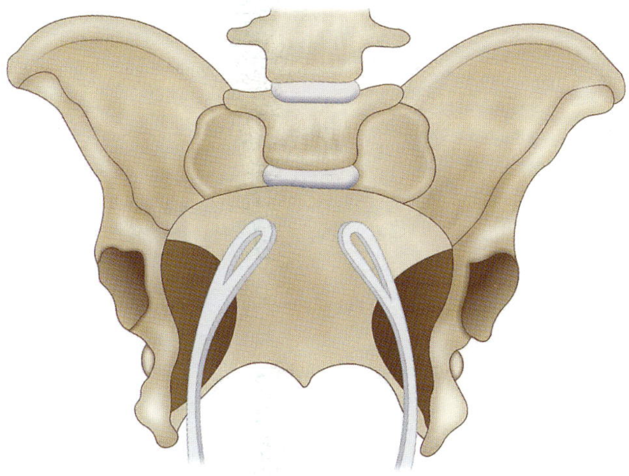

Fig. 20: Pelvic application.

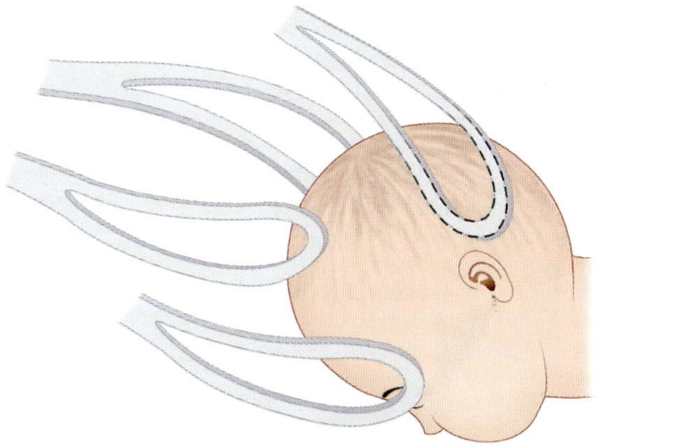

Fig. 21: Malapplication—one blade is applied over the brow and other blade over the occiput. Hence, blades cannot be locked and head gets extended during traction and eventually blades slip off. There is also the chance of injury over fetal head.

Indications of Operative Vaginal Delivery

In second stage of labor, OVD is indicated in situations of threatening the maternal and/or fetal conditions. The indications are fetal and maternal.

Indications of Forceps Delivery

Fetal compromise: Thick meconium-stained liquor, pathological continuous cardiotocography (CTG) [abnormal fetal heart rate (FHR)], scalp blood abnormal pH, and cord prolapse. Aftercoming head of the breech, occipitoposterior, and face presentation are other indications.

Maternal:

- Prolonged second stage [definition of prolonged second stage nulliparous >3 hours with or >2 hours without regional anesthesia. In multiparous women it is >2 hours and >1 hour (ACOG, 2012)]. However, exact total duration of second stage is not yet defined beyond which OVD is done (ACOG, 2019).
- To cut short second stage to avoid prolonged pushing in some maternal conditions such as eclampsia, severe preeclampsia, heart disease, and postcesarean section pregnancy, cerebrovascular disease, cerebrovascular malformation, and spinal cord injury.
- Maternal exhaustion and inadequate expulsive force.

Combined: When maternal and fetal factors may coexist.

Prophylactic Forceps

Prophylactic forceps is the type of forceps operation which is applied to cut short the second stage of labor in anticipation of maternal and fetal distress. This term was introduced by De Lee. Prophylactic forceps are applied in postcesarean section pregnancy, heart disease, eclampsia and severe preeclampsia, painful second stage patients under epidural analgesia, and low birth weight baby.

Classification of Forceps Delivery

Delivery procedures by forceps/ventouse are categorized into *outlet forceps*, *low forceps* **(Fig. 22)**, and *midforceps* **(Fig. 23)** procedures in relation to the level of ischial spines. Leading point of the skull at the level of ischial spines is considered as "zero" station. Station is measured from –5 cm to 0 to +5 cm. High forceps procedure which means application above 0 station has no place in present obstetrics. Two most important determinants of risk to both mother and neonate are station and rotation. Classification of OVD is given in **Table 1**.

Low forceps and outlet forceps are performed in majority (90%) of the cases. Midforceps is attempted not so frequently. High forceps is completely obsolete.

Prerequisites of Forceps Application (Safety Criteria)

- Cervix must be fully dilated, i.e., patient is in second stage of labor.
- Membranes must be ruptured.
- Presentation is essentially cephalic.
- Head must be engaged.
- Station of the head is determined and at desired level.
- Position of the presenting part should be known with certainty.
- For cephalic and pelvic applications together, the sagittal suture must be in the AP diameter of the pelvis.
- Fetal weight is estimated with ultrasound (USG) and clinically.
- There should not be fetal coagulopathy.
- Pelvis seems to be adequate for vaginal birth. There should not be cephalopelvic disproportion (CPD not suspected).
- Bladder should be emptied before application.
- Adequate anesthesia

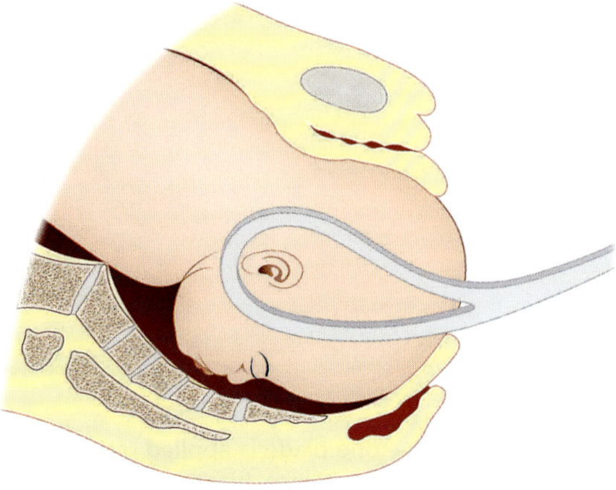

Fig. 22: Low forceps operation.

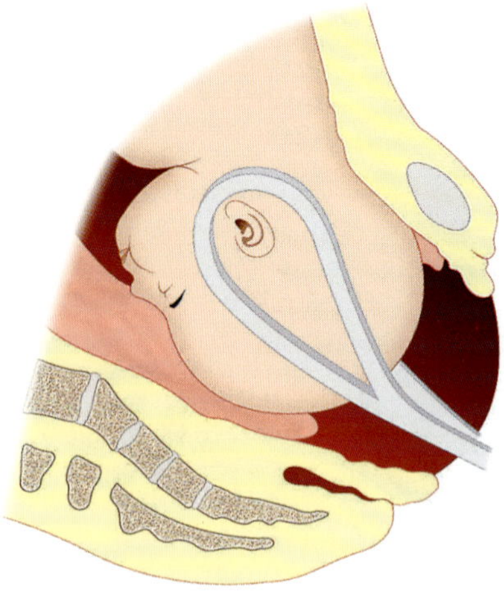

Fig. 23: Midforceps operation.

TABLE 1: Classification of forceps deliveries (ACOG, 2020).

Type	*Definition*
Outlet	• Fetal scalp visible without separating the labia • Fetal skull has reached the pelvic floor • Fetal head is at or on the perineum • Sagittal suture is in the anteroposterior diameter or right or left occiput anterior or posterior position • Rotation does not exceed 45°
Low	• Leading point of the skull is at station plus 2 cm or more and not on the pelvic floor • Two subdivisions: (a) Without rotation—rotation is 45° or less (right or left occiput anterior to occiput anterior, or right or left occiput posterior to occiput posterior) or (b) With rotation—rotation is more than 45°
Mid	Station is between 0 and +2 cm. But head is engaged
High	Not included in classification (applied above O station)

NB: Classification of ventouse (vacuum extractor) delivery is same as forceps delivery except rotation is not considered in vacuum extractor.

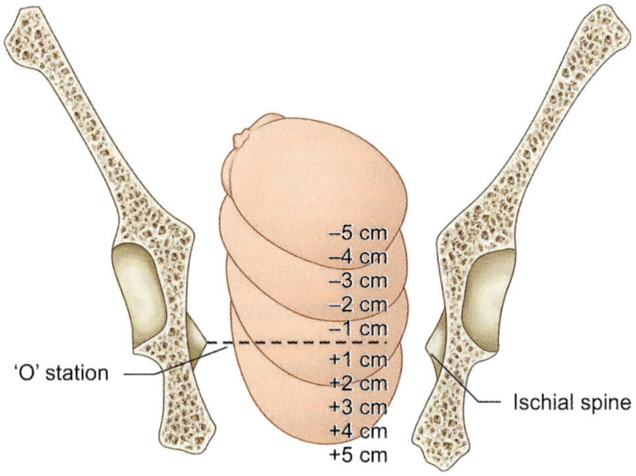

Fig. 24: Assessing station of fetal head in relation to ischial spine in centimeter.

- Counseling and informed consent of risks and benefits are mandatory.
- Willingness to abandon trial of operative vaginal birth and back-up plan if delivery fails.
- Operator must have enough training and experience.

Assessment before forceps application should be done very carefully to ascertain the fulfillment of criteria.

Presentation—most of the cases is vertex presentation; forceps delivery is also possible in face presentation and after coming head of the breech.

Station is the relation of the presenting part with the ischial spines. Prior forceps application, it is determined by per vaginal examination **(Fig. 24)**. In the current system, station is considered ranging from: "0"—presenting part at the level of ischial spines. –1 cm, –2 cm, –3 cm, –4 cm, and –5 cm and floating—the presenting part is above the ischial spines. +1 cm, +2 cm, +3 cm, +4 cm, and +5 cm and on the perineum—the presenting part lies below the ischial spin. Stations range from 5 to 0 to +5. Upper limit of midforceps operation is station "0".

Position: Position is determined by palpating the sutures and fontanels with fingers by vaginal examination. Sutures and fontanel may be difficult to palpate in excess caput formation. The direction of ear pinna identifies the side of occiput. Anterior fontanel (Bregma) is a diamond-shaped area measuring 3 × 3 cm, meeting place of four sutures—frontal suture, two coronal sutures, and sagittal suture. Posterior fontanel (lambda) is Y-shaped triangular, small measuring 1.2 cm × 1.2 cm and joining of three suture lines, sagittal suture, and two lambdoid sutures. Correct determination of position is essential for cephalic application of forceps. Excess molding and excessive caput formation are features of prolonged labor and/or CPD and careful assessment is needed. Currently, sonographic determination of position has been attempted, but yet to come for regular practice. Fetal orbits and nasal bridge can be identified using sonography in difficult cases.

Degree of *Asynclitism*, which is the deflection of sagittal suture away from transverse diameter of pelvic inlet should be assessed before application. Forceps with sliding lock is useful for correction of asynclitism.

Estimation of fetal weight clinically and with sonography is done to detect large fetus. However, relative size of fetus and capacity of pelvis is pertinent for outcome of vaginal delivery.

Clinical assessment of the pelvic capacity and to determine the CPD should be done in a systematic manner to know the pelvic adequacy and to rule out fetopelvic disproportion before application of forceps for success of OVD with less complications.

Contraindications of Forceps Operation

- Incompletely dilated cervix
- Floating head, application of forceps in station above zero (high forceps) is obsolete
- Obstructed labor due to contracted pelvis
- Some malpresentation (brow, mentoposterior face).

Determination of the Side of the Forceps Blades (Das Forceps)

If two blades are together **(Fig. 25)**, the blades are articulated in front of the maternal pelvis with cephalic curve facing each other and convex pelvic curve looking forward and pointing the tip of the blades upward. The blades corresponding to the left half of the maternal pelvis is the left blade and the blade lying on the right side is the right blade.

The fixation screw is usually present in the left blade in Das forceps.

When one blade is provided **(Fig. 26)**, the tip of the blade is directed upward, convex side of pelvic curve forward, and cephalic concave curve inward. The convexity of the cephalic curve directs the side to which it belongs (in relation to maternal pelvis).

Anesthesia in Forceps Delivery

In outlet forceps, pudendal block is sufficient. Regional analgesia is better in low forceps or midforceps delivery.

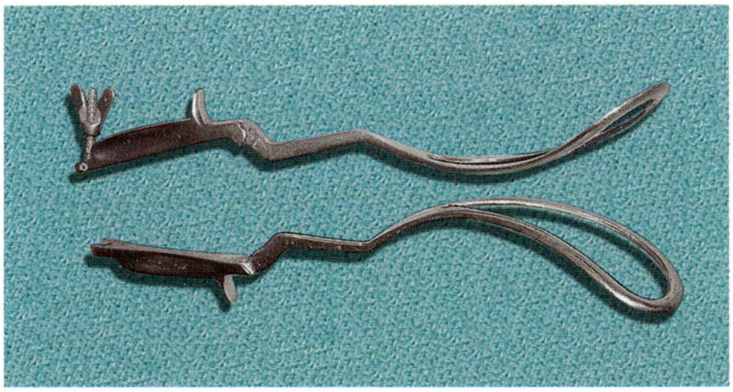

Fig. 25: Determination of side after articulating two blades.

Procedures

Steps of low forceps, outlet forceps, midforceps, and Kielland forceps are described one by one. **Table 2** shows types of forceps delivery and which instruments to be used.

Steps of Low Forceps Delivery Using Das Forceps

Low forceps is done when leading point of the skull is at station plus 2 cm or more and not on the pelvic floor.

Patient is made lithotomy position. The operator will be ready with a gown, gloves, and mask. Antiseptic dressing and draping are done. Catheterization is done to make the bladder empty (rubber catheter). Internal examination is done to ascertain finally about the fulfillment of conditions. Mediolateral episiotomy with local infiltration of lignocaine (1%) or pudendal block is given; however, episiotomy is not mandatory and currently restrictive episiotomy is preferred to routine. Mediolateral episiotomy is protective against obstetrical anal sphincter injuries (OASIS) than midline episiotomy. Episiotomy can also be given later, i.e., after application of forceps and just before traction. Regional or general anesthesia may also be given in low- or midfoceps delivery. Identification of the side of forceps blades (as above) is determined.

Left blade is introduced first **(Figs. 27 to 29)**. The left blade is held vertically in front of the introitus by the left hand in pen holding fashion keeping it almost parallel to right inguinal ligament. Four fingers of the right hand (semisupinated) are introduced in between the fetal head and the left pelvic wall keeping the thumb outside. With movement of the left hand, the left blade is introduced in between the fetal head and the four fingers of the right hand. The thumb of the right hand is placed over the convex edge of pelvic curve (near the shank) and the blade is pushed by the thumb with a passive movement of left hand. Blade goes easily without any resistance in correct application. The left blade can be kept in this position without the help of any assistant in low forceps operation.

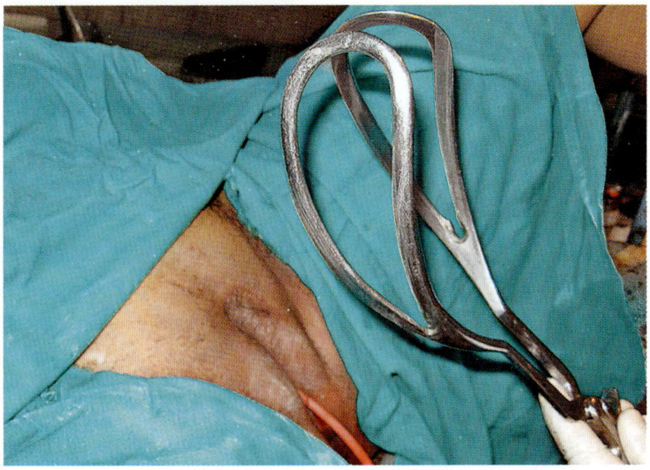

Fig. 26: When single blade is given.

TABLE 2: Types of delivery and instrument used.

Types of delivery	***Instrument used***
Outlet forceps delivery	Wrigley's forceps, Das forceps, Simpsons forceps, Elliot forceps
Low forceps delivery	
<45° rotation	Das forceps, Simpsons forceps, Elliot forceps
>45° rotation	Das forceps, Simpsons forceps, Elliot forceps, Kielland, Tucker–MacLane
Midforceps delivery	Kielland, Tucker–MacLane
Breech delivery	Piper forceps
Cesarean section	Vectis (single blade), Das forceps, Simpsons forceps, Elliot forceps

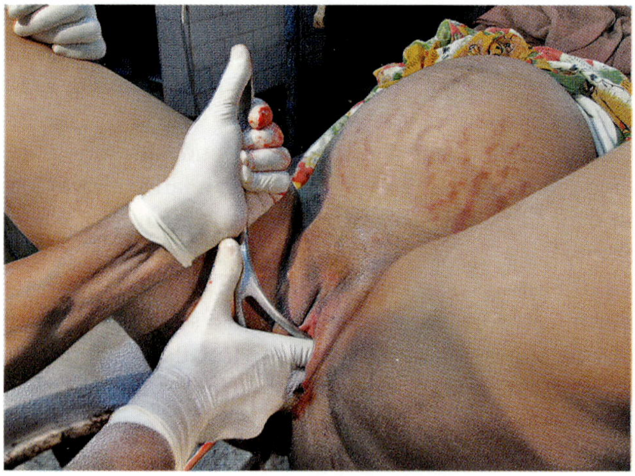

Fig. 27: Introduction left blade. Posterior margin of the blade is pushed by right thumb.

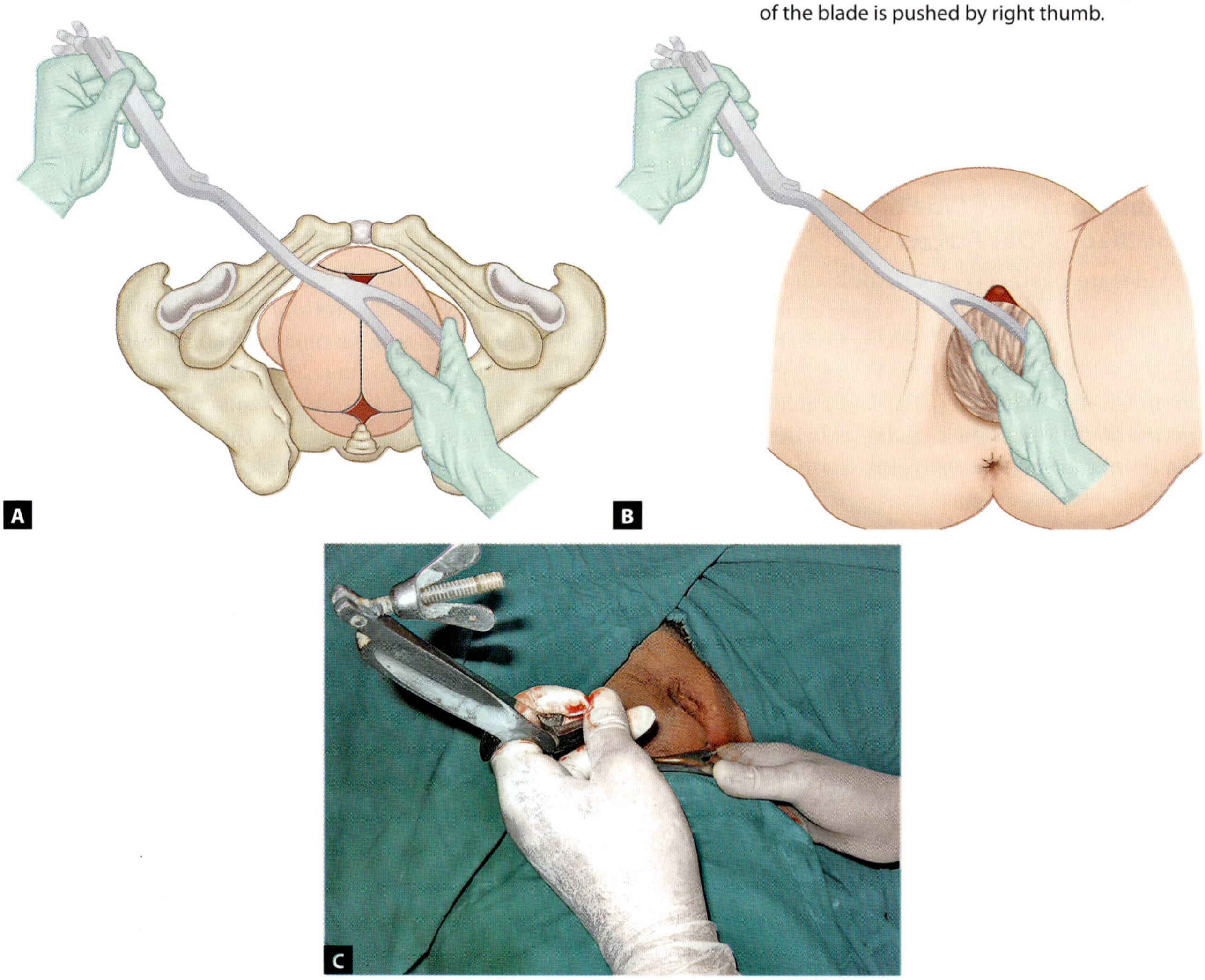

Figs. 28A to C: (A) Introduction of left blade (diagrammatic); (B) Introduction of left blade (diagrammatic); (C) Introduction of left blade.

Right blade **(Figs. 30A to C)** is introduced in the same way. Four fingers of the left hand are introduced in between the right pelvic wall and the fetal head, and the right blade is introduced with the help of the thumb of left hand holding it parallel to the left inguinal ligament.

Blades should be placed properly so that the distance of both the blades from sagittal suture and lambdoid suture are equal.

The locking of the blades **(Figs. 31A to D)**—usually in correct application (cephalic and pelvic application

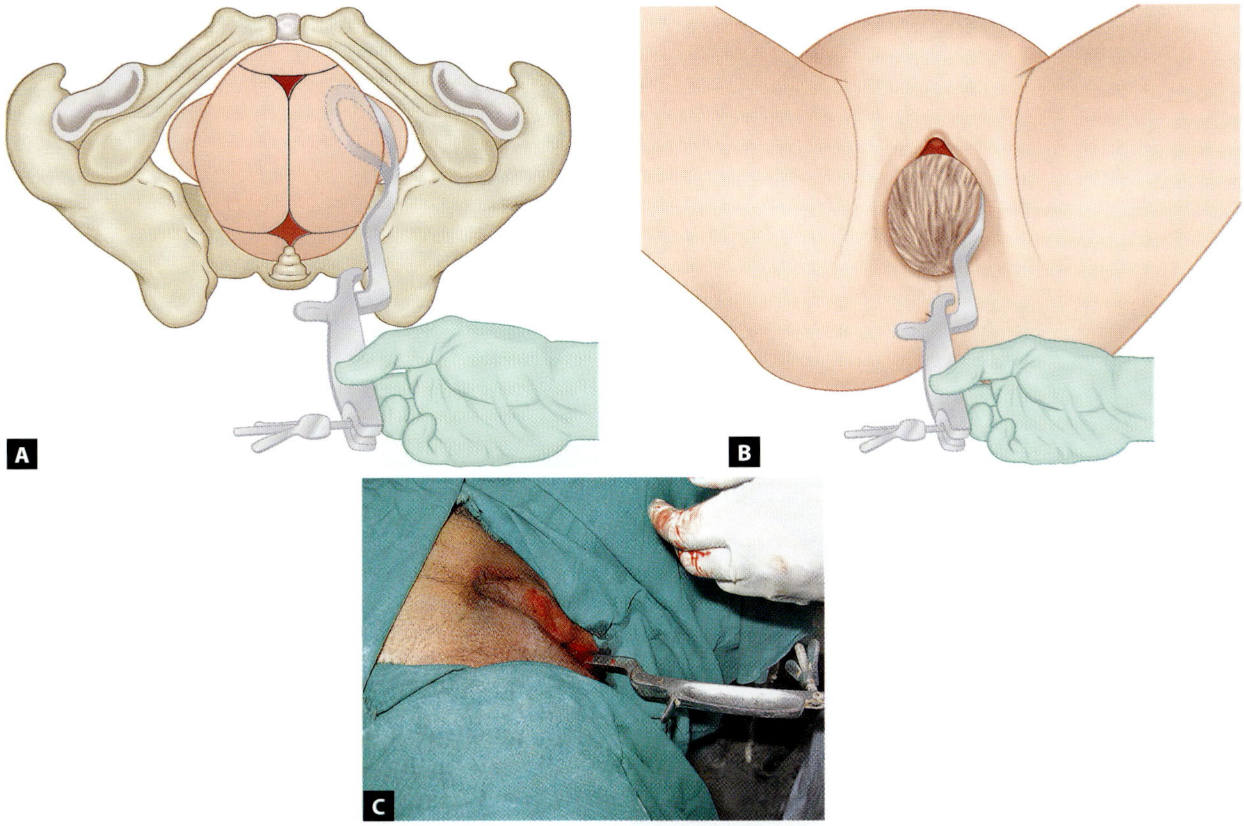

Figs. 29A to C: (A) Left blade is placed (diagrammatic); (B) Left blade is placed (diagrammatic); (C) Left blade in position.

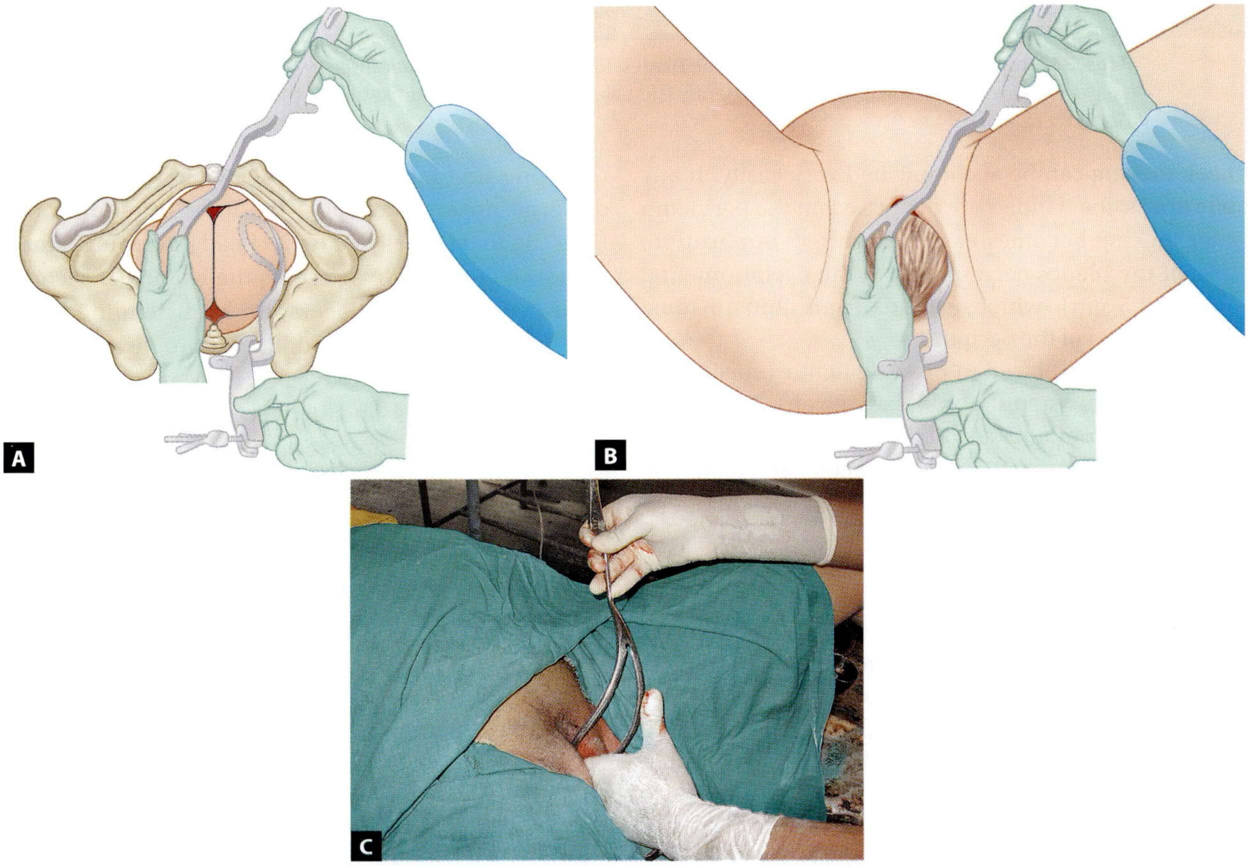

Figs. 30A to C: (A) Introduction of right blade (diagrammatic); (B) Introduction of right blade (diagrammatic); (C) Introduction of right blade.

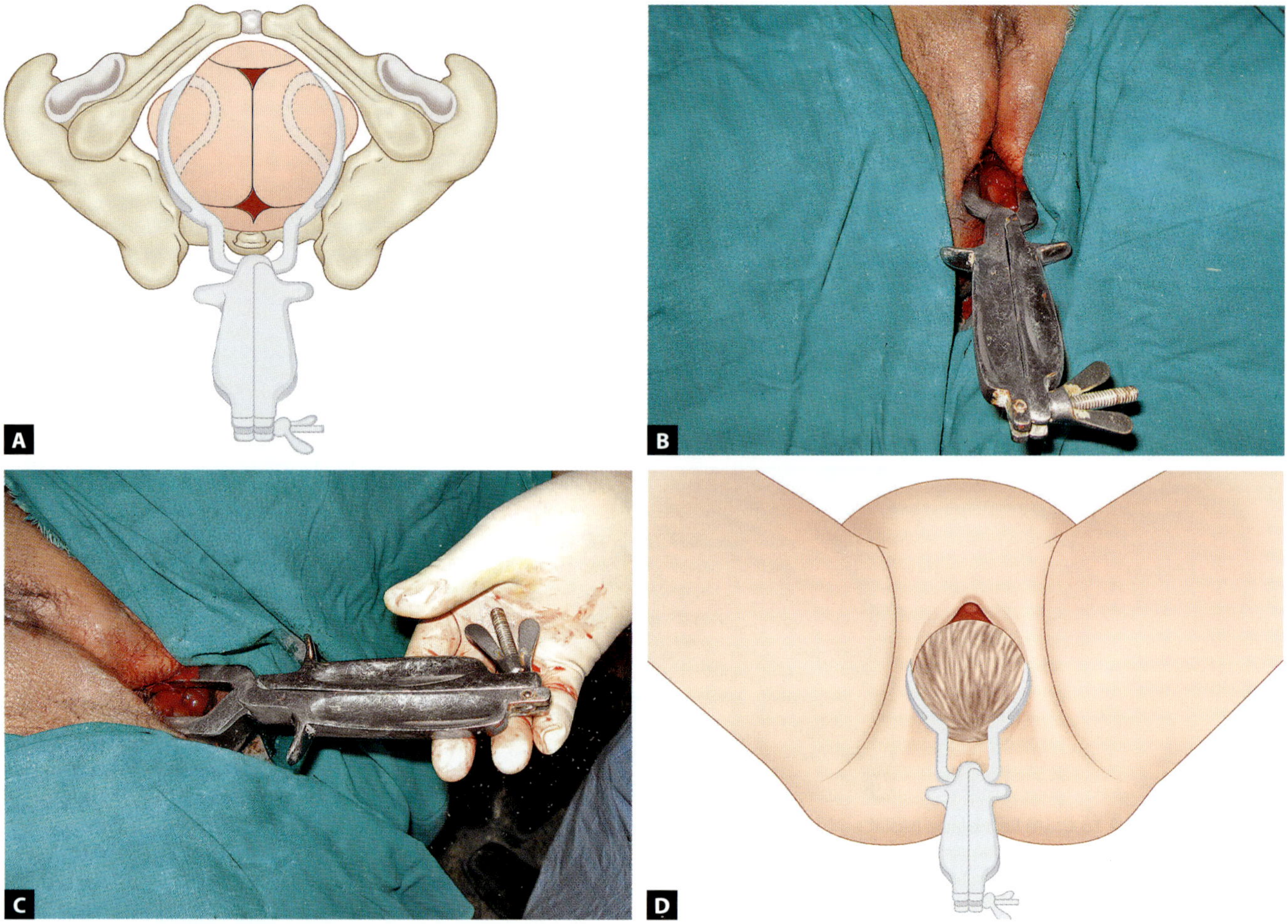

Figs. 31A to D: (A) Locking and fixation of the blades; (B) Fixation of the fixation screw gently (front view); (C) Fixation of the fixation screw gently (side view); (D) Locking and fixation of the blades.

together), locking can be accomplished very easily. If any difficulty arises, the handles are depressed on the perineum and later locking becomes easier. In correct application, long axis of the blades corresponds to the occipitomental diameter (12.5 cm), which extends from chin to most prominent portion of the occiput.

Fixation screw is placed in position lightly (episiotomy can be given in this step if not already given). Traction is given by intermittent and steady, slow and gentle pull and is given preferably during uterine contraction and along the axis of birth canal.

Pull and delivery of head **(Figs. 32 and 33)**—with low forceps operation, the pull is first given downward and backward to bring the head to the perineum and then the pull is given horizontally toward the operator till the head is toward crowned. Thereafter, the pull is changed to upward and forward toward the mother's abdomen and thus head is delivered by extension. The traction is slow, deliberate, and gentle to prevent undue decompression.

Removal of blades is done before the delivery of head. The fixation screw is released and the blades are removed, right one first followed by left. Rest of the procedures is done as normal delivery (modified Ritgen maneuver) **(Figs. 34 to 36)**. Delivery of the head (crowning) along with forceps blades inside increases the chance of second- and third-degree perineal laceration by distending perineum. Just before delivery of head, blades are disarticulated and removed. Mother is asked not to bear down during the removal of blades and delivery of head. Simultaneous application of pressure over perineum by an assistant also prevents the advanced perineal tears. However, too early removal and disarticulation may cause receding of the head causing delayed delivery.

Injection oxytocin 10 IU IM is given after delivery of the baby. Following removal of the placenta, cervix, and vaginal walls are inspected thoroughly for presence of any tear or laceration. Cervix is inspected with the help of two sponge holding forceps and Sims speculum pushing down the fundus of the uterus per abdominally by the assistant **(Fig. 37)**. Careful examination is done to examine any extension of perineal laceration and OASIS. Episiotomy and any other tears if present are repaired.

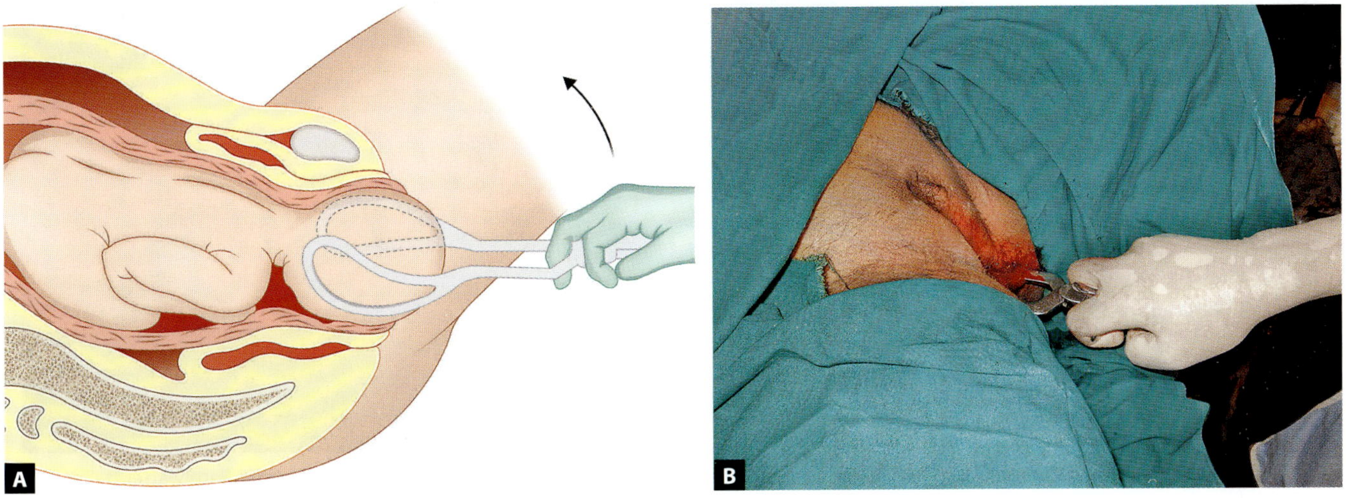

Figs. 32A and B: (A) Traction is given first downward and backward, then horizontally and finally upward and forward (diagrammatic); (B) Traction is given first downward and backward, then horizontally and finally upward and forward.

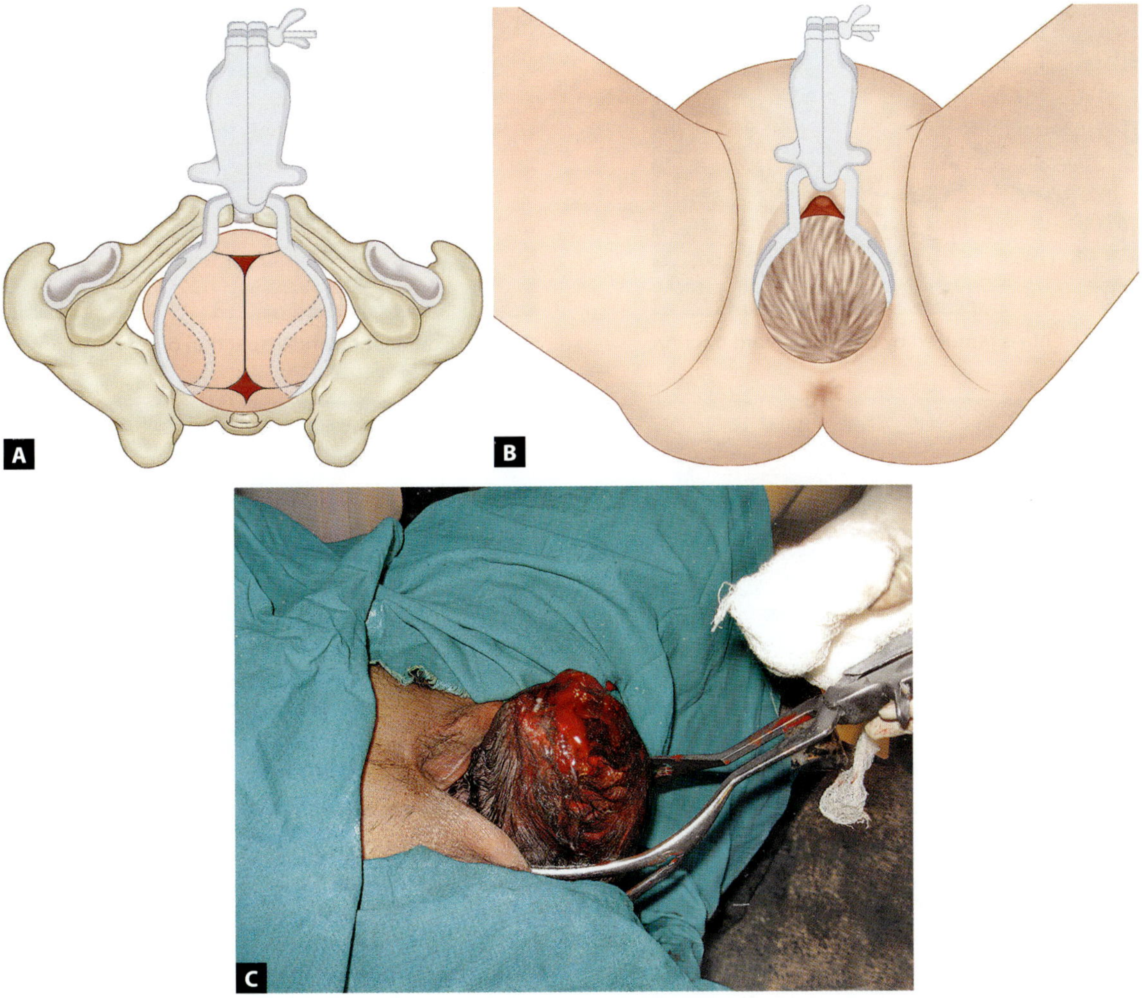

Figs. 33A to C: (A) Head is delivered by pulling upward and forward toward the mother's abdomen (diagrammatic); (B) Head is delivered by pulling upward and forward toward the mother's abdomen (diagrammatic); (C) Head is delivered by pulling upward and forward toward the mother's abdomen.

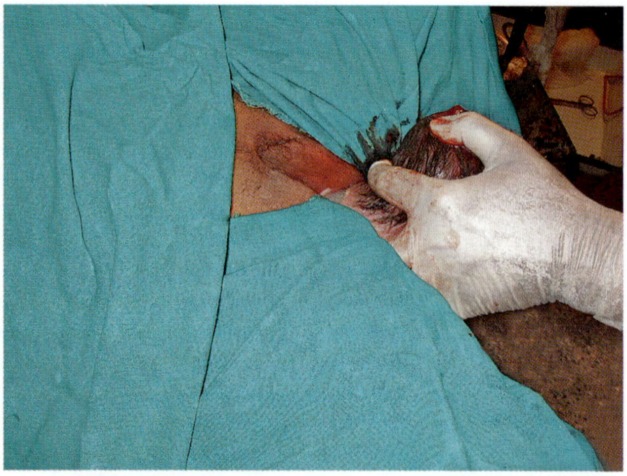

Fig. 34: After removal of the forceps baby's head is grasped.

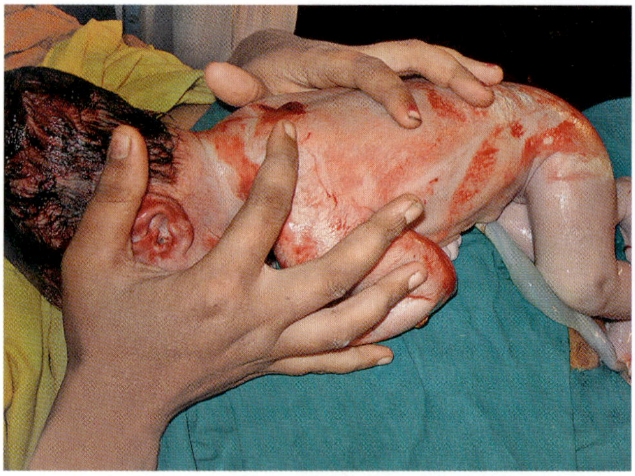

Fig. 35: Baby is on mother's chest immediately after delivery.

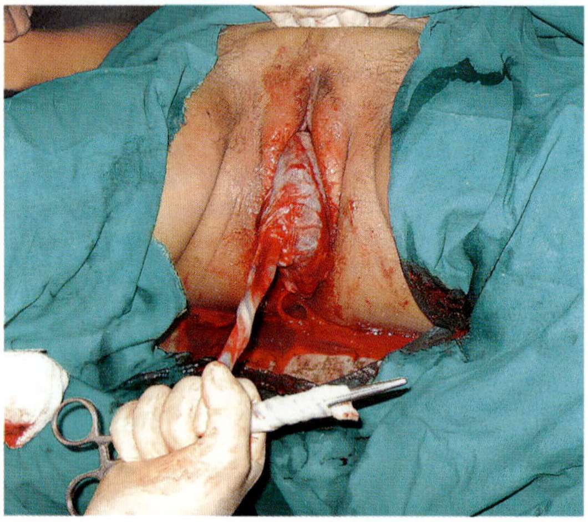

Fig. 36: Placenta is removed by controlled cord traction.

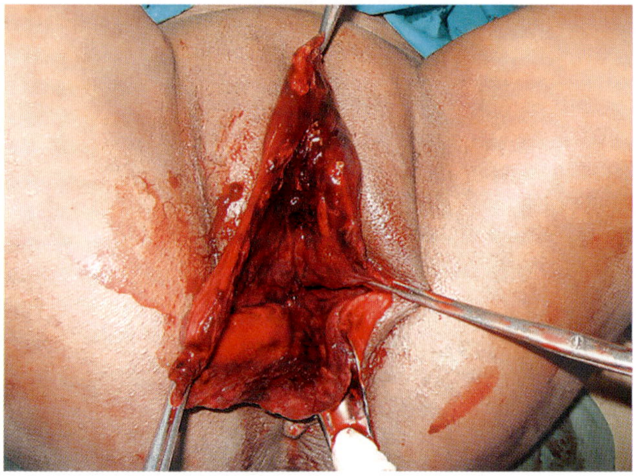

Fig. 37: Examination and inspection of cervix for any laceration.

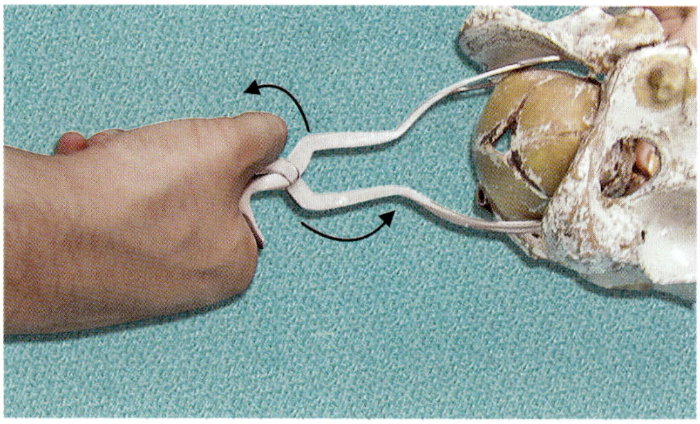

Fig. 38: Head is at left occiput anterior (LOA), rotated anticlockwise 45° to make occiput anterior (OA) (see next Figure 39).

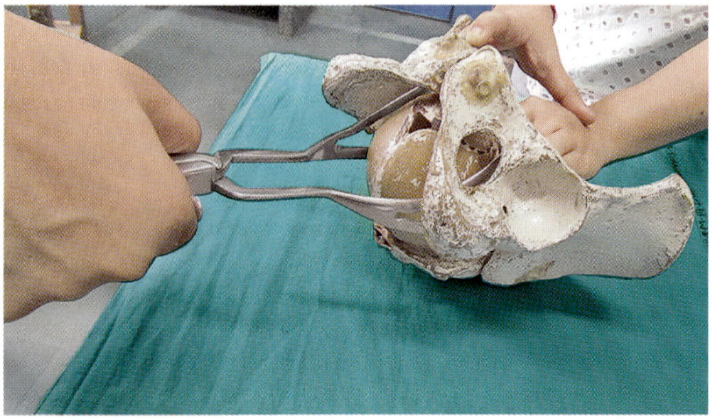

Fig. 39: Head is brought to occiput anterior (OA) after rotation of anticlockwise 45°. Traction in outlet forceps delivery.

In incomplete rotation: In right or left occipitoanterior position forceps is applied on the side of head (cephalic application) and lower of the two blades applied first, articulated, and then rotation to occipitoanterior to make direct occipitoanterior before traction is applied. If articulation is done in left occiput anterior (LOA) position of head, head is rotated to occipitoanterior prior to traction and the arc of rotation is 45° anticlockwise by swinging the handle **(Fig. 38)**. Once the head is made occipitoanterior position **(Fig. 39)**, head is flexed by lowering the handle. Before traction, application is checked carefully.

Steps of Outlet Forceps (Figs. 40A to C)

Here, fetal skull has reached the pelvic floor, fetal scalp visible without separating the labia, and fetal head is at or on the perineum.

Short-curved obstetric forceps like Wrigley's forceps are used. Application in the same way but it is easier. Instead of four fingers only two fingers are introduced. Direction of pull is as first straight horizontal and then upward and forward toward the mother's abdomen **(Figs. 40A to C)**. Just like low forceps operation, no backward pull is needed here.

Reasons of application of left blade first: Left blade is applied first for easy application of the right blade from the front side, and to facilitate locking.

Rarely, right blade is applied first in right occiput posterior (ROP) or right occiput transverse (ROT) positions of head following manual rotation of fetal head done by full hand method which is rarely performed now. In that case, the left blade is applied from behind after application of right blade.

Steps of Midforceps Delivery

This type of operation is done when station is between 0 and +2 cm. Usually, there is incomplete rotation (sagittal suture does not lie direct anteroposteriorly and/or head is high up. Position of patient and preliminaries are similar to low forceps operation. Manual rotation is done to make the sagittal suture anteroposteriorly (regional anesthesia is preferred in midforceps operations). The blades are introduced like low forceps operation. Following application of left blade here support is mandatory by an assistant to hold the blade in position. Pull is like low forceps operation, but here more downward and backward pulls are needed to bring the head in perineum.

Application of Forceps Along with Axis Traction Device (Figs. 7 and 41)

The corresponding traction rods are attached with the blades before application of blades. The blades are applied holding the forceps and axis traction rods together thus keeping parallel to each other. After application of right blade, the

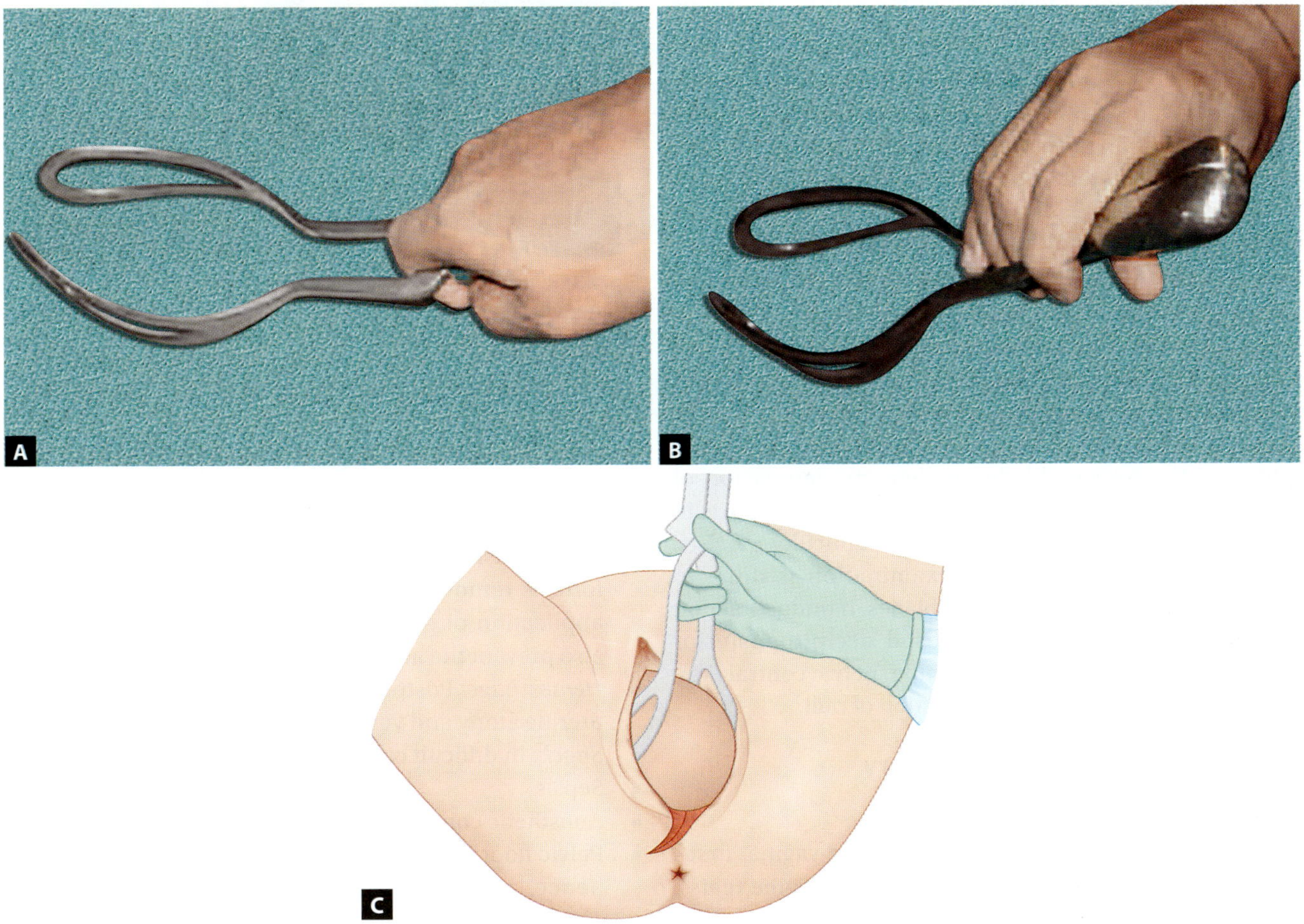

Figs. 40A to C: (A) Index finger is kept in middle, thumb one side and other four fingers other side; (B) Traction in outlet forceps delivery; (C) Traction in outlet forceps delivery. Note the change of position of fingers with change of pull.

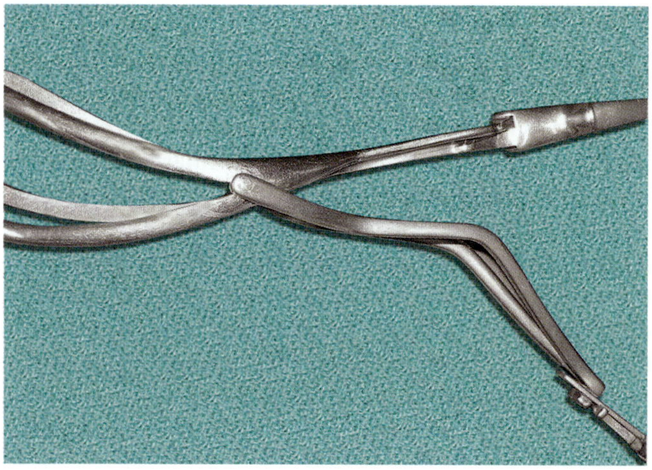

Fig. 41: Axis traction rod fitted with long-curved obstetric forceps.

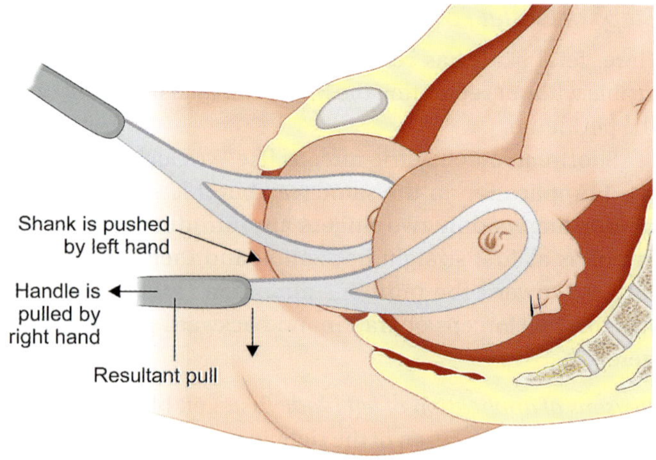

Fig. 42: Pajot's maneuver.

axis traction rods are kept in front to facilitate locking of the blades. Following locking the forceps blades and fixing the fixation screw, axis traction handle is attached with the axis traction rods from behind. Traction is given by grasping the handle of axis traction device and the direction of pull is given in such a manner that during descend of head, the shank of forceps and middle part of the axis traction rods always remain parallel to each other.

Pajot's maneuver **(*Fig. 42*)***:* This is the maneuver by which traction is given without using axis traction device. The accoucheur pulls on the handles of the forceps with his right hand, while with his left he presses the shanks downward.

Difficulties Encountered during Forceps Operation

Difficulties may be during application, locking, traction, and delivery of the fetus.

In application, difficulty probably preassessment was wrong, and cervix was undilated, and/or rotation was not complete. The reasons of difficulty in locking may be unrotated head, lack of cephalic application, incomplete pushing of the forceps blade, inadequate depression of the blades over the perineum and inclusion of fetal parts in between the blade and fetal head. If the difficulty persists, blades are withdrawn. Vaginal examination is done to reassess before reapplication of the blades. If undue traction is needed, think about undiagnosed occipitoposterior position, improper cephalic application, pelvic contraction, constriction ring, and/or wrong direction of pull.

Complications of Forceps Delivery

Maternal

- *Injuries*: Laceration of the perineum and vagina, first-, second-degree, OASIS (third- and fourth-degree tears), cervical tear, rarely bladder injury, uterine rupture **(Fig. 43)**, nerve injury (femoral and lumbosacral nerve), and bony pelvic injury (fracture dislocation of coccyx).

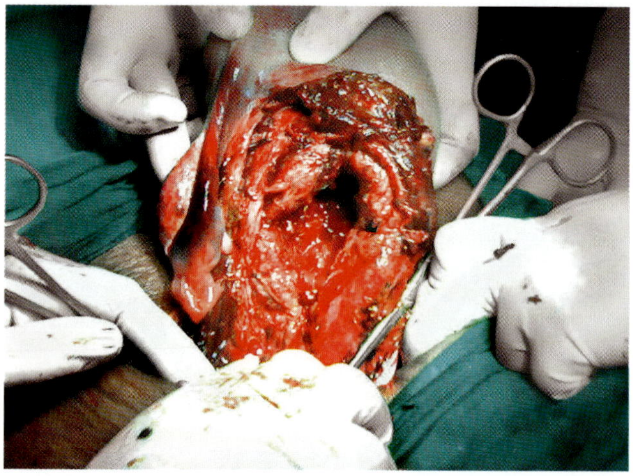

Fig. 43: Rupture uterus following forceps delivery in a primigravida mother which was repaired successfully by preserving the uterus—an uncommon complication.

- Second- and third-degree tears (OASIS) occur more commonly in forceps than ventouse particularly in median episiotomy. Removal of blades before the delivery of head, asking mother to prevent bearing down during forceps removal, and head delivery and simultaneous application of pressure over perineum by an assistant also prevent the advanced perineal tears (OASIS).
- *Hemorrhage:* Postpartum hemorrhage due to trauma or uterine atony and vulval hematoma.
- *Shock:* In difficult cases
- Sepsis
- Anesthetic complications
- Pelvic floor injuries (urinary incontinence, anal incontinence, and pelvic organ prolapse) are more in OVD. The causes are specific structural damages and nerve damages due to traction force.
- Dyspareunia.

Fetal Complications following OVD (Forceps Delivery)

Fetal injury is more common in instrumental vaginal delivery than cesarean section (CS) or normal vaginal birth.

Injuries are facial nerve injury, brachial plexus injury, bruises and abrasion over skin and cornea, and scalp injury **(Fig. 44)**, depressed skull fracture, cervical spine injury, cephalhematoma, subgaleal hemorrhage, retinal hemorrhage, intracranial hemorrhage, and neonatal jaundice due to hemorrhage.

There are more facial and brachial nerve injuries, skull fracture, corneal abrasion in forceps delivery whereas cephalohematoma, subgaleal hemorrhage, retinal hemorrhage, neonatal jaundice, and scalp injury is more in ventouse delivery. Incidence of intracranial injury is similar with both methods which occur either due to vessel injury for depressed skull fracture and/or due to vessels tear due to force applied. Facial nerve paralysis occurs due to compression of seventh cranial nerves over facial bones by forceps blades and brachial plexus injury is as a result of stretching of brachial plexus.

Cerebral or spastic palsy is rare following OPD. Long-term neurodevelopment outcome is reassuring in most of the studies. No relation between OVD and development of epilepsy was found in large studies.

Examination of cervix and management of cervical tear: Cervix is inspected with the help of two sponge holding forceps and Sims speculum pushing down the fundus of the uterus per abdominally by an assistant, with bladder is emptied. The circumference of the whole cervix is inspected in good light by holding with two sponge holding forceps and changing their positions. If there is any tear (bleeding will occur) it is repaired with interrupted catgut stitches (see chapter of genital tract injuries).

Management of Complete Perineal Tear (OASIS)

Following forceps delivery [see Chapter 15 of Episiotomy, Obstetric Anal Injuries, Perineal Tear (OASIS)]:

It should be repaired immediately in the operation theater under general anesthesia by a senior person (see Chapter 15). But if it is significant delayed and infected then it is repaired after 3 months following resolution. Currently, early repair is advocated after 7 days if the primary repair is delayed. Postoperatively, patient is kept in low-roughage diet at least for 3 days followed by laxative.

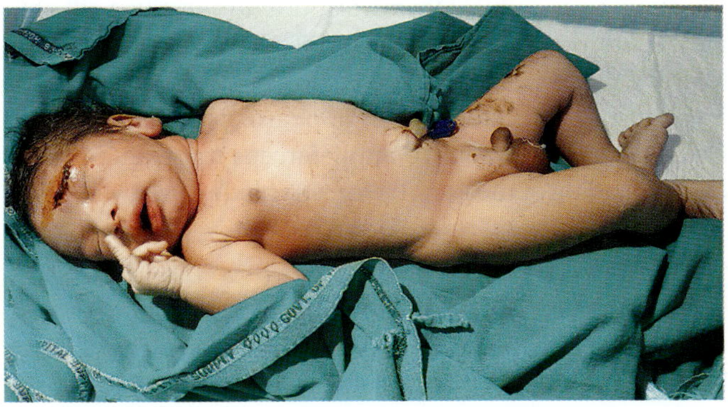

Fig. 44: Superficial injury over forehead near eyebrow. There was no trauma over eye. Uneventful healing took place.

Management of facial palsy of baby following forceps applications: No active treatment is needed and spontaneous recovery occurs almost in all cases. The most important thing is the counseling of the parent.

Caput Succedaneum

It is the localized swelling over the fetal scalp outside the periosteum which appears during labor **(Figs. 45A and B)**. This occurs due to the interference of the venous and lymphatic drainage of the area of the scalp by the pressure of the adjacent birth canal such as cervix and vulval ring. The site of the caput varies depending on the position of the head. In LOA position, caput is formed on right parietal bone and in ROA position, it is found on left parietal bone. Caput is formed usually after rupture of membranes.

Clinical importance of caput succedaneum: Small caput is a normal finding. Caput denotes the static position of the head for a significant period of time. Large caput indicates significant disproportion, and occurs in prolonged labor and usually associated with excess molding. Site of caput gives an idea about the position of head. Determination of station may be misguided by the formation of caput. Abdominal method (fifth formula) of determination is preferred in that case. "Chignon" is artificial molding created during ventouse application.

Management of caput succedaneum: It needs no treatment and spontaneously regresses within 24–48 hours.

Subgaleal Hemorrhage

It is the accumulation of blood in between the galeal aponeurosis and periosteum **(Fig. 46)** due to rupture of emissary veins, mostly associated with operative delivery, but may occur following spontaneous delivery. As the bleeding occurs in subgaleal space outside the periosteum and not limited by sutures significant blood volume can be collected in large area which may extend from neck of the orbit to temporal fascia above the ears resulting significant morbidity (anemia) and even mortality. In that case active management is needed. Majority of the cases are treated by conservative management.

Cephalhematoma

Cephalhematoma is the collection of blood in between the periosteum and the bone of the skull **(Fig. 47)**. It is due to rupture of small emissary veins from the scalp. It is usually caused by forceps delivery but may be found following normal labor also. It appears within a few hours to days after delivery and is never present at birth. The swelling is

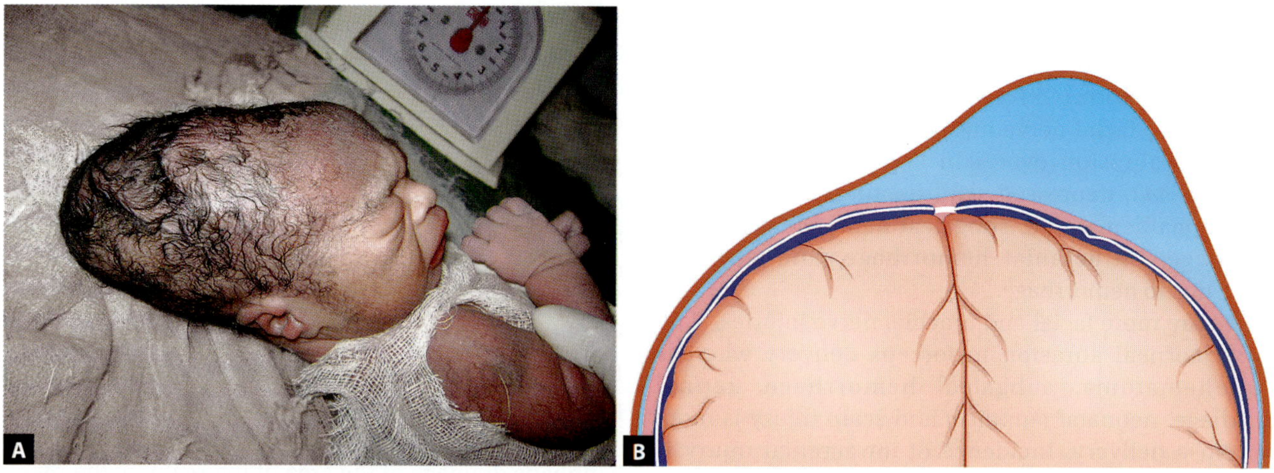

Figs. 45A and B: (A) Caput succedaneum in a newborn following vaginal delivery; (B) Caput succedaneum—localized swelling over the fetal scalp outside the galea aponeurotica and periosteum.
Courtesy: (A) Dr Anirban Mondal, Associate Professor, Bankura Sammilani Medical College and Hospital, Bankura, West Bengal, India.

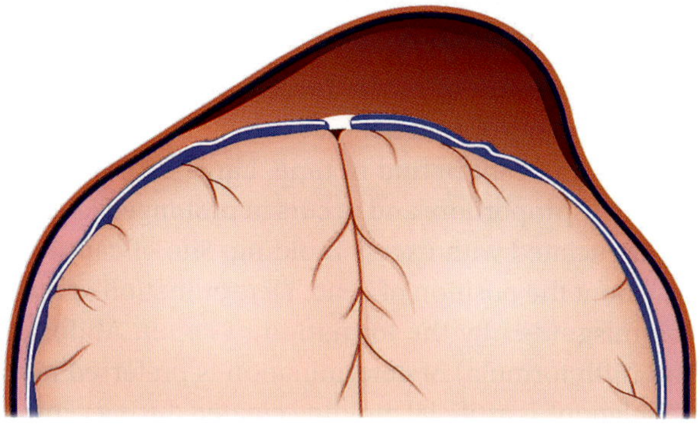

Fig. 46: Subgaleal hemorrhage—accumulation of blood in between the galea aponeurotica and periosteum.
Courtesy: Arunima Majhi, NIFT.

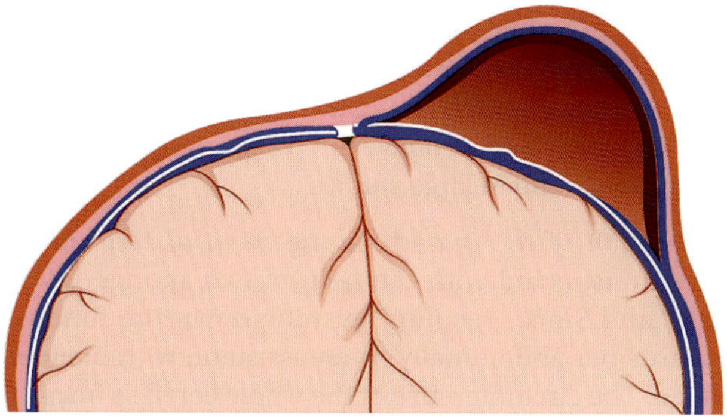

Fig. 47: Cephalhematoma—collection of blood in between the periosteum and the bone of the skull.
Courtesy: Arunima Majhi, NIFT.

well defined and limited by suture lines in contrast to caput succedaneum and subgaleal hemorrhage.

Management of cephalhematoma: No active treatment is necessary and should never be drained. The swelling spontaneously regresses within 6–8 weeks of delivery.

Forceps in Occipitoposterior Position (Face to Pubis) (Figs. 48 and 49)

Diagnosis of the condition is the most important. In face to pubis delivery, there is more chance of perineal laceration and episiotomy is needed. During forceps delivery, the pull is given by remembering the mechanism of face to pubis delivery. The direction of pull is as follows—horizontal and backward traction till the root of the nose is brought under the pubes which act as a fulcrum. Next, pull is changed to upward and forward to deliver the vertex and occiput by flexion. Lastly, by downward traction, face is delivered by extension. There is more chance of brachial (upper trunk) and facial nerve palsies in newborn delivered by forceps in face to pubis.

Application of Forceps in Face Presentation (Figs. 50A and B)

Forceps delivery is possible only in mentoanterior face (in mentoposterior face, vaginal delivery is not possible except in very small fetus). Forceps are applied as in occipitoanterior position. The direction of pull is same as given in anterior vertex. Here submentum hinges under the symphysis pubis. Downward traction is given till chin appears under the symphysis pubis, then with upward and forward movement the face is slowly extracted, with the nose, eye, brow, and occiput appearing in the perineum. One should be cautious to apply forceps more anteriorly to avoid grasping of the neck by forceps blades.

Application of Forceps in Aftercoming Head of the Breech (Fig. 51)

Long curve forceps or Piper forceps are used. Trunk of the baby is lifted up by the assistant (not too much to avoid extension). Forceps blades are applied from below. The pull is given along the axis of the pelvis. The head is delivered very

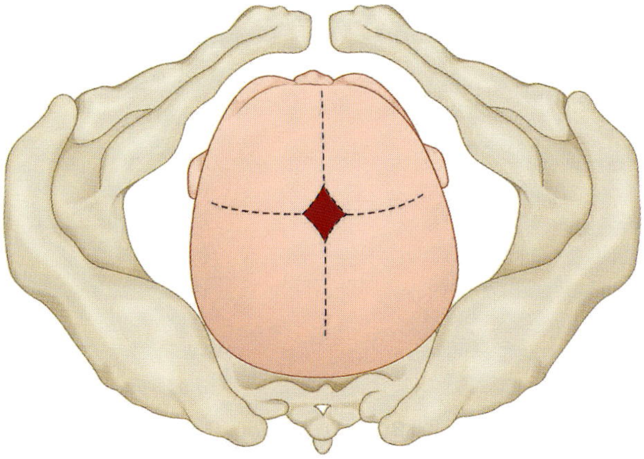

Fig. 48: Face to pubis delivery in occipitoposterior position.

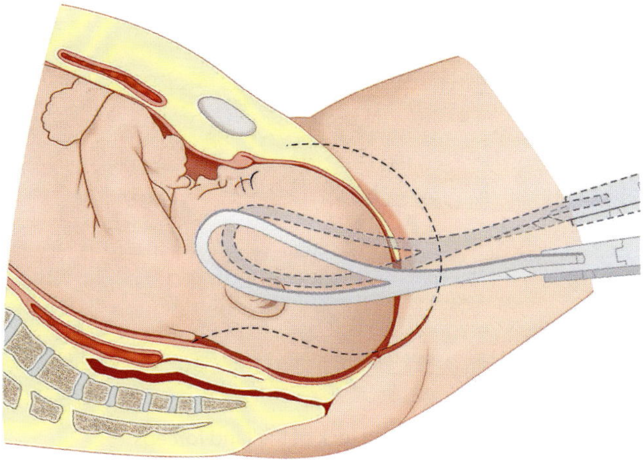

Fig. 49: Forceps application in occipitoposterior position.

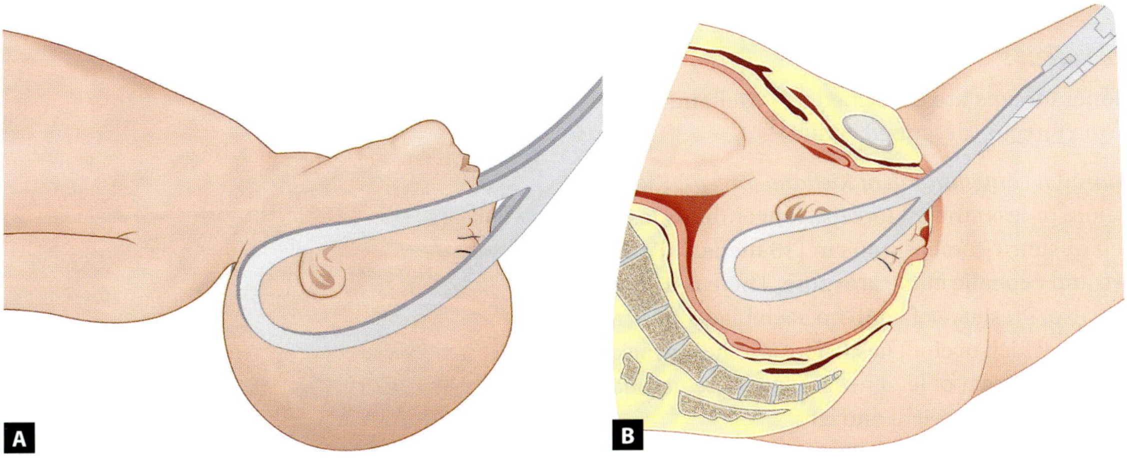

Figs. 50A and B: (A) Forceps application in face presentation; (B) Forceps application in face presentation (relation to pelvis).

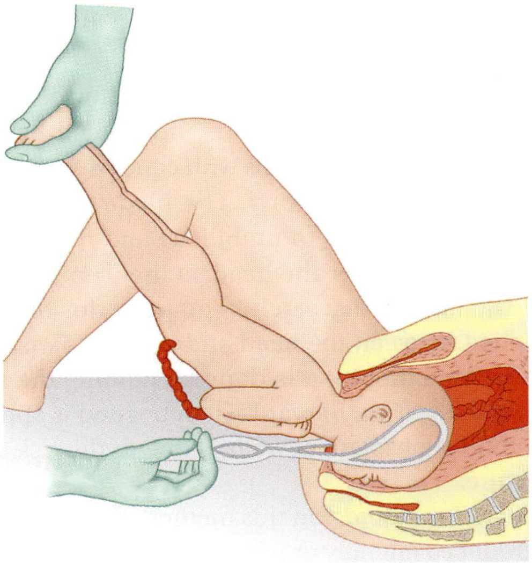

Fig. 51: Forceps in aftercoming head of the breech.

slowly as sudden decompression following delivery of head may cause intracranial hemorrhage. The details of delivery of aftercoming head of breech are described in Chapter of Breech, Chapter 8. Direction of pulls in different forceps operation are described in **Table 3**.

TABLE 3: Direction of pulls in different forceps operations.

Outlet	Direction of pull is as first straight horizontal and then upward and forward
Low forceps	First downward and backward to bring the head to the perineum and then horizontally toward the operator. Thereafter upward and forward toward the mother's abdomen.
Midforceps	Pull is like low forceps operation, but here more downward and backward pulls are needed to bring the head in perineum
Occipitoposterior (face to pubis delivery)	First horizontal and backward traction till the root of the nose is brought under the pubes. Next, pull is changed to upward and forward to deliver the vertex and occiput by flexion
Face delivery	Lastly, by downward traction, face is delivered by extension
Aftercoming head of breech	The direction of pull is same as given in anterior vertex (low forceps)
Traction with axis traction device	The pull is given along the axis of the pelvis. This can be achieved by keeping the middle part of axis traction rod parallel to shank of forceps.

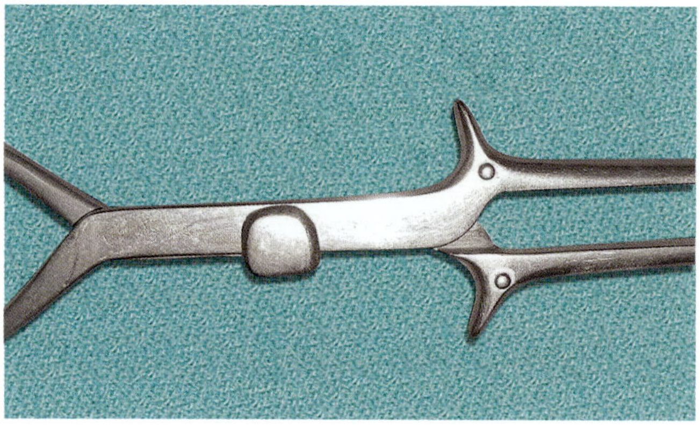

Fig. 52: Sliding lock of Kielland forceps.

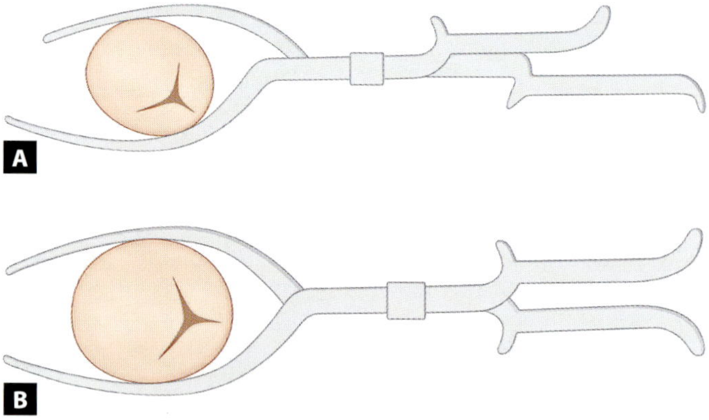

Figs. 53A and B: (A) Correction of asynclitism; (B) Correction of asynclitism.

Rotational Forceps

Two rotational forceps are described: (1) Kielland forceps and (2) Burton forceps (described earlier)

Special features in configuration of Kielland forceps: Kielland forceps is more or less straight forceps, longer than classical long-curved obstetric forceps—40 cm (16 inches). Radii of pelvic curve and cephalic curve are more. There is a reverse pelvic curve also. Presence of knob on each blade indicates the side towards which occiput lies. There is a sliding lock for correction of asynclitism of fetal head. Blades are named as anterior and posterior, not right and left.

Kielland forceps is indicated in arrested occipitoposterior position. It can also be used in face presentation.

The advantages of Kielland forceps over manual rotation and forceps extraction are: (1) Both rotation and extraction can be performed with the instrument; (2) Head is not displaced above the brim during rotation which may occur when it is done manually; (3) There is a provision of correction of asynclitism on the sliding lock **(Figs. 52 and 53)**; and (4) In experienced hand, it is safer. Manual rotation and forceps delivery is appropriate when the arrest is due to deflexed head and not due to abnormal pelvic shape.

The disadvantages of Kielland forceps are: (1) It should be used always by an experienced and skilled person; (2) Grip is not so firm and there is chance of slipping; and (3) Chance of fetal and maternal trauma is more. Kielland forceps is contraindicated in deep transverse arrest in flat pelvis where Burton forceps is useful.

Procedures of application of Kielland forceps: Side determination: Blades are articulated and held in front of the vulva. Forceps are held with the knobs directed to the occiput. The upper blade is the anterior blade which is to be applied first. Lower blade is the posterior one **(Fig. 54)**.

There are three methods of application: (1) classical method; (2) wandering method; and (3) direct method.

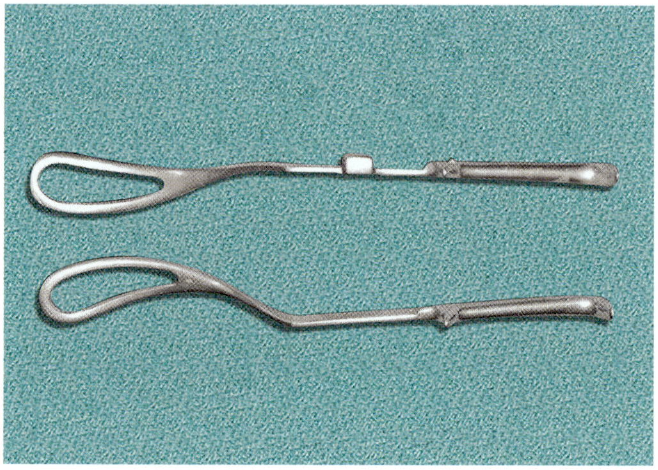

Fig. 54: Blades of Kielland forceps shown separately.

- *Classical method:* This method is performed in floating head. The anterior blade is introduced between the head and symphysis pubis with concavity of the cephalic curve keeping anteriorly. The blade is pushed above the head about up to umbilicus and rotated 180° and pushed down over the head so that cephalic curve fits on the head transversely. The posterior blade is then applied between the head and sacrum. Two blades are articulated. Rotation is done by holding the shanks to bring the occiput forward. Then traction is applied. This method is obsolete nowadays due to the risk of uterine rupture.
- *Wandering method:* In this method, the anterior blade is introduced laterally or posteriorly under the guidance of the two fingers over the face and then pushed over the fetal head so that it comes in front of anterior parietal eminence. The blade is supported by assistant and the posterior blade is introduced between the head and sacrum. Asynclitism is corrected with the help of sliding lock. Rotation is done at different levels depending on the pelvic architecture and ease of the method. Head

is finally delivered by pulling in the direction to which the handles are pointing. This is the method which is commonly employed.

- *Direct method:* It is suitable when head is in low down position. The blades are applied directly, with operator being seated in very low level.

Rotation may be done at three levels depending on the pelvic architecture and the degree of force needed. (i) Above the level of arrest—head is pushed up at higher level and then rotated; (ii) At the same level of arrest; (ii) Below the level of arrest—head is pulled down first then rotated. Accordingly, traction is given before or after rotation. But traction and rotation should never be done simultaneously to prevent spiral tear of birth canal.

Management of Unrotated or Malrotated Occipitoposterior

Diagnosis of Occipitoposterior Position in Vaginal Examination

Vaginal examination by palpating the sutures and anterior fontanel which should be easily palpable in absence of caput. In presence of excessive caput which usually occurs in cases of occipitoposterior position with prolonged labor, the side of occiput is determined by palpation of ear (root of the pinna).

Currently, sonography is used to diagnose position of fetal head but not widely used in practice.

The delivery options are: (1) ventouse—autorotation and extraction; (2) forceps rotation and forceps extraction; (3) manual rotation and forceps extraction; (4) cesarean section if vaginal delivery is contraindicated; and (5) craniotomy in dead baby.

Steps of manual rotation and forceps extraction: This can be done either by half hand method or full hand method.

Preliminary steps like forceps application—lithotomy position. General anesthesia, antiseptic dressing, draping, and catheterization are done.

In *half hand method* right hand is always used. Rotation is done by tangential pressure applied on the side and the parietal eminence of the head. In ROP or ROT, fingers are placed anterior to the head and pressure is given by ulnar border on right hand. In left occiput posterior (LOP) or left occiput transverse (LOT), fingers are introduced on the posterior aspect of head and pressure is exerted by radial border of right hand. Left hand is used abdominally to rotate the shoulder of the fetus from flank to midline. Left blade is applied first and supported by assistant and then right blade is introduced followed by locking. Tractions are given like midforceps operations **(Fig. 55)**.

In *full hand method*, four fingers and the thumb are introduced to grasp the fetal head. In ROP and ROT, the left hand is introduced and in LOP and LOT the right hand is used.

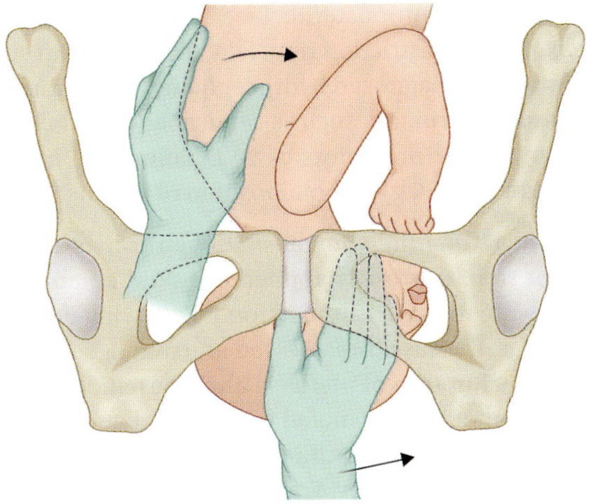

Fig. 55: Manual rotation of the head from right occiput posterior/right occiput transverse (ROP/ROT) (half hand method).

The half hand method is preferred as there is more chance of displacement in full hand method.

Trial of Operative Vaginal Delivery (Trial Forceps)

It is a tentative attempt to expedite the fetus with forceps application in a case of doubtful midpelvic contraction keeping everything ready for cesarean section to deliver the baby if there is failure with reasonable traction. If with moderate traction fetal head can be descended without any harm to mother and fetus, process is continued otherwise the procedure is abandoned in favor of cesarean section. Vacuum extraction can be done, but if no descent with traction, CS is performed. Trial of forceps is attempted only in well-equipped center where a facility of cesarean section is available and it should be performed in operation theater. The aim of trial forceps is to reduce the cesarean section; however, it should not be attempted in an expense of maternal and fetal health. Trial of OVD is supported by ACOG (2015) if the operator feels that chance of success is high. ACOG (2020) warns that attempt for trial OVD should only be done if successful outcome is likely as judged by clinical assessment. Failed trial of forceps is not synonymous with failed forceps (see below), the latter is due to the improper judgment of the clinician. In trial forceps there is a preamble declaration that it may be converted to abdominal delivery.

Failed Forceps

Failure to deliver the fetus following an attempt of forceps applications is known as failed forceps. Failure may be in the form of (a) failure in application, (b) failure in locking, and (c) failure in completion of delivery with traction. Failed forceps is due to the improper judgment and wrong preassessment of the operator.

Causes of failed forceps: Undiagnosed occipitoposterior position—(the most common). Other malpresentations such as brow, mentoposterior face, incomplete dilatation of cervix, CPD, constriction ring, fetal malformation such as monster and undiagnosed hydrocephalus. Other rare cause is soft tissue obstruction such as cervical fibroid and ovarian tumor. Important predictors of OVD failure are increased birth weight (>4,000 g) and malposition of fetal head.

Management of failed forceps: Prevention is the most important step. If wrongly applied it should be abandoned as soon as the mistake is understood. Following withdrawal of the blades, the case is reassessed and managed according to the cause. Rupture of uterus is always excluded. In every case, the mother is resuscitated with IV fluid and antibiotics. Management is done according to the cause. In incompletely dilated cervix, one may wait for full dilatation in an expectation of vaginal delivery if situation permits. In case of unrotated head, manual rotation and forceps delivery are done. In case of CPD, cesarean section is done. If the baby is dead destructive operation (craniotomy) can be considered. In case of constriction ring, deep anesthesia is given to relax the ring and to manage accordingly.

Triple Obstetric Tragedy

Princess Charlotte, daughter of King George IV who at the age of 21 in 1817 went into labor in her first pregnancy which was postdated. Labor was prolonged for 50 hours. Unborn, "would be prince", was born as stillborn boy after 24 hours in second stage. The placenta was retained and removed after 3 hours of delivery. Princess Charlotte died of hemorrhage, thus leaving the King without an heir and Royal line of succession was broken.

The whole episode had strong impact on the life of obstetrician in-charge, Sir Richard Croft. Three months later he shot himself with pistols on temple. Death of Princess Charlotte, stillbirth of the baby, and suicidal death of obstetrician Sir Richard Croft are called "triple obstetric tragedy".

These tragic deaths were highly criticized. The consensus was that this "triple obstetric tragedy" could have been avoided by a timely forceps delivery which could not be applied due to Hunterian/Denman (William Hunter and Thomas Denman) legacy of conservatism and this conservatism was about to be challenged after this event. Sir Richard Croft was husband of one of the twin daughters of Denman.

By middle of 18th century, obstetric forceps was used abundantly due to wider availability, even by unskilled personnel resulting huge catastrophy both for mother and baby. To avoid this, a guideline was imposed at the time of Smellie and Hunter to restrict the use of forceps. This guideline of conservatism (Hunterian/Denman conservatism) stated that it would be used only on the most urgent occasions, head on the perineum for 6 hours and if the head advances, no matter how slowly, no interference would be done unless the baby be dead. By the early 19th century, forceps had been almost abandoned till the happening of Princess Charlotte tragedy in 1817. This tragedy in part accounted for resurgence in forceps use that lasted for >100 years.

Sir Kedarnath Das

Sir Kedarnath Das (1867–1936) **(Fig. 56A)** was a great obstetrician from Calcutta. He designed a special type of forceps which is long but lighter and suitable for Indian babies. Primarily, the forceps were named as "Bengal forceps" and were available from 1912. He developed both ordinary type and axis traction type. The description of the forceps was published in his own language in the journal "The Indian Medical Gazette" in June 1923 issue. Professor Das wrote a treatise on obstetric forceps titled "Obstetric forceps—its history and evolution" published in 1929 (**Fig. 56B**). He compiled the book with 878 illustrations including obstetric forceps of different models. He wrote two other valuable books at that time namely, "Handbook of Obstetrics" (1914) and "Textbook of Midwifery" (1921). He also invented few other obstetric instruments of which cervical dilator is very popular. Das collected hundreds of

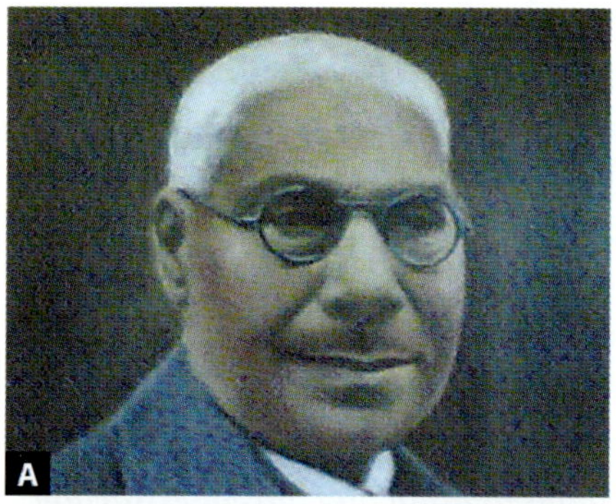

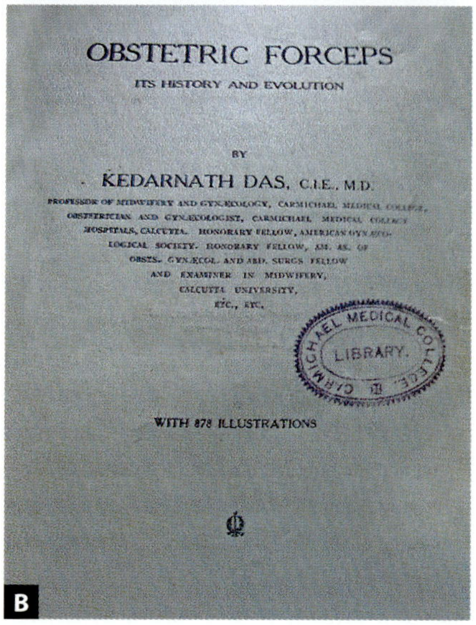
OBSTETRIC FORCEPS

ITS HISTORY AND EVOLUTION

BY

KEDARNATH DAS, C.I.E., M.D.

PROFESSOR OF MIDWIFERY AND GYNÆCOLOGY, CARMICHAEL MEDICAL COLLEGE, OBSTETRICIAN AND GYNÆCOLOGIST, CARMICHAEL MEDICAL COLLEGE HOSPITALS, CALCUTTA. HONORARY FELLOW, AMERICAN GYNÆCOLOGICAL SOCIETY. HONORARY FELLOW, AM. AS. OF OBSTS. GYNÆCOL. AND ABD. SURGS. FELLOW AND EXAMINER IN MIDWIFERY, CALCUTTA UNIVERSITY, ETC., ETC.

CARMICHAEL MEDICAL COLLEGE LIBRARY.

WITH 878 ILLUSTRATIONS

Figs. 56A and B: (A) Sir Kedarnath Das (1867–1936). (B) Front page of the book "Obstetric forceps—its history and evolution" (1929) written by Professor KN Das.

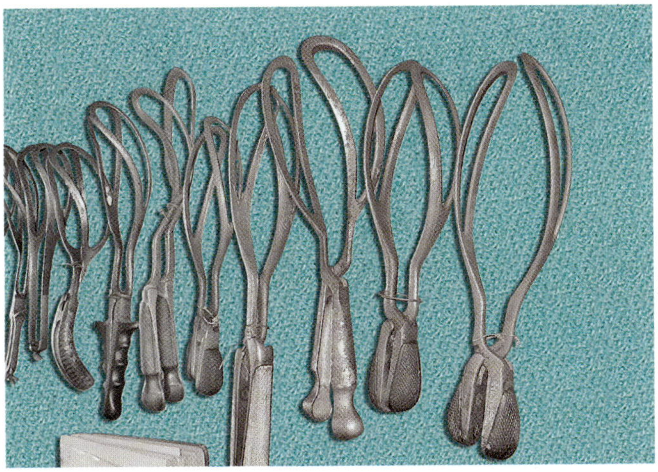

Fig. 57: Few collections of various models of obstetric forceps collected by Professor KN Das displayed at Gynecology and Obstetrics Department Museum, RG Kar Medical College, Kolkata. *Courtesy:* Ex-students Association, RG Kar Medical College (previously named as Carmichael Medical College), Kolkata.

obstetric forceps of different models from various parts of the world and many of them have been kept in forceps gallery at RG Kar Medical College, Kolkata **(Fig. 57)**.

Some the forceps collected by Sir Kedarnath Das are shown here.

Frequency of Use of Forceps Through the Centuries

1. From 1600 to 1720—restricted to Chamberlen family
2. From early 18th century—increasing trend and later widely used till Smellie-Hunter guideline of applying forceps was imposed.
3. From Hunter-Denman conservatism to Princess Charlotte's tragedy (1813)—almost abandoned
4. From 1813 Charlotte's tragedy to first half of 19th century—liberally used, then declined gradually
5. Sharply declined after 1950

Incidence of Forceps Delivery Rises till 1950

The reasons are: (1) Introduction of obstetric anesthesia in mid-19th century (1853 by Simpson) increased the popularity of forceps and patient acceptance and (2) Prophylactic use of forceps, introduced by DeLee (1920) contributed to a nearly 70% incidence of forceps deliveries by the late 1940s.

Use of Forceps Declined Steadily since 1950

The reasons are: (1) Risks of traumatic delivery in association with forceps delivery for both mother and baby; (2) Pelvic floor injury (anal incontinence, urinary incontinence, and pelvic organ prolapse) is a real concern; (3) Increase in litigation is nightmare to obstetrician; (4) Reservation and refusal of patient is practical problem; (5) Liberal use of cesarean section led to a generation of obstetricians inexperienced and uncomfortable with obstetric forceps use; and (6) Introduction of ventouse results the decrease of forceps use.

Present Incidence of Forceps Delivery

In UK, present incidence is consistent to 10–15%. The incidence of forceps delivery steadily declined in the USA from 5% (total instrumental delivery—9%) of 1990 to 0.5% at 2019 (total Instrumental delivery—3%).

VACUUM EXTRACTION/VENTOUSE

Ventouse or vacuum extractor is a suction-traction instrumental device to deliver the fetal head by creating a negative pressure between the instrument and scalp of the fetus in labor. Ventouse literally means "soft cup" in French. The term vacuum extractor is popular in the United States, whereas the term ventouse is familiar in Europe.

History

James Young Simpson developed the first vacuum extractor in 1849 which was very simple with a metal syringe attached to a soft rubber cup, but not popular. Malmstrom from Sweden, in 1954 developed vacuum extractor with a metal cup of varying sizes 40, 50, and 60 mm diameters connected to a handheld vacuum pump machine. Since then, it is modified with various designs with various soft cups.

Basic Principle

A suction cup is placed and fixed over the fetal scalp resulting in artificial caput by creating vacuum in between the scalp and the suction cup, which through connecting shaft, is attached with vacuum generating system where negative pressure is created. And then by giving traction, the fetal head is delivered. The main advantage of vacuum extractor over forceps is the ease of application and it does not occupy space between the fetal head and vaginal wall.

Parts of Ventouse

Old design ventouse had the following parts **(Fig. 58)**:

- Suction cup
- Traction chain fitted with steel plate within the cup
- Traction tube which contains the traction chain
- Metallic traction bar
- Connecting rubber tube
- Wide mouth vacuum glass bottle fitted with rubber cork containing three channels, one is for manometer and of the other two, one is fitted with connecting rubber toward the suction cup and other channel with a hand or electric pump for evacuation of air.

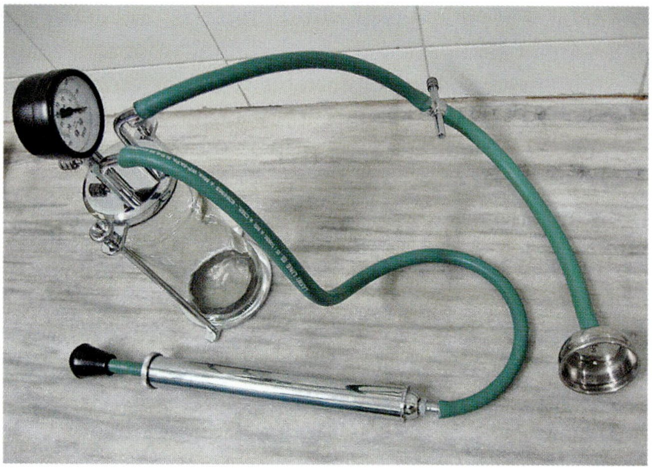

Fig. 58: Ventouse (vacuum extractor, old model).
Courtesy: Dr Pradipta Sanyal, RG Kar Medical College, Kolkata, West Bengal, India.

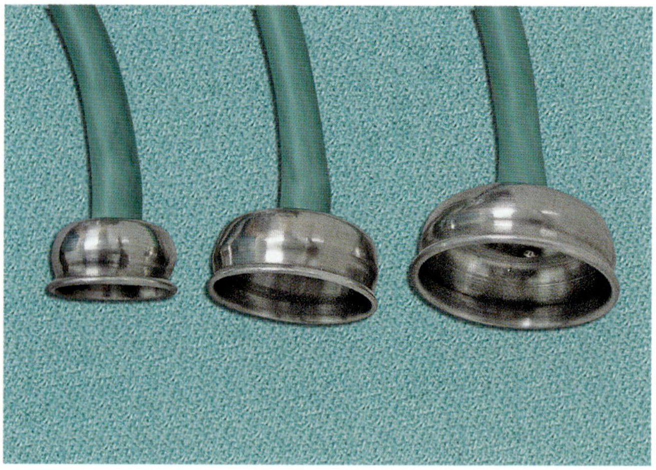

Fig. 59: Metallic suction cup of different sizes.

Suction cups may be of metallic variety **(Fig. 59)** or made of silicone rubber or plastic materials **(Fig. 60)**. This can be of different sizes (40, 50, and 60 mm diameter) and the depth of each metal cup is about 20 mm. After introducing this cup inside the vagina, it is placed over the fetal scalp where vacuum is created. Inside the metallic cup there is a metallic plate which is fitted with the traction chain and the cup is also fitted with a rubber tube inside which the chain is passed. In some varieties, there is a knob over the outer surface of the suction cup to indicate the direction of occiput.

Metallic traction bar is fitted with the suction cup by the chain. Traction is given by holding this traction bar in between the fingers.

There are three connective rubber tubes, one connects the suction cup and traction bar, second one connects traction bar and vacuum bottle, and third one between the vacuum bottle and the pump.

Vacuum glass bottle is fitted with an airtight rubber cork on which there are three openings, two for connective tubes and the other is for manometer. With the help of hand pump or electric pump, vacuum is created inside the glass bottle to create negative pressure in between the suction cup and the scalp. The manometer (vacuum gauze) records the pressure inside the glass bottle and is graduated either in kg/cm^2 ranging from 0.1 kg/cm^2 to 0.8 kg/cm^2 or in mm Hg ranging from 0 to 760 mm Hg.

Newer Design Ventouse

In the newer system, malleable silicon cup is used instead of the originally used metal cup. The cups are of different diameters like metal cup **(Fig. 60)**. Commonly 60 mm cup is used. The cup may be of soft bell cup, dome-shaped, or rigid mushroom-shaped cup which are firm and flattened with ridge around. Rigid mushroom cup is suitable for occipitoposteror positions or with asynclitism where placement over flexion point is difficult. Soft bell cups are

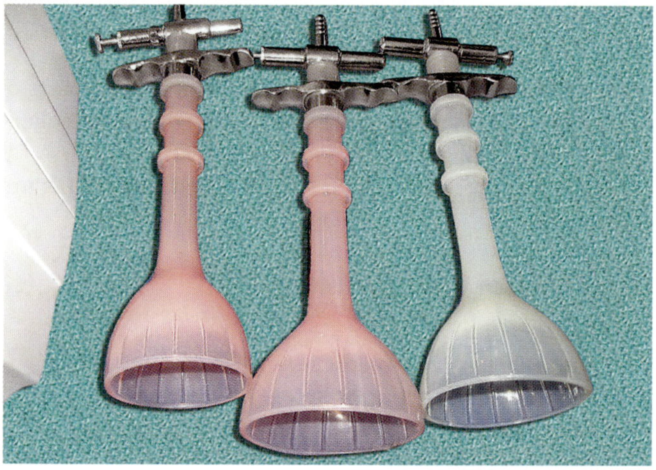

Fig. 60: Three different sizes of silicon rubber cup (soft cups are bell-shaped dome which are pliable).

suitable for occipitoanterior delivery. Success with metal cup is higher but scalp injury and hematoma is more. Traction force is created more in mushroom cup, but is associated with higher scalp laceration. Soft bell cup has a lower rate of scalp injury but has less success rate. The electric pump has replaced the traditional hand pump which is cumbersome **(Figs. 61 and 62)**. Instead of bicycle-type pump, other varieties of manual pumps are also popular in various countries. The example is Mityvac pump **(Fig. 63)**, which remains attached to a disposable MitySoft Bell vacuum-assist delivery cup with tube and filter.

Another completely disposable vacuum-assisted fetal delivery device is very popular in European countries. The PalmPump's integral design **(Fig. 64)** provides a simple hand vacuum pump, thumb, or finger-activated vacuum release valve and an accurate vacuum indicator gauge all in an ergonomic hand. The *PalmPump* is designed for complete control without an assistant and provides a safe and effective

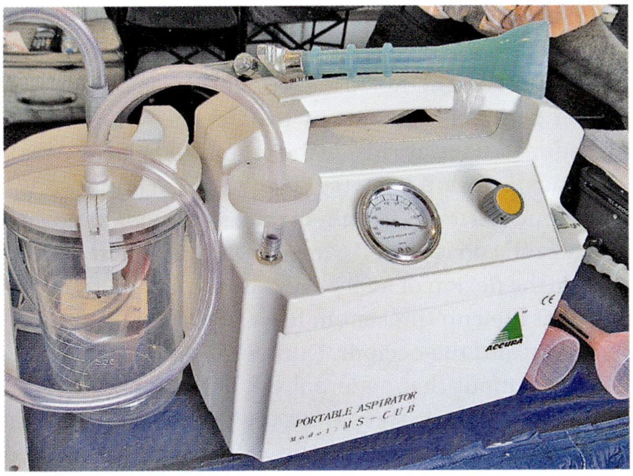

Fig. 61: Newer vacuum extractor with electric pump.

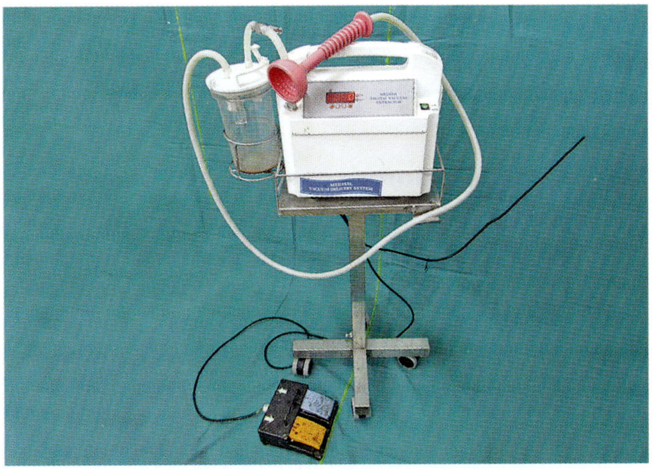

Fig. 62: Electric vacuum extractor with foot pedal used today.

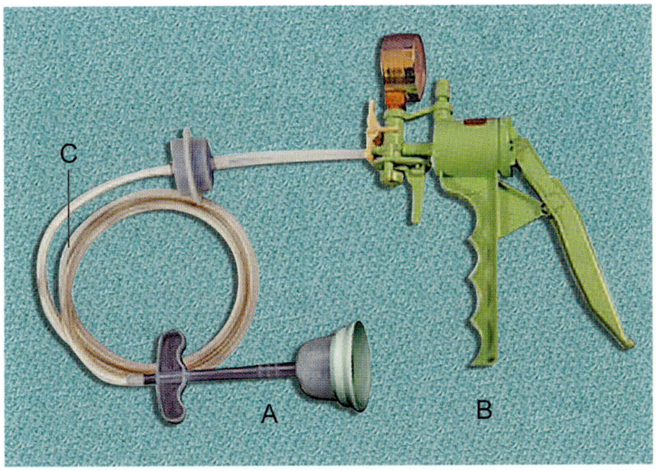

Fig. 63: MitySoft cup (A) Soft bell cup, Mityvac pump (B), and Tube with filter (C).

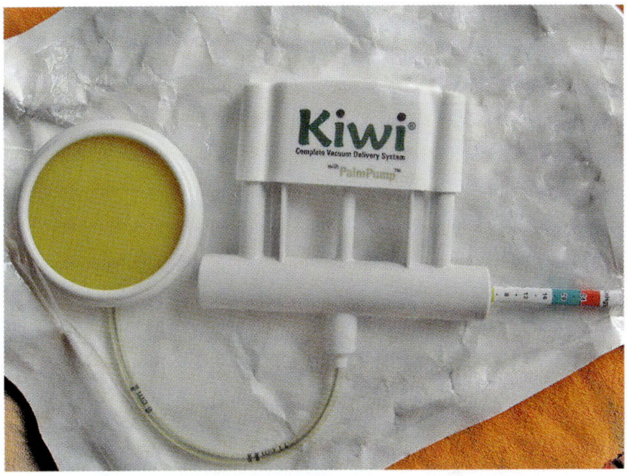

Fig. 64: Vacuum delivery system with PalmPump (Kiwi ProCup), Rigid Mushroom cup.

system in the palm of hand. It has the advantages of using in cesarean section.

The malleable silicon cup produces a much less marked "chignon" over the scalp. The negative pressure can be created with more speed.

The original system is still used with few failures. In original hand pump, the chance of excessive vacuum creation is less and so, scalp damage, cephalhematoma, and serious subaponeurotic bleeding are claimed to be less.

Indications of Ventouse

Delay in the late first stage of labor due to uterine inertia not corrected by oxytocics is an important indication. In case of incomplete rotation (occipitoposterior or occipitotransverse position), ventouse is used as an alternative to rotational forceps delivery. Trial of ventouse instead of trial of forceps, second baby of twins in vertex presentation—where there is delay in descent and head is in high up position are other indication. Vacuum delivery system (the PalmPump) also can be used in cesarean delivery.

Contraindications

Some contraindications of ventouse applications are face presentation, aftercoming head of the breech, premature baby, and acute fetal distress where immediate delivery is needed and can be better performed by forceps. Another contraindication is suspected fetal coagulopathy. Before 34 weeks' gestation ventouse delivery should not be attempted due to increase chance of intracranial hemorrhage in premature baby.

Criteria (Prerequisites) for Ventouse Applications

Patient should be at least in the late first stage of labor (>6 cm cervical dilatation), better the cervical os is fully dilated. There should not be any pelvic contraction. Head should be in low down position in singleton pregnancy.

Classification of Operative Vaginal Delivery

In vacuum delivery, it is same as forceps delivery except rotation.

Steps and Procedures

The basic steps of application of ventouse are application of suction cup, creation of chignon, and final negative pressure and delivery of head by traction. Chignon is an artificial caput succedaneum containing fat and fluid produced after ventouse application which fills the cup. The chignon disappears spontaneously within 12–48 hours.

Procedures of Ventouse Applications (Figs. 65 and 66)

Patient is in lithotomy position. Episiotomy is given following perineal infiltration or pudendal block anesthesia with 1% lignocaine. The proper size of suction cup (larger size depending on the dilatation of cervix) is chosen and all the instruments are assembled and airtightness is tested.

After perineal retraction by two fingers, the suction cup is introduced sideways inside the vagina and placed over the fetal head on flexion point (see below) which is more toward the occiput. Posterior margin of cup is adjacent to posterior fontanel and cup is placed centering sagittal suture. This will facilitate the flexion of fetal head during traction. If there is a knob over the cup (present in few metal cups), it should be pointed toward the occiput. During the cup placement one must be cautious that maternal soft tissue is not entrapped that may cause maternal tissue laceration and also predisposes to cup detachment, called "pop off". To avoid this, whole cup circumference is palpated before and after the creation of vacuum and also prior to traction. Disk cup is superior to silastic cup or bell-shaped cups in presence of occipital malposition and asynclitism.

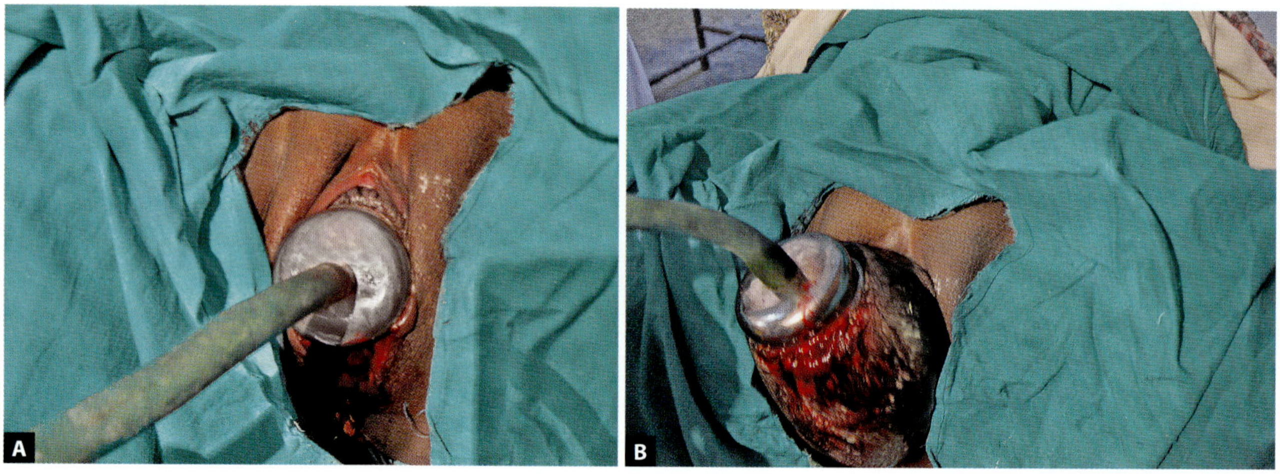

Figs. 65A and B: (A) Delivery by ventouse using metallic cup; (B) Delivery by ventouse using metallic cup (Head is just delivered).

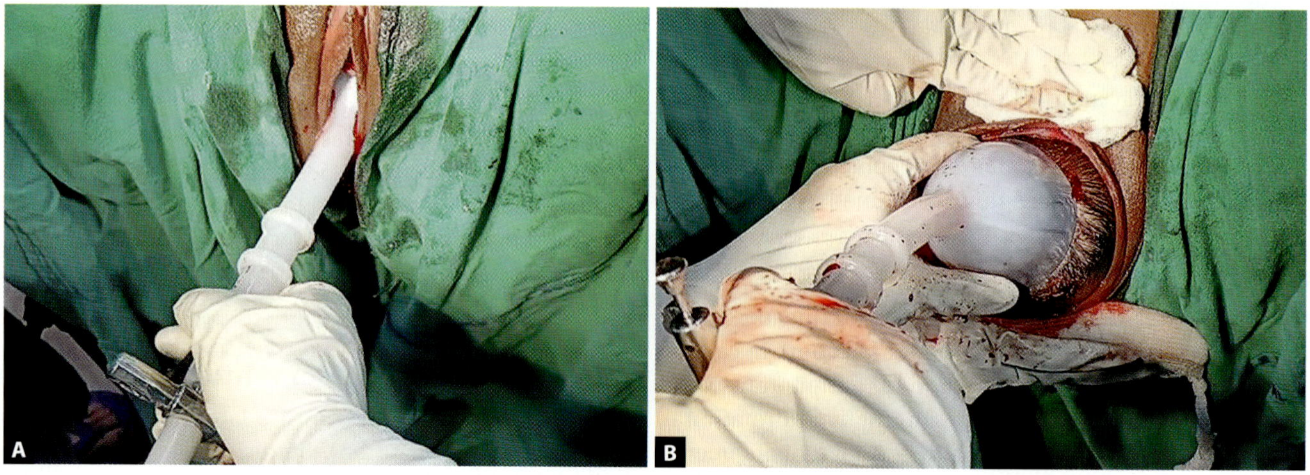

Figs. 66A and B: (A) Delivery by ventouse using silicone rubber cup; (B) Delivery by ventouse using silicone rubber cup (Head is about to deliver).

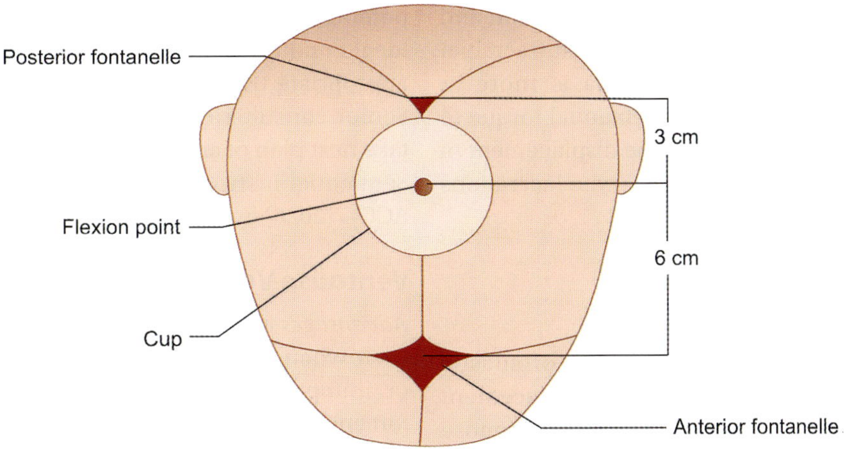

Fig. 67: Placement of cup over flexion point.

Flexion Point

Flexion point is situated along the sagittal suture, 3 cm in front of posterior fontanel and 6 cm away from anterior fontanel **(Fig. 67)**. Proper placement over flexion point facilities maximum traction, flexion, minimizes cup detachment, prevents twisting of fetal head, and allows smallest diameter of head during delivery.

Creation of chignon and final effective negative pressure: An assistant will initially create a vacuum of 0.2 kg/cm^2 (152 mm Hg as 1 kg/cm^2 is equal to 760 mm Hg) very slowly, taking at least 2 minutes. The scalp is checked surrounding the cup to exclude any inclusion of any cervical or vaginal tissue in between the cup and scalp. By giving mild traction it is also checked whether negative pressure has been created inside the cup. Thereafter, the pressure is gradually raised at the rate of 0.1 kg/cm^2 (76 mm Hg)/minute till 0.8 kg/cm^2 (608 mm Hg) is achieved (for conversion of different units of vacuum pressure from one unit to other **(Table 4)**. The time needed to produce effective vacuum is about 6–8 minutes. Chignon is an artificial caput succedaneum **(Fig. 68)** produced during the ventouse applications. The chignon spontaneously disappeared within 12–48 hours.

TABLE 4: Conversion of vacuum pressure from one unit to other.

mm Hg	*kg/cm^2*	*lb/in^2*
100	0.13	1.9
200	0.27	3.9
300	0.41	5.8
400	0.54	7.7
500	0.68	9.7
600	0.82	11.6

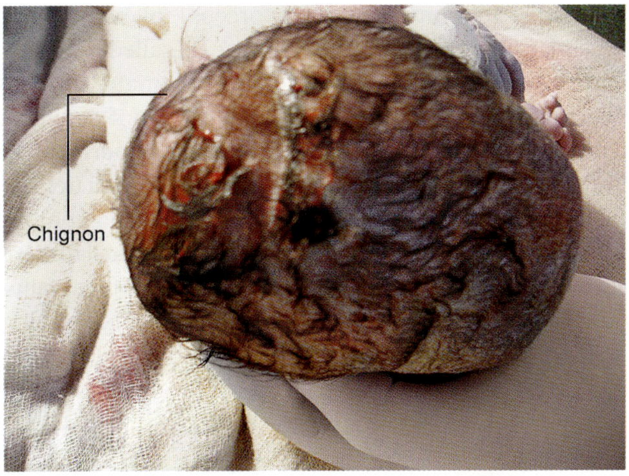

Fig. 68: Formation of Chignon and note the mark of Ventouse cup.

Traction: Traction is given intermittently during each uterine contraction. Traction should always be at right angle to the plain of the cup by dominant hand, with simultaneous placement of nondominant hand inside the vagina, thumb on extractor cup and one or two fingers on scalp to monitor descent of presenting part that will guide to change the axis of traction. Cup separation can also be detected with the vaginal fingers which are at the junction of cup margin and scalp.

Head is gradually delivered with autorotation of the head with traction. Rotation can be observed by seeing the change of position of knob over suction cup if it is present. Usually, 3–4 tractions and not >30 minutes are needed to expedite the fetus. Cup is not detached till the head is delivered in contrast to forceps delivery. As the head comes out, negative pressure is released by losing valve screw.

If there is no descent of fetal head with successive tractions and within 30 minutes, the procedure is discarded in favor of either forceps or cesarean section.

Complications of Vacuum Extractor

Maternal complication is less and occurs only if the tissues are entrapped in between suction cup and scalp.

Fetal complications are cephalhematoma, abrasion and sloughing of the scalp, subgaleal hematoma, and intracranial hemorrhage. Risk of subgaleal hematoma is more in ventouse than in forceps. During traction manual torque to the cup is avoided otherwise there may be displacement of cup, cephalhematomas or "Cookie-cutter" type lacerations with metal cup.

Reasons of Failure to Accomplish Delivery with Ventouse

These are wrong choice of instrument—use of silastic cup ventouse for rotational delivery, incorrect placement of cup, e.g., over anterior fontanel and failure to diagnose position—occipitoposterior is wrongly identified as occipitoanterior.

The action to be taken after failure depends on reasons of failure. Options are forceps application (sequential use of instruments) or cesarean section. If failure is due to cup detachment and the head is low down occiput anterior (OA) low forceps delivery (sequential use) is better than cesarean delivery. If no descent on pull after correctly applied ventouse CPD is likely and is delivered by cesarean delivery. If failure is due to wrong diagnosis of position safer is cesarean section or rotational instrument delivery can be tried.

Sequential Use of Instruments

Use of other instrument (usually forceps) following failure of first instrument (most often ventouse) is called sequential use of instruments. It is observed that neonatal outcome is worse in sequential use of instrument than if delivery is accomplished by single instrument. Chance of perineal tear (third and fourth degree) is also more in sequential delivery. One must balance the risk of CD following failed ventouse with the risk of use of sequential instrument (forceps) (RCOG, 2011). If cup detachment is due to technical failure or improper placement trial of forceps is justified to avoid potentially complex cesarean delivery. But detachment in ideal conditions of cup placement, vacuum creation, and appropriate traction cesarean delivery is the safer option. Senior consultation and re-evaluation should be done to take next plan of action and every case to be individualized. Sequential instrumental delivery is not recommended by ACOG (2020) except in compelling and justifiable cause.

Ventouse Versus Forceps

Advantages of ventouse over forceps: Ventouse can be used even when there is no full rotation of the fetal head. In occipitoposterior position and occipitotransverse position, forceps can be applied after manual rotation or following oblique application, baby is delivered by forceps rotation. Both the procedures are difficult and may be traumatic but with the help of ventouse, delivery occurs safely with autorotation of head during traction. It is not a space-occupying devise, so chances of maternal injury are less. Ventouse can be used even if the head lies at a higher level. Due to malapplication of the forceps, severe types of fetal complications may occur. The requirement of traction force (10 kg) is needed less.

Advantages of forceps over ventouse: Chance of mechanical failure is less in comparison to ventouse where failure occurs commonly due to lack of proper airtightness. Delivery of preterm baby is safer as forceps acts as protective cage for fetal head. Forceps can be applied in nonvertex presentations such as in face and aftercoming head of breech. In suspected pelvic contraction, forceps are the better choice than ventouse as there is more chance of failure in the latter. Chance of cephalhematoma is less than the ventouse.

ODON (FIGS. 69 AND 70)

The odon device is a new device designed for instrumental vaginal delivery such as forceps and ventouse. This device

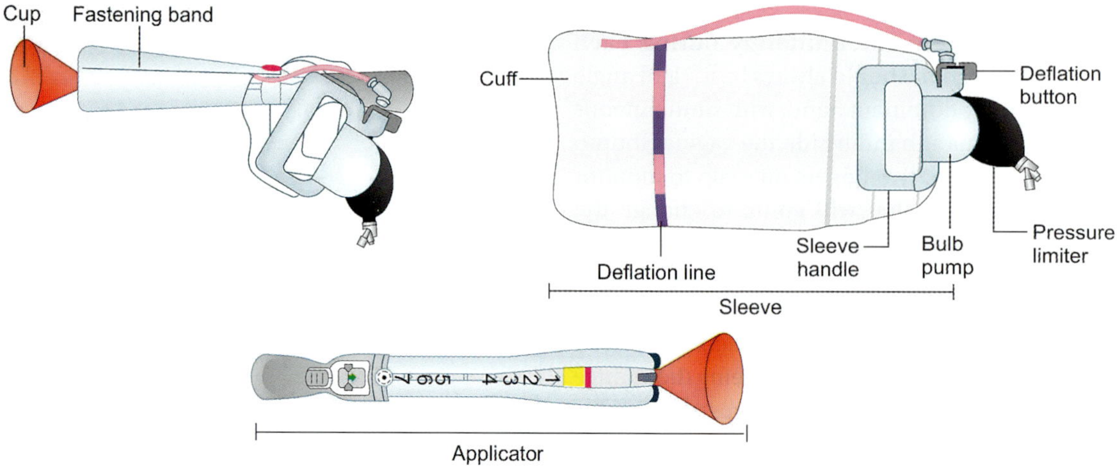

Fig. 69: Components of Odon device.

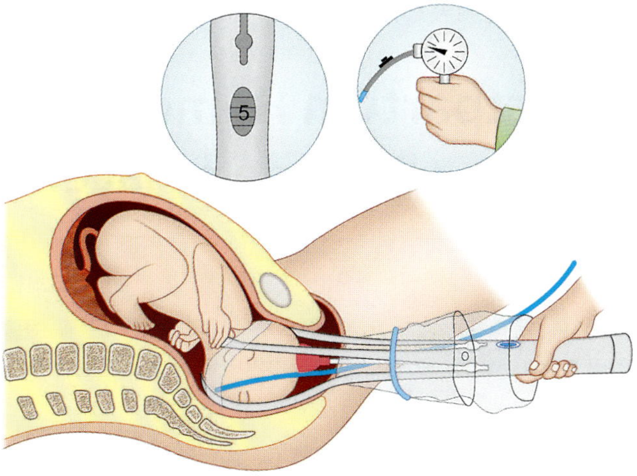

Fig. 70: Application of Odon device (diagrammatic).

is made of two components: (1) A polythene sleeve and (2) A plastic applicator (**Figs. 69**). Polythene sleeve looks like a plastic bag which is inserted with the help of the plastic applicator (inserter). The inserter has four pronged flexible spatulas arising from a handle. These spatulas surround the fetal head to place the sleeve in position. To verify the accurate depth of applicator it is provided with a progress indicator. With the sleeve there is a circumferential air chamber which is inflated around fetal head. Traction is given to pull, after the applicator inflating around the baby's head. The air chamber is supposed to minimize the pressure and its harm which is associated with the use of forceps. As there is no negative pressure which is implicated to cause hematoma formation associated with ventouse application is also eliminated with use of this device. It is claimed to be safer and simpler than forceps and vacuum extractor and a safe alternative of second stage cesarean section with limited surgical capacity and human resource constraints. Odon device was studied first on clinically indicated cases in prolonged second stage/fetal distress, etc. by the ASSIST study (October 2018 to April 2019). ASSIST II study is a follow-on clinical study to investigate the efficacy and safety of the device and also for making strategy for future study. Studies on Odon device so far indicate that this device does not pose higher risk than present obstetrics care. The Odon device has potential for wide application in resource poor settings even by mid-level providers. However, its safety and efficacy needs to be proved before wider applicability. The Odon Device is invented by Mr Jorge Odón, a car mechanic from Argentina.

CHAPTER 19

Postpartum Hemorrhage Including Retained Placenta

Learning Objectives

Postpartum Hemorrhage

- Types and Classification
- Etiology and Risk Factors (Predisposing Factors) for Obstetric Hemorrhages
- Causes of Primary Postpartum Hemorrhage
- Dangers of Postpartum Hemorrhage
- Measures to Prevent Death from Postpartum Hemorrhage
- Management of Atonic Postpartum Hemorrhage
- Pelvic Pressure Packing (Transvaginal)
- Internal Iliac Artery Ligation
- VP Paily's Vascular Clamps for Management of Postpartum Hemorrhage
- Samartha Ram's SR Vacuum Suction Cannula for the Management of Atonic Postpartum Hemorrhage
- Hysterectomy in Postpartum Hemorrhage
- Secondary Postpartum Hemorrhage
- Management of a Case of Secondary Postpartum Hemorrhage
- Oxytocics

Retained Placenta

- Causes of Retained Placenta
- Management of a Case of Retained Placenta
- Steps of Manual Removal of the Placenta

POSTPARTUM HEMORRHAGE

INTRODUCTION

Postpartum hemorrhage (PPH) complicates 1–10% of all deliveries [the International Federation of Gynecology and Obstetrics (FIGO), 2022]. PPH is a serious emergency and the leading cause of maternal morbidity and mortality in most countries of the world. It is the most common cause of maternal mortality which contributes more than one-fourth [29.6%—World Health organization (WHO)] of all maternal deaths worldwide. About 80,000 maternal deaths occurred due to PPH in 2015. The most tragic part is that majority of the deaths from PPH are preventable if timely and prompt interventions are taken.

DEFINITION

Postpartum hemorrhage is defined as bleeding from or inside the genital tract after delivery of the baby up to the end of the puerperium, the amount is such that it threatens the hemodynamic stability of the mother.

Any blood loss of >500 mL in vaginal delivery or >1,000 mL in cesarean section is classically called PPH. The American College of Obstetricians and Gynecologists (ACOG, 2017) defined PPH as blood loss of >1,000 mL or the amount of blood loss that was accompanied by signs or symptoms of hypovolemia within 24 hours of delivery irrespective of mode of delivery. Alternatively, PPH is defined as either a 10% drop in hematocrit (Hct) and/or need for red blood cell (RBC) transfusion (ACOG). The Royal College of Obstetricians and Gynecologists (RCOG, 2017) defined PPH as minor PPH (500–100 mL) and major PPH (>1,000 mL).

TYPES AND CLASSIFICATION

Postpartum hemorrhage is classified as primary PPH and secondary PPH.

Primary PPH: WHO defines primary PPH as blood loss of >500 mL following vaginal delivery or >1,000 mL following cesarean delivery in the first 24 hours of postpartum. Most primary PPH occurs within first 4 hours of delivery.

Third stage hemorrhage: Postpartum hemorrhage before the delivery of the placenta is called third stage hemorrhage. Third stage hemorrhage is included under primary PPH. *True postpartum hemorrhage* is the type of primary PPH which occurs following expulsion of placenta but within 24 hours of delivery of the baby (primary PPH after delivery of placenta).

Secondary PPH: Abnormal or excessive bleeding from the genital tract after 24 hours of delivery but within 6 weeks is called *secondary PPH*. Some authorities extend it to 12 weeks (ACOG, 2017). Secondary PPH is also called *late or delayed PPH* occurring from 24 hours to 12 weeks after delivery. *Late PPH* sometimes causes worrisome problems in 1% cases.

Classification of PPH According to the Amount of Blood Loss (Volume Deficit)

This can be done by *Benedetti's classification*:

- *Class 1:* <900 mL* (15% loss)—no symptoms and signs → no acute treatment is needed.
- *Class 2:* 1,200–1,500 mL (20–25% loss)—pulse↑, blood pressure (BP)↓, respiratory rate (RR)↑, no classic cold clammy extremities.
- *Class 3:* 1,800–2,100 (30–35% loss)—overt hypotension—severe tachycardia, cold clammy extremities.
- *Class 4:* 2,400 mL (40% loss)—profound shock, BP, and pulse difficult to record. This is called massive obstetric hemorrhage. If not managed urgently with volume replacement, case may be fatal.

For all practical purpose, *massive PPH* is defined as blood loss ≥1,500 mL after delivery and should be treated aggressively. It is seen in cases of severe abruption, fulminant hepatic failure due to acute fatty liver in pregnancy, hepatitis E infection, and sepsis.

Postpartum hemorrhage has been also classified as:

- *Minor PPH:* Blood loss 500–1,000 mL
- *Major PPH:* Blood loss >1,000 mL which is further subdivided into:
  - *Moderate:* 1,000–2,000 mL
  - Severe >2,000 mL.

Classification of PPH is done also according to rapidity of blood loss. When blood loss is >150 mL/min (>50% loss of blood volume within 20 minutes) or sudden blood loss of >1,500–2,000 mL (uterine atony, 25–35% loss), hemorrhage is classified as *severe hemorrhage*.

Estimation of Blood Loss

Estimation of blood loss is done by (a) visual method (qualitative) which is not accurate; (b) counting the pieces of blood-soaked cloths and subtracting these after weighing the swabs; (c) collection of blood in receptacles, such as in a bag, and adding the increased weight of sponges or linen; (d) using bedpan to collect blood and blood clots after drainage of liquor; (e) laboratory technique (photometric method)—blood pigment collected from the linen is converted to acid or alkaline hematin and compared with patient's blood; and (f) calculation of blood loss by colorimetric analysis using a tablet device camera, which is an emerging tool (Venkatesh 2020). Quantitative method for detection of severe hemorrhage is recognized by ACOG (2019).

Prevalence of Postpartum Hemorrhage

Prevalence of PPH is 1–10% of all deliveries. Incidence is double in cesarean delivery than vaginal. In Africa, prevalence is highest (5.1–25.7%) and it is 1.9–8% in Asia.

ETIOLOGY AND RISK-FACTORS (PREDISPOSING FACTORS) FOR OBSTETRIC HEMORRHAGES

- High risk patients—obesity, anemia, and chronic renal insufficiency
- Obstetric factors—antepartum hemorrhage, pre-eclampsia/eclampsia, history of PPH in previous pregnancy, and sepsis
- Defect in placentation—placenta previa, abruptio placentae, placenta accreta spectrum (PAS), ectopic pregnancy, hydatidiform mole
- Uterine atony (described later)
- Traumatic—injuries to birth canal (detailed later)
- *Coagulation disorders—itself or intensifying other causes*: Congenital coagulopathy, abruptio, acute fatty liver of pregnancy, HELLP syndrome, sepsis, massive transfusions, amniotic fluid embolism, prolonged intrauterine fetal death (IUFD), and intra-amniotic hypertonic saline-induced abortion.

The important causes of obstetric hemorrhages responsible for maternal death are placental abruption, retained placenta, uterine atony, laceration/rupture uterus, PAS, disseminated intravascular coagulation (DIC), ectopic pregnancy, abortion, and placenta previa.

CAUSES OF PRIMARY POSTPARTUM HEMORRHAGE

- Atonic PPH
- Traumatic PPH
- Partially retained placenta and fragments
- Coagulation disorder
- Mixed variety
- Placenta accreta.

Etiology of PPH is referred in "4Ts" mnemonic—(1) tone (poor uterine contraction after delivery), (2) trauma (to genital tract), (3) tissue (retained products of conception or blood clots), or (4) thrombin (coagulation abnormalities). Atonic uterus is the most common cause of PPH. It is responsible for 75–90% cases of primary PPH.

Atonic Postpartum Hemorrhage—Pathology and Predisposing Factors

Normally, following delivery of the placenta, hemostasis occurs by myometrial contraction which acts as

*Considering a 60-kg woman possesses 6,000 mL blood at 30 weeks gestation.

"physiological sutures" or "living ligature". Atonicity results in failure of the living ligature to stop bleeding.

Predisposing factors for atonic PPH:

- Overdistended uterus—multiple pregnancy, polyhydramnios, and macrocosmic baby
- Primipara and grand multipara
- Anemia and malnutrition
- Prolonged labor and precipitate labor
- Antepartum hemorrhage
- Induction or augmentation of labor
- Retained clots
- Uterine fibroids
- Uterine anomaly
- Prior history of atonic PPH
- Obesity
- Anesthesia specially halothane and regional with hypotension
- Mismanaged third stage of labor
- Chorioamnionitis.

Traumatic Postpartum Hemorrhage—Types and Predisposing Factors

Traumatic PPH contributes 10–20% of all PPH. The various types of trauma may be:

- Laceration of the cervix, vagina, and perineum (vulval hematoma), extension of episiotomy, and paraurethral tear
- Ruptured uterus
- Extension of cesarean section wound
- Broad ligament hematoma
- Uterine inversion.

Important predisposing factors for traumatic PPH are delivery through undilated cervix such as precipitate labor or delivery caused by excessive fundal pressure, instrumental delivery, occipitoposterior (face to pubis) delivery, delivery of large baby, and vaginal delivery after cesarean section.

Traumatic PPH is discussed in detail in Chapter 21.

Coagulation Disorder as a Cause of Postpartum Hemorrhage

This is a rare cause of PPH, may be acquired or inherited. Various acquired causes of coagulation disorder are placental abruption, severe preeclampsia, HELLP syndrome, abnormal placentation, uterine inversion, amniotic fluid embolism, massive blood transfusions, severe intravascular hemolysis, retention of dead fetus, sepsis, infection-associated hemophagocytic syndrome (IAHS), and anticoagulant therapy. Inherited disorders are von Willebrand disease, idiopathic thrombocytopenic purpura, and hemophilia.

DANGERS OF POSTPARTUM HEMORRHAGE

Postpartum hemorrhage contributes to 29.6% of all maternal deaths (WHO estimate). Various morbidities are shock, acute kidney injury, DIC, anemia, puerperal sepsis, Sheehan syndrome, and lactational failure.

Disseminated intravascular coagulation occurs in 25–35% cases in massive PPH. Hypoxic injury resulting liberation of tissue factors along with consumption of coagulation factors trigger DIC. Rapid transfusion of stored red cells which are usually deficient of coagulation factors leads to dilutional coagulopathy.

Sheehan syndrome is a pituitary failure due to massive intrapartum or early PPH, which is a rare complication. It is characterized by failure of lactation, amenorrhea, breast atrophy, loss of pubic and axillary hair, hypothyroidism, and adrenal cortical insufficiency. Earliest manifestation is lactation failure.

MEASURES TO PREVENT DEATH FROM POSTPARTUM HEMORRHAGE

Postpartum hemorrhage contributes more than one quarter of deaths (29.6%, WHO estimate). Majority of deaths occur within 24 hours of delivery. Most of the deaths can be avoided by (1) using prophylactic uterotonic [active management of the third stage of labor (AMTSL)] and (2) by timely and proper management of PPH (see below).

In majority of the cases, risk factors are not identified. The following measures will reduce the incidences of PPH or reduce the number of deaths due to PPH.

- Regular antenatal care (ANC)
- Correction of anemia
- Identification of high-risk cases
- Delivery in hospital with facility of emergency obstetric care (EmOC)
- Otherwise transport to the nearest large hospital at the earliest. Speedy transport available is kept. Large caliber needle is placed routinely during labor.
- *Routine active management of the third stage of labor.*
- Fourth stage of labor—observation, oxytocin
- Quick and effective application of first response *bundle* [uterotonics, uterine message, fluid replacement, and tranexamic acid (TXA)] in PPH.

Active Management of the Third Stage of Labor

Active management of the third stage of labor consists of interventions which facilitate the expulsion of the placenta by increasing uterine contractions to prevent PPH by averting uterine atony. AMTSL shortens the duration of the third stage about half and also reduces the blood loss by fifth.

Components of Active Management of the Third Stage of Labor

It consists of:

- Administration of *uterotonic agents* immediately (within 1 minute) after the birth of the baby. WHO updated the use of uterotonics for the prevention of PPH in 2018 which has been accounted in FIGO recommendation 2022.
- *Controlled cord traction* (CCT) by Brandt Andrew's method—should be done in settings where skilled birth attendants are available and contraindicated in settings without a skilled birth attendant.
- *Assessment of uterine tone* is done by abdominal palpation and if the uterus is not well contracted, uterine massaging is done. Continuous uterine massage after delivery of placenta is not routinely recommended now (WHO, 2012), where prophylactic oxytocin is given. Uterine massage helps to contract atonic uterus.

Late cord clamping (approximately 1–3 minutes after birth) is recommended. Early cord clamping (<1 minute after birth) is not recommended unless the newborn is asphyxiated and needs immediate resuscitation.

In summary, the main intervention within the (AMTSL) is the use of uterotonics.

FIGO recommendations for prevention of postpartum hemorrhage (2022): FIGO has released the updated recommendation for prevention of PPH in 2022 synthesizing updates of evidence from literature. Recommendations are summarized here.

- For all births, use of uterotonics is recommended during the third stage of labor to prevent PPH (WHO). 10 IU of *oxytocin* is administered intravenously or intramuscularly in both vaginal and cesarean delivery for prevention of PPH. Attention should be paid to the oxytocin cold chain.
- In settings where oxytocin is not available or the quality is not guaranteed the other injectable uterotonics (*ergometrine/methylergometrine 200 µg* intravenous/intramuscular (IM/IV) if appropriate; hypertensive disorders can be safely excluded prior to its use) or *oral misoprostol* (400–600 µg orally) or *carbetocin* 100 µg IM or IV is recommended for prevention of PPH (WHO).
- The *combinations of ergometrine with oxytocin* or *misoprostol with oxytocin* may be more effective uterotonic drug strategies compared with the current standard, oxytocin for prevention of PPH ≥500 mL. This is at the expense of adverse effects, vomiting and hypertension with ergometrine, and fever with misoprostol.
- The administration of misoprostol (400–600 µg orally) by community health workers and lay health workers is recommended for prevention in settings where skilled birth attendants are not present to administer injectable uterotonics and oxytocin is unavailable (WHO).
- Controlled cord traction is not recommended in settings where skilled birth attendants are unavailable (WHO).
- Continuous uterine massage is not recommended as a measure to prevent PPH in women who have been given prophylactic oxytocin (Cochrane Database Syst Rev. 2013)
- *Assessment of postpartum uterine tone* is done by abdominal palpation is recommended for all women for early identification of uterine atony (WHO).
- *Intravenous or intramuscular oxytocin* is the recommended method for removal of the placenta for prevention of the prevention of PPH in cesarean delivery.

As per WHO recommendation (2018), any of the oxytocics are administered within 1 minute of birth (a) oxytocin, (b) carbetocin, (c) misoprostol, (d) ergometrine/methylergometrine, or (e) oxytocin and ergometrine fixed-dose combination. Oxytocin (10 IU, IM/IV) is the recommended uterotonic agent (of choice) for the prevention of PPH for all births. Fixed-dose combination means oxytocin (5 IU) and ergometrine (500 µg) which is given intramuscularly.

Injectable prostaglandins are not recommended for the prevention of PPH.

Approach to a Case of PPH When Profuse Vaginal Bleeding Occurs after Expulsion of Placenta and Membranes Following a Term Delivery

Principles of management are:

- Immediate resuscitation—fluid replacement
- To detect the cause of bleeding
- Measures to control the bleeding

The priority is to stop the bleeding to prevent coagulation problems and organ damage by hypoperfusion. Conservative approaches should be tried first followed by rapid switching over to invasive procedures in failure (FIGO, 2022).

Sequences of the Steps of Management

- Always ask for help
- An IV channel is made with large caliber needle and IV fluid (crystalloids) like normal saline or ringer lactate is rapidly infused (with oxytocin as atonicity is the most common cause). Isotonic crystalloids are recommended in preference to the use of colloids for IV fluid resuscitation.
- Blood loss should be accurately assessed and crossmatch blood is given as quickly as possible. Colloids may be given till blood is available.
- Oxygen inhalation given at a rate of 10–15 L/min.
- Continuous catheterization of urinary bladder with Foley catheter is done. This will facilitate uterine contraction and urine output measurement will also be possible.

- Monitoring of vital parameters—blood pressure, pulse, respiration, oxygen saturation, urinary output, electrocardiogram (ECG), central venous pressure (CVP) measurement, maintenance of input and output chart, complete hemogram, blood grouping, coagulation profile, blood gas analysis, serum electrolytes, urea, and creatinine are sent.
- Examinations are done to find out the cause of bleeding (see below).
- Examination of the placenta and membranes are also done for their intactness (if available), and to know whether there are any left out portions inside the uterus.
- If the cause is uterine atonicity (as in majority of the cases), the procedures are done one after another (details given below) if the previous method fails are: (a) administration of uterotonic agents (medical methods); (b) mechanical methods like uterine massage and bimanual compression, uterine packing, and balloon tamponade; and (c) surgical methods—stepwise uterine devascularization, internal iliac artery ligation (IIAL), B-Lynch or brace suture, embolization of the uterine artery and internal iliac artery, and hysterectomy.
- If the cause seems to be traumatic, immediate exploration is done.

Detection of Cause of Bleeding

Hand is kept over the uterus to palpate it. If it is persistently relaxed and not well contracted, the cause of bleeding is *atonic* with or without associated trauma to genital tract. If the uterus is found contracted and still bleeding, the cause is probably *trauma to genital tract* and if the uterus is well contracted and following exploration no injury is found, the cause is likely to be *coagulopathy* which is very rarely encountered.

Assessment of Severity

Rule of 30

Rule of 30 has been proposed for the general acute management of PPH. If the patient's systolic blood pressure (SBP) drops by 30 mm Hg, heart rate (HR) increases by 30 beats/min, RR increases to >30 breaths/min, and a fall of 30% hemoglobin (approximately 3 g/L) or Hct drops by 30% and/or her urinary output is <30 mL/hour then the patient is most likely to have lost at least 30% of her blood volume and is in moderate shock leading to severe shock.

Shock Index

Reduction in tissue perfusion which is not sufficient to meet the metabolic demands of tissue and organs is called shock, which is clinically identified by lactic acidosis, altered mental status, oliguria, and tachycardia. Changes in vital signs do not occur till a large amount of bleeding occurs, in healthy postpartum mother it needs loss of >1,000 mL blood volume. The use of conventional vital signs (pulse and BP) lack accuracy for assessment of hypotension, but a simple combination of both of them gives an accurate information of hypovolemia, such as shock index (SI). SI refers to heart beat divided by the systolic BP. The normal value is 0.5–0.7, however, with significant hemorrhage it increases to 0.9–1.1. SI is valuable in monitoring and the general management of women with PPH. The change in SI of an individual patient appears to be a better correlation in identifying early acute blood loss than the HR, SBP, or diastolic blood pressure (DBP) used in isolation. SI has inverse linear relationship with left ventricular stroke work in acute circulatory failure. A threshold of SI ≥0.9 should be taught to the health worker in community level to transfer the patient to higher center.

The SI combined with the rule of 30 helps to determine the amount of blood loss and the degree of hemodynamic instability in an emergency.

The Golden Hour

The golden hour is the time at which resuscitation must be commenced to ensure the best chance of survival. The chance of survival decreases sharply after *the first hour* if the patient is not resuscitated effectively.

Volume Replacement and Treatment of Hypovolemia in General

Restore fluid balance: Choice of fluid is crystalloids before blood and blood products are available. Principle is to transfuse volume 2–3 times more than the estimated blood loss.

For the treatment of hypovolemia due to catastrophic hemorrhage compatible whole blood is the ideal but may not be readily available. Shelf life of whole blood is 24 days. 70% remain functioning for 24 hours after transfusion. 3–4 volume percent of Hct increases (equivalent to 1 g% Hb) for one unit of whole blood. After 5 units or more transfusion of RBC platelet count, clotting tests and fibrinogen should be evaluated. Massive transfusion means ≥4 units of PRBC, according to other it is ≥10 units of packed red blood cell (PRBC) in 24 hours or replacement of 50% blood in 3 hours. To replace coagulation factors in consumptive coagulopathy and transfusion are also needed in acute bleeding. The guideline is in the ratio of 1:1:1 of fresh frozen plasma (FFP), PRBC transfusion and platelets due to the resemblance with whole blood. It is done in multiple rounds, in each typical round consists 6 U PRBCs, 6UFFP, 6 U platelets, and 10 U cryoprecipitate and can be repeated. FFP is started immediately to correct coagulation in bleeding patient irrespective of Rh type. Cryoprecipitate in a dose of 10–15 mL/kg is given to correct hypofibrinogenemia, commonly found in DIC. At least 10 units of cryoprecipitate is needed when fibrinogen level is <100 mg/dL to raise >200 mg/dL.

MANAGEMENT OF ATONIC POSTPARTUM HEMORRHAGE

- Medical methods
- Nonsurgical mechanical methods
- Surgical methods

Medical Methods

- Intravenous *oxytocin* alone is the recommended uterotonic for treatment of PPH (FIGO 2022, WHO). Oxytocin infusion is given by adding 10 units in 500 mL of normal saline to start with 15 drops/min and rapidly increasing up to 60 drops/min, if still bleeding, 60 drops/min is continued for till 1,000 mL is infused, then followed by 40 drops/min, another 1,000 mL as maintenance dose. Not >3 L of IV fluid containing oxytocin is given.

  In 24 hours not >100 units oxytocin is administered.

  If IV oxytocin is not available or bleeding continues IV ergometrine, oxytocin—ergometrine fixed dose, or a prostaglandin drug including sublingual misoprostol (800 μg) is given (FIGO 2022, WHO).
- Methergine 0.2 mg or ergometrine 0.25 mg are given IV and may be repeated after 15 minutes if not contraindicated like severe hypertension and then can be repeated 4 hourly.
- Injection *15 methyl PGF2α* (250 μg) is given intramuscularly (*never intravenously*). It can be repeated every 90 minutes or earlier but not before 15 minutes. It can be given a maximum of 8 doses. But in repeated doses it may cause diarrhea, vomiting, tachycardia, and pyrexia. Before administration history of bronchial asthma is taken as it precipitates bronchospasm and is contraindicated in a patient with bronchial asthma. It can also be given intramyometrially.
- *Misoprostol* [methyl ester of prostagladin E1 (PGE1)] can be given sublingually up to a maximum of 800 μg. There is no evidence of safety and efficacy of additional 800 μg of misoprostol if already 800 μg given prophylactically. ACOG (2019) recommends 600–1,000 μg orally, sublingually, or rectally.

  Dinoprostone, a PGE2 suppository 20 mg can be used as off-label per rectum or per vagina repeated every 2 hours. One adverse effect is diarrhea which is problematic for rectal use. Prostagladin E2, sulprostone is used intravenously in some country.
- Intravenous *TXA* is recommended early as soon as PPH is diagnosed but within 3 hours of birth in addition to standard care of PPH following vaginal birth or cesarean delivery. Dose is 1 g (100 mg/mL) IV at 1 mL/min (i.e., administered over 10 mL), followed by a second dose of 1g IV if bleeding continues after 30 minutes, or if bleeding restarts within 24 hours of the first dose.

Details of the Oxytocics and TXA are discussed at the end of this chapter.

Postpartum Hemorrhage Bundle Care

Postpartum hemorrhage bundle care is the multimodal strategies that involve multiple intervention points and actions called "bundles" to control mortality from pathologies like PPH. The bundle consists of four action domains: (1) readiness, (2) recognition and prevention, (3) response, and (4) reporting and systems learning comprising total 13 key elements.

WHO (2017) developed bundles care of PPH in 2017 and defined two care bundles: (1) First response PPH bundle and (2) Response to refractory PPH bundle.

First response PPH bundle is comprised of administration of uterotonic drugs, isotonic crystalloids, TXA, and application of uterine massage. Fluid resuscitation and IV administration of uterotonics are performed simultaneously. In unavailability of IV uterotonic sublingual misoprostol or other parenteral uterotonics are given along with fluid resuscitation. In case of retained placenta, placenta is removed and a single dose of antibiotics is given. Lacerations, if any are repaired.

Response to refractory PPH bundle is compressive measures (aortic compression or bimanual uterine compression), intrauterine balloon tamponade (UBT), and NASG. Uterotonics (e.g., oxytocin diluted in isotonic crystalloids) are continued and a second dose of TXA is administered along with this bundle.

It must be assured that first response PPH bundle is implemented at both the primary healthcare facility and hospital levels. Incorporation of the PPH bundle care approach in the management of PPH is recommended by FIGO (2022).

Nonsurgical Mechanical Methods

When bleeding is not controlled by medical management, following mechanical procedures are recommended (FIGO, 2022).

(1) Uterine massage; (2) Bimanual uterine compression; (3) Uterine balloon tamponade with a Sengstaken-Blakemore tube, Bakri balloon, or Rusch hydrostatic balloon catheter or condom inside the uterus (after ruling out retained products and uterine rupture); (4) Uterine artery and internal iliac artery embolization—if facility available, besides (5) External aortic compression as a temporary measure; and (6) Nonpneumatic antishock garment, especially if transfer is required are effective lifesaving measures; (7) Uterine packing, an age old procedure is not recommended for the treatment of PPH for uterine atony following vaginal birth (FIGO 2022, WHO).

If bleeding does not stop using uterotonic and other available nonsurgical mechanical methods surgical intervention is recommended (FIGO 2022, WHO).

Surgical Methods

Various surgical procedures to arrest bleeding in uterine atony are: (1) Stepwise uterine devascularization, (2) Internal iliac artery ligation, (3) Compression sutures including B-Lynch or brace suture (1997) and "Cho multiple square" suturing technique, cervicoisthmal suture, Cho circular sutures, and (4) Hysterectomy as a last resort.

Bimanual Compression of Uterus for Uterine Atony (Fig. 1)

Uterine massaging is the first action to prevent atony and PPH. If not sufficient enough with simple massaging even after uterotonics bimanual compression is done.

One hand is made into fist and introduced into the vagina by separating the labia and pressing the uterus through the anterior fornix. The other hand fixes the uterus abdominally and massages the posterior aspect of the uterus. Thus, uterus is firmly pressed in between the two hands. This compression is done for a prolonged period.

This method is a very effective first-line measure to reduce bleeding. If bleeding is not controlled by oxytocic, bimanual compression is done.

Packing of the Uterus (Fig. 2)

Tight intrauterine packing with about 5 m long gauze is given under previously given epidural anesthesia or IV sedation and can be done in labor room. General anesthesia is seldom needed.

The gauze is soaked in antiseptic solution and introduced in high-up position of the uterus completely and uniformly starting from fundus to downward and from side to side without leaving any dead space for blood to accumulate. Technique of insertion is very important for efficacy. Intrauterine insertion with single thirst is not effective. Instead after unrolling, the gauze is evenly placed with the help of sponge holding forceps with repeated thrust in all aspects of uterus. If more than one roller gauze is needed knot to be secured tightly. A separate pack is used for the vagina. Not more than few minutes are needed for the entire procedure. Following insertion soakage of the pack is observed. In case of failure, bleeding through the gauze occurs immediately after insertion. Normally, in case of success, gauze is soaked with blood but there will be no trickle of blood externally other than mild soakage.

It is kept for 24–36 hours following which it is removed. The gauze is removed slowly. Before removal of the pack patient should be hemodynamically stable, for which removal can be delayed balancing the risk of infection.

Uterine packing can be useful for women both who have delivered abdominally and vaginally. In case of placenta previa, it is useful after placental removal. It is helpful for transferring a patient to a reference center, when surgical treatment either not available or the patient is unsuitable for surgery for the time being.

Broad-spectrum antibiotic is given and continued till the pack is not removed.

It is a simple, safe, and useful procedure to control PPH in appropriate circumstances. The disadvantage is that it might conceal ongoing hemorrhage and it may also cause infection. In properly performed packing, concealed hemorrhage is unlikely. Uterine packing is not effective in fibroid uterus, müllerian anomaly where uterine cavity is distorted and is not a good choice in presence of infection.

Packing is practiced in PPH since 1800 AD.

The uterine packing is not recommended (FIGO 2022, WHO) for the treatment of PPH due to uterine atony after vaginal birth (weak recommendation).

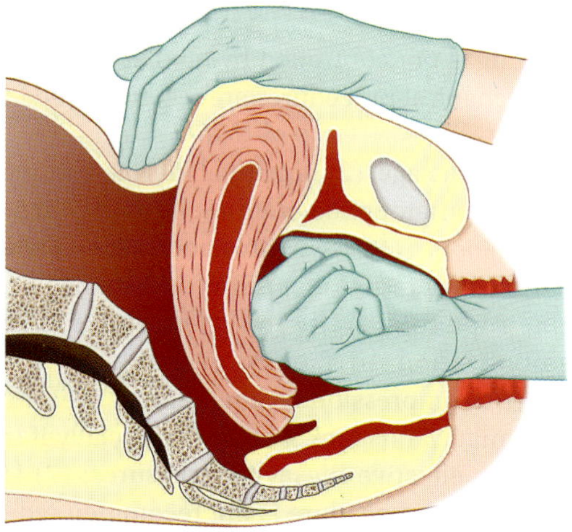

Fig. 1: Bimanual compression of uterus. Note that one hand is in the anterior fornix and other hand over the posterior aspect of uterus.

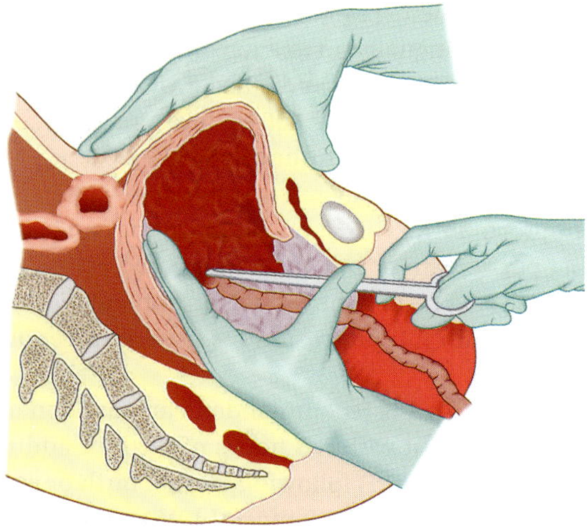

Fig. 2: Packing of uterus with gauze.

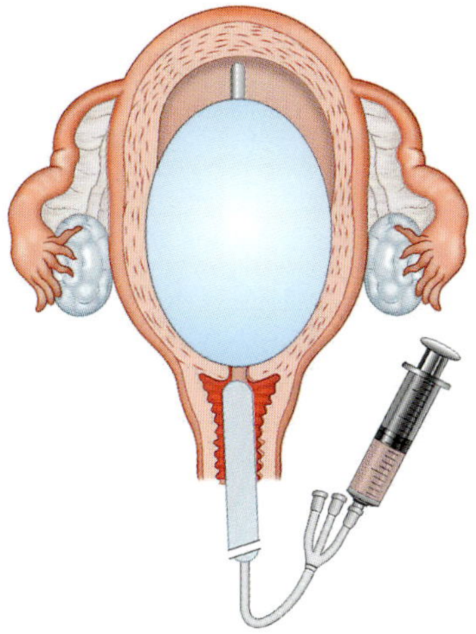

Fig. 3: Sengstaken–Blakemore tube diagrammatic placement.

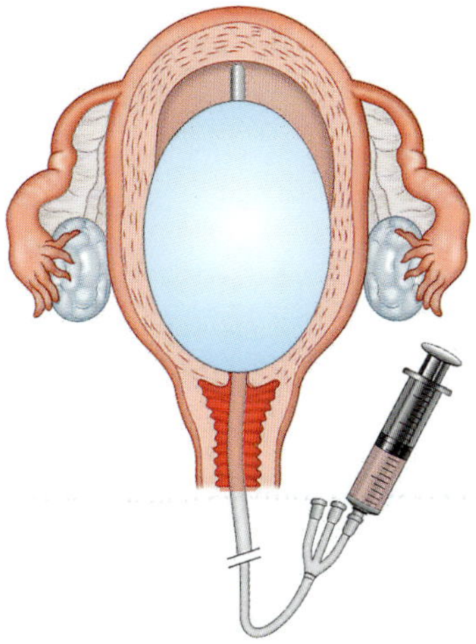

Fig. 4: Bakri balloon diagrammatic placement.

Uterine Balloon Tamponade

The concept of balloon tamponade is not new. Foley catheter is used for many years after inflation of bulb with normal saline. Later various devices are introduced for this purpose. UBT devices can be divided in two groups: (1) Fixed volume devices such as condom uterine balloons, Bakri balloon, Rusch balloon, and Ebb system and (2) Free flow devices such as the glove balloon, Ellavi UBT, and Zukowski balloon. They allow intrauterine pressure control according to SBP.

The mechanism how the UBT works is likely multi-factorial. Device stimulates the receptors which in turn stimulates uterine contraction and by applying hydrostatic pressure directly against the bleeding sinuses.

Sengstaken-Blakemore esophageal catheter **(Fig. 3)** is inserted inside the uterine cavity and inflated with 75–500 mL warm saline. The tube is usually kept for 24 hours. It is effective to control hemorrhage like intra-uterine plugging, and success varies between 70 and 100%.

Rusch hydrostatic balloon or *Bakri* balloon **(Figs. 4 and 5)** has also been used with great success. Bakri balloon device consists of a silicon catheter with a balloon of 500 mL capacity. It may be placed under ultrasound guidance. Displacement and expulsion may occur occasionally. However, it may not be affordable in resource-poor countries.

Multiple Foley catheter (5–6 in number) inflated with normal saline is still used. Foley catheter 24 F to 30 F with 30 mL balloon is introduced and inflated with 60–80 mL normal saline. As there is rupture of balloon with 50 mL 34 F Foley catheter with 60 mL balloon is safer use.

Catheter fitted with *condom* (Bangladesh) is a good choice for resource poor countries (see below).

Prophylactic antibiotic using cefazolin 1 g 8 hourly is given till the removal.

Intrauterine balloon tamponade is an effective non-surgical technique in context of PPH bundle care and improves survival of women with refractory PPH.

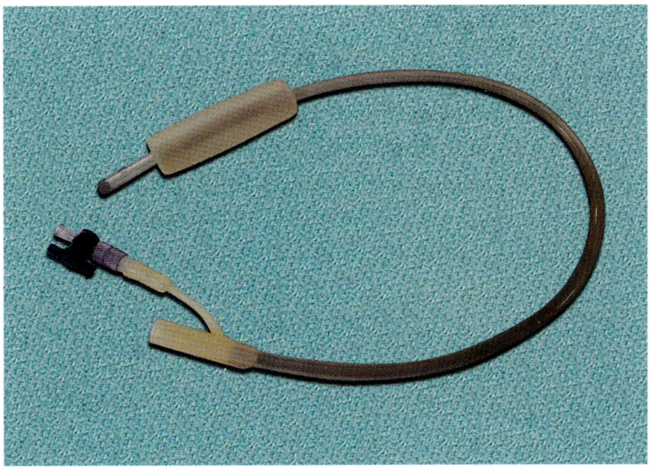

Fig. 5: Bakri balloon.

Tamponade Test

Sengstaken-Blakemore esophageal catheter is inserted in uterine cavity and inflated. If no or minimal bleeding is observed through the cervix, or in the gastric lumen of the catheter, surgical intervention is avoided. This is called "tamponade test". If significant bleeding continues, it means the tamponade test has failed and laparotomy is performed. The tamponade test has a positive predictive value >87% in PPH management.

Condom emponade technique: A condom is inflated with isotonic saline through a rubber catheter, and is used to create tamponade (**Fig. 6**) within the uterus to arrest massive PPH. A sterile catheter is inserted within the condom and tied near the mouth of the condom with a silk thread, and the outer end of the catheter is connected to a saline set. Cervical lips are held by sponge holding forceps. Fitted condom is inserted inside the uterus. The mouth of cervix and vagina is then packed by ribbon gauge pack or sterile sanitary pads to prevent slippage of condom from the uterine cavity. Normal

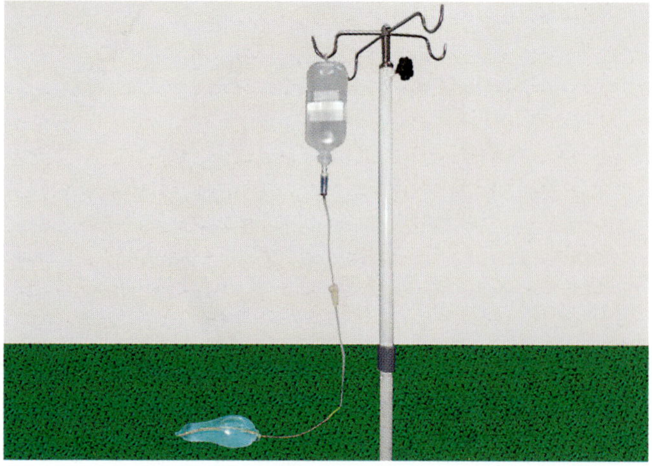

Fig. 6: Condom tamponade.

saline is allowed to pass inside the uterine cavity from height to inflate the uterine cavity initially by 250–500 mL of fluid.

In severe atony, even 1,500 mL of saline may be needed and can be introduced without any harm. When flow of saline stops, saline bottle is compressed to push saline in pressure. Feeling of resistance indicates formation of tamponade. Cessation of bleeding indicates positive temponade test. Then outer end of catheter is folded and tied after detaching from saline set when bleeding has ceased. In most of the cases bleeding stops within 0–15 minutes. Vulval pad is applied tightly. Patient's vital signs are monitored, oxytocin IV infusion continued for at least 6 hours and antibiotic is administered. Condom catheter is kept for 24 hours and sometimes for 48 hours when deflation is done gradually and stepwise and not suddenly at a time. Finally, pack and catheter with condom is removed. This method is cheap, simple and quick intervention which may prove invaluable in, especially, in resource-poor countries.

Other than atonic PPH, UBT is used in molar-pregnancy associated hemorrhage, placenta accreta, placenta previa, cervical pregnancy, and uncontrolled bleeding from lacerations by placing over vagina and cervix. Other than vaginal delivery, UBT is used after cesarean delivery.

External Aortic Compression (Fig. 7)

Compression of aorta as a temporary measure is an effective method to reduce blood loss. With a closed fist downward pressure is applied over the aorta (a point just above and left to the umbilicus where aortic pulsation is felt) through the abdominal wall, with the other hand femoral artery is palpated to check adequacy of compression **(Fig. 8)**. If the pressure is adequate, the femoral pulse is not palpable. Compression is maintained until bleeding is controlled or alternative measures can be taken. This is very useful in thin patients.

Aortic compression by an assistant is also effective method during surgical procedure (in laparotomy) to prevent blood loss and allowing surgeon providing more time to work with a drier field specially in managing cases like morbidly adherent placenta.

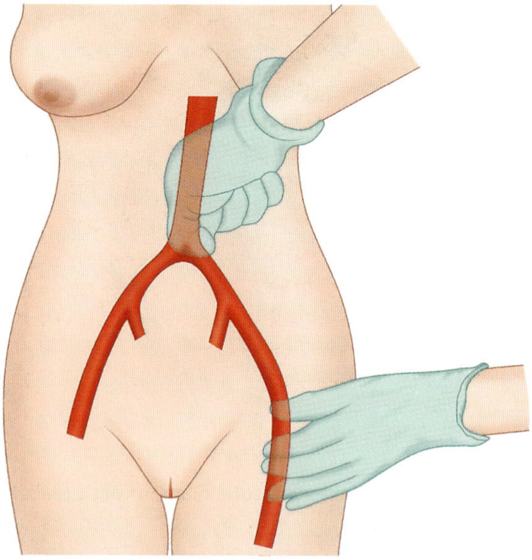

Fig. 7: External aortic compression—compression of abdominal aorta by right feast and palpation of femoral pulse by left fingers. Courtesy: Arunima Majhi, NIFT, Kolkata.

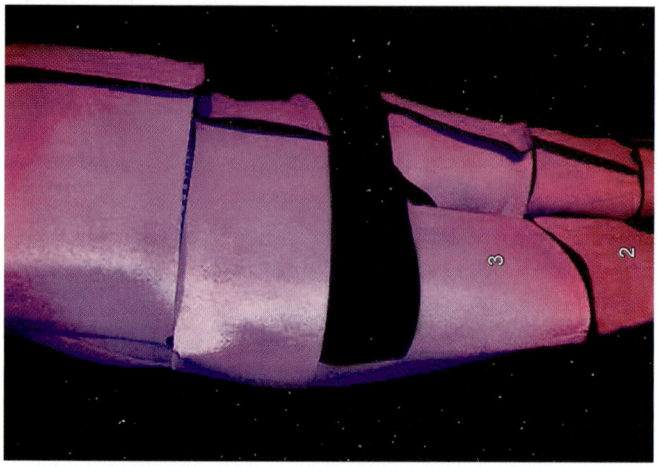

Fig. 8: Non-pneumatic anti-shock garment (NASG).
Courtesy: Dr Sheela Mane, Bengaluru, Karnataka, India.

Nonpneumatic Antishock Garment (NASG) (Fig. 8)

The NASG is nonpneumatic antishock garment that is made up of neoprene used in patients with severe PPH.

Nonpneumatic antishock garment is indicated in patients with PPH developing clinical signs or laboratory findings compatible with shock or hemodynamic instability. It is used as a temporary measure to recover hemodynamic stability for the management and *safe transfer of severe ill patient* to higher centers for a long distance.

The garment can exert 30–40 mm Hg of circumferential counter pressure over the lower extremity from the ankles up to the level of the diaphragm by using the three-way elasticity of neoprene and the tight grip of the Velcro fasteners. This pressure helps in shunting blood from lower extremity to the vital organs.

There are six articulated segments (1–6 from below upward) in the NASG. The three segments cover the lower extremities, independent and bilateral: ankles, calves, and thighs. The upper three circumferential segments are placed over the pelvic and abdominal areas. Initially, it is unfolded and placed behind the patient's body. For proper fitness the upper margin of superior segment (segment 6) over the lower rib is confirmed. Each segment is applied by stretching and closing as tightly as possible starting from the ankle with segment 1 and continued with the successive segments one after another. However abdominal part is not binded too tightly to maintain adequate respiration. The garment can be adjusted to all heights and sizes, like in short height patient segment 1 can be folded over segment 2 to put the first segment over the ankle. It is desirable that both knees are uncovered by the leg segments to maintain joint mobility. Symphysis pubis is used an anatomical reference point for placement of segment 4 and umbilicus as placing of segments 5 and 6. Abdominal segments may need to be loosened, not completely opened if signs of respiratory distress are observed. In case of need of urgent surgical intervention, abdomen and pelvic segments are temporarily opened keeping the leg segments closed. Hypotension may be expected during this procedure which can be tackled with appropriate procedures.

The device can be kept for up to 48 hours until control of bleeding or hemodynamic stability is achieved. During the NASG use, the patient is closely monitored for HR, BP, and optimal fluid resuscitation. For safe removal, some criteria are maintained, e.g., blood loss, <50 mL/hour. Heart rate is <100 beats/min and systolic BP is ≥100 mm Hg (rule of 100) at least for 2 hours. The segments are opened in the same sequence of starting. That said, first segment will be opened first, ending with 6. After opening of each segment 15 minutes time is allowed to reassess the vital signs before opening the next. If HR increases by 20 beats/min and systolic BP drops by 20 mm Hg and fresh bleeding starts, all the segments are quickly closed. It takes about 1 hour 15 minutes for removal of whole garment. After removal NASG is placed in a biohazard container for send to cleaning, drying, and refolding. It is washable, reusable (50 times) and light weighted.

Selective Arterial Embolization (Interventional Radiology)

In 1979, Brown first reported the method of angiographically guided arterial embolization for the treatment of PPH. Selective arterial embolization can be done alternative to laparotomy or hypogastric artery ligation. High success (85–95%) has been claimed using this method.

Indications are uterine atony (in most of the cases), vaginal wall hematoma, broad ligament, and retroperitoneal hematoma, abdominal pregnancy, placental abnormality including placenta accreta, and obstetrics hysterectomy hemorrhage. Angiographic embolization may be indicated either before delivery, in cases of placental abnormality, or after delivery in hemorrhagic patient.

Uterine artery or internal iliac artery embolization is usually done through the femoral artery catheterization. Under local anesthesia, femoral artery catheterization is done and anatomy of pelvic vessels and site of hemorrhage are detected by an angiogram in fluoroscopic guidance. Bleeding vessel is catheterized selectively and occluded. Contrast media at extravascular site and blush appearance indicates bleeding area. Anterior division of internal artery is occluded alternatively.

Various embolizing agents are used. For larger vessel metal wire coils and for small vessels absorbable gelatine sponge, polyurethane foam or polyvinyl alcohol particles are used for short-term occlusion of 10–20 days. Metal oil coils are made of steel or platinum of various sizes and may be provided with fibers for thrombus formation and are used for permanent occlusion. Micro coils are also available for small vessels.

It should be the choice of treatment prior to surgical intervention. Collateral circulation preserves the uterine function. Internal artery ligation works by reduction of pulse pressure but embolization directly blocks the specific bleeding vessels. No general or regional anesthesia is needed and morbidity is less than surgical occlusive methods.

It needs interventional radiological setup and expert which may not be available in emergency and need to transfer the patient to radiology department which is the most disadvantage. Surgical approach is better to radiological interventional in life-threatening PPH. Femoral puncture is contraindicated in coagulopathy. Important complications, though rare, are uterine necrosis due to ischemia, for which hysterectomy may be needed and the other is massive buttock necrosis. In internal artery embolization following PPH future fertility is not severely hampered. Uterine artery embolization is a relatively safe technique where preservation of fertility is priority.

PELVIC PRESSURE PACKING (TRANSVAGINAL) (FIG. 9)

Following a postpartum hysterectomy or in case of placenta percreta or abdominal pregnancy sometimes control of bleeding becomes difficult with diathermy coagulation or with sutures. In these situations, pelvic pressure packing is a lifesaving measure. This concept and method was originally described by Logothetopulos (1926) following which several workers have described its successful use with little variable technique. Several cloth laparotomy mops (sponges) tied together or multiple (8–10) roller gauzes tied end to end are packed in any bag like X-ray cassette bag made of plastic or plastic instrument bag. The ends of the sponges or roller gauzes should be protruded for accessibility through the vaginal cuff opening or separate opening in POD. After tying the vaginal end is connected with any weight, like 1 L of filled IV fluid bottle by a tube and is allowed to hang toward the foot end of the bed. This umbrella or "parachute pack" **(Fig. 9)** will arrest bleeding by pressure by the weight of the fluid bottle. The pack is removed after 24–48 hours through the vagina during which period the patient is expected to be clinically stable. This method is seldom done today, but is a lifesaving procedure when all other methods fail and particularly useful in low resource setting (Obstet Gynecol Survey 2018).

Surgical Treatment

Uterine Artery Ligation

For control of PPH uterine artery ligation has been known from 1960. It is very simple, fertility preserving surgery and can be done rapidly. To do uterine artery ligation the suture is given at the junction of the upper and lower uterine segment 2 cm medial to the uterine artery *through myometrium* **(Fig. 10)**.

Bilateral uterine artery ligation is effective in 70–80% cases of uterine atony.

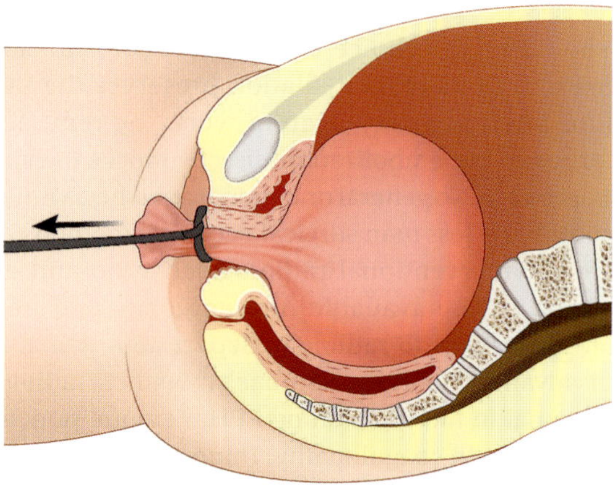

Fig. 9: Pelvic pressure pack (transvaginal).

Uterine artery versus Internal Iliac Artery Ligation

Nineteen percent of the blood supply of uterus in pregnancy is from uterine arteries. Uterine artery ligation should be attempted prior to IIAL if bleeding is from the uterus. Uterine artery ligation is technically easier and associated with less morbidity.

Stepwise Uterine Devascularization (Fig. 10)

Stepwise uterine devascularization was first reported in Egypt. It is effective in controlling PPH in 80% of the cases. Devascularization is done in the following sequences:

- Unilateral uterine vessel ligation at the upper part of lower uterine segment
- Uterine vessels ligation on both sides
- Ligation of low uterine vessel to include the cervicovaginal branches and the vaginal artery (independent branch of internal iliac artery) after pushing the bladder down and avoiding ureteric injury (may need more than one stitches)
- Unilateral ovarian vessel ligation (near utero-ovarian anastomosis)
- Bilateral ovarian vessels ligation
- Unilateral or bilateral IIAL may become necessary as a further step to stop massive PPH.

INTERNAL ILIAC ARTERY LIGATION

Ligation of internal iliac artery was first performed by Kelly in 1894 and an effective strategy in controlling obstetric hemorrhages to save the life of the mother and also to prevent maternal morbidity. Sometimes it is also performed in some

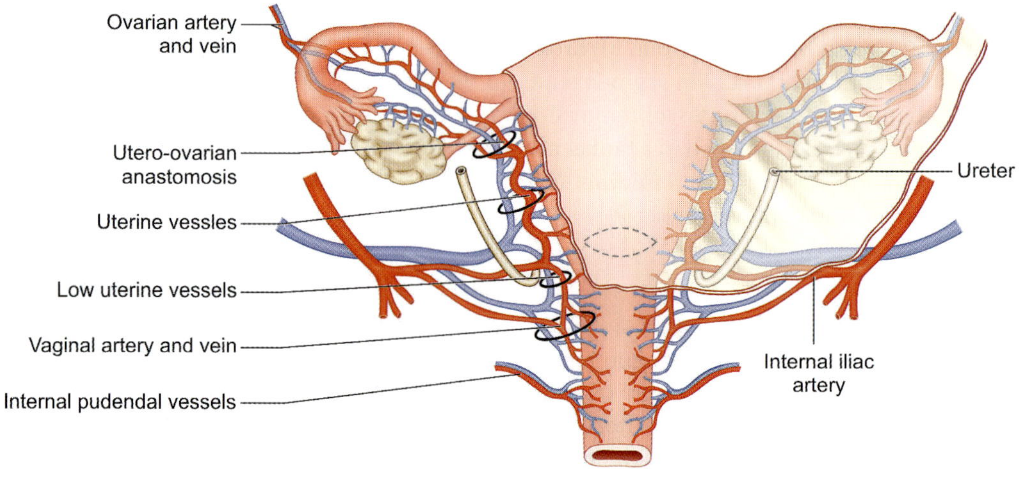

Fig. 10: Stepwise devascularization (view from behind the uterus).

gynecological conditions. In spite of its efficacy in controlling hemorrhage, this method is unused due to the apprehension of adjacent structures injury (vessels and ureter).

Indications of Internal Iliac Artery Ligation

Internal iliac artery ligation is indicated in uterine atony, midline perforation, large broad ligament or lateral pelvic hematoma, multiple cervical tears, lower segment bleeding (placenta previa), abruptio placentae, and placenta accreta. It is less effective in placenta accreta. In uterine atonic PPH, it avoids hysterectomy and in traumatic PPH it clears the operative field to facilitate hysterectomy.

Mechanism of Controlling Hemorrhage

The outcome of bilateral IIAL is 85% reduction in pulse pressure in the arteries distal to the tie, and this converts an arterial pressure system into one with pressure that approaches those in the venous circulation and results hemostasis by simple clot formation. It reduces pelvic blood flow by 50%. After ligation of internal iliac artery, collateral circulation is established within 45–60 minutes and hemostasis are achieved by this time.

Effectiveness and Advantages of Internal Iliac Artery Ligation

It is successful in controlling hemorrhage in between 40 and 100% cases (FIGO, 2022). It is particularly useful in traumatic PPH (like rupture of uterus). It has no adverse effect on subsequent fertility and pregnancy outcome. This procedure should always be considered for women who are very young and nullipara to preserve the uterus.

Internal iliac artery ligation is commonly done in both sides (bilateral) particularly in cases of atonic PPH and can be done unilateral in broad ligament hematoma, by which only ipsilateral blood flow can be minimized.

Steps of Internal Iliac Ligation (Figs. 11 to 18)

This can be done in two approaches, (1) anterior and (2) posterior. In anterior approach, peritoneum is opened in between round ligament and infundibulopelvic ligament to reach the retroperitoneal space. In posterior approach, retroperitoneal space is reached behind the infundibulopelvic ligament. Posterior approach is relatively easier.

In anterior approach, an 8–10 cm incision is made on the peritoneum with fine scissor gently after lifting the loose peritoneum, lateral and parallel to ureter at the level of sacral promontory/sacroiliac joint. Ureter enters into the pelvis by crossing over the bifurcation of common iliac artery or the proximal part of external iliac artery and lying medial to ovarian vessels and is retroperitoneal. It follows the course of internal iliac artery for a short distance slightly in front and medial to it until it passes near the ischial spine where it changes its direction. The peritoneum flap is retracted medially along with the ureter attached to it.

Common iliac artery is found to bifurcate into external iliac artery which goes laterally along the psoas and internal iliac artery which lies medially and slight posteriorly **(Fig. 11)**. These vessels are identified by palpation of pulsation. The loose areolar tissue **(Fig. 12)** in front of external iliac artery, external iliac vein, internal iliac artery, and internal iliac vein (from lateral to medial) is cleared off with the peanut sponge stick (small galley). Internal iliac artery is exposed clearly 5 cm distally. A common thin fascia lies in front of external iliac vein, internal iliac artery, and internal iliac vein. Clearing fascia in between the vessels to make cleavage between the vessels will ease the introduction of the tips of Mixter right-angle clamp. Tip of the small curve artery forceps (or any other instrument like lymph node dissector) may be used very gently to make the cleavage. The forceps is kept parallel to vessels and horizontal and the tip should be more toward the surface of internal iliac artery to avoid injury of thin venous wall. Now the right-angle clamp **(Figs. 13 and 14)** is passed beneath the artery at a distance 2–3 cm from the bifurcation. This can also be done with the help of aneurism needle **(Fig. 15)** with preloaded sutures. A nonabsorbable suture (like silk, 0 or 1) is grasped by the tips of right-angled clamp or by aneurism needle **(Figs. 16 to 18)** with preloaded sutures, which passed beneath the artery and double ligated without division of the artery. Instead of double ligatures few surgeons do single ligature. In ligation of internal iliac artery below 2–3 cm from origin, posterior

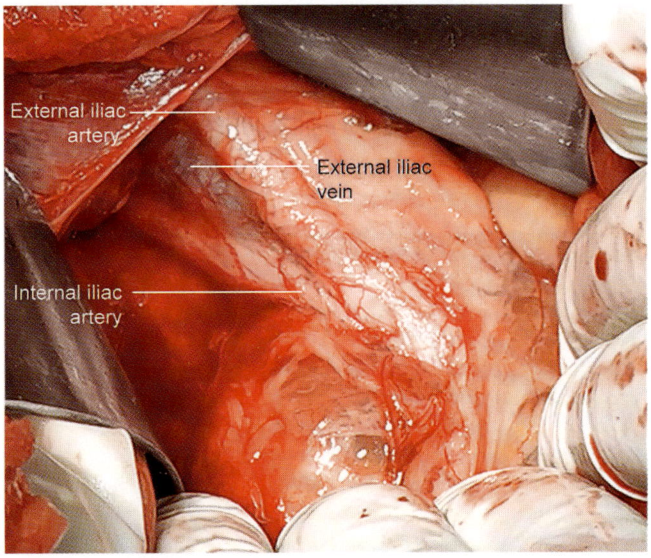

Fig. 11: Relation of the iliac vessels (right side). Common iliac artery is found to bifurcate into external iliac artery which goes laterally along the psoas and internal iliac artery which lies medially and slight posteriorly. External iliac vein lies between the external iliac artery and internal iliac artery. Internal iliac vein lies just medial and along with internal iliac artery is not visible here. Ureter along with the medial flap of peritoneum is retracted medially and not visible.

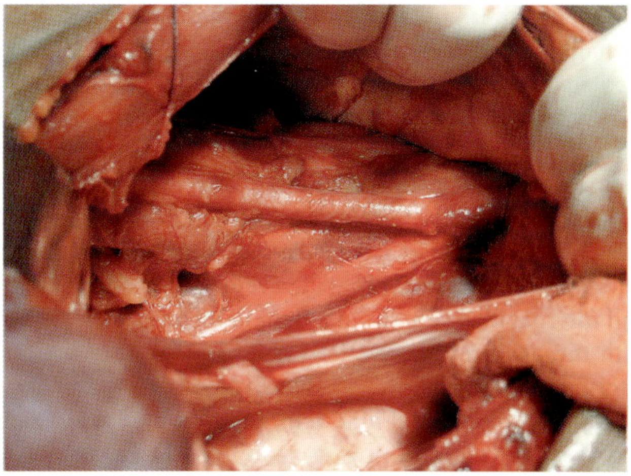

Fig. 12: Loose areolar tissue in front of external iliac artery, external iliac vein, internal iliac artery, and internal iliac vein from lateral to medial (right side) should be cleaned.

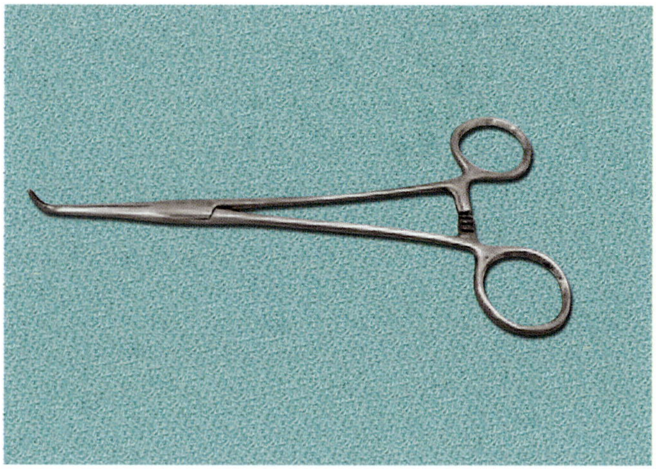

Fig. 13: Right-angled forceps (Meigs–Navratil forceps).

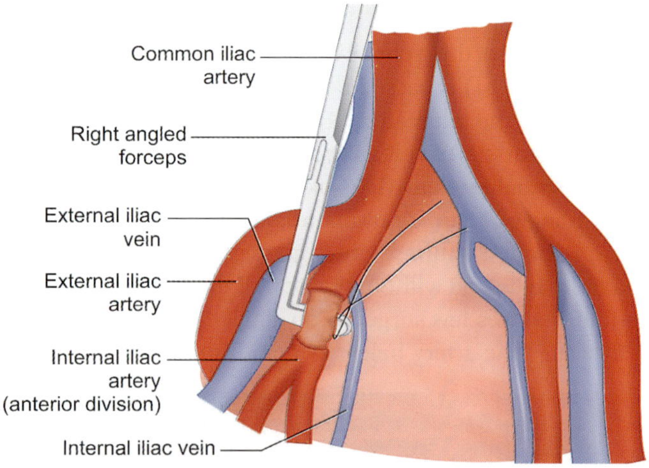

Fig. 14: Diagrammatic figure of internal iliac artery ligation on both side using right-angled forceps.

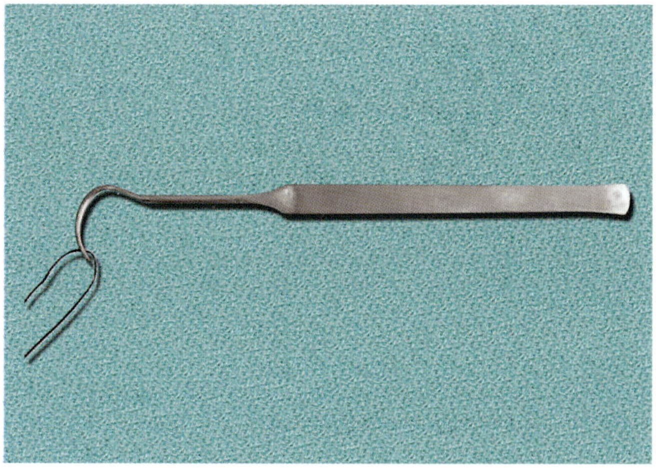

Fig. 15: Aneurysm needle with thread.

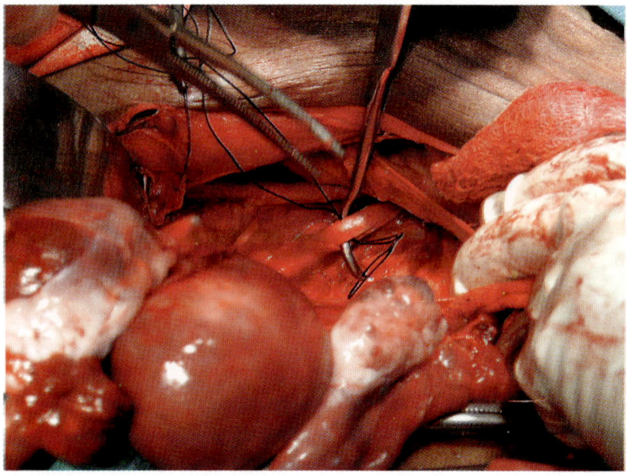

Fig. 16: Aneurysm needle with thread is passed behind the right internal iliac artery.

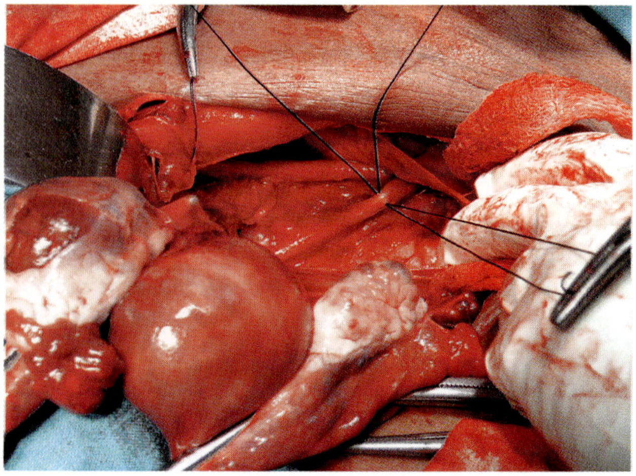

Fig. 17: Aneurysm needle is withdrawn leaving the threads.

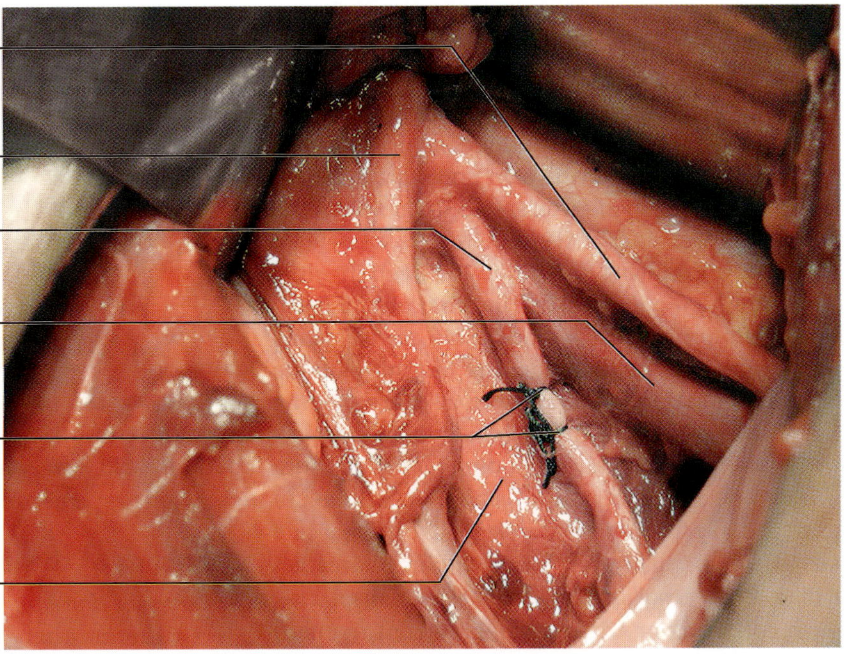

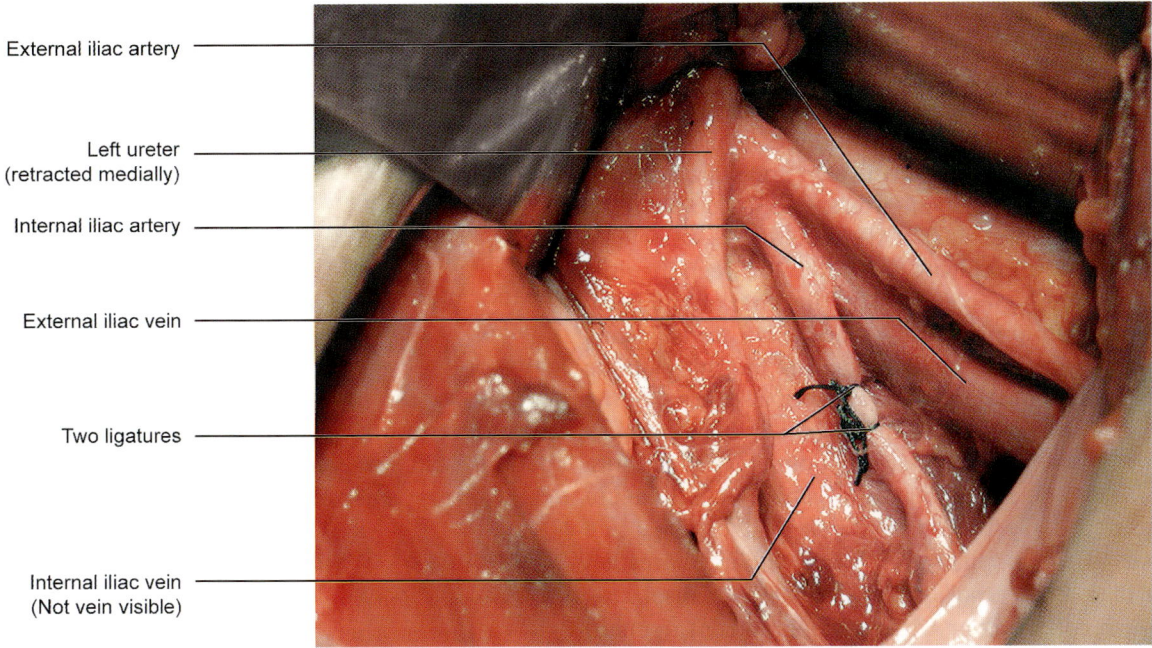

Fig. 18: Ligation of internal iliac artery I (left side) with double ligature is shown.

division will be escaped. Femoral pulse over the inguinal region and arterial dorsalis pedis over the dorsum of foot on respective side should be palpated before and after ligation to make assured that external iliac artery is not wrongly ligated.

Complications of Internal Artery Ligation and Prevention

- *Injury to internal iliac vein and external iliac vein:* Laceration may occur during exposure of the place or during passage of right-angle clamp. Severe hemorrhage may occur, may be difficult to control, catastrophy may occur specially in injury of external iliac vein and help of vascular surgeon is sought. Injury by the right-angled clamp can be prevented by keeping the tip against the artery and elevating it during its introduction. Passage of the clamp from lateral to medial is suggested in order to avoid injury to external iliac vein. Lateral to medial or medial to lateral which one is better remains disputed. However, beginners should perform from lateral to medial **(Fig 14)** to avoid injury to large external iliac vein.
- *Inadvertent ligation of external iliac artery:* This can be prevented by careful identification of the arteries from bifurcation of external iliac artery and palpation of femoral pulse and arterial dorsalis pedis before and after ligation.
- *Injury to ureter:* It is avoided by identifying the ureter by seeing the peristalsis of a tubular structure and retracting it medially along with the peritoneum flap.
- Very rarely, ischemic damage to the pelvis with lower motor neuron damage results weakness of lower extremities.

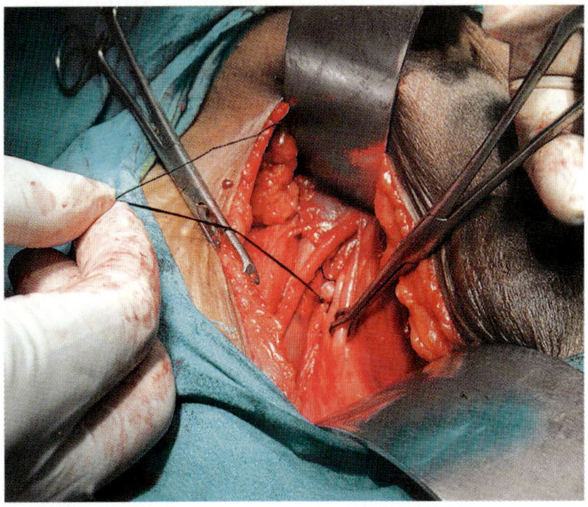

Fig. 19: Internal artery ligation through extraperitoneal approach. Internal iliac artery is double ligated with silk thread. Ureter is shown by Babcock's tissue forceps in the medial peritoneal flap.

- Sometimes retroperitoneal hemorrhage may occur which can be controlled by pressure and topical hemostatic agents.
- Long-term buttock pain (due to gluteal muscle ischemia) as a result of inadvertent ligation of the artery above the point where the posterior branch of internal artery arises.

Internal Iliac Artery Ligation through Extraperitoneal Approach (Fig. 19)

Subodh Mitra from Kolkata (1954) popularized pelvic lymphadenectomy through extraperitoneal approach in radical hysterectomy in cancer cervix, popularly called Mitra's operation. The approach is technically very easy and the vessels are well visualized and no much separation of fascia is needed to access the internal iliac artery **(Fig. 19)**. There is variation of techniques.

An incision is given from the pubic tubercle to a point at the junction of lateral one-third and medial two-thirds of spinoumbilical line. After incising skin and subcutaneous tissue, external oblique aponeurosis is split along the line of incision and lower end of which ends in superficial inguinal ring. By introducing finger into the deep inguinal ring through the inguinal canal the internal oblique and transversus abdominis muscle and fascia transversalis are separated from the peritoneum. The internal oblique transversus abdominis and fascia transversalis are cut by the scalpel keeping a flat small instrument, like posterior part of dissecting forceps (Mitra devised a director called Mitra director). Psoas major muscle is now visible and peritoneum is displaced medially from lateral wards. On the medial side of the psoas, common iliac artery along with its bifurcation (external iliac and internal iliac artery) is seen. By displacing the ureter medially along with peritoneum (not opened) internal iliac artery is ligated as done in intraperitoneal approach. Internal oblique and transversus abdominis muscles are repaired with interrupted stitches. External oblique aponeurosis, subcutaneous tissues, and skin are repaired in layers. One must be cautious not to injure the inferior epigastric vessels which lie medial to the deep inguinal ring which may cause severe bleeding and may need to be ligated if needed.

Internal Iliac Artery Ligation versus Hysterectomy

The problem of IIAL is that surgeon should be experienced and well conversant with pelvic surgery. And in emergency, quick surgery is needed. Surgeon should also be experienced with tackling the external and internal vein injury which is more dangerous that arterial injury to repair. Vascular surgeon's availability is preferable. Taking prolonged time in an already compromised patient may increase the chance of mortality; hence hysterectomy is the preferred method in absence of skilled surgeon and in life-threatening emergency. Switching to hysterectomy after unsuccessful attempt of IIAL results severe hemorrhage, cardiac arrest, and ureteric injury. IIAL is justified in relatively stable patient, skill surgeon is available and necessity of future child bearing is a strong factor.

Branches of the Internal Iliac Artery

- *Anterior division:*
  - Uterine artery
  - Obliterated umbilical artery
  - Obturator artery
  - Internal pudendal artery
  - Superior vesical artery (from patent part of umbilical artery)
  - Inferior gluteal artery
  - Middle rectal artery
  - Vaginal artery

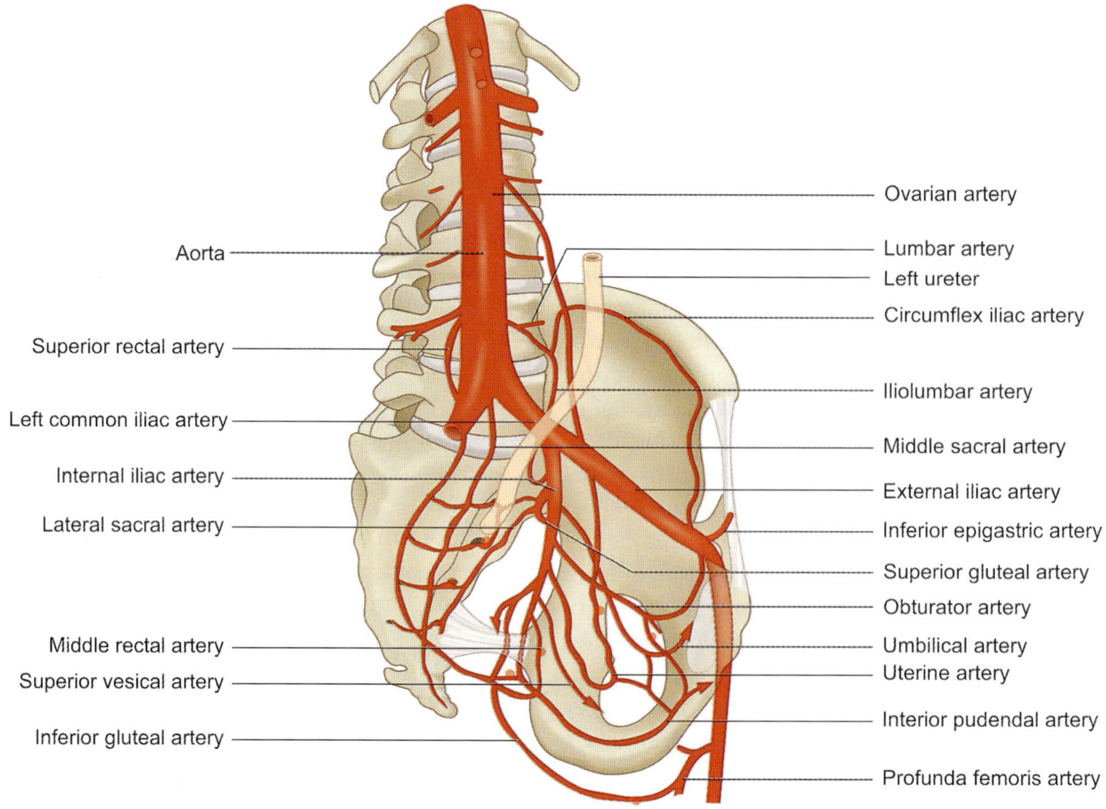

Fig. 20: Common iliac artery, external iliac artery, internal iliac artery, their branches and anastomosis of pelvic vessels, ureter crosses near the bifurcation of common iliac artery.

- *Posterior division:*
  - Superior gluteal artery
  - Lateral sacral artery and
  - Iliolumbar artery

Anastomosis of Internal Iliac Arteries (Collateral Circulation of Pelvic Vessels) (Fig. 20)

Branches of internal iliac artery:

- Uterine arteries with right and left ovarian arteries (direct branches of aorta)
- Inferior and middle rectal with superior rectal artery (branch of inferior mesenteric)
- Obturator pubic branches with inferior epigastric (branch of external iliac)
- Inferior gluteal with circumflex and perforating branches of the deep femoral artery
- Superior gluteal with lateral sacral (posterior branches)
- Iliolumbar with lumbar artery (from aorta)
- Lateral sacral with middle sacral
- Vesical arteries with branches of uterine and vaginal arteries

Besides, the vessels of each side anastomose with one another horizontally such as:

- Branches of vesical arteries for each side
- Pubic branches for obturator from each side.

Uterine Compression Sutures

Hemostatic suturing technique is a conservative surgery to control the bleeding in uterine wound. Compression suture can be done satisfactorily after a cesarean delivery or after vaginal delivery. If the medical and other nonsurgical methods fail to control bleeding, placement of compression suture is an effective tool to slow the bleeding, stabilize the patient, and hysterectomy can be avoided. Three most used compression suture techniques are B-Lynch, Hayman, and Pereira techniques for PPH. Bakri balloon can be used along with these three suture techniques additionally as tamponade. Other compression sutures described are Cho multiple square suture, Hackethal, Quahba, and Massuba sutures.

For placental bed bleeding transverse cervicoisthmic suture, longitudinal suture, endouterine square hemostatic suture, and U-suture are described.

Injections of vasopressin (4 units in 20 mL saline) in placental bed following removal of placenta reduce the bleeding significantly.

B-Lynch Compression Suture (Figs. 21 to 24)

Christopher B-Lynch introduced this simple surgical treatment in 1997. This technique involves the use of vertical brace sutures which will approximate the anterior and posterior walls of the uterus. And thus it works by tamponade to control hemorrhage. It is commonly done during cesarean section but can also be done following vaginal delivery. In case of vaginal delivery following laparotomy uterus is delivered through abdominal incision. Transverse incision is made over anterior wall of lower segment after displacing the bladder downward. The major advantage is that this is very simple to apply and fertility is preserved avoiding hysterectomy. Modified B-Lynch stitch is much simpler.

Steps of B-Lynch suture (1997) ***(Figs. 21 to 24):*** A 70–80-mm round body needle with mounted number 2 chromic catgut is introduced 3 cm below the incision on left side, which is passed through uterine cavity and taken out 3 cm above upper cut margin of 4 cm from lateral border of uterus. Then the suture is continued on outside uterus over the fundus to posterior side about 4 cm from uterine cornu. On the posterior surface, it is taken through posterior uterine wall from back to front on left side at the level of uterine incision.

Thereafter, suture is taken out from front to back through posterior wall on right side and brought over the fundus 4 cm from uterine cornu on right side.

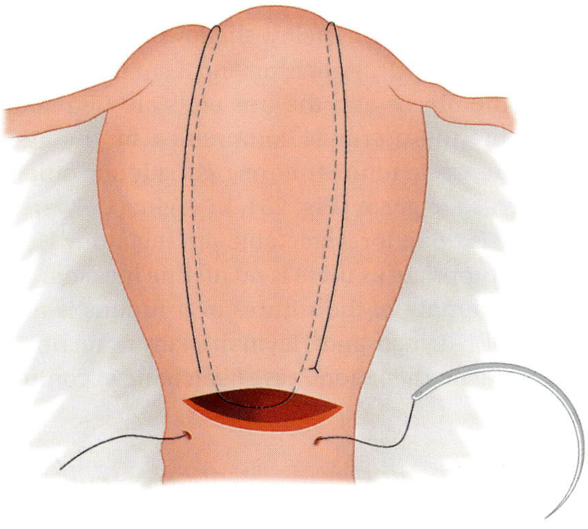

Fig. 21: Diagrammatical representation of B-Lynch compression suture—anterior view.

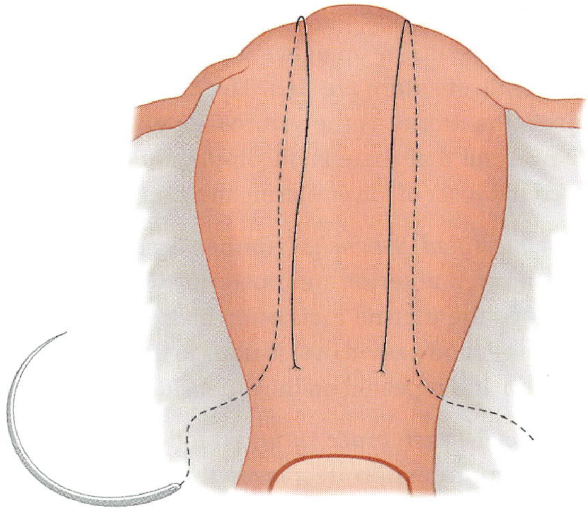

Fig. 22: Diagrammatical representation of B-Lynch compression suture—posterior view.

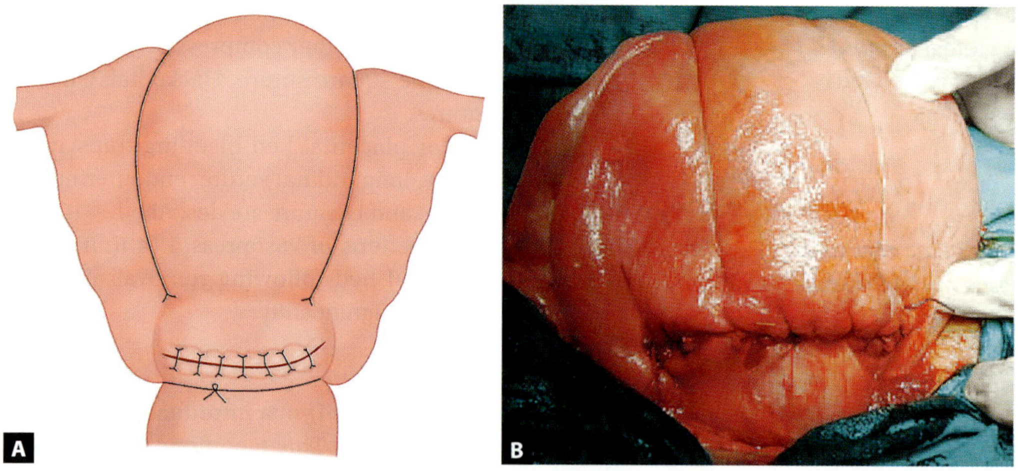

Figs. 23A and B: (A) Diagrammatical representation of B-Lynch compression—anterior view after completion of suture; (B) B-Lynch compression suture—anterior view after completion of suture.

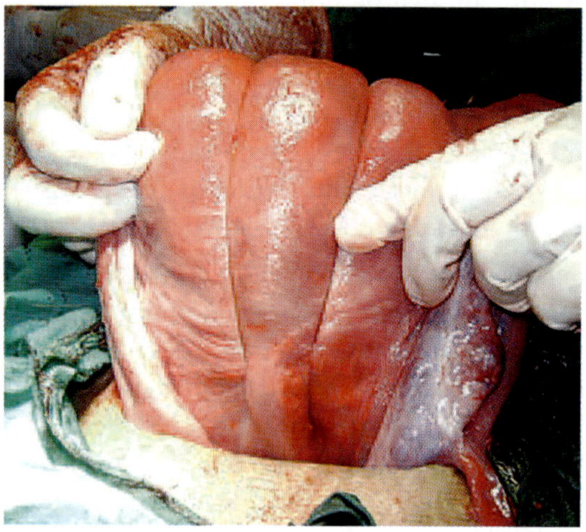

Fig. 24: B-Lynch compression suture—posterior view after suture. *Courtesy:* Dr Debjani Deb, Associate Professor, Bankura Sammilani Medical College and Hospital, Bankura, West Bengal, India.

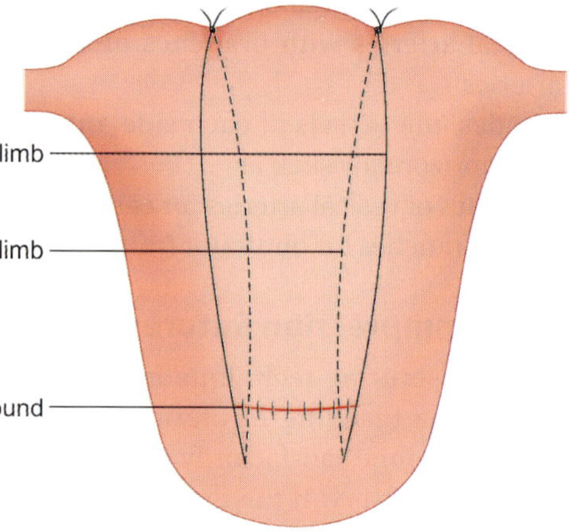

Fig. 25: Hayman's suture.

Needle is passed in the same way as on left side, i.e., through anterior wall 3 cm above the incision and 4 cm from lateral border into uterine cavity and then taken out 3 cm below the incision line on right side.

Two ends of suture are tied. The assistant continues to compress the uterus as the sutures are given and tied and also be careful that there is no slipping of the sutures. It is followed by closer of lower uterine incision.

Steps of modified B-Lynch: Number 2 chromic catgut is passed through anterior and posterior walls of the uterus 3 cm above the uterine incision, which is 4 cm medial to lateral border and passed over fundus to the anterior surface and tied up. It is repeated on the other side.

Criteria for B-Lynch brace suture: If following laparotomy, bimanual compression decreases the amount of uterine bleeding on inspection of vagina then brace suture will be successful and can be applied.

Hayman's Suture Technique (2002) (Fig. 25)

In Hayman's technique, suture is passed anterior to posterior through the uterus 3 cm below the lower uterine segment cesarean section (LUCS) incision and 3 cm medial to lateral border of the uterus and the free ends are tied above the fundus while the uterus is compressed by the assistant. Hence two separate sutures one on right side and other on left side of uterus are given **(Fig. 25)**. In vaginal delivery, when laparotomy is done for intractable uterine atony Hayman's suture is appropriate as there is no uterine incision.

Lateral slipping of the sutures over fundus is the main weakness of B-Lynch and Hayman's suture technique for which several modifications have been done in compression suture.

Pereira Compression Suture Techniques (2005)

In Pereira technique five sutures, combining two longitudinal sutures and three transverse sutures are placed. In this

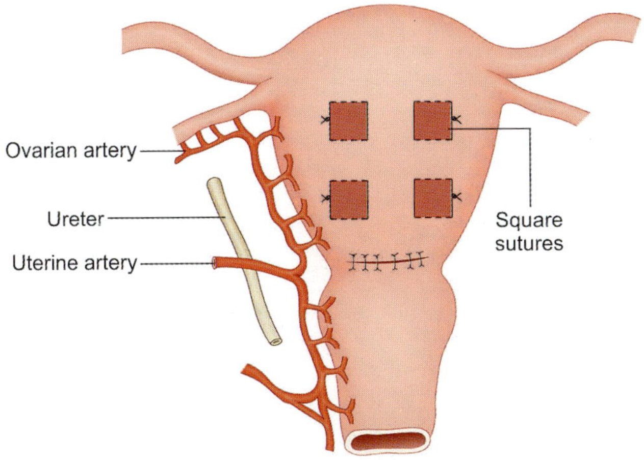

Fig. 26: Cho multiple square sutures.

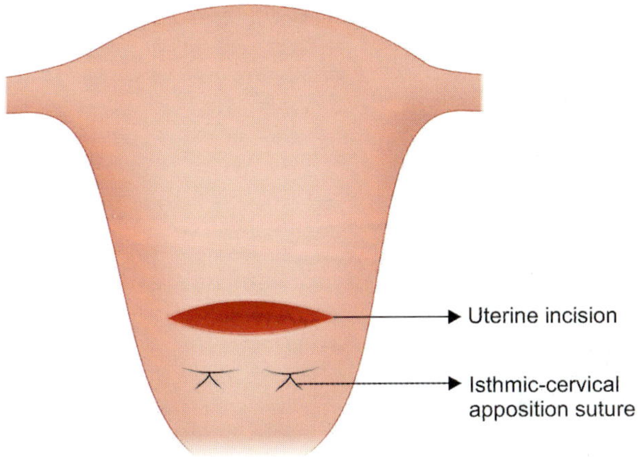

Fig. 27: Cervicoisthmal suture.
Courtesy: Professor Chandana Das, NRS Medical College, Kolkata, West Bengal, India

technique, sutures are passed through submucosal region avoiding endometrial cavity. During placement of transverse sutures one must be careful not to injure uterine vessels and ureter.

Steps of Cho Multiple Square Suture Technique (Fig. 26)

The anterior and posterior uterine walls are approximated with multiple square sutures until no spaces are left. This will compress and control the bleeding. This is very simple, relatively safe to perform, and can be carried out by less experienced surgeons.

Cervicoisthmic Suture (Fig. 27)

This is indicated when there is persistent bleeding in placental bed even after oxytocics and direct pressure over the lower uterine segment in cesarean section. After pushing down the bladder number 2 chromic catgut suture fitted with straight needle is passed through the uterus from anterior wall to posterior wall 2 cm medial to the lateral edge of lower segment and 3 cm below the lower margin of uterine incision and brought back from posterior wall to anterior wall about 1 cm medial to entry of the suture and tied anteriorly. A pair of artery forceps in closed condition is kept in cervical canal through the uterine incision during suturing so that accidental closure of the cervical canal does not occur.

Success Rate of Compression Suture

Overall success rate of compression suture is reported to be 91.7%. Reported success rate of original study of B-Lynch, Hayman, and Pereira are 100% (B-Lynch—5/5, Hayman—3/3, and Pereira—7/7 cases).

Complications of Compression Suture

Complications are less. Uterine synechia is one potential complication, which limited in methods that traverse the uterine cavity. Rarely, ischemic necrosis of uterus may occur following compression suture.

VP PAILY'S VASCULAR CLAMPS FOR MANAGEMENT OF POSTPARTUM HEMORRHAGE

For management of PPH VP Paily from Kerala, India has contributed few innovative techniques introducing some devices, e.g.,

- *Transabdominal uterine artery clamp* is used mostly for controlling bleeding during cesarean section **(Fig. 28)**.
- *Atraumatic aorta clamp* ***(Figs. 29A and B)****:* This atraumatic clamp was initially developed to occlude the common iliac arteries or the aorta during surgery for placenta accreta spectrum.
- *Uterine artery occlusion clamp* is used to apply vaginally. The clamp was desired to occlude the uterine artery at the side of the isthium of the uterus. It is applied vaginally with one blade in the cervical canal and the other in the lateral fornix **(Fig. 30)**. These devices are very useful to save the mother in life-threatening situations.

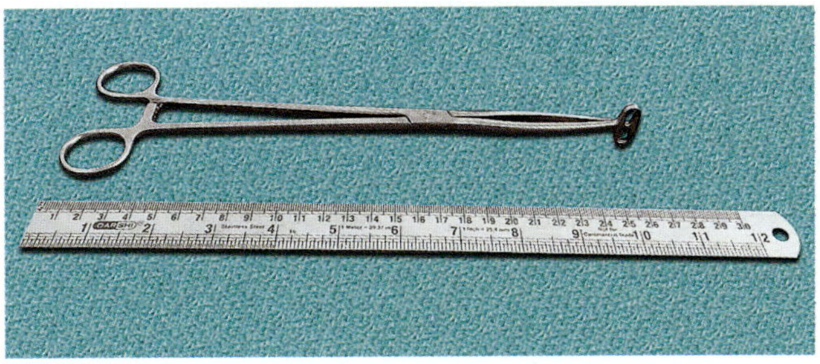

Fig. 28: VP Paily's transabdominal uterine artery clamp used mostly for controlling bleeding during cesarean section.
Courtesy: Dr VP Paily, Kerala, India.

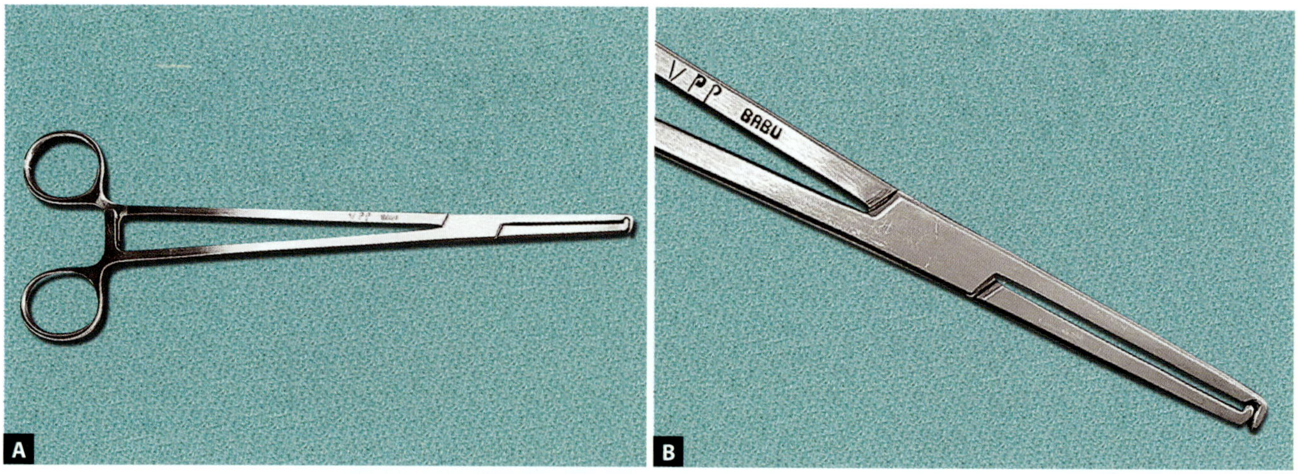

Figs. 29A and B: (A) VP Paily's atraumatic aorta clamp; (B) VP Paily's atraumatic aorta clamp (close view).
Courtesy: Dr VP Paily, Kerala, India.

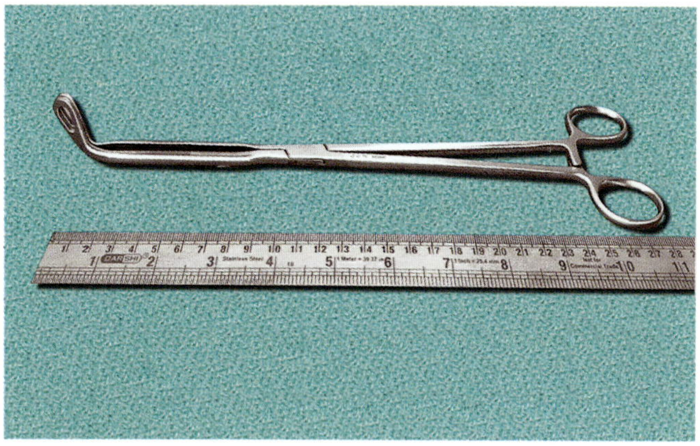

Fig. 30: VP Paily's uterine artery occlusion clamp for application in vaginal approach.
Courtesy: Dr VP Paily, Kerala, India.

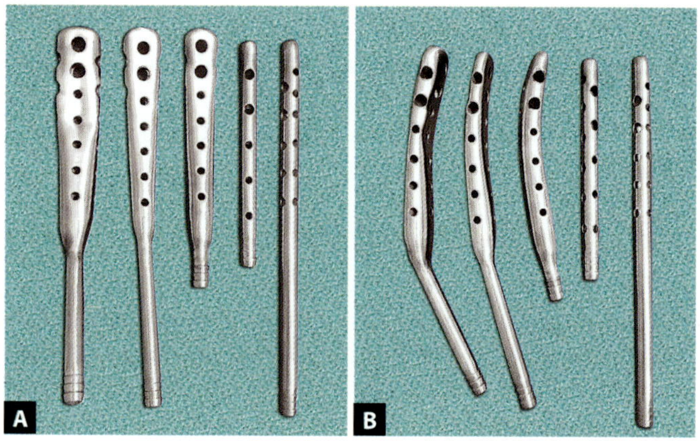

Figs. 31A and B: (A) SR vacuum suction cannula—anteroposterior (AP) view (A) and SR vacuum suction cannula—lateral view (B).
Courtesy: Dr Samartha Ram, Kerala, India.

SAMARTHA RAM'S SR VACUUM SUCTION CANNULA FOR THE MANAGEMENT OF ATONIC POSTPARTUM HEMORRHAGE

Samartha Ram from Kerala, India has devised PPH suction cannula of different sizes for creating uterine suction tamponade to prevent and treat atonic PPH **(Figs. 31A and B)**.

This specially designed suction cannula by creating negative pressure inside the uterine cavity, results in shrinking of uterus which in turn helps natural physiological process of contraction and retraction and effectively controls atonic PPH.

HYSTERECTOMY IN POSTPARTUM HEMORRHAGE

Indication of Hysterectomy in Postpartum Hemorrhage

It is considered as a last resort in the treatment of PPH. It is a lifesaving measure where all conservative methods fail to arrest bleeding. In multipara, there is no reason to delay the hysterectomy in uncontrolled hemorrhage. Total hysterectomy or subtotal hysterectomy may be done depending on the situation. In placenta previa, as the bleeding is from lower uterine segment, total hysterectomy should always be done.

Hysterectomy is indicated in persistent uterine atony **(Fig. 32)**, extension of uterine incision where bleeding could not be controlled by uterine artery ligation or other method, PAS, placenta previa in postcesarean pregnancy, ruptured uterus, severe type of broad ligament hematoma with lacerated cervix, vagina, and uterine trauma following any obstetric manipulation.

The most common indications of peripartum hysterectomy are placental pathology (38%) (PAS, placenta previa, and placental abruption), uterine atony (27%), and rupture uterus (26%) (FIGO, 2022).

When all conservative measures fail, early resort to hysterectomy is lifesaving.

The best is to save both—life and uterus. But, losing a life in an attempt to preserve the uterus is the greatest tragedy in obstetrics.

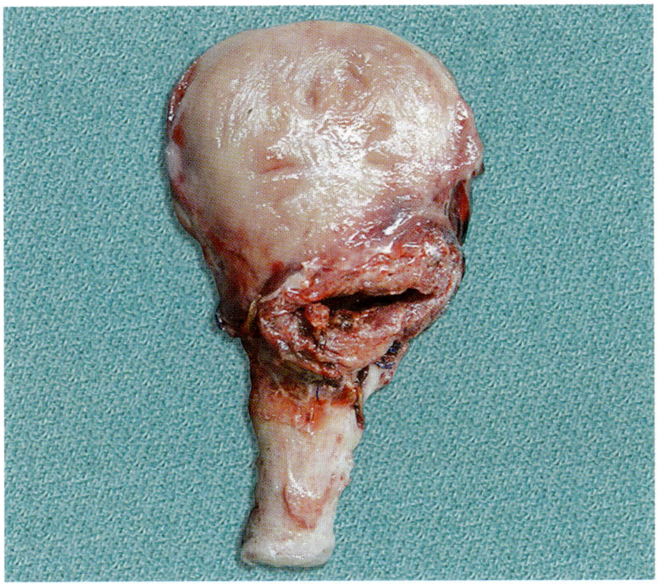

Fig. 32: Specimen of uterus after subtotal hysterectomy done after relaparotomy in a case of atonic postpartum hemorrhage (PPH) following cesarean section.

BOX 1: Hemostasis algorithm.

General Medical Management

H: Ask for help
A: Assess (vital parameters, blood loss) and resuscitate
E: Establish etiology, ecbolic, ensure availability of blood
 Establish etiology: "4Ts"—tone, tissue, trauma, thrombin
 Ecbolics (syntometrine, ergometrine, bolus oxytocin)
 Ensure availability of blood and blood products
M: Massage the uterus
O: Oxytocin infusion, prostaglandins (IV, rectal, IM, intramyometrial)

Specific Surgical Management

S: Shift to operating theater
 Bimanual compression
 Antishock garment, especially if transfer is required.
 Balloon therapy
T: Tissue and trauma to be excluded and proceeded to tamponade balloon, uterine packing
A: Apply compression sutures
S: Systematic pelvic devascularization (uterine, ovarian, internal iliac)
I: Interventional radiology, uterine artery embolization
S: Subtotal or total abdominal hysterectomy

Stepwise management of PPH can be demonstrated with the mnemonic HAEMOSTASIS as shown in **Box 1**. Management protocol of postpartum hemorrhage is given in **Flowchart 1**.

SECONDARY POSTPARTUM HEMORRHAGE

Causes of Secondary Postpartum Hemorrhage

The important causes are retained bits of placenta and membranes and uterine artery pseudoaneurysm, puerperal sepsis, infection of the cesarean section wound, coagulopathies—von Willebrand disease, etc. Choriocarcinoma and placental site trophoblastic tumor are very rare cause.

Late PPH sometimes causes worrisome problems in about 1% cases. Severe hemorrhage may occur within 1–2 weeks mostly for incomplete involution of the placental site. Retained bits of placenta or uterine artery pseudoaneurysm are mostly responsible for late PPH. In very rare cases, placental polypoidal mass **(Fig. 33)** is formed by vascularization of necrotic placental bits after fibrin deposition and severe hemorrhage may occur in some of the cases. Color Doppler shows hypervascularity of endometrium embedding inside myometrium.

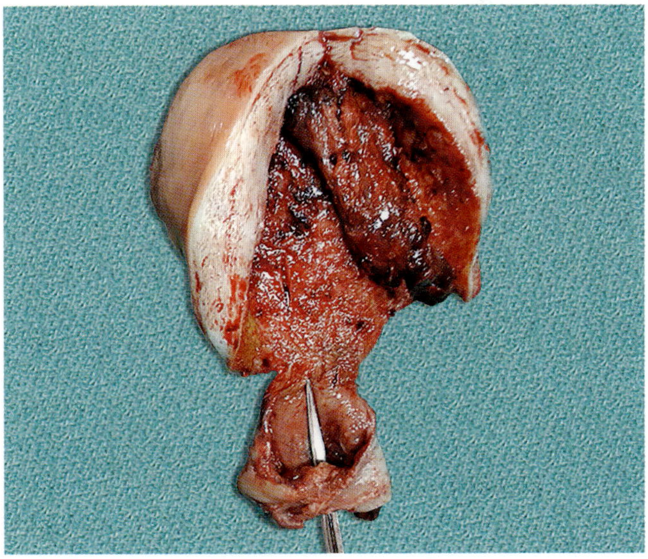

Fig. 33: Hysterectomy specimen to cut open to show a large placental polyp (histology proved) in multiparous woman with living tissue there came with persistent secondary hemorrhage.

MANAGEMENT OF A CASE OF SECONDARY POSTPARTUM HEMORRHAGE

Immediate blood transfusion if the blood loss is moderate to severe. Broad-spectrum antibiotic is administered. Ultrasonography is done to detect any placental bit inside the uterus. Uterine curettage under anesthesia if uterine cavity contains any bit of placental tissue as detected by ultrasound (USG). It should be done very gently. The material is sent for histopathological examination to exclude trophoblastic tumor. In a rare case, if bleeding is recurrent, in spite of curettage laparotomy followed by ligation of bilateral internal iliac artery is done. Very rarely, hysterectomy is needed.

Management of a Case of Secondary PPH Following Cesarean Section

Incidence of secondary PPH following CS is rare—0.1%. Conservative treatment with broad-spectrum antibiotics, IV fluid, and blood transfusion are done first. Ultrasonography

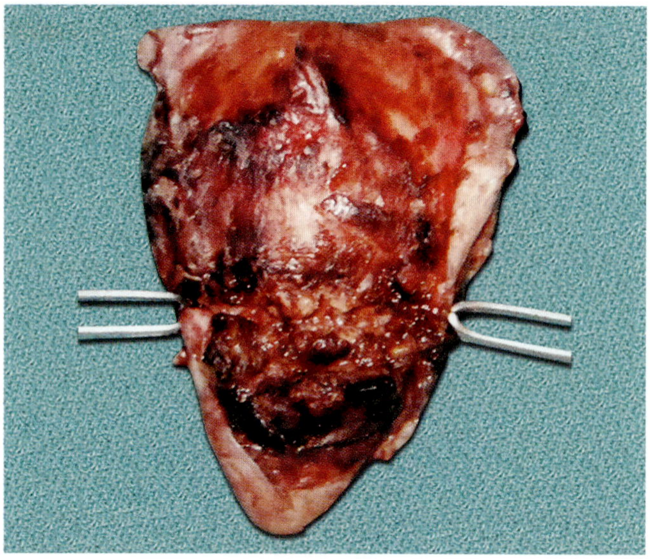

Fig. 34: Hysterectomy specimen showing unhealthy scar tissue at cesarean section wound, this hysterectomy was performed 6 weeks after cesarean section. A multiparous patient came with three episodes of postpartum hemorrhage (PPH) following cesarean section.

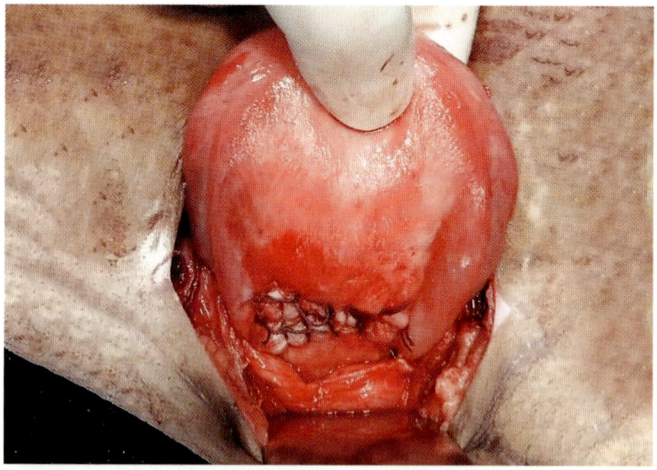

Fig. 36: After debridement the wounds were repaired in two layers. There was no further bleeding in follow up. Primipara 22 years, first episodes of postpartum hemorrhage (PPH) occurred after weeks, second episodes after 1 month of lower uterine segment cesarean section (LUCS) following which laparotomy decision was taken. *Courtesy:* Professor Abhijit Rakshit; Dr Ajanta Samanta, Assistant Professor, G&O.

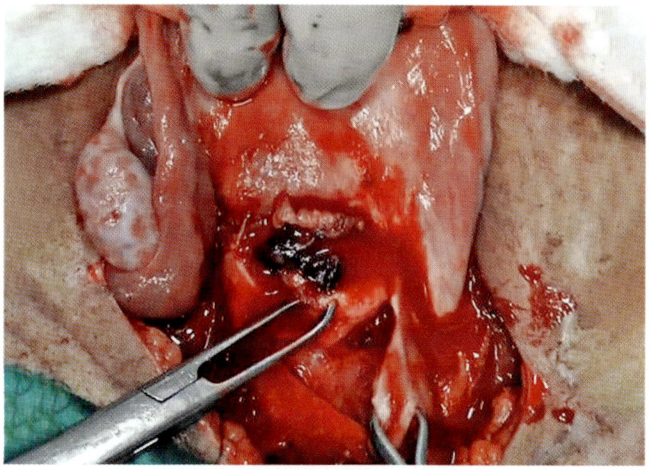

Fig. 35: Unhealthy uterine wound—debridement of wound was done to make the margins healthy.

is performed to detect any retained placental bit. If there is any retained bit, curettage is done very gently by an expert surgeon to avoid injury of the cesarean section scar. If the uterus is empty yet bleeding continues, laparotomy is indicated. Bilateral IIAL is done and sometimes, *hysterectomy* may be required **(Fig. 34)**.

Uterus preserving surgery: In a significant number of patients, conservative surgery with *scar excision and repair with delayed absorbable sutures* **(Figs. 35 and 36)** with or without IIAL is effective to control bleeding. In these cases, instead of normal healing, uterine wound was replaced by unhealthy necrotic tissue resulting in erosion of blood vessels by granulation tissue producing severe bleeding. Scar separation and echogenic debris are identified around the region of lower segment scar by USG.

On opening the abdomen, bladder is slightly retracted downward after incising the uterovesical fold of peritoneum to expose the cesarean section wound adequately. Unhealthy uterine wound is seen **(Fig. 34)**, which is easily opened by the tip of the artery forceps, tip of scissors, or using scalpel blade **(Fig. 35)**. Debridement of the unhealthy wound margin is done to remove the unhealthy tissue making the margin fresh and healthy. Wound is repaired in two layers with interrupted stitches using delayed absorbable suture **(Fig. 36)**. Angles are secured first. Result is very good and recurrence rate of PPH is less.

Damage Control Resuscitation in Postpartum Hemorrhage (FIGO, 2022)

The concept of damage control resuscitation (DCR) is introduced by trauma surgeons and it is applied also in obstetrics both in traumatic and atraumatic scenarios as hemorrhagic shock is most common type of shock in obstetrics. DCR refers to combined methods of resuscitation and surgical interventions with an aim to restore hemostasis and normal physiology (FIGO, 2022).

Damage control resuscitation measure consists of series of strategies to reduce hemorrhage, maintain hemostasis, and thus preventing the deadly triad of coagulopathy, acidosis, and hypothermia by maintaining oxygen saturation, minimizing organ dysfunction and thus averting death. This is achieved by fluid resuscitation, blood products

Flowchart 1: Management protocol of PPH.

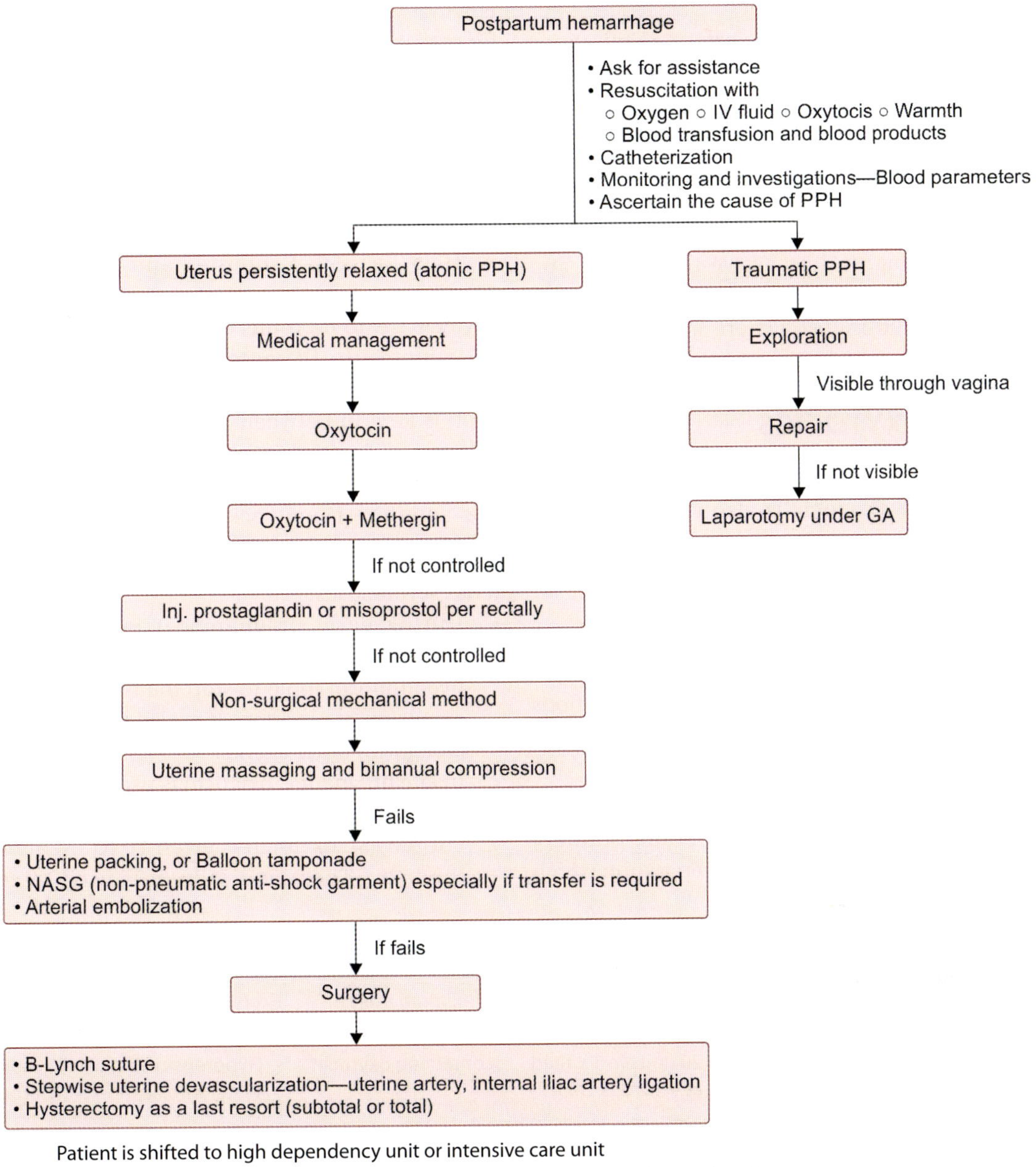

(GA: general anesthesia; PPH: postpartum hemorrhage)

transfusion, use of massive transfusion protocols, limited use of crystalloids, and staged surgical approach [damage control surgery (DCS)], and stabilization in intensive care unit (ICU) for physiological and biochemical stabilization. DCS is a therapeutic approach for the management of severe PPH where conventional treatment fails. DCS is possible in higher level care facilities.

For fluid resuscitation there are two approaches: (1) *aggressive approach* and (2) *hypotensive approach*. In aggressive approach effective circulating volume is restored rapidly with large amounts of crystalloids to achieve normal BP. It has several disadvantages of coagulopathy and hemorrhage due to increase hydrostatic pressure, dilution of coagulation factors, and resulting more hypothermia with deterioration of triad of death. Hypotensive resuscitation which is also called *permissive hypotension* involves restrictive crystalloid resuscitation in early stage of hemorrhagic shock maintaining BP lower than normal systolic or mean BP, optimal for organ perfusion until the bleeding stops. Balanced crystalloid solution (Ringer's lactate) is recommended and preferred over chloride-rich solution in small boluses of 500 mL, with monitoring clinical improvement. Target BP is 80–90 mm Hg or mean BP is 50–60 mm Hg. In *hemostatic reanimation,* fewer crystalloids are given, instead an early and aggressive blood product replacement is started with transfusion ratio of PRBC, FFP, and platelet in 1:1:1 ratio due to the resemblance with whole blood.

Hypotensive resuscitation and *hemostatic reanimation* are fundamentals of DCR. Massive transfusion means ≥4 units of PRBC, according to other it is ≥10 units of PRBC in 24 hours or replacement of 50% blood in 3 hours. It is done in multiple rounds, in each typical round consists 6 U PRBCs, 6 U FFP, 6 U platelets, and 10 U cryoprecipitate according to hospital protocol and can be repeated. Target for serum fibrinogen is 150–200 mg/dL in massive transfusion and usual dose of cryoprecipitate is 10 U. This will increase the serum fibrinogen by 100 mg/dL. There are also several complications of massive transfusion and should be tackled.

OXYTOCICS

An oxytocic is a drug which stimulates the contractions of uterine musculature. Oxytocic is also called "ecbolic". The different varieties are:

- Oxytocin
- Ergometrine
- Prostaglandins
- Carbetocin
- Doses, routes, precautions of use and contraindications of oxytocics are given in **Table 1**.

OXYTOCIN

Sir Henry Dale discovered oxytocin from crude pituitary extract in 1909. Syntocinon is a synthetic preparation which has only oxytocic effect but without vasopressor effect. For AMTSL oxytocin is given 10 IU IM after delivery of the baby for prevention of PPH. It is used in IV routes and IM routes, and also as buccal tablets or nasal solution. Most commonly it is used in IV route. Oxytocin is available in ampoule—2 IU/mL or 5 IU/mL. It can be given directly to uterus (per abdominally/per vaginally) to control atonic PPH.

Along with ergometrine it is called syntometrine (syntocinon 5 IU and ergometrine 0.5 mg).

Half-life is 3–4 minutes and duration of action is 20 minutes approximately and quickly metabolized by oxytocinase. In IM route, the action becomes evident within 2.5 minutes. In IV route, the action starts immediately. The action of oxytocin is quick, pronounced, and short lived.

It is kept in between 2 and 8°C temperature. Hence, a refrigerator is needed for its preservation and cold chain maintenance is mandatory for transport. Water intoxication and antidiuresis may occur in high doses. There is risk of hypotension in bolus dose.

It has several uses:

- During early pregnancy it is used in abortions—inevitable, incomplete and missed varieties, and in hydatidiform mole to stop the bleeding and to expedite expulsion of products. It is also used to induce abortion along with other agents.
- In late pregnancy, oxytocin is used for induction of labor and in labor for augmentation of labor.
- For AMTSL oxytocin is given 10 IU IM after delivery of the baby. Therapeutically, it is used to control PPH.

TABLE 1: Oxytocics and TXA in atonic PPH.

	Route and doses	***Maintenance dose***	***Maximum dose***	***Precautions/contraindications***
Oxytocin	Intravenous (IV) infusion of 20 units in 1 L fluid at fastest flow rate possible IM: 10 units	IV infusion of 20 units in 1 L fluid at 40 drops/min	Not >3 L of IV fluids containing oxytocin	• IV bolus is avoided • Hypotension if given by rapid IV bolus. Water intoxication with large volumes
Methylergometrine or ergometrine	IM or IV slowly 0.2 mg	Repeat 0.2 mg IM after 15 minutes. May be repeated 0.2 mg IM or IV slowly every 4 hours	5 dose (total 1.0 mg)	Preeclampsia, hypertension, heart failure, severe anemia, nausea, vomiting, dizziness
15 methyl prostaglandin F2α	IM 250 µg (never IV, may be fatal in IV route)	Repeat IM 250 µg every 15 minutes	8 doses (total 2 mg)	Bronchial asthma or severe renal, hepatic or cardiac disease
Misoprostol PGE1	Sublingual: 800 µg	Repeat 200–800 µg	Not >1,600 µg	Minor side effects are nausea, vomiting, diarrhea, chills, shivering, and fever
Tranexamic acid	1 g (100 mg/mL) IV at 1mL/min (i.e., administered over 10 mL)	Second dose of 1 g IV if bleeding continues after 30 minutes, or if bleeding restarts within 24 hours of the first dose	Not >10 mg/kg body weight 3–4 times daily	History of convulsion, coagulopathy or active intravascular clotting

(PGE1: prostaglandin E1; PPH: postpartum hemorrhage; TXA: tranexamic acid)

For diagnostic purposes oxytocin can be used for oxytocin challenge test and oxytocin sensitivity test.

METHYLERGOMETRINE

Methylergometrine is available as Methergin. The different ergot alkaloids are ergometrine (ergonovine), ergotoxin, and ergotamine.

It is used in management of PPH and can also be used in AMTSL in context-specific situations. Ergometrine is available in 0.5–1 mg tablet or ampoules of 0.25 or 0.5 mg. Methergin is available in 0.5–1 mg tablet or ampoule of 0.2 mg. Syntometrine is available in ampoule containing combination of 0.5 mg ergometrine and 5 units oxytocin. It can be used orally, intramuscularly and intravenously. In early pregnancy, it is used to control uterine bleeding in case of any type of abortion or after evacuation of the products of conception and also in hydatidiform mole.

Contraindications are severe preeclampsia and eclampsia, heart disease, multiple pregnancy following birth of the first baby in Rh negative mother. Adverse effects are nausea, vomiting, rise of BP, and interference in lactation.

Storage and transport of methylergometrine: Injectable ergometrine and methylergometrine are kept in <8°C as much as possible. However, it can be stored or transported in room temperature not exceeding 30°C for a short period of time (usually not >1 month). The duration of keeping in room temperature may be extended up to 60 days or even more depending on manufacturer's instruction. Methylergometrine must always be kept protected from light.

Onset and duration of actions of different preparations:

- *Ergometrine:* In oral route, onset occurs after 10–12 minutes, in IM 7 minutes and in IV within 1 minute and action lasts for 3 hours.
- *Methergin:* In oral route, onset occurs after 10 minutes, in IM 7 minutes and in IV within 1.5 minutes and action lasts for 3 hours.
- *Syntometrine:* It is used only in IM route and action starts within 2.5 minutes and lasts for 3 hours.

MISOPROSTOL

Misoprostol is a methylester of PGE1. It is cheaper, has a longer shelf-life, is stable at room temperature, no refrigeration is needed, easy to administer, and no injection is needed, the patient has no need to stay in bed during administration. It is ideal for low resource settings, particularly for developing countries.

Minor side effects are nausea, vomiting, diarrhea, chills, shivering, and fever. For active management of third stage misoprostol 600 µg tablet orally (in home delivery) or rectally is given alternative to oxytocin (oxytocin is the first-line agent). In atonic PPH, misoprostol is given rectally 800 µg, not >1,600 µg. Evidence is lacking in use of higher doses.

Different uses of misoprostol are medical abortion, second trimester abortion, incomplete abortion, missed abortion, cervical ripening and induction of labor for IUFD, induction of labor for live baby (>28 weeks), and to treat PPH.

CARBETOCIN

Carbetocin is a synthetic oxytocin analog. It possesses combined property of quick onset action of oxytocin and long-acting effect of ergometrine. It has fourfold longer uterotonic activity. Onset of action is 1.2 minutes in IV route, 2.3 minutes in IM route. Duration of action is 60 minutes in IV route and 120 minutes in IM route. Half-life is 40 minutes. It has shelf life of 36 months at 30°C and 75% humidity. It has side effects such as nausea, vomiting, abdominal pain, metallic taste, chest pain, dizziness, chills, sweating, tachycardia, respiratory distress, and hypertension. However, overall side effects are lesser than oxytocin. Overdosage or repeated use in pregnancy can cause uterine hyperstimulation, uterine rupture, placental abruption, fetal distress, or fetal death. Hence, it has no antenatal use, neither for induction nor for augmentation of labor. It is contraindicated in cardiovascular disorder, liver disease, renal disease, epilepsy, in case known allergy to carbetocin, or oxytocin homologous. Its use is restricted in prevention of PPH only (AMTSL) immediately after birth of the baby. Carbetocin is given 100 µg in IV bolus single dose over 1 minute or in IM route. At present, available formulation of carbetocin is heat stable, hence there is no cost for refrigerated storage and transport.

Prostaglandin F2α (PGF2α): Prostaglandins are oxytocic agent containing 20-carbon carboxylic acids with a cyclopentane ring. Carboprost is a synthetic 15-methyl analog of PGF2α (250 µg/mL). This is commonly used for arrest of PPH. It is used in IV route (should never be used through IV route). Carboprost (250 µg) can be given in 15 minutes interval and up to maximum of eight doses can be administered. History of bronchial asthma is important because it precipitates the bronchial asthma for which it is contraindicated in woman with history of bronchial asthma. Carboprost tromethamine is methyl analog of PGF2α which is available in 1 mL vial containing 250 µg and 10 mL vial containing 2.5 mg for injectable use. PGF2α is available in injectable form and also as vaginal suppository. Other than atonic PPH it is used in incomplete abortion, inevitable abortion, missed abortion, for medical termination of pregnancy (MTP), in hydatidiform mole. It is not used prophylactically in prevention of PPH.

Adverse effects are nausea, vomiting, diarrhea, and exaggeration of bronchial asthma.

TRANEXAMIC ACID

Tranexamic acid which is a synthetic analog of the amino acid lysine that inhibits fibrinolysis by reducing the binding of plasminogen and tissue plasminogen activator (tPA) to fibrin. As hyperfibrinolysis and fibrinogen depletion are common in the early stages of major PPH, TXA is useful. TXA is cost-effective, heat stable, with a long shelf life and is widely available. Evidence for role of TXA for prophylactic use is limited. TXA has some adverse effects like headache, body ache, nasal symptoms, fatigue, muscle spasm, etc.

The WOMAN trial (World Maternal Antifibrinolytic trial 2017): This multicentric trial aimed to explore role of antifibrinolytic agent TXA in treating PPH involving 193 hospitals in 21 countries using about 10,000 patients in each group (either 1 g IV TXA or matching placebo).

Maternal death due to bleeding is significantly reduced in women receiving TXA. WHO (2017) recommends tranexamic as second-line agent in PPH, once uterotonics have failed.

RETAINED PLACENTA

INTRODUCTION

Retained placenta is defined as a condition when placenta is not expelled after 30 minutes of birth of the baby. Retained placenta is one of the important causes of PPH. There may not be severe bleeding in all cases of retained placenta. When third stage lasts for >20 minutes there is significant chance of hemorrhage and if it lasts longer than 30 minutes there is sixfold increase risk of PPH.

CAUSES OF RETAINED PLACENTA

- *Trapped placenta*: Placenta separated but not expelled due to lack of expulsive force.
- Placenta simply adhered with the uterine wall but not separated and expelled—mostly due to uterine atony.
- *Morbid adhesion of the placenta*: Accreta, increta, and percreta.
- Hourglass contraction with formation of constriction ring.

MANAGEMENT OF A CASE OF RETAINED PLACENTA

It can be done through manual removal of placenta with simultaneous resuscitation of the patient. Before attempt of manual removal it should be assured that injection oxytocin 10 IU IM administered and control cord traction has been attempted [i.e., active management of third stage is done (WHO)]. In absence of profuse bleeding, shock is corrected before attempt of manual removal.

STEPS OF MANUAL REMOVAL OF THE PLACENTA (FIGS. 37 AND 38)

Patient is brought to the operation theater. Patient is lie in lithotomy position. Usually general anesthesia is administered. In remote places where general anesthesia is not available it can be done with slow IV diazepam (10 mg) and injection morphine (not in the same syringe) with caution or using ketamine. Antiseptic dressing, draping, and catheterization are done.

A right-handed person introduces the right hand in the vagina in a *cone-shaped fashion* **(Fig. 37)** inside the uterus through the cervix by tracing the umbilical cord after separating the labia with the left hand. If cord is torn previously the hand is directly inserted into the uterine cavity. Now the *left hand is kept over the fundus* of the uterus abdominally to fix the uterus and to give counter pressure **(Fig. 38)**. The inner hand is now brought to the margins

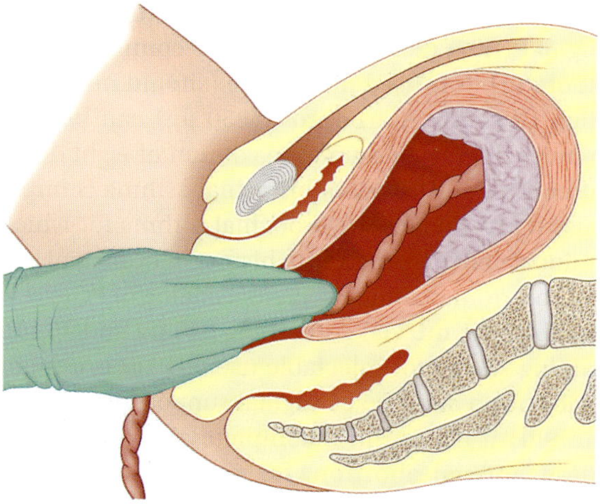

Fig. 37: Manual removal of placenta—one hand is introduced in the vagina in a cone-shaped fashion inside the uterus through the cervix by tracing the umbilical cord.

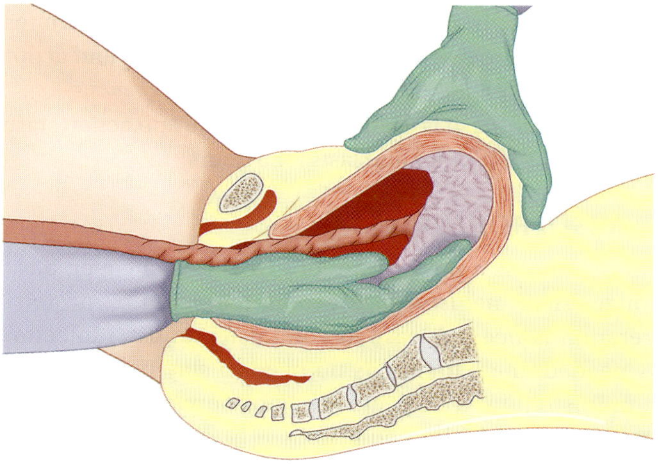

Fig. 38: Manual removal of placenta—other hand is kept over the fundus of the uterus abdominally to fix the uterus and to give counter pressure. The inner hand is now brought to the margins of the placenta and placenta is made separated.

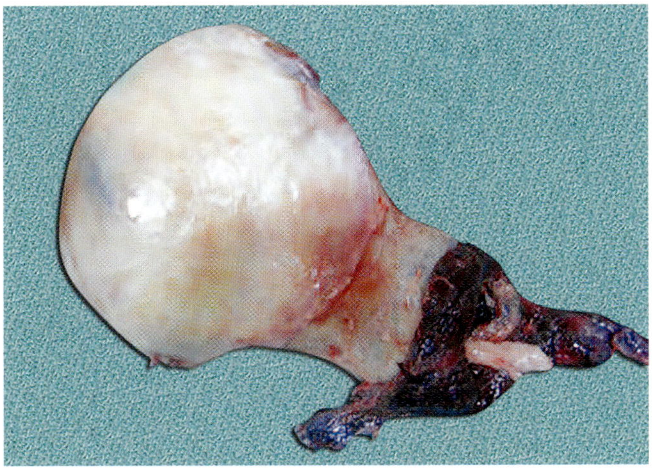

Fig. 39: Total hysterectomy done in retained placenta following failure of removal of placenta.

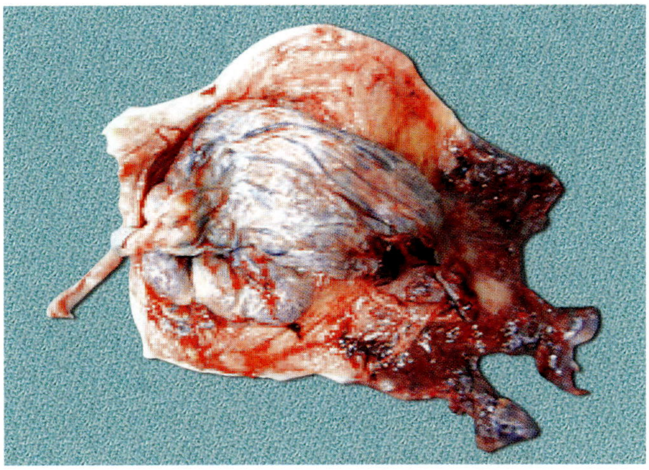

Fig. 40: Same specimen as in Figure 39 to cut open to show the adhered placenta.

of the placenta and placenta is made separated from the uterine wall by the fingers of the right hand through the plane of cleavage between placenta and uterine wall moving by *slicing movement*. The inner hand is moved from below upward, above downward, and side to side to separate the placenta entirely from the uterine wall keeping the dorsal side of the hand toward the uterine wall. Following complete separation, the placenta is gradually slowly extracted by grasping with the internal hand. Uterine cavity is palpated to ensure that all placental tissue has been removed.

If there is difficulty in separation of placenta from the uterine surface intact placenta is removed in fragments. If very adherent placenta accreta is suspected and needs laparotomy for hysterectomy, subtotal or total **(Figs. 39 and 40)**.

Intravenous ergometrine (0.25 mg) or infusion of 10 units of oxytocin in 500 mL of Ringer lactate 60 drops per minute is given. Alternatively, it can be given before removal of the placenta to make the uterus contracted, thus avoiding more bleeding and to prevent uterine inversion. An assistant is asked to massage the fundus of the uterus to stimulate uterine contraction. In case of continued heavy bleeding, give ergometrine 0.2 mg IM is repeated or prostaglandins administered.

Whenever the manual removal of the placenta is done, a single dose of prophylactic antibiotics (ampicillin 2 g IV or cefazolin 1 g IV) is administered.

If there is uterine inversion reposition of the uterus is done first before manual removal.

After manual removal the placenta and membranes are examined thoroughly to search for any missing parts. Fundus is palpated to see that uterus is well contracted and contour is normal. If not, fundal massage is given and oxytocic are increased. The genital tract is examined to exclude any injury and excessive bleeding. Always exclude the rupture of uterus. Postoperatively patient is vital.

CHAPTER

20

Inversion of Uterus

Learning Objectives

- Incidence
- Classification and Degrees
- Causes of Inversion of the Uterus
- Differential Diagnosis
- Diagnosis of Uterine Inversion
- Management of Uterine Inversion
- O'sullivan's Hydrostatic Method (1945)
- Huntington Technique (1928)
- Haultain Technique (1901)
- Newer Techniques

INTRODUCTION

Inversion of the uterus is one of the disastrous conditions in obstetrics and failure to manage properly in time results severe hemorrhage and may be life threatening. Though not all, but majority are preventable.

Inversion is defined as the turning inside out of the uterus. It is extremely rare but a life-threatening complication of third stage.

INCIDENCE

It varies from 1 in 500 to 1 in 20,000 vaginal deliveries in reported series. The incidence is not less following cesarean delivery.

CLASSIFICATION AND DEGREES

Classification is based on timing of diagnosis and magnitude of the inversion.

Clinical Varieties of Uterine Inversion

- *Acute* (***Fig. 1***), which is diagnosed within 24 hours of delivery.
- *Subacute:* When it occurs after 24 hours but within less than 4 weeks postpartum.
- *Chronic:* When it is diagnosed after 4 weeks postpartum.

Degrees of the Uterine Inversion (Figs. 2 to 5)

- *First degree or incomplete* (***Fig. 2***)*:* Fundus is depressed while reaching up to the internal OS, not coming out through cervix.
- *Second degree or complete* (***Fig. 3***)*:* The fundus comes out through the external OS.
- *Third degree (prolapse)* (***Fig. 4***)*:* The fundus protrudes to or beyond the vaginal introitus.
- *Fourth degree (total)* (***Fig. 5***)*:* Inversion of uterus and vagina.

Inversion may be with or without placental attachment. Majority are acute and second or third degree.

CAUSES OF INVERSION OF THE UTERUS

Uterine atonicity: Inversion of the uterus occurs in 40% cases due to atonicity of the uterus which is found more in multipara.

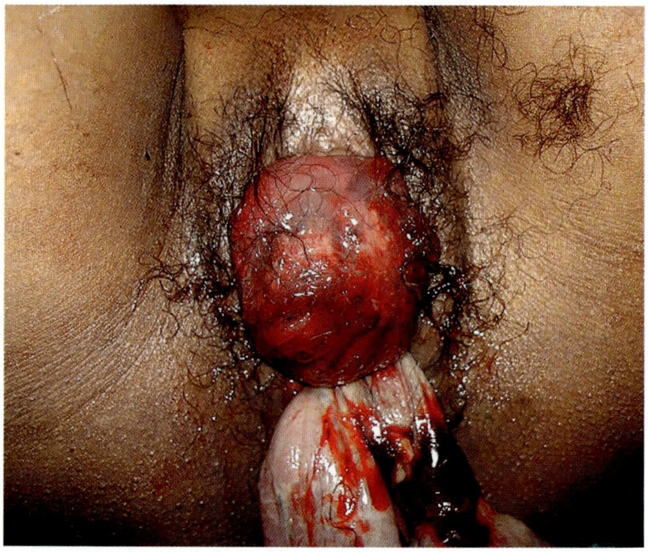

Fig. 1: Uterine inversion (acute) with placenta.

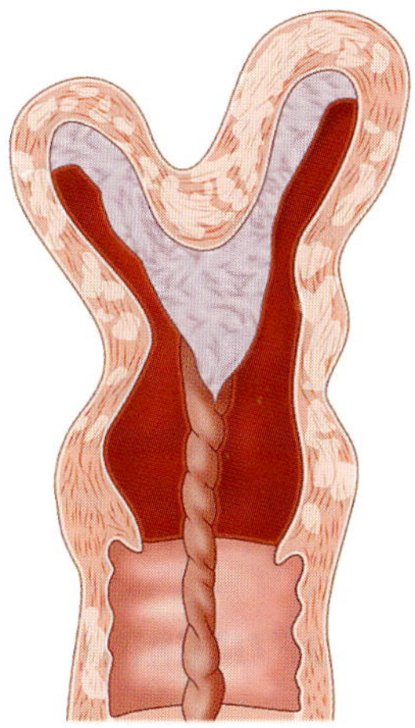

Fig. 2: First-degree or incomplete uterine inversion with placenta.

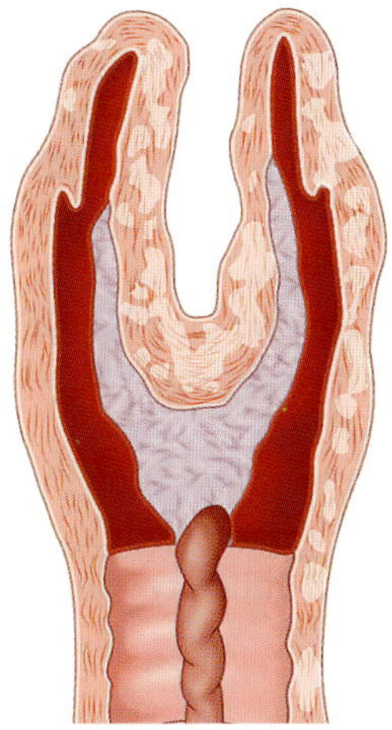

Fig. 3: Second-degree or complete uterine inversion with placenta.

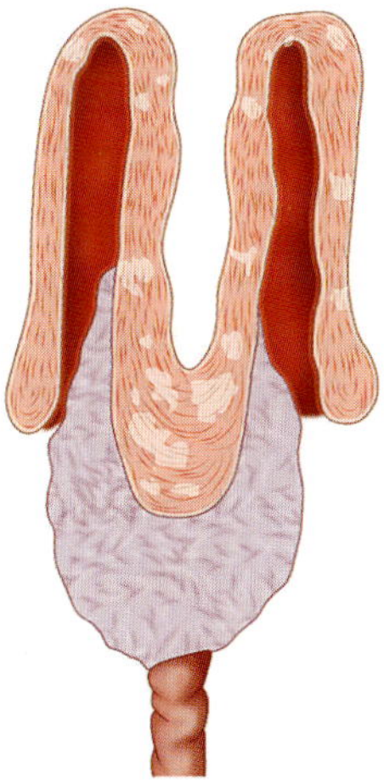

Fig. 4: Third-degree (prolapse) uterine inversion with placenta.

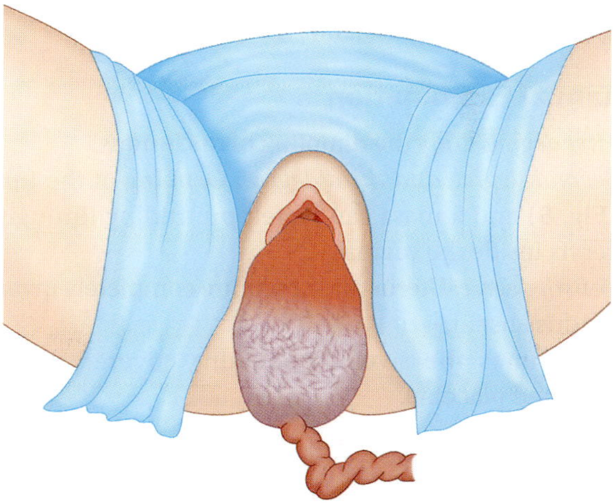

Fig. 5: Fourth-degree (total) uterine inversion with placenta.

Mismanaged third stage of labor: Pulling off the cord before the separation, especially the uterus is atonic.

Excessive fundal pressure (Crede maneuver): In this method fundus is grasped by one hand keeping the thumb anteriorly and fingers on posterior part of fundus and steady pressure is given inferiorly toward the pelvis for expulsion of placenta. However, in recent days it is not practiced.

Adherent placenta (placenta accreta spectrum), short cord, congenital weakness of the uterine wall, fundal insertion of placenta, and fibroid polyp are other factors.

Active management of the third stage of labor (AMTSL) is protective and incidence of inversion is reduced fourfold.

Dangers of Uterine Inversion

Uterine inversion is a life-threatening condition with severe morbidity and mortality if not managed urgently. Important morbidities are shock in acute inversion; may not be proportionate to blood loss, cardiac arrest, profuse bleeding, transfusion related complications, pulmonary embolism, and infection. Cardiac arrest may be due to severe hemorrhage, neurogenic, or air embolism. Acute inversion, if not addressed may turn into chronic inversion. Mortality may range from 10 to 40% in resource poor settings. Death is less in well-equipped center.

DIFFERENTIAL DIAGNOSIS

- Cervical fibroid polyp
- Uterine prolapse
- Elongated and hypertrophic cervix.

DIAGNOSIS OF UTERINE INVERSION

Uterine inversion is mostly diagnosed clinically and treatment should start based on clinical diagnosis. Symptoms and signs depend on the type and acuity of inversion.

Symptoms

In acute inversion, following delivery of placenta, there may be something coming down from vagina followed by shock and hemorrhage. In majority of cases, inversion is acute, and in advance degree there will be severe hemorrhage with hypotension with development of features of shock, especially in advanced degree. Shock may be out of proportion to blood loss. In incomplete variety, diagnosis is not obvious as bleeding is less, large vaginal mass is not seen vaginally and fundus may be palpable abdominally. Incomplete variety may present with subacute or chronic type.

In subacute or chronic variety, the symptoms are—something coming down per vagina, vaginal bleeding, pain in lower abdomen, and difficulty while passing urine.

Signs

In acute variety, there are features of shock which is disproportionate to the vaginal bleeding. Anemia is evident.

Per abdominal examination: Fundus is not palpable. There is cupping in the fundus of uterus.

Bimanual Examination

- *First degree:* Only the dimpling of the fundus.
- *Second degree and third degree: Cupping* of the fundus **(Fig. 6)** and a mass can be felt protruding through the cervix inside the vagina.
- *Fourth degree:* Uterus and cervix are completely inverted, fundus absent.

Sometimes the swelling remains covered with the unseparated placenta.

Imaging

Ultrasonography (USG): There are several characteristic findings in sonography. "Mirror sign" is found in both incomplete and complete varieties where uterus becomes U-shaped cavity due to inverted fundus extending to cervical OS. Serosal surfaces face each other and form "pseudostrip". Hyperechoic inverted fundus surrounded by hypoechoic lower uterine segment makes "target sign". Ovaries on two sides at the folding sites of uterine inversion are also visible by sonography. With the help of magnetic resonance imaging (MRI) detailed anatomical changes of uterus and surrounding structures are found. Sonography is also helpful for completeness of uterine reposition after the procedure.

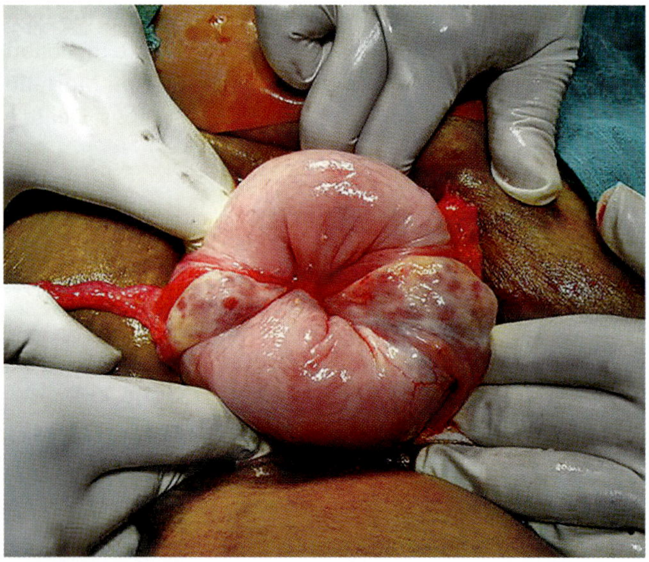

Fig. 6: Inverted uterus (cupping of fundus) seen following laparotomy.
Courtesy: Dr Prabhat Mondal, Associate Professor and Dr Debmalya Maity, Assistant Professor, BSMC, Bankura.

MANAGEMENT OF UTERINE INVERSION

Preventive

Third stage should be managed properly. Traction of cord should only be done after separation of the placenta. Crede maneuver for delivering the placenta is not encouraged now. Routine AMTSL which is now standard recommended practice is preventive of uterine inversion to some extent.

Curative

Principle of management is immediate recognition, to know the degree of inversion, simultaneous resuscitation and quick management. Crossmatching and blood requisition is done. Intravenous infusion with crystalloid is started with two large-bore needles to combat hypovolemia till blood and blood products arrive. Anesthetist is consulted.

Acute Inversion

If the patient has not developed shock quick *manual reposition* **(Figs.7 to 9)** is done under general anesthesia (GA) or with intravenous drugs (injection morphine and injection diazepam—should not be mixed in the same syringe). Resuscitative measures are taken simultaneously.

If the patient is in severe shock, shock is treated first and then patient is brought to the operation theater, thereafter, reposition is done under GA.

Uterotonics if started are stopped before manual removal.

Inverted uterus is compressed with wet, warm sterile towel till the procedure starts. If the inversion is very recent and uterus is atonic and placenta separated, it is easy to repose immediately with two fingers pressing over fingers upward, care must be taken so that perforation of uterus does not occur with finger tips.

Manual Repositions

Inverted uterus is grasped with sterile gloved hands and pushed though the cervix toward the direction of umbilicus to repose its normal anatomical position **(Figs. 7 to 9)**. This is called Johnson manoeuver. Other hand is used to support the uterus abdominally. Grasping and traction with sponge holding forceps on cervical ring may act as countertraction.

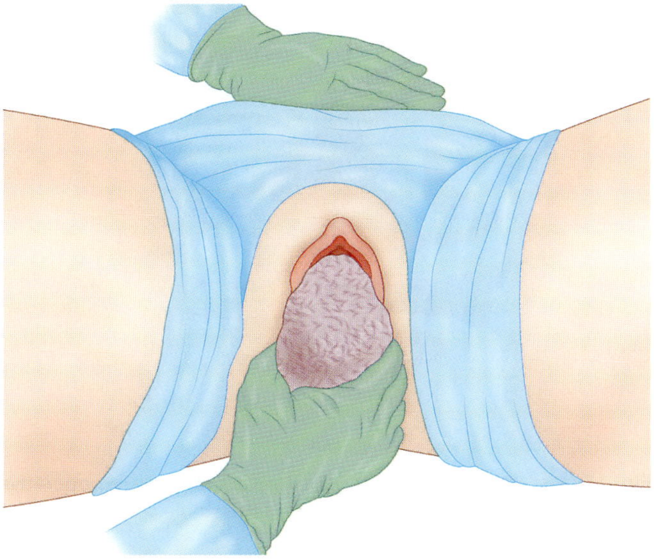

Fig. 7: Manual replacement of uterus: Inverted uterus is grasped with sterile gloved hands and pushed though the cervix to repose its normal anatomical position.

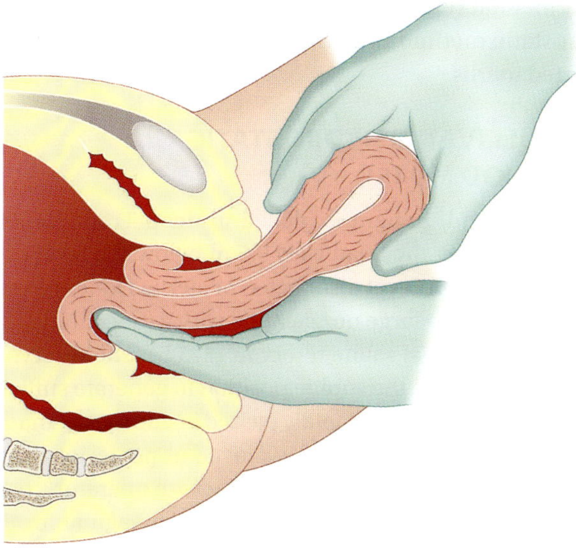

Fig. 8: Manual replacement of uterus: The part of the uterus which was inverted last (the part closest to the cervix) goes in first.

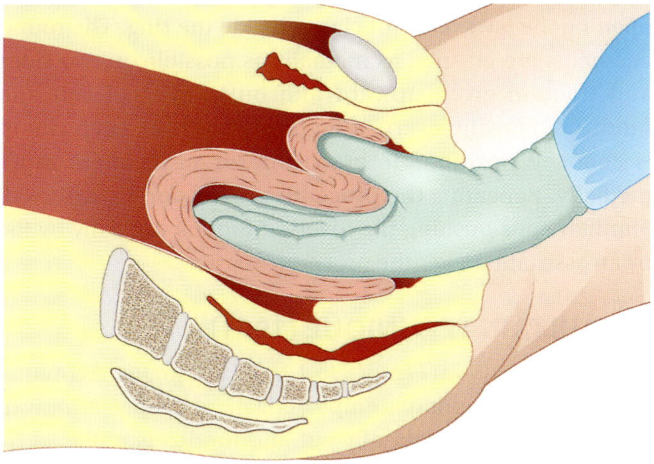

Fig. 9: Fundus is replaced in position.

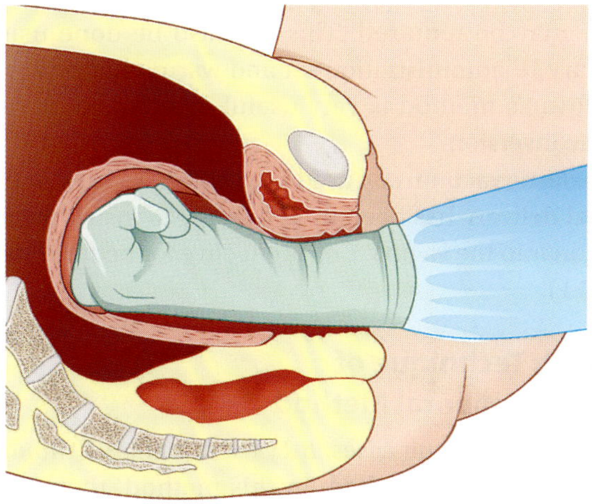

Fig. 10: Fist of the hand is placed inside the uterus till the uterus is contracted after oxytocin is given.

It is important that the part of the uterus which was inverted last (the part closest to the cervix) goes in first even if the placenta is attached. After replacement, manual removal of placenta is done if it is present. If reposition is not possible with attached placenta peeling off placenta is done and then manual reposition is attempted. However, one should be very cautious that prior placental removal may cause torrential hemorrhage sometimes.

If it becomes unsuccessful in first attempt, a tocolytic may be helpful and further manipulation is done. The tocolytics are ritodrine (0.15 mg IV), terbutaline (0.25 mg IV or IM), nitroglycerine (100 μg IV), or magnesium sulfate (2–4 g IV over 5–10 minutes). In repeated failure, GA is administered. Rapid-acting halogen anesthesia is very effective for relaxation and reposition.

After reposition the hand is kept inside the uterus **(Fig. 10)**, tocolytics stopped if any and removed with contraction of uterus after oxytocin administration (20 units in 2 L ringer lactate solution), or injection methergin 2 mg IM every 2 hours) or injection carboprost 250 μg IM 15–90 minutes interval.

Use of Balloon Tamponade after Reposition

Following reposition balloon tamponade may be used additionally to prevent reinversion and to control postpartum hemorrhage. Bakri balloon and Rusch balloon are used, which are removed within 24–48 hours. Antibiotic prophylaxis is given.

In majority of cases, above technique is successful for repositioning of uterus.

If manual replacement has not succeeded, O'Sullivan's hydrostatic method under GA is performed to replace the inverted uterus.

O'SULLIVAN'S HYDROSTATIC METHOD (1945)

In this method, patient is placed in deep Trendelenburg position keeping the head level 0.5 m below the level of the perineum. A high-level disinfected or sterile Douche system is prepared with a large nozzle fitted with a long tubing (2 m) and a warm normal saline reservoir (3–5 L). The reservoir is elevated 2 m above the supine position to generate sufficient gravity. Normal saline is rapidly passed inside the vagina with the help of the Douche nozzle placed at posterior vaginal fornices by blocking the vaginal orifice with operator's palms over the labia to prevent leakage. Posterior vaginal fornix is easily identified in incomplete inversion. In advanced cases, the posterior fornix is identified by the demarcation where the rugose vagina becomes the smooth. The vagina becomes distended with fluid, and increased intravaginal pressure replaces the uterus in normal position. Up to 6–10 L normal saline may be required. This can also be done using an ordinary IV administration set and warmed normal saline. O'Sullivan's method is very useful in subacute variety of uterine inversion.

A silastic vacuum cup used for vacuum-assisted operative vaginal delivery has been used recently to install the sterile solution into the vagina. Cup is effective for better water seal **(Fig. 11)**.

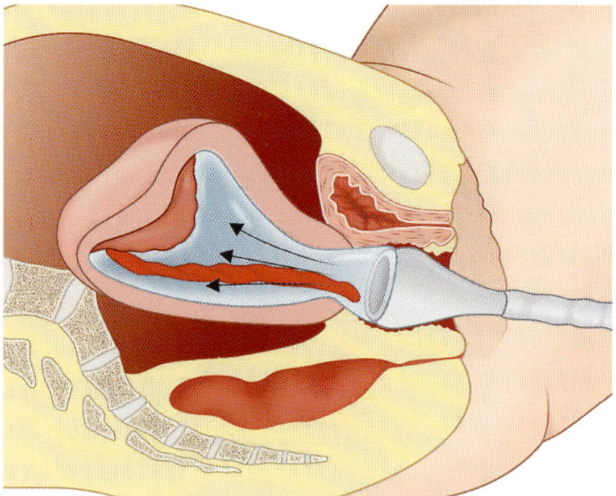

Fig. 11: A silastic vacuum cup used for vacuum-assisted operative vaginal delivery has been used to install the sterile solution into the vagina.

B-Lynch Technique of Noninstrumental Method

In extremely difficult cases, *B-Lynch technique of noninstrumental method* is applied. In this method, the patient is dropped in Lloyd Davies (frog-legged) position with head down (Trendelenburg) tilt and the inversion is corrected after midline laparotomy. After packing of bowels upward, the surgeon places his or her hands in front and back of the lower segment with the finger tips between and below the level of the inverted fundus. By giving pressure gradually by the fingertips of both hands, the internal dimple is replaced by the ascending uterine fundus. Uterine perfusion returns progressively.

HUNTINGTON TECHNIQUE (1928)

Huntington technique: In this technique, patient is made low dorsal position so that with laparotomy simultaneous vaginal manipulation can be done. On opening abdomen traction is given by holding round ligaments bilaterally as medial as possible by using atraumatic clamps such as Babcock's clamp or ring forceps while the assistant exerts upward pressure on the inverted parts from the vagina below. Tight myometrial ring above the cervix is the main hindrance for replacing the uterus. To get more space taut myometrial ring may be stretched with fingers or by introducing and opening the jaws of a stiff clamp inside the ring. The round ligaments are grasped as medially as possible on two sides and traction given upward and outward to elevate the fundus. Following every attempt of elevation, each clamp is changed positions to grasp the round ligament more medially. Repeating the procedures inversion is corrected. Simultaneous pushing the inverted fundus vaginally by fist by an assistant makes the procedure easier.

HAULTAIN TECHNIQUE (1901)

Haultain technique ***(Figs. 12 to 14)****:* If Huntington technique fails, Haultain method is employed where the posterior wall of the ring is longitudinally cut and fundus is replaced by hooking and then suturing is done. Vaginally, a malleable vaginal wall retractor is pushed along posterior vaginal wall as upward as possible. A longitudinal incision is given over the posterior ring. Rectosigmoid is pushed laterally to prevent its injury. Following opening of the ring depressed fundus is elevated by hooking by finger and by Huntington technique. Cut myometrium is repaired with absorbable or delayed absorbable suture. In Ocejo technique, incision is given over anterior cervix instead of posterior cervix.

In chronic variety **(Fig. 15)**, uterus is replaced commonly by this surgical method or vaginally by *Spinelli technique* through anteriorly or by *Kustner technique* posteriorly (Details in Author's Bedside Clinics in Gynecology, 2nd edition 2023 published by Jaypee Brothers).

NEWER TECHNIQUES

Use of ventouse: A silastic cup is applied over the inverted uterus vaginally during correction through laparotomy

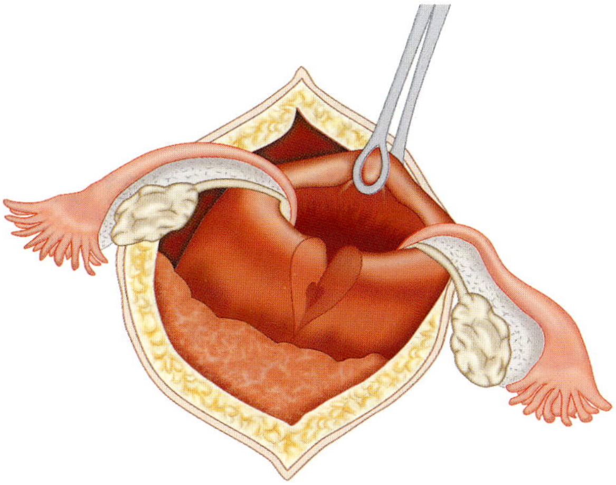

Fig. 12: Diagrammatical representation of surgical method through abdominal route (Haultain's technique).

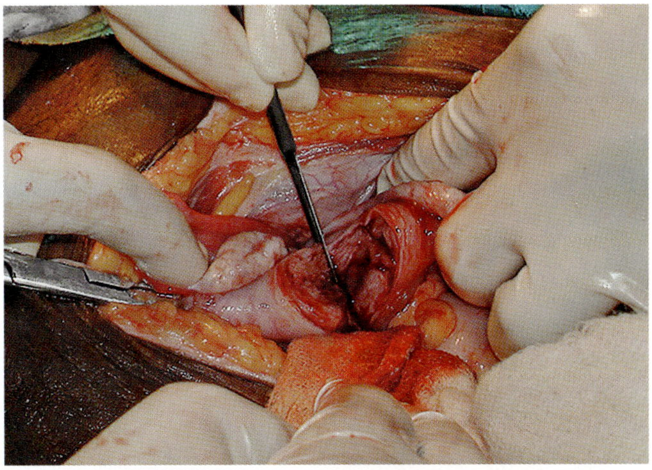

Fig. 13: Surgical method through abdominal route (Haultain's technique—clinical picture).

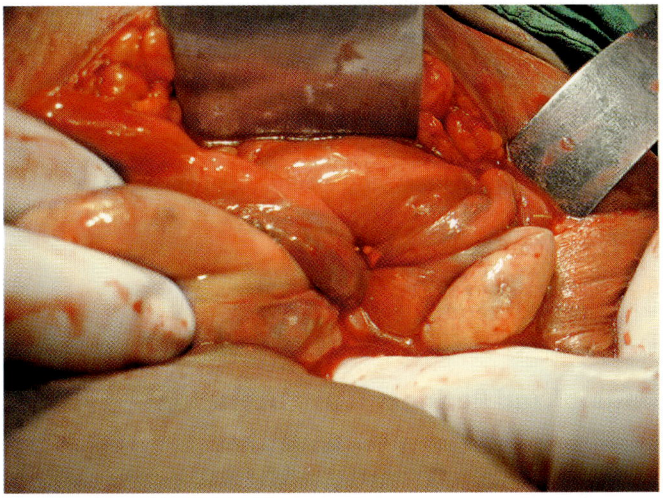

Fig. 15: Chronic inversion of uterus due to large cervical fibroid polyp.

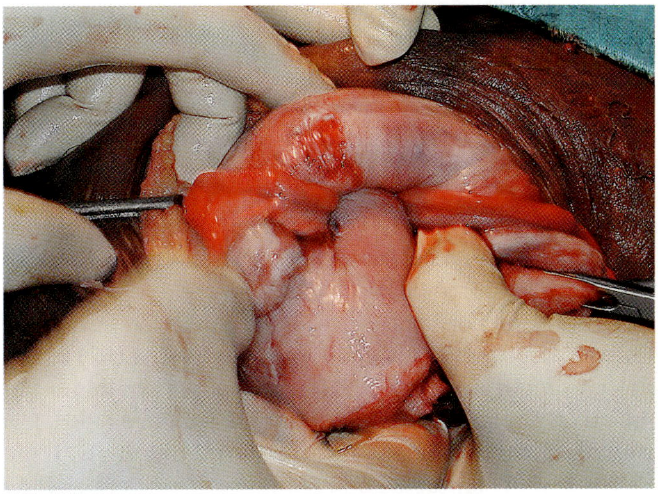

Fig. 14: Reposition of the fundus introducing the fingers through the incision wound (Haultain's technique).
Courtesy: Professor D Santra and Dr Prabhat Mondal, Associate Professor BSMC, Bankura.

(Antonelli 2006). This technique is an adjunctive procedure during Huntington technique when it is failed, before switching to the Haultain procedure where incision is needed.

Compression suture: After successful fundal reposition during laparotomy compression suture is given to prevent hemorrhage and uterine reinversion by through and through longitudinal sutures from anterior surface to posterior surface of the uterus followed by two transverse sutures using no. 1 delayed absorbable sutures (Matsubara 2009). B-lynch or Hayman suture may also be applied alternate to this suture.

Transabdominal *cervical cerclage* is sometimes used to treat chronic recurrent inversion for prevention of reinversion.

Laparoscopic approach has been described recently for correction of both acute and chronic inversion.

Antibiotic prophylactic, though role is unclear, is administered.

Recurrence Risk and Future Pregnancy Outcome

Recurrence risk in future pregnancy is not known. Regarding mode of delivery following inversion and reposition vaginal delivery is not contraindicated. Pregnancy following surgical correction of inversion involving cervix and uterus obviously needs special consideration and cesarean delivery is done in most of the cases.

CHAPTER

21

Genital Tract Injuries and Puerperal Hematomas

Learning Objectives

- Risk Factors for Traumatic Postpartum Hemorrhage
- Sites of Laceration
- Perineal and Vaginal Tear
- Cervical Tear
- Puerperal Hematomas
- Broad Ligament Hematoma
- Rupture uterus—causes, classification, diagnosis, management and prevention

INTRODUCTION

Genital tract injuries are very common during childbirth. Statistically up to 80% cases in childbirth some type of injuries occurs ranging from minor vaginal mucosal injury to life-threatening hemorrhages, revealed or concealed [American College of Obstetricians and Gynecologists (ACOG) 2020]. Postpartum hemorrhage (PPH) is almost present in most of the cases. Traumatic PPH contributes 10–20% of all PPH. It is very pertinent to differentiate from the uterine atony. If the uterus is well contracted and hard persistence of bleeding indicates traumatic PPH. Red blood indicates arterial bleeding. However, atonic PPH and traumatic PPH may coexist, especially following instrumental vaginal delivery. Routine examination of cervix and vagina should be done following instrumental vaginal delivery to see the source of bleeding. If on local examination no laceration is detected, uterus is hard and contracted injury of uterus may be suspected. Rarely, bleeding due to coagulation disorder may occur in absence of uterine atony and laceration.

RISK FACTORS FOR TRAUMATIC POSTPARTUM HEMORRHAGE

Important predisposing factors for traumatic PPH are episiotomy, delivery through undilated cervix like precipitate labor, delivery caused by excessive fundal pressure, instrumental delivery, occipitoposterior (face to pubis) delivery, delivery of large baby, shoulder dystocia, obesity, short stature, cesarean delivery, and vaginal delivery after cesarean section (CS).

SITES OF LACERATION

- Paraurethral tear/laceration
- Vulva, perineal tears, and extension of episiotomy
- Vaginal laceration (above and below the levator ani)
- Levator ani lacerations
- Cervical lacerations and tear
- Ruptured uterus
- Extension of CS wound.

Vaginal and Perineal Tear/Laceration

Paraurethral tear/laceration on anterior vaginal wall is very common and mostly superficial, bleeding is absent or less. If small, superficial, and there is no bleeding no suturing is needed or a few absorbable suturing is needed. In presence of bleeding and of large size, paraurethral tear is repaired with 1-0 interrupted catgut stitches and continuous bladder drainage is given for few days.

Perineal tear/laceration: If it is confined to lower one-third of vagina and extension of episiotomy wound depending upon the degree. Third-degree or fourth-degree [obstetric anal sphincter injuries (OASIS)] involving the anal sphincters are described in detail in the chapter of episiotomy and OASIS (Chapter 15).

Vaginal lacerations in middle or upper third of vagina: Usually associated with perineal laceration or cervical laceration/tear either following spontaneous delivery or commonly with instrumental vaginal delivery. This may involve deeper tissues with upward extension and needs experienced surgeon to repair. Absorbable suture is used to repair with proper visualization under good anesthesia securing hemostasis to prevent paravaginal hematoma formation. Patient should be resuscitated well. Vaginal vault tear may extend deeply, even involving peritoneum either opening of peritoneal and/or retroperitoneal hemorrhage.

Associated extensive cervical tear needs to exclude uterine injury including rupture. In suspected cases of uterine and peritoneal involvement laparotomy is indicated.

With deep vault laceration levator ani muscles (pubococcygeus, puborectalis, and iliococcygeus muscles) are involved which needs identification for repair, otherwise pelvic relaxation may result in future as well as anal and urinary incontinence.

Cervical Tear/Laceration

Types and Extension

In >50% cases, superficial laceration of cervix is found following vaginal delivery. Only in few cases repair is needed. Cervical tear up to 1 cm or even up to 2 cm in absence of bleeding no repair is needed for which proper inspection is needed to visualize bleeding or oozing from the cervix using sponge holding forceps (see below). There may be partial or complete avulsion of cervix resulting annular tear (bucket handle tear) **(Figs. 1 and 2)** or circular detachment which usually occurs following forceps delivery when cervix is entrapped wrongly inside the blades. Cervix may be avulsed entirely or partially from vagina in the fornices involving the vagina which is called *colporrhexis* (see details later). There may be spiral tear involving the vagina. Bucket handle tear of cervix occurs when part of the circumference of cervix is avulsed. Sometimes, cervical tear may extend upward to lower uterine segment involving uterine vessels, its branches, and formation of *broad ligament hematoma*. Hence, all tears are not possible to repair through vaginal approach and laparotomy is needed. Sometimes, cervix becomes edematous entrapped between pubis symphysis and fetal head which mostly subsides, but in few cases ischemic necrosis occurs.

Diagnosis of Cervical Tear

Excessive arterial bleeding in third stage and thereafter in presence of hard contracted uterus is suspicious of cervical laceration. For diagnosis, proper exposure by lithotomy position with empty bladder and with good light is mandatory. Cervix is inspected by holding the lips of cervix and exerting traction with sponge-holding forceps (two forceps at a time) and changing the positions throughout its circumference **(Fig. 3)**. Mere palpation of cervix is not sufficient to diagnose cervical tear. Presence of bleeding indicates laceration as normally at this stage cervix becomes thin, floppy, and irregular **(Fig. 4)**.

Repair of Cervical Tear (Fig. 5)

In suspected case of cervical lacerations patient is best managed at operation theater. Patient is made lithotomy position. Antiseptic dressing and draping are done. Catheterization is done. Posterior wall of vagina is retracted with Sims posterior vaginal speculum or right-angled vaginal retractor.

The deep cervical tear or any tear with bleeding needs repair. The procedure is done in *good exposure with light* and *uterus is pushed down* by an assistant abdominally. The site for repair is identified by the presence of bleeding point on sites of tear. Tear is repaired from inside outward with interrupted or continuous 0-0 or 2-0 chromic catgut or polyglactin stitches **(Fig. 5)**. Uppermost stitch is given first just above the apex of tear. Any other vaginal tear and/or episiotomy is pressed with gauze to prevent bleeding. These are repaired later. Overzealous suturing in an attempt to restore the normal cervical appearance is avoided to prevent stenosis. Cervical tears have bad impact on future pregnancy outcome. Optimal repairing is important to prevent miscarriage, cervical incompetence, and preterm labor.

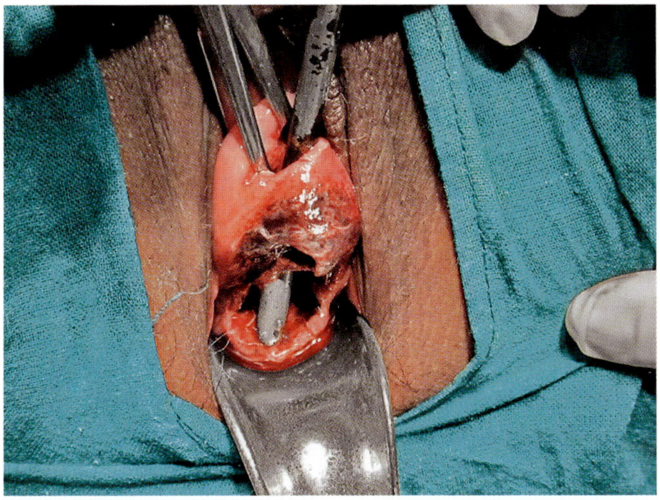

Fig. 1: Bucket handle tear (old) of cervix at the junction of vault of the vagina and cervix. Following home delivery patient reported much later.

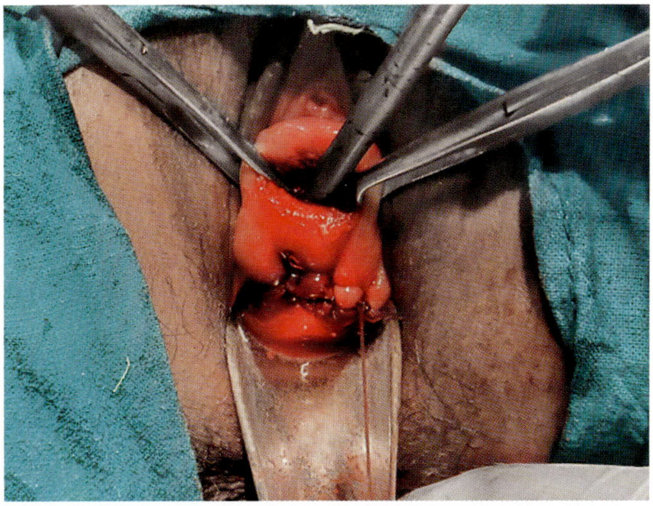

Fig. 2: Repair was done with absorbable suture of bucket handle tear in the patient as shown in Figure 1.

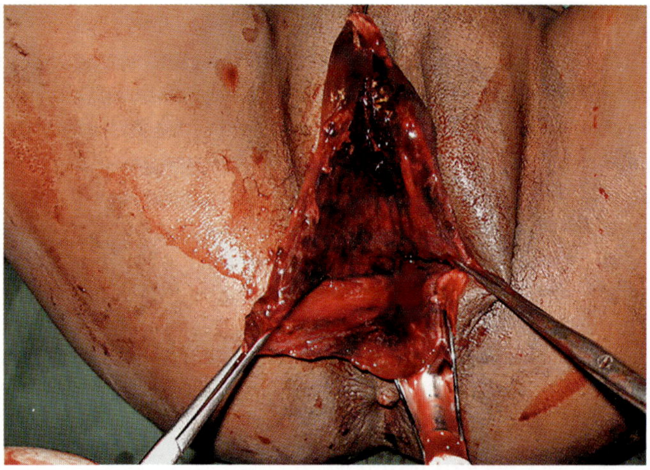

Fig. 3: Examination of cervix following delivery for detection of any tear with the help of sponge-holding forceps.

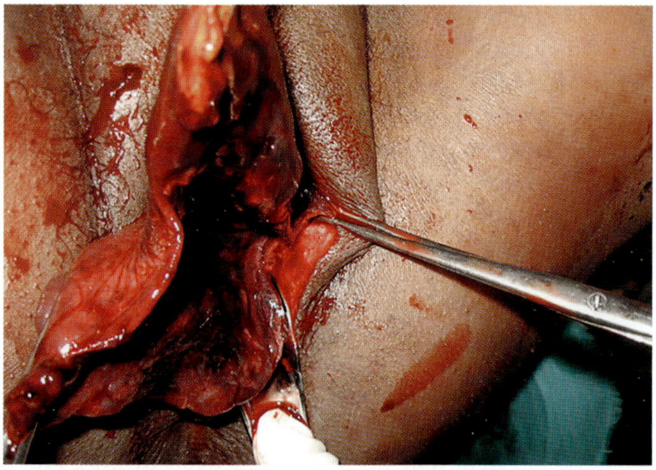

Fig. 4: Cervix becomes thin, floppy, and irregular as shown immediately after delivery.

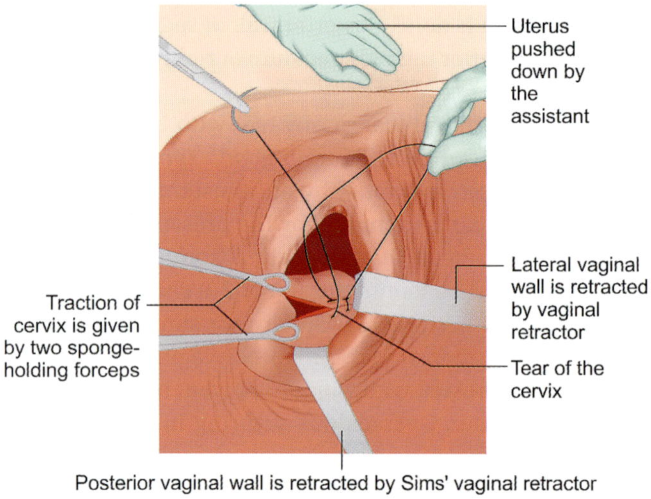

Fig. 5: Repair of cervical tear—assistant gives downward pressure over the uterus abdominally by one hand and retracts the posterior vaginal wall with the Sims speculum with other hand.

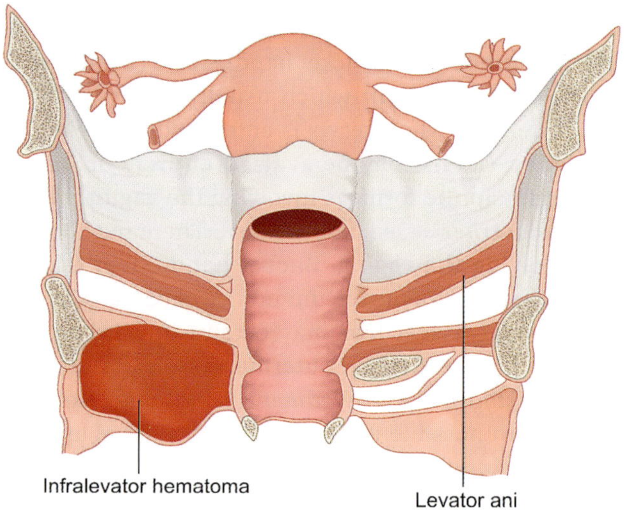

Fig. 6: Infralevator hematoma—diagrammatic.

Any deep cervical lacerations should be properly examined to exclude the uterine involvement and in uterine extension laparotomy may be needed and/or angiographic procedure is applied.

PUERPERAL HEMATOMAS

Pelvic hematoma is a common problem of childbirth. In most of the cases, these are mild-to-moderate varieties and prognosis is good, but few cases may be severe and life-threatening.

Types of Puerperal Hematoma

According to anatomical location, hematomas may be:

- Vulval
- Vulvovaginal
- Paravaginal
- Retroperitoneal

According to relation with levator ani muscles and fascia are:

- Infralevator hematoma
- Supralevator hematoma.

Hematomas mostly occur following laceration, episiotomy, and instrumental delivery. Occasionally, hematoma may occur following rupture or stretching of blood vessels without any visible laceration, especially following forceps delivery. Hematoma may rarely occur due to coagulation disorder.

Infralevator Hematoma (Fig. 6)

Infralevator hematoma lies below the levator ani muscle. It includes those of vulva, perineum, paravaginal space, and ischiorectal fossa. It is repaired from below. Vaginal packing using gauze may be necessary to achieve hemostasis. Sometimes it may extend upward causing supralevator hematoma.

Vulvovaginal Hematoma

It is one type of infralevator hematoma. It may involve vestibular bulb and branches of pudendal artery (inferior rectal, perineal and clitoral arteries).

Vulvovaginal hematoma is managed according to the location, size, progression, and duration after delivery. A nonprogressive small-to-moderate hematoma without bleeding may sometimes be managed expectantly with cool packs and analgesics and spontaneous absorption may occur. As there is concealed hemorrhage in puerperal hematoma and clinical estimation is not always possible, it should never be underestimated.

Diagnosis of vulvovaginal hematoma: Vulvar hematoma usually occurs after repair of episiotomy **(Fig. 7)**, but may also occur following spontaneous vaginal delivery **(Figs. 8 to 10)** due to tear of submucosal vessels. Patient gives the history of increasing pain, pelvic pressure, increase swelling of vulva, and sometimes retention of urine. Patient may develop tachycardia, pallor, and hypotension. In unattended situation, patient may present with features of shock. Abdominally, no swelling is palpable other than gravid uterus and unevacuated bladder in absence of supralevator hematoma. On vulva and perineal examination, there is a tense bluish color, cystic, gradually increasing, tender swelling almost obliterating vaginal introitus. There may not be any outside vaginal bleeding. Per rectal examination reveals a tense mass in front of the rectum. Sonography and computed tomography (CT) scan are helpful to measure the exact extent and size of the hematoma.

Management of vulvovaginal hematoma: Management depends on site, size, and duration after delivery and progression. Management consists of resuscitation, immediate drainage of hematoma, repair with or without drain. Intravenous (IV) fluid, antibiotic, blood grouping, cross matching, and blood requisition is done. Immediate drainage of hematoma in operation theatre under general anesthesia is undertaken. An incision is given over the most prominent point over the hematoma. After incision

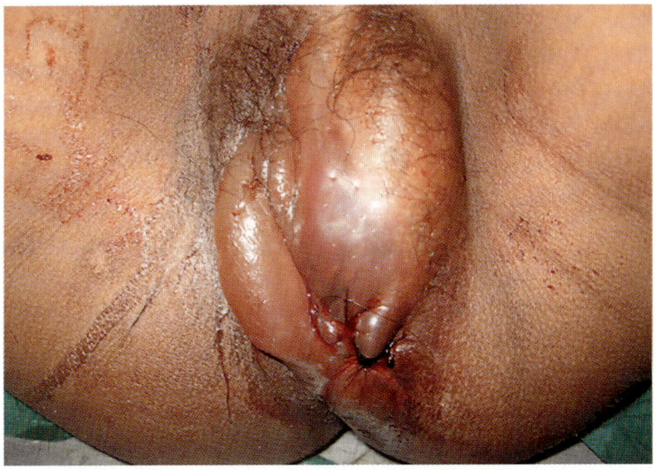

Fig. 7: Vulvar hematoma following episiotomy repair.

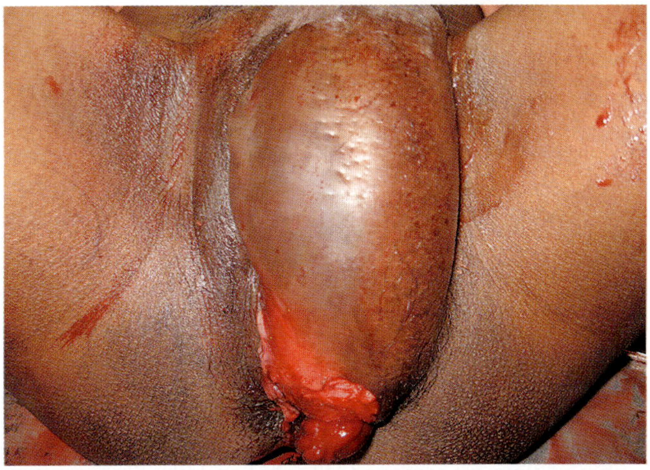

Fig. 8: Spontaneous vulvar hematoma following vaginal delivery without episiotomy.

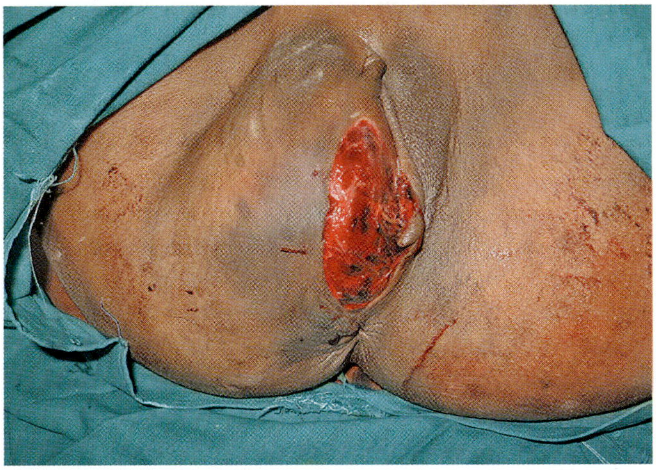

Fig. 9: Spontaneous vulvar hematoma following vaginal delivery without episiotomy.

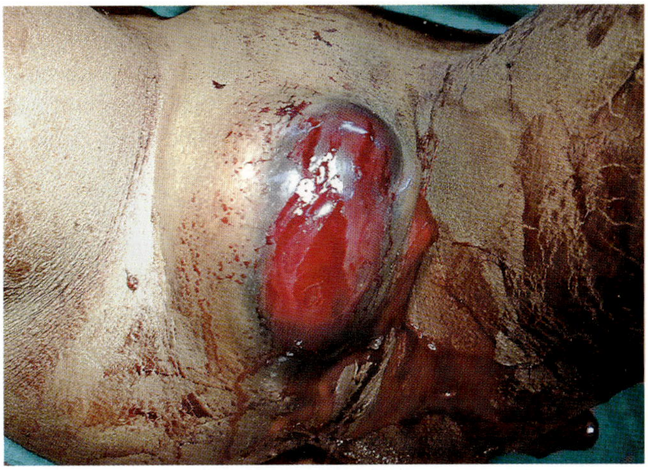

Fig. 10: Spontaneous vulval hematoma following vaginal delivery without episiotomy.

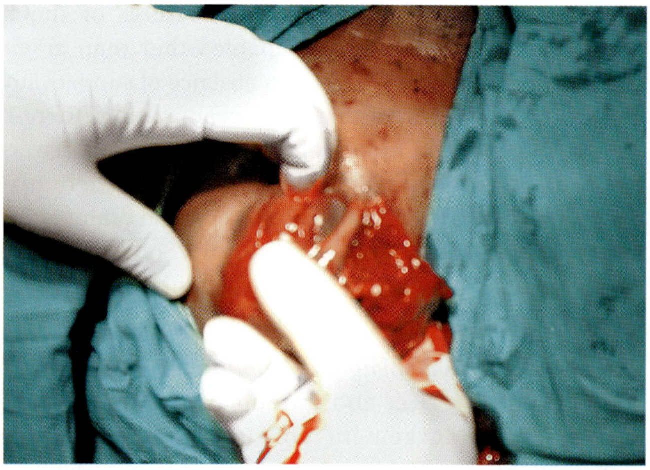

Fig. 11: All blood clots are removed in operation theater and repaired done.

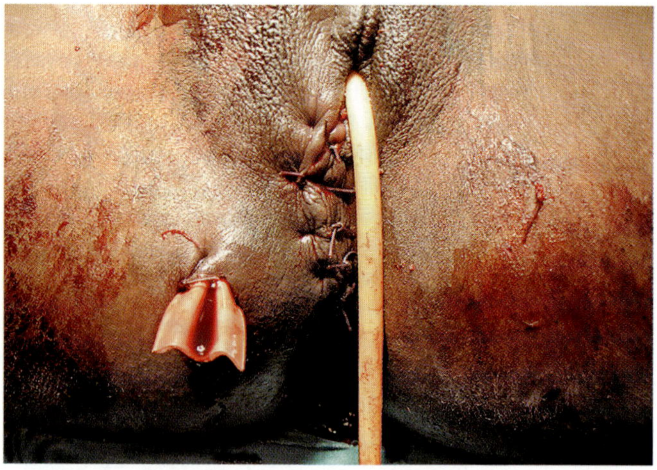

Fig. 12: Rubber drain has been given and continuous bladder drainage is given following repair of vulvar hematoma.

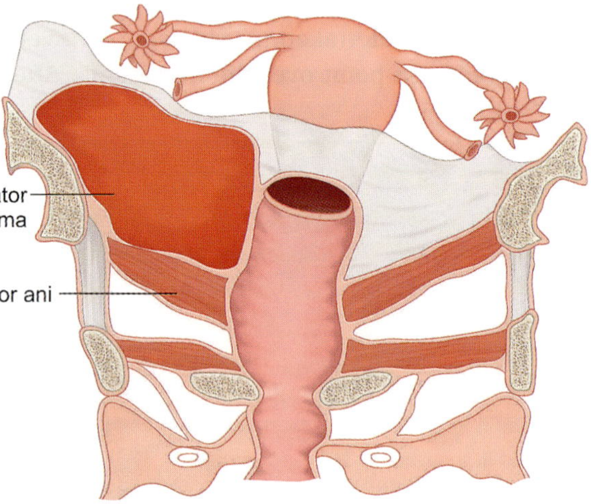

Fig. 13: Supralevator hematoma—diagrammatic.

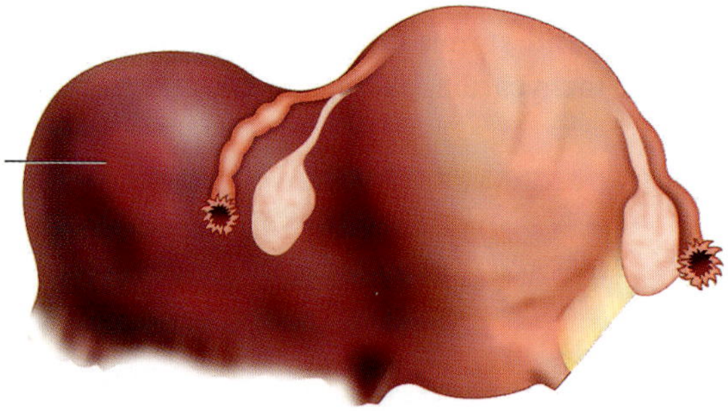

Fig. 14: Broad ligament hematoma.

all blood clots are removed **(Fig. 11)** and bleeding points, if any are secured. In most of the cases, the spurting vessel is not found. The cavity is repaired with deep mattress stitches in layers obliterating the cavity with absorbable or delayed absorbable sutures 0-0 or 2-0 size. Vaginal hematoma may need to be packed in 12–24 hours. A suction rubber drain is kept for 24 hours **(Fig. 12)** when there is doubt about tight cavity obliteration and continuous bladder drain is given.

Supralevator Hematoma (Fig. 13)

Supralevator hematoma lies above the levator ani and spreads upward into the broad ligament. Supralevator hematoma is dangerous; very difficult to diagnose and control the bleeding, massive retroperitoneal bleeding may also occur. It may escape detection till abdominally palpable or patient develops hypovolemia. In undetected cases, patient may be fatal. Sonography or CT scan is useful for diagnosis. Laceration high in the vaginal vault and extending up from the cervix may involve uterus or be the cause of *broad ligament* and *retroperitoneal hematoma*. This may extend behind the ascending colon to the hepatic flexure below the diaphragm.

For management of supralevator hematoma, laparotomy is needed in most of the cases. Few cases can be evacuated through vulvar or vaginal incisions. Drainage can be easier under ultrasound guidance. During repair, proximity of ureter and base of the bladder should be kept in mind. Following laparotomy, drainage, bilateral internal iliac ligation, and even hysterectomy may be needed. Angiographic embolization of bleeding vessels is alternate method and becoming popular where it is available.

BROAD LIGAMENT HEMATOMA (FIG. 14)

Broad ligament hematoma is one sequel following lower uterine segment rupture. Broad ligament hematoma formation may also occur during CS due to extension of wound or commonly develops in postoperative period, or sometimes as result of extension of laceration of cervix and vaginal vault. Diagnosis is based on clinical parameters, hematocrit value, and imaging findings. Urgent laparotomy is needed. In few cases, it can be managed vaginally or by arterial embolization. Bladder base hematoma is described in the chapter of Rectus sheath hematoma following cesarean delivery (Chapter 17).

RUPTURE UTERUS

Rupture of the uterus is one of the threatening condition resulting catastrophic hemorrhage. With the increase of CS rate from the beginning of later half of last century the incidence of secondary uterine rupture has increased, though primary rupture has been decreased. Due to decrease of multiparity and decrease of injudicious use of oxytocics primary scar rupture has been decreased.

Definition

Rupture of uterus means separation of the uterine wall in pregnant condition with or without expulsion of the product of conception, fetus, placenta, and membranes resulting catastrophic hemorrhage. However, dissolution of the uterus in early months of pregnancy is called perforation of uterus instead of rupture. Primary rupture is defined as rupture in intact or unscarred uterus and secondary means preexisting scar, or anomaly. Uterine rupture may be upper-segment rupture and lower-segment rupture **(Figs. 15 and 16)**.

It was Bandl who described first the condition in 1875. Pathological retraction ring or Bandl's ring is named after Bandl.

Prevalence and Risk of Rupture of Uterus

The prevalence of uterine rupture depends on obstetric care. In developed country, it ranges at the rate of 3/10,000 births and that of unscarred uterus is 0.6/10,000 births and post-CS is 22/10,000 births [International Network of Obstetric Survey Systems (INOSS) 2019]. The risk of scar rupture in lower-segment cesarean section (LSCS) scar uterus is 0.5% (0.2–1.5), in classical variety it is three to four times "more" than LSCS. Following myomectomy, the chance of rupture is very rare.

Causes of the Rupture of Uterus

Scarred or Damaged Uterus

- Previous CS scar **(Fig. 17)** (risk of rupture following one lower transverse CS is 0.2–0.9% and 2–9% after classical CS).
- Scars of previous operations in the uterus—hysterotomy, myomectomy, and metroplasty
- History of previous rupture uterus
- History of operative hysteroscope, endometrial ablation, previous vigorous dilatation, and curettage and uterine perforation
- Manual removal of the placenta in previous pregnancy.

Spontaneous Rupture

- Obstructed labor due to malpresentation (like transverse lie), contracted pelvis, cephalopelvic disproportion (CPD), hydrocephalus, and other fetal anomaly.
- *Grand multipara:* Its lower incidence has reduced the primary rupture recently.
- Placenta accreta spectrum due to local myometrial weakness.
- Gestational trophoblastic neoplasia (GTN)
- Adenomyosis
- Uterine over distension—polyhydramnios and multifetal pregnancy
- Advanced maternal age
- Abdominal cerclage

Iatrogenic or Traumatic Rupture

- Obstetric operations—forceps application **(Fig. 18)**, destructive operation
- Oxytocics/prostaglandin—inappropriate stimulation, sequential stimulation may increase the risk of rupture.
- Internal podalic version
- Breech extraction

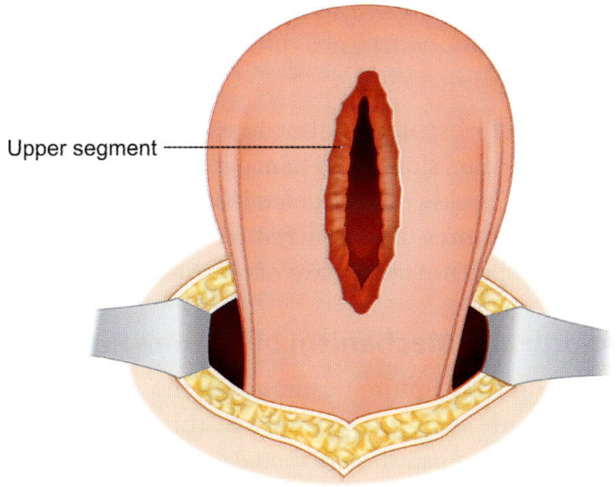

Fig. 15: Diagrammatic representation of uterine rupture—upper uterine segment rupture.

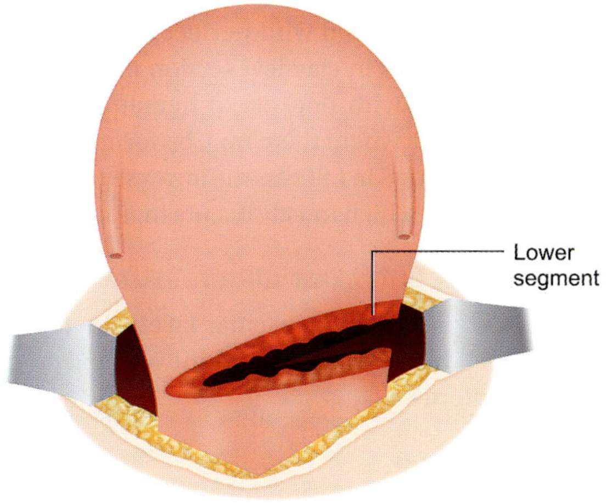

Fig. 16: Diagrammatic representation of uterine rupture—lower uterine segment rupture.

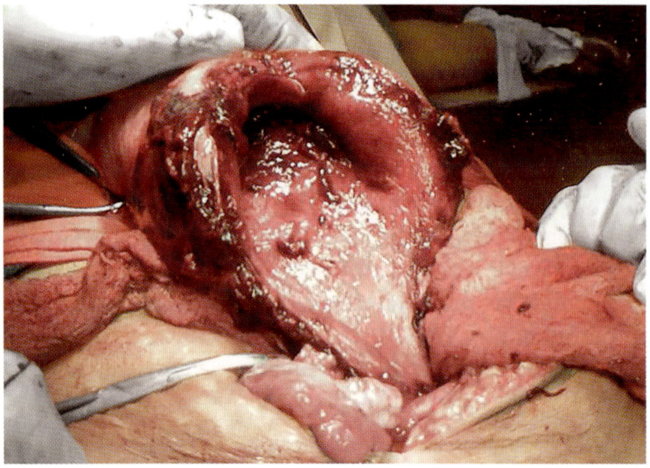

Fig. 17: Rupture of uterus in a postcesarean pregnancy at term where only the posterior wall of uterus was intact.
Courtesy: Professor Sudhir Adhikary, Medical College, Kolkata.

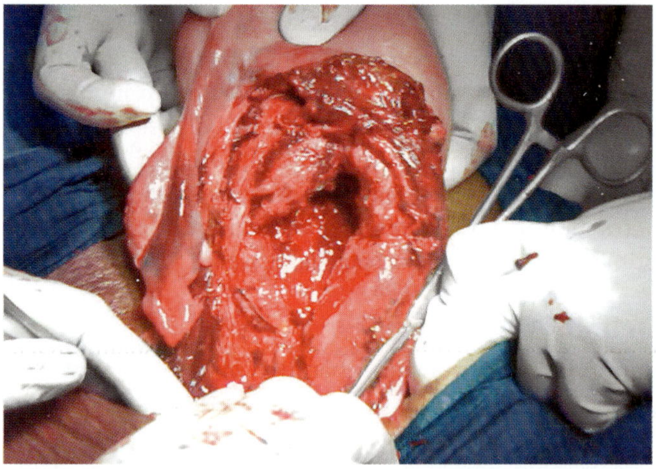

Fig. 18: Rupture of uterus following forceps delivery in a primigravida mother which was repaired successfully preserving the uterus—an uncommon complication.
Courtesy: Dr G Mukhopadhyay, RG Kar Medical College, Kolkata, West Bengal, India.

- External version
- Manual removal of the placenta
- Blunt trauma over the pregnant uterus and/or following an accident, sharp trauma, e.g., knife.

Congenital

- Rudimentary horn pregnancy
- Connective tissue disorder—Marfan syndrome, systemic lupus erythematosus (SLE), Elhers-Danlos syndrome.

Previous CS is the most common cause of rupture of uterus. Previously, it was the obstructed labor. The change in cause is due to improvement of intranatal care and increase in post-CS pregnancies. However, in developing countries, rupture following obstructed labor still occurs.

Reasons of More Chance of Scar Rupture in Classical Cesarean Section than in LSCS Scar

Scar following classical CS becomes weaker than that of LSCS scar.

Anatomical apposition with perfect hemostasis occurs in LSCS scar, whereas in classical section thick margins are opposed unevenly with pockets of hematoma formation followed by abscess where there may be formation of gutter inside. Healing is good in LSCS as the lower segment does not contract or retract, which mostly occurs in upper segment.

Reasons of More Chance of Rupture in Grand Multipara

With repeated pregnancy, muscular layers are replaced by fibrous tissues which weaken the uterine wall and predispose to rupture of uterus.

Traumatic Rupture

Gravid uterus due to presence of amniotic fluid can sustain blunt trauma to some extent, but possibility of uterine rupture should always be remembered following blunt trauma. Pregnant mother is monitored closely. Abruptio placentae is an important complication following a trauma. Uterine rupture is more common in pregnancy with prior cesarean delivery. CT scan may be useful to diagnose traumatic rupture if fetus is dead.

Timings of Rupture

Rupture uterus commonly occurs during labor (intranatal). During pregnancy (antenatal), the chance of rupture of uterus is rare but may occur in some conditions, e.g., (1) silent rupture in a post-CS pregnancy (classical variety), (2) violent rupture in underdeveloped horn or a rudimentary pregnant horn—usually included under ectopic pregnancy, (3) traumatic rupture following sudden blow or accident, and (4) spontaneous rupture in placenta percreta.

Differences of Clinical Sequence between Scar Rupture Following LSCS and Following Obstructed Labor

The rupture of obstructed labor is usually dramatic but that of LSCS occurs slowly and hence it is sometimes called silent rupture. In case of obstructed labor, rupture is always preceded by features of obstructed labor but in LSCS scar rupture there may not be features of obstruction always.

Pathology and Mechanism of Uterine Rupture

In scarred uterus, rupture occurs along the scar. In intact uterus, rupture occurs commonly in thinned out lower uterine segment, mostly in obstructed labor.

Mechanism of rupture in obstructed labor—with the progress of labor the upper uterine segment contracts and retracts, and the lower uterine segment passively dilates to give passage to the fetus. This process goes on. As a result, the upper uterine segment becomes thicker and thicker, and lower uterine segment gradually becomes thinner and a formation of ring (*pathological retraction ring*) occurs in between the two segments known as *Bandl's ring* which is visible and palpable abdominally. This ring is usually oblique in position and ascends gradually. With time, if the patient is *multigravida*, lower uterine segment ruptures. When it occurs near cervix rent occurs transversely or obliquely. When it extends to broad ligament the rent is longitudinal to one side involving upper segment and extending downward involving cervix and vagina. Sometimes, bladder may be involved in the process of rupture.

Tear of the vaginal vault is called *colporrhexis*. It may be along with rupture of uterus or without rupture of uterus. This type of rupture usually takes place when the vagina is distended by the fetal head and more common along the posterior fornix. Features are like rupture of uterus and the diagnosis is done on routine examination of vagina following delivery. Examination under anesthesia, and repair of wound is attempted from below. If not approachable from below laparotomy is done and sometimes hysterectomy is needed.

In obstructed labor in case of *primigravida mother*, uterus becomes inert and the patient becomes exhausted and also develop the features of sepsis. In extreme rare occasion, rupture may occur in primigravida.

Classification of Uterine Rupture (Figs. 19A to C)

Rupture may be complete variety, incomplete variety, and uterine dehiscence.

Complete rupture means all the layers of the uterus including the peritoneum are torn, and uterus is opened and its contents come outside the cavity. If the rupture is not large and head is engaged only apportion of fetus comes out of the uterus. Complete ruptures occur more commonly in case of spontaneous rupture.

A rupture is said to be incomplete when the peritoneum is intact and part of some thickness of myometrium may be there and the contents of the uterine cavity lies inside the cavity. There is possibility of hemorrhage inside broad ligament and huge retroperitoneal hematoma, which becomes evident during laparotomy. Traumatic ruptures are commonly of incomplete variety. Incomplete rupture is also commonly referred as uterine dehiscence. *Scar dehiscence* is the separation along the previous scar. In scar dehiscence, the unscarred tissue is usually not involved.

Diagnosis of Rupture of Uterus

History: Patient either multipara or with history of previous CS pregnancy is usually in advanced stage of labor, and she experiences excruciating abdominal pain followed by cessation of pain and feeling of something giving away inside the abdomen. There may be sudden increase of vaginal bleeding. Patient may sometimes complain pain in chest and right shoulder as a result of irritation of the diaphragm due to hemoperitoneum. However, pain may be masked due to analgesia including epidural used in labor.

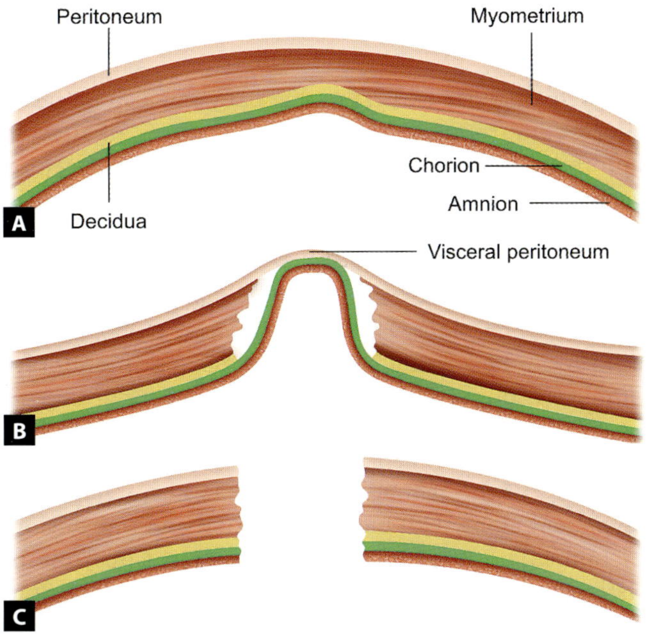

Figs. 19A to C: Uterine scar following cesarean section (normal)—(A) Schematic diagram; (B) Incomplete rupture (scar dehiscence). Visceral peritoneum is intact—schematic diagram; (C) Complete rupture—all layers of the uterine wall are separated—schematic diagram.

General examination: Features of shock may be evident—tachycardia, hypotension, sweating, and marked pallor.

Per abdominal examination: Outline of the gravid uterus is lost and contraction of the uterus is absent. Fetal parts are palpable superficially. A firm contracted uterus may be felt separately from the fetus (like two fetal heads). Flanks may be full due to intraperitoneal hemorrhage. Fetal heart sound is absent.

Per vaginal examination: There may be excessive and fresh vaginal bleeding provided the impacted fetal head does not block the birth canal. Cervix is felt like a curtain-like structure (reformation of the cervix). Presenting part ascends higher in comparison to previous station. Hematuria may be present. However, all symptoms and signs are not typically found in every case. Findings depend on whether it is a complete or incomplete rupture or if in a scarred uterus or unscarred uterus.

Abruptio placentae and amniotic fluid embolism sometime may be confused with rupture uterus and should be considered for differential diagnosis.

Diagnosis of Rupture Uterus during Trial of Labor after Cesarean Section

Aim is to diagnose earliest so that baby can also be saved before compromised stage. Acute features of uterine rupture are variable which may include fetal bradycardia, increased or decreased uterine contractions, new onset severe abdominal pain, finding of blood in the urine or urine collection bag, vaginal bleeding, and ascend of fetal presentation. *The most common sign indicative of uterine rupture is abnormality of fetal heart tracing (70%).* Uterine rupture can occur suddenly in spite of close monitoring without warning resulting in fetal compromise or death.

Management of a Case of Uterine Rupture

Principles of the management are: (1) Resuscitation of the patient along with blood requisition and transfusion; (2) Immediate laparotomy—either repair if possible or hysterectomy; and (3) Preliminary measures are IV fluid with crystalloid (ringer lactate solution), blood transfusion, continuous catheterization, and antibiotic prophylaxis. Patient is being prepared to send to the operation theater.

Steps of Laparotomy

- Patient is made to lie in supine position. Catheterization, antiseptic dressing, and draping are done. General anesthesia is administered.
- A midline vertical incision is given to open the abdomen.
- Blood and blood clots are removed quickly.
- Fetus is delivered first whether it is outside the uterus, partly or fully (in incomplete variety) inside the uterus. Placenta and membranes are removed.
- Peritoneal cavity, uterus, nature of wounds, and adjoining structures such as broad ligament hematoma, extension of retroperitoneal hemorrhage are thoroughly examined and decision is taken whether repair of the wound with preservation of the uterus **(Figs. 20A to C)** or hysterectomy **(Fig. 21)**.
- If hysterectomy decision is taken, then *subtotal hysterectomy* **(Figs. 22A and B)** is usually done because total hysterectomy takes longer time. Complete hemostasis is secured.
- If there is any broad ligament hematoma, it is drained and the bleeding vessels if visible are ligated individually. In uncontrolled bleeding, sometimes bilateral ligation

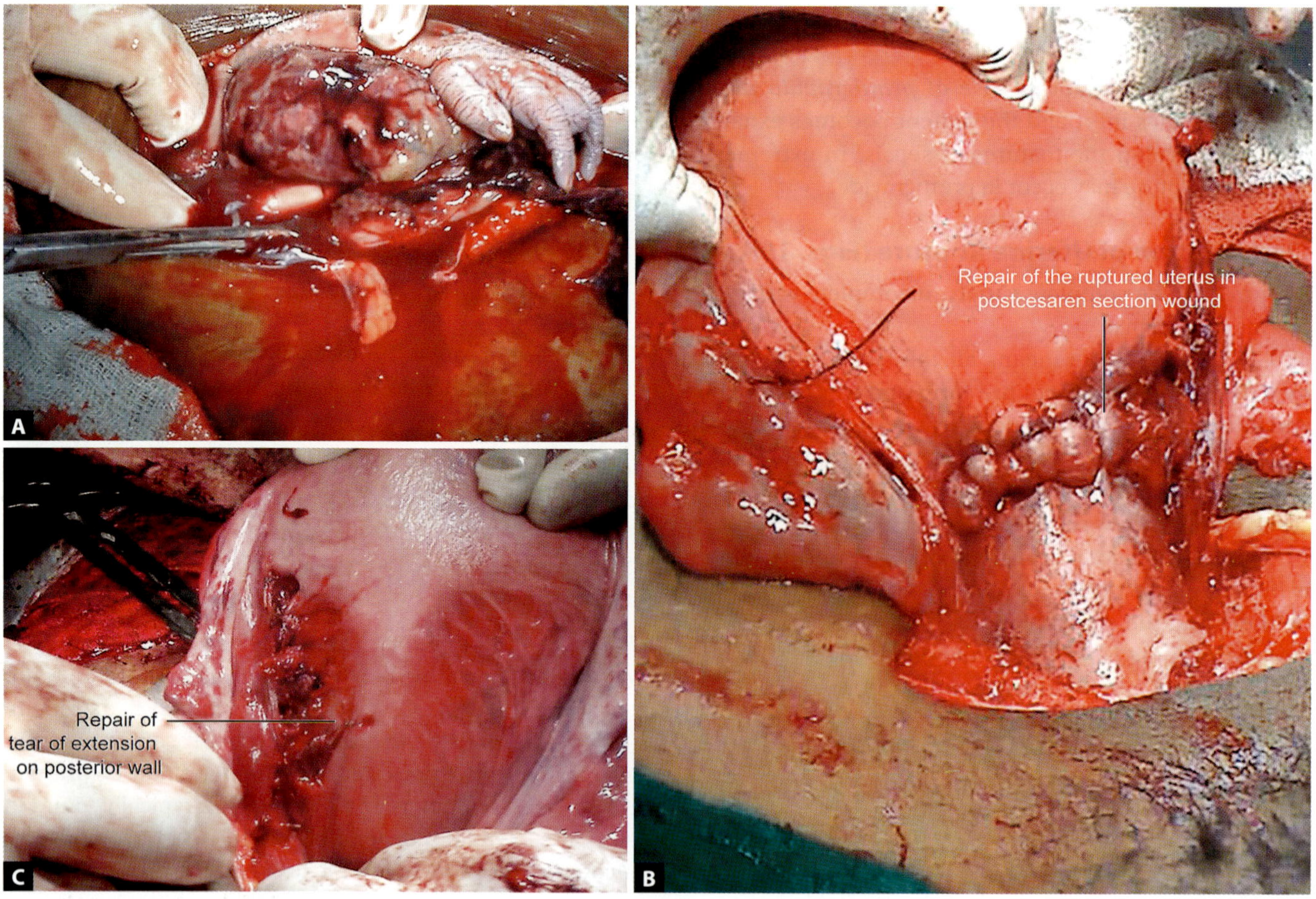

Figs. 20A to C: (A) Ruptured uterus in a second gravida postcesarean section mother with no living issue at 32 weeks. Uterine wound was repaired along with left-sided internal iliac ligation. The baby was dead; (B) Wound repaired in the patient as shown in Figure 20A; (C) Extension of wound and repaired in the patient as shown in Figure 20A.
Courtesy: Professor Sudhir Adhikary, Professor Mandira Dasgupta, Medical College, Kolkata, West Bengal, India.

of internal iliac artery is needed. If there is rupture of bladder, then it is repaired and a continuous drainage is given at least for 10 days postoperatively.

- Abdomen is closed in layers.

Scope of Conservative Surgery following the Rupture of Uterus

If the patient is primigravida or multigravida with no living issue, repair of the uterine wound in layers is attempted. Even if the patient has living issue but young, repair of uterine wound is attempted if possible. Subsequent rupture in next pregnancy is a possibility. However, in that case, ligation of fallopian tubes may be considered to prevent future pregnancy and scar rupture with prior counseling.

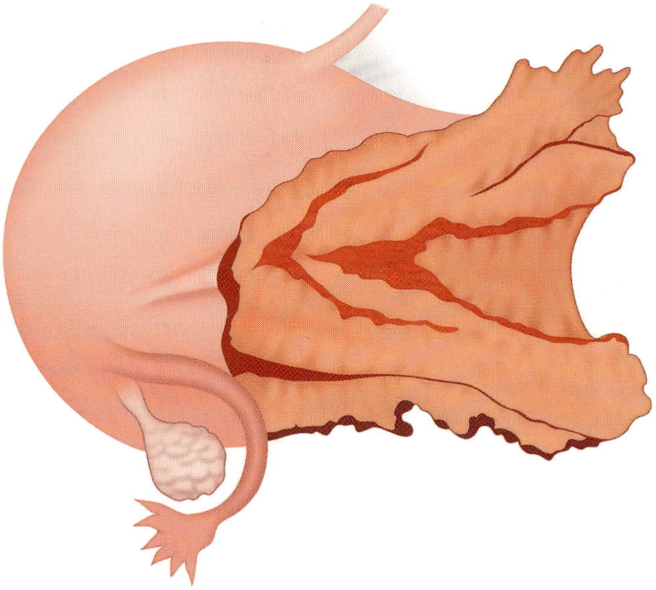

Fig. 21: Hysterectomy following uterine rupture—schematic diagram.

Prevention of the Rupture of Uterus

Anticipation of obstructed labor is made in some conditions such as CPD, malpresentation, and trial of labor after cesarean (TOLAC).

Close monitoring is done during administration of oxytocin and prostaglandin for augmentation. For attempt of vaginal birth in after cesarean section (VBAC) pregnancy proper selection of the cases is done.

All the VBAC cases should be done in institution and closely monitored during labor. Application for forceps are done only when all the criteria are fulfilled. Destructive operation (very rarely done and almost abandoned today) should be performed only by an experienced surgeon. It is safer to deliver abdominally than to perform destructive operation by an inexperienced person. Manipulation inside the uterus like internal podalic version is only performed when there is adequate amniotic fluid. In impending rupture, it is always justified to deliver the baby by CS.

Impending Rupture or Threatened Rupture

Before rupture of the uterus, there may be some symptoms and signs which will indicate that rupture of uterus is imminent with features of obstructed labor. These are identified by—complain of excruciating pain, features of obstructed labor with dry tongue, lesser amount of urine, raised temperature, and tachycardia. Per abdominally uterus becomes tonically contracted and Bandl's ring appears. Alteration of fetal heart rate (FHR) (fetal bradycardia) also occurs. In previous CS pregnancy, tenderness develops over the scar. Vaginal finding is dry vagina with offensive discharge. There will also be excessive caput formation, molding, and meconium-stained liquor.

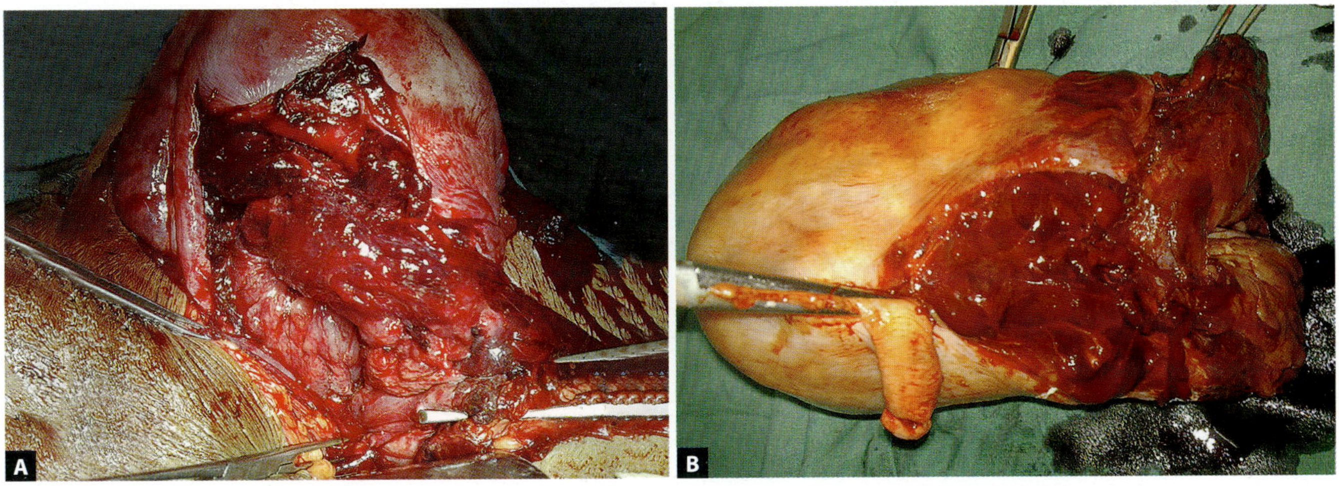

Figs. 22A and B: (A) Rupture of uterus in a postcesarean pregnancy; (B) Specimen of subtotal hysterectomy in the patient as shown in Figure 22A.

Courtesy: Professor Anindya Das, Bankura Sammilani Medical College, Bankura, West Bengal, India.

Unexplained tachycardia with features of obstructed labor in unscarred uterus and in post-CS pregnancy is highly suggestive of impending rupture of uterus.

Maternal and Fetal Outcome Following Uterine Rupture

Maternal Outcome

Maternal death following uterine rupture has become less nowadays but still happens. In developed countries, the incidence is <0.2%. In developing countries, the maternal mortality ratio (MMR) caused by uterine rupture is much higher.

Uterine rupture contributes up to 10% all hemorrhagic deaths in USA (2011–2013). Hysterectomy is the most common morbidity, other is bladder injury. Pregnancy with previous rupture is recommended for cesarean delivery.

Some other maternal morbidities following birth trauma are: "Pelvic relaxation syndrome" is a condition where woman complains of pain and discomfort due to separation and softening of ligaments of pelvic girdle during process of birth. "Coccygodynia" is a fracture and dislocation of coccyx, a potentially disabling obstetric injury, caused by pressure of fetus. Spontaneous symphysis pubic injury is extremely rare condition and intentional symphysiotomy is performed in some special situations discussed elsewhere. Injury of urinary tract and fistula formation is not uncommon in developing countries.

Fetal and Neonatal Prognosis

Prognosis depends on the size of the rent, whether fetus is outside or inside the uterus, degree of placental separation, maternal status, and how much rapidly diagnosis is done and action taken. Perinatal morbidity and mortality are high. Mortality rate ranges as high as 75%. Severe neonatal neurological abnormality is a serious concern among survivors.

CHAPTER 22

Obstetric Hysterectomy

Learning Objectives

- History of Obstetric Hysterectomy
- Varieties and Classification of Obstetric Hysterectomy
- Indications of Cesarean Hysterectomy
- Variations in Type of Obstetric Hysterectomy
- Variations in Technique in Total Hysterectomy
- Postoperative Management
- Complications of Obstetric Hysterectomy
- Peroperative Complications
- Ureter and Bladder Injury
- Postoperative Complications
- Mortality

INTRODUCTION, DEFINITION, AND INCIDENCE

Obstetric hysterectomy or peripartum hysterectomy is one lifesaving procedure mostly for uncontrollable bleeding from uterine atonicity, trauma, and placental abnormal attachment.

Obstetric hysterectomy means removal of gravid or recently pregnant uterus.

During last few decades the incidence of obstetric hysterectomy has been increased abruptly, the main reason of which is cesarean delivery rate, its complications, and defective placental attachment in future pregnancies.

Due to changes in anatomy, physiology, increase vascularity, and relation to adjacent structures of pelvic genital organs, hysterectomy is more difficult in comparison to gynecological hysterectomy. Besides it is done mostly in a compromised situation due to hemorrhage or patient is vulnerable to hemorrhage when a quick procedure is needed by skilled surgical team avoiding the injury of adjacent vital structures like bladder, ureter, and sigmoid colon. For these reasons, detailed discussion of the topics with the technical details are needed and will be helpful especially for the beginners.

HISTORY OF OBSTETRIC HYSTERECTOMY

History of obstetric hysterectomy is related to the history of development of techniques of cesarean delivery. It was Eduardo Porro from Italy who introduced the subtotal or supravaginal hysterectomy in obstetric surgery in 1876 to lower the death rate from cesarean section (CS). Before that cesarean delivery was almost fatal with >80% death rate. In Porro's technique, after delivering the baby amputation of the body of the uterus was done and the cervical stump was made fixed to the lower angle of abdominal wound where bleeding could be controlled by pressure. Maternal mortality came down to half, and due to removal of the uterus possibility of bleeding from the unstitched uterus was removed and infection also greatly lessened. Porro published in 1876 the first case report of survival of woman who was undergone hysterectomy following cesarean delivery of a large baby (3,300 g female). Cesarean hysterectomy is referred to as Porro operation by many.

First documented peripartum hysterectomy on woman was in the year 1868 by Horatio Robinson Storer (Boston). This was a case of obstructed labor with dead baby caused by large uterine tumor and destructive operation could not be performed due to the tumor. The woman died after 3 days. Much before that in 1768, Joseph Cavallini (Florence) developed the concept of obstetric hysterectomy based on the animal experiment. Blundell from Guy's Hospital, London, successfully performed the operation on rabbits (1834). After the Porro obstetric hysterectomy, the death rate had come down. In that era, the indication was mostly contracted pelvis due to rickets which was very common at that time. Following improvement of anesthesia and aseptic techniques, indications widened. Other than life-threatening emergencies, elective cesarean hysterectomy was also performed gradually. Nonemergent indications are some gynecological conditions associated with pregnancy and need hysterectomy, e.g., fibroid, cervical intraepithelial neoplasia (CIN)/cervical malignancy. Severe uterine infections were an important indication at that time, the incidence of which has gradually reduced. Subtotal (supracervical) hysterectomy has been largely replaced by total hysterectomy. Now radical obstetric hysterectomy has been introduced. Obstetric hysterectomy is mostly done during CS or immediately after CS. It is also done following vaginal delivery due to intractable postpartum hemorrhage (PPH), mostly atonic. Obstetric hysterectomy is rarely done during antenatal period.

VARIETIES AND CLASSIFICATION OF OBSTETRIC HYSTERECTOMY

Categorization of obstetric hysterectomy is done according to the time in relation to gestation, extent of removal of uterus, and adjacent structures and whether emergency or nonemergency.

Classification in Relation to Gestation

Obstetric hysterectomy in relation to gestation is classified as follows:

- Antepartum hysterectomy (fetus inside)
- Peripartum hysterectomy

Peripartum hysterectomy is further subdivided into:

- Cesarean hysterectomy **(Fig. 1)** which is done after cesarean delivery
- Postpartum hysterectomy which is performed within a short time after vaginal delivery.

Cesarean hysterectomy is comprised of 80% cases and postpartum hysterectomy is needed in rest 20% cases only. Antepartum hysterectomy is rarely needed.

Classification According to the Extent of Removal

Obstetric hysterectomy according to the extent of removal is classified as follows:

- Subtotal (supracervical) with or without salpingo-oophorectomy **(Fig. 2)**
- Total hysterectomy with or without salpingo-oophorectomy **(Fig. 1)**
- Radical hysterectomy with or without salpingo-oophorectomy.

Total or subtotal hysterectomy is done in both antepartum and peripartum hysterectomy cases.

Surgery for cancer cervix early in second trimester (antepartum hysterectomy) may be treated by radical hysterectomy with fetus in situ which is commonly performed with lymph node dissection. Sometimes, modified radical hysterectomy is also performed in peripartum hysterectomy for safe surgery without removal of lymph nodes.

Obstetric hysterectomy may be emergency or indicated nonemergency.

INDICATIONS OF CESAREAN HYSTERECTOMY

The indications have been widened and the incidence has increased. The most common indication is to stop hemorrhage.

Emergency:

The important emergency indications are:

- Hemorrhage with intractable uterine atony
- Placenta previa with lower segment bleeding
- Placental abruption
- Morbid adhesion of placenta **(Fig. 3)**
- Traumatic bleeding—cervical or uterine laceration
- Rupture uterus—prior CS, myomectomy scar, intact uterus, rudimentary horn pregnancy (uterine anomaly) **(Fig. 4)**
- Large myomas during CS.

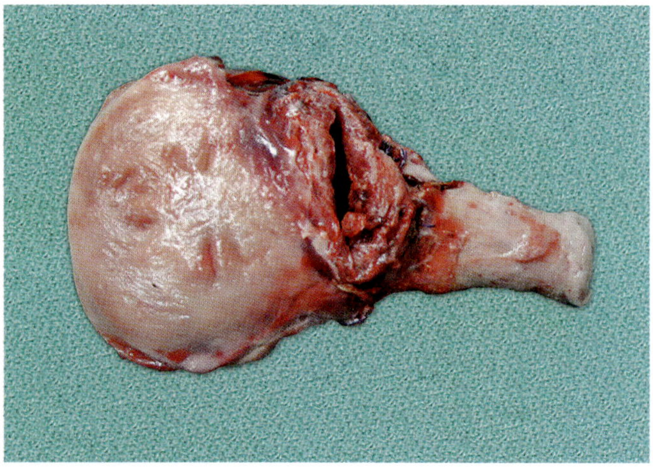

Fig. 1: Cesarean hysterectomy (total) due to uncontrolled bleeding performed in a case of second gravida postcesarean section pregnancy with anterior placenta previa at 34 weeks.

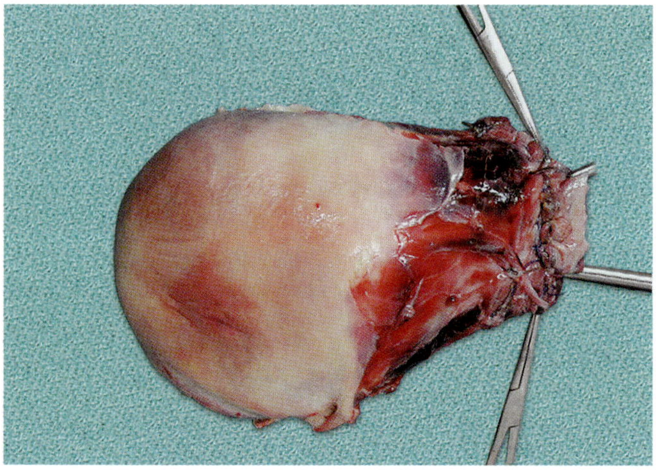

Fig. 2: Subtotal hysterectomy in immediate postoperative period due to intractable postpartum hemorrhage.

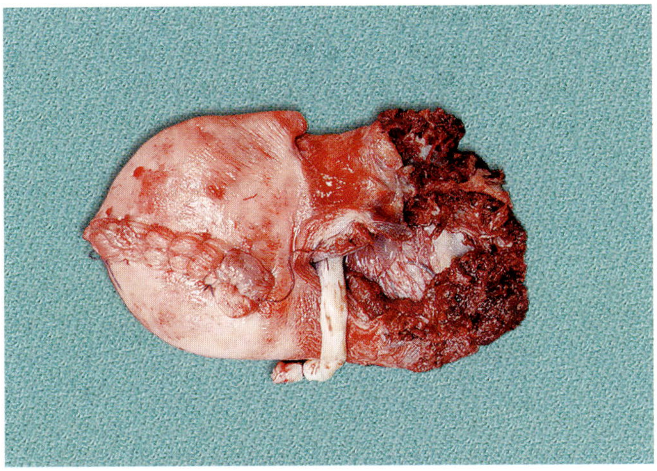

Fig. 3: Hysterectomy in morbid adhesion of placenta.

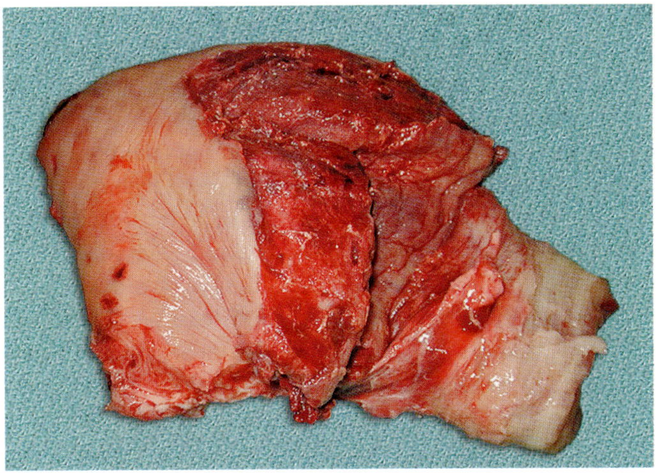

Fig. 4: Hysterectomy specimen following cornual rupture. Initially cornual resection done to preserve the uterus. Hysterectomy decision was taken due to uncontrolled bleeding.
Courtesy: Professor RP Ganguly, R.G. Kar Medical College, Kolkata, West Bengal, India.

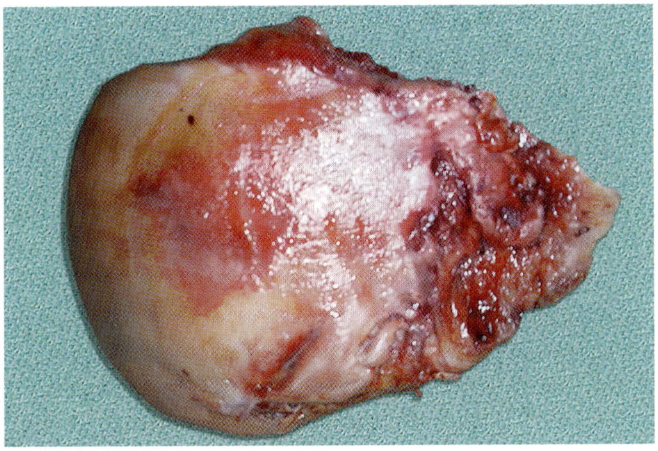

Fig. 5: Postabortal sepsis hysterectomy specimen in a 22-year-old P2+0 woman with two living issue, referred from a remote place with severe sepsis following an attempt of midtrimester abortion (the method not clear) by quack about 4 weeks back.

Nonemergency:
- Pregnancy associated with gynecological disorders which need hysterectomy, e.g., genital malignancy associated with pregnancy—CIN, uterine fibroids.
- Puerperal/postabortal severe uterine infections **(Fig. 5)**

Elective cesarean hysterectomy merely for sterilization is not recommended.

The most common indication for obstetric hysterectomy in recent days has been placenta accreta spectrum (PAS) in prior CS pregnancy which has dramatically increased in the last few decades. The other indication is PPH due to uterine atony.

Technical Difficulties of Obstetric Hysterectomy in Comparison to Gynecological Hysterectomy

Technical difficulties of obstetric hysterectomy in comparison to gynecological hysterectomy are:
- Surgery is done either in compromised or hemorrhagic environment, hence skill experienced surgeon, expert anesthetic team should be available and it should be done in well-equipped center.
- Gravid uterus is hugely enlarged, hypervascular, edematous, and friable; pelvic vessels become wide caliber and tortuous and collaterals are well developed and quick surgery is needed to cut off all vascular supply at the earliest.
- As the pedicles are often large and thick in pregnancy, surgeon becomes very cautious that the tissue containing the vessels are occluded properly. Clamps should not be manipulated or twisted rather only supported otherwise the tissues will be torn due to friability and edema. Very quick ligature tightening may cut the friable tissues, on the other hand, too much delay may cause bleeding, hence optimal time is given to secure the pedicle.
- To prevent retrograde blood loss (back bleeding), routine extra clamp is needed in pregnant uterus.
- Choice of suture is also important. Many use 1 or 0 chromic catgut, as 1 or 0 Vicryl has disadvantage of cutting through the soft tissue of pedicle. On the other hand Vicryl has advantage of long half-life.
- Double ligature is preferable for vascular pedicle as the pedicle shrinks and become loosen as edema subsides. Principle is to give one free tie and another transfixation suture proximal to free tie (circumferential sutures). Proximal placement will avoid hematoma if any vessel puncture occurs.
- Every pedicle should be inspected and secured after final ligature. The pedicle of utero-ovarian ligament, fallopian tube, and utero-ovarian anastomosis is very vulnerable to bleed due to its thickness and improper tightness.
- Traction and manipulation of gravid uterus is another difficulty, as in nongravid uterus traction is given by two large clamps on two cornu, the area which are very

vulnerable to be lacerated in pregnant uterus. One good practice is to grasp the fundus with tumor tenaculum along with retraction with the help of Deaver or Richardson retractor for good exposure.

- Another area of concern is separation of edematous and friable bladder and its retraction during hysterectomy. The bladder is separated very gently and carefully with sharp dissection by fine (Metzenbaum) scissors rather than blunt dissection. The assistant will avoid to retract the bladder directly with pressure; instead, he/she can use a laparotomy sponge between bladder and the retractor. In the presence of dense adhesion in uterovesical space as found in one or more prior cesarean delivery, it is better to reflect the bladder up to the cervix before the uterine incision and avoids bladder opening which is a possibility if separation is attempted after cesarean delivery.
- Bladder and ureter are vulnerable to be injured in obstetric hysterectomy due to more close proximity for enlarged uterus, obscured vision, and softness and edematous nature in pregnancy. The precaution taken, detection, and management of bladder injury are described below.
- Vagina is often edematous, friable and vascular for which during closure of vaginal cuff proper hemostasis is maintained and one should be very careful that no hematoma is entrapped in vaginal layers, a potential site of infection and secondary hemorrhage.

Preoperative Steps

Preoperative steps of obstetric hysterectomy in comparison to gynecological hysterectomy are:

- Health status of the women, hemodynamic stability, complications, and coagulation status are assessed.
- Counseling regarding severe hemorrhage and risks of urinary tract injury is done. Consent for hysterectomy is taken.
- It should preferably be done in a tertiary care center (level III or IV) equipped with adult intensive care unit (ICU) and neonatal ICU. The surgical team should consist of experienced obstetric surgeon, oncosurgeon, senior anesthetist, and urological surgeon. Availability of blood and blood products should be assured. It is better to have interventional radiologist if there is facility. Many prefer ureteric stenting (cystoscope).
- At least two large intravenous (IV) cannulas should be placed.
- Prophylactic antibiotics is administered. Thromboprophylaxis is considered.

Surgical Steps (Figs. 6 to 15)

Technique of surgery differs depending on the indications. Steps in postpartum uterine atony following vaginal delivery are definitely not so difficult than placenta accreta syndrome with distorted anatomy, and uterine rupture with extension, and steps are modified according to the individual case.

- Infraumbilical midline vertical skin incision **(Fig. 6)** is always preferable in planned hysterectomy.
- Hysterectomy starts with the clamping and cutting of round ligament (**Figs. 7A** and **B**) if it is for atonic postpartum hysterectomy. In rupture uterus, fetus is delivered first whether it is outside the uterus, partly or fully (in incomplete variety) inside the uterus. Placenta and membranes are removed. If there is any bleeding vessel in the rupture site, especially in the angle, it is grasped with sponge holding forceps to stop bleeding; then hysterectomy (if decision taken against the repair) is proceeded with clamping of round ligament. If CS is done concurrently as in placenta accreta, uterine wound is closed after pushing the ligated cord inside the uterus following delivery of the baby; then hysterectomy is started.
- Many prefer to extend the incision of uterovesical fold up to two to three to the round ligament and bladder is retracted after creating uterovesical space before hysterotomy (cesarean delivery).
- Any of the round ligament (say left) is clamped with straight or curved Kocher clamp 2–3 cm lateral to uterus and cut with scissors or scalpel and retroperitoneal space is opened where ureter is visible. Cut end of distal part is ligated with double threads, commonly 0 or 1 Vicryl. The thread is held with artery forceps for traction or made short to keep the area clear.
- Now, an avascular area is selected in the broad ligament below the fallopian tube and ovarian ligament at medial part and is opened **(Fig. 8)** with help of a sharp pointed artery forceps or Kelly clamp. If the tip of index finger

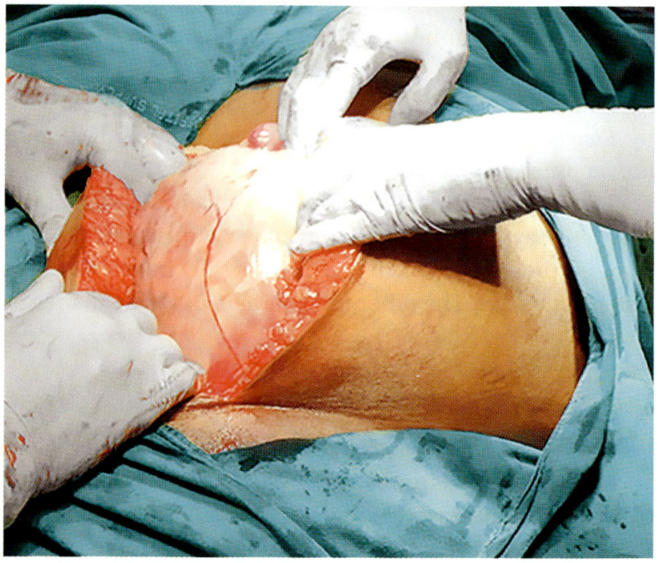

Fig. 6: Abdomen is opened through vertical incision.

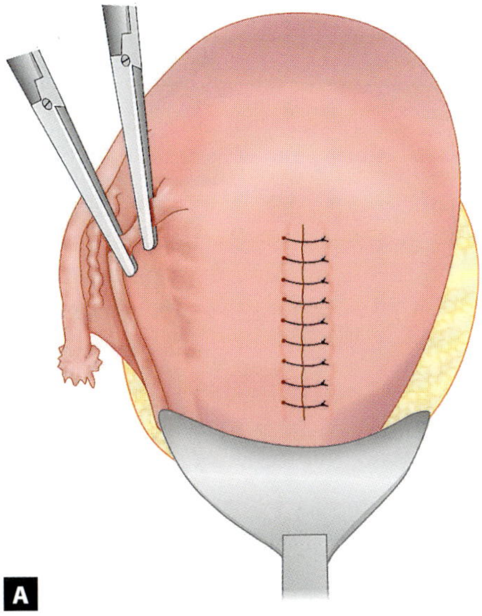

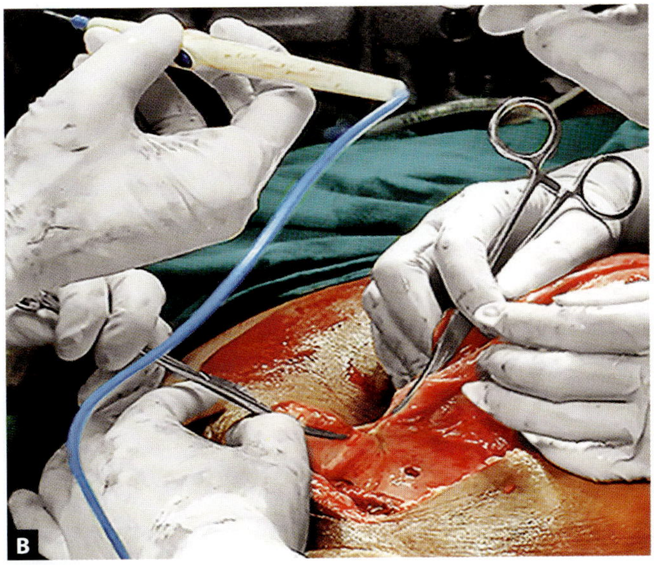

Figs. 7A and B: (A) Round ligament is clamped (right side); (B) Round ligament is cut (right side).

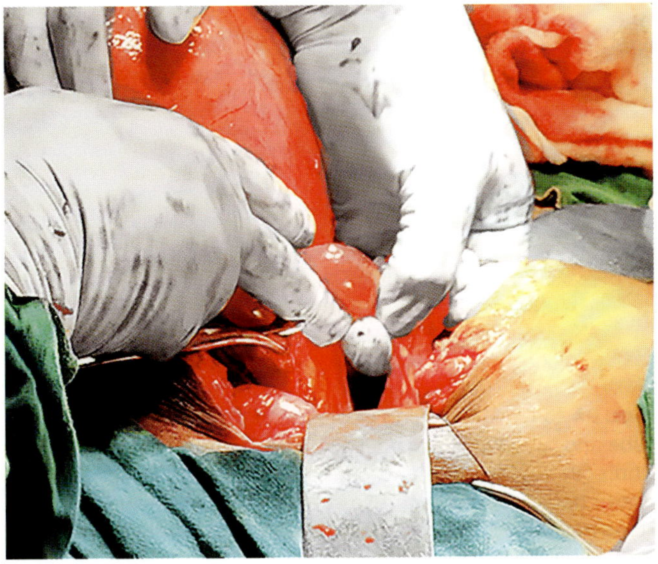

Fig. 8: Opening an avascular space in broad ligament.

is kept in the avascular area from behind and pressed, the opening of the broad ligament gets easier without injuring any vessel or bleeding. Scissors can also be used for opening the broad ligament.

- Now, medial end of fallopian tube and ovarian ligament **(Figs. 9A and B)** is clamped with uterine clamps (Kocher or Ochsner) one medially and another laterally. For more security two clamps are used medially. If the index finger is introduced in the rent and slightly stretched laterally upward, the pedicle becomes stretched and clamp placing becomes easy. The pedicle is then divided with scalpel or scissors or cutting diathermy. The pedicle **(Fig. 9C)** is tied with two sutures one free tie and another transfixation. Transfixation will prevent slipping of the tie.
- Now uterovesical fold of peritoneum is incised from one round ligament to other **(Fig. 10)** if the space is not already opened. Bladder is retracted downward as far as possible. Sharp dissection is preferable to blunt dissection for bladder separation in this step to prevent inadvertent injury of bladder. Now uterus is retracted to the opposite side to visualize the uterine vessels for clamping.
- Posterior leaf of broad ligament is now cut from the previous opening and incision extends along the lateral margin of the uterus to reach the uterosacral ligament. This will allow displacement of ureter more laterally to a safer site.
- Skeletonization which is the removal of the connective tissue around the uterine vessels makes better griping. However, overenthusiasm on clearing of tissue may cause bleeding. Here, ureter can be easily identified as a tubular structure with peristalsis at the medial leaf of broad ligament, if anyone tries to see.
- During pregnancy diameter of ureter increases and becomes thick and edematous. In case of difficulty ureter can be traced from bifurcation of common iliac artery downward.
- Now uterine vessels are clamped with long uterine clamp (Heaney) at the level of junction of cervix and body of uterus **(Fig. 11)**. Another clamp (Kocher or Henry) is placed on the uterus above the first clamp to prevent retrograde blow. The vascular pedicle is incised by scalpel, scissors, or cutting diathermy. Level of incision is so that some part of the tissue proximal to the distal clamp so that suture does not slip. Tip of the lower clamp is slightly freed for placing of suture well. A suture with needle is passed beneath the tip of this proximal clamp. Surgical knot is given and gradually the clamp is released slowly to prevent retraction and hematoma formation.

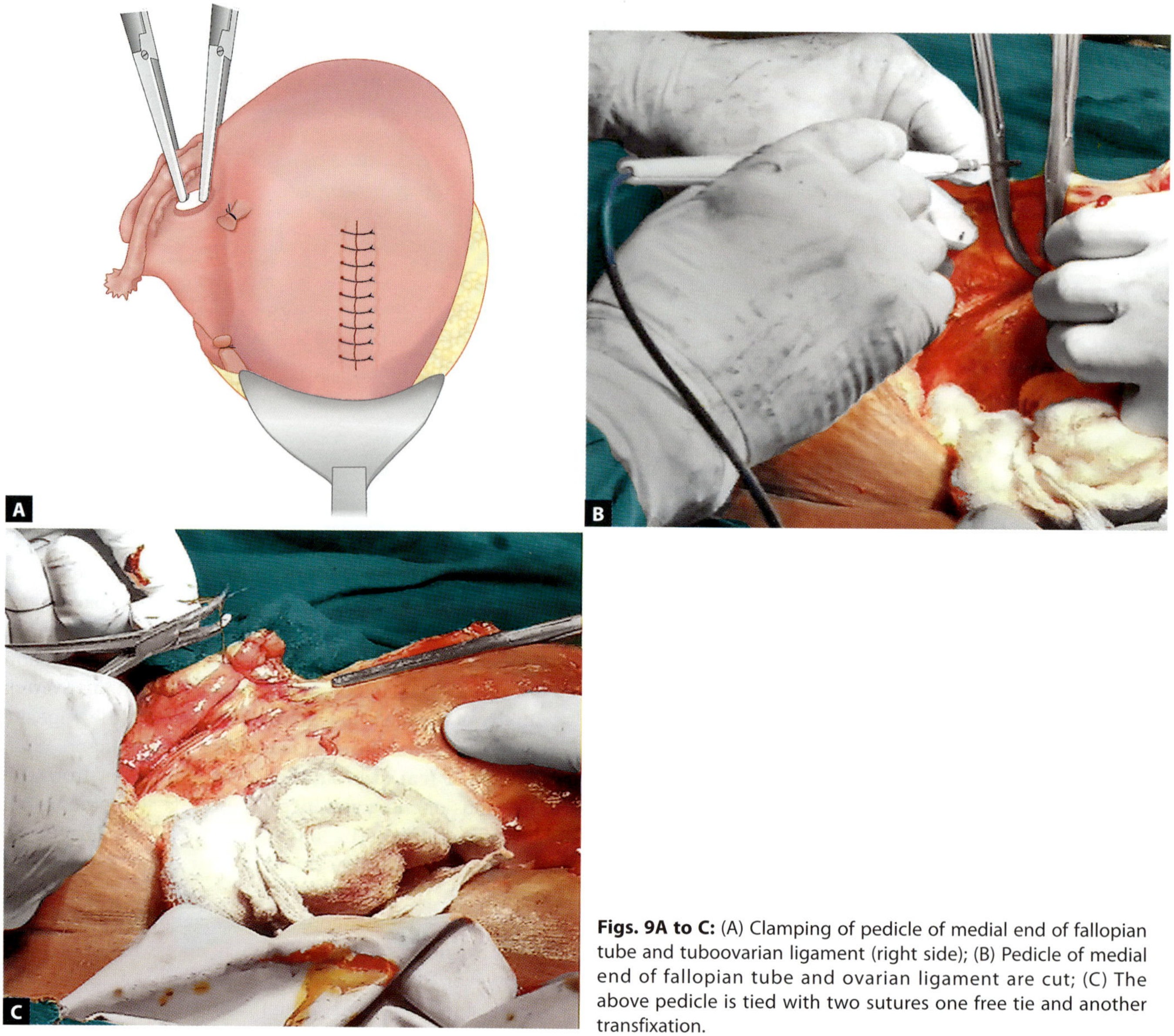

Figs. 9A to C: (A) Clamping of pedicle of medial end of fallopian tube and tuboovarian ligament (right side); (B) Pedicle of medial end of fallopian tube and ovarian ligament are cut; (C) The above pedicle is tied with two sutures one free tie and another transfixation.

Many prefer to give a free tie and another transfixing suture in the uterine vessel pedicle.

- In the same way, pedicles of the opposite side—round ligament, tubo-ovarian pedicle, and uterine vessels—are clamped, cut, and ligated.
- Now, more mobilization of bladder **(Fig. 12A)** is needed from the cervix. It should be done very gently with the help of fine scissors. Dissection is done in midline avoiding the lateral side dissection may cause severe venous bleeding.
- Now uterus is elevated with the help of two clamps on two sides on cornu or by grasping the uterine fundus in the midline by tumor tenaculum.
- The cardinal ligaments **(Fig. 12B)** are clamped as medial as possible slipping over the cervix not too holding much of tissue at a time. Scalpel or fine curve scissors is used to incise the tissue. Needle with suture is passed along the tip of the clamp and tightened and clamp is released slowly. In this way, two to three pedicles are created for cardinal ligaments successively. Lower clamp is always placed medial to the upper clamp and chance of ureteric injury will be less.
- The uterosacral ligaments which lie posteriorly just above the vaginal vault may need clamping separately or may be included in the clamps of cardinal ligaments.
- Cardinal and uterosacral ligaments are clamped, incised, and sutured on the opposite side in the same manner.
- Now cervix becomes free from its attachment on all sides. Just beneath the cervix at the level of cervicovaginal junction two curved hysterectomy clamps are placed **(Fig. 13A)** one on each side along the lateral fornix

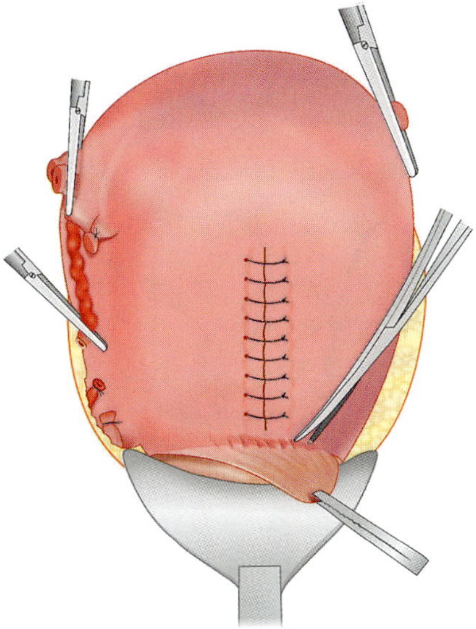

Fig. 10: Vesicouterine fold of peritoneum is cut from one end to other and vesicouterine space is dissected.

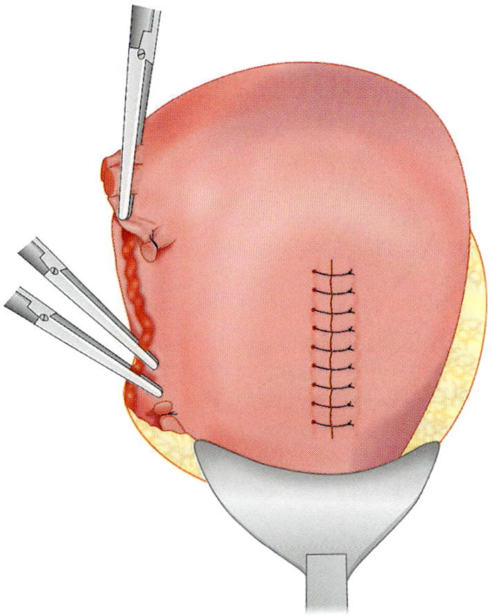

Fig. 11: Uterine vessels are clamped with long uterine clamp at the level of junction of cervix and body of uterus.

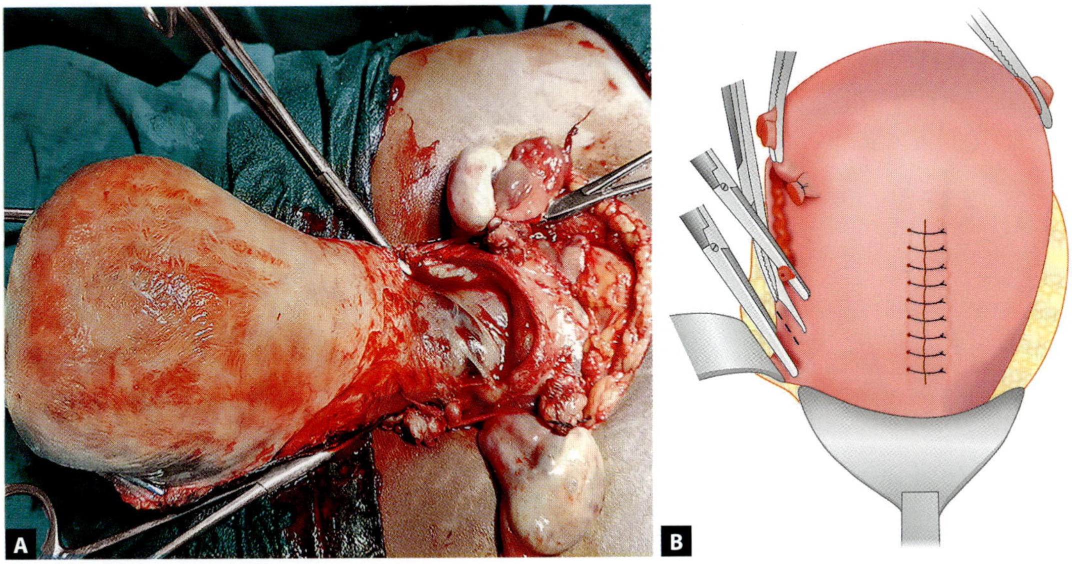

Figs. 12A and B: (A) More mobilization of bladder and clamping of cardinal ligament; (B) Cardinal ligament clamped after securing uterine vessels. Two to three pedicle may be needed to clamp and cut successively.

over the vaginal vault and proceeded for vault opening. As in pregnancy the vault becomes wider the tip of the opposite clamps may not touch each other.

- Another difficulty in pregnancy is to locate the cervicovaginal junction if the cervix is effaced and the os is dilated due to labor. One method is to palpate by finger through the hysterotomy opening if present or to make a small vertical slit to open the cavity and to palpate the cervicovaginal junction. This is done before application of clamps on lateral vaginal vault (fornices) laterally. The contaminated glove is changed.
- Now vaginal vault above the transversely placed clamps is cut (**Fig. 13B**) from lateral to midline on each side. The specimen removed is examined for full removal of cervix. If some part is left removal of that part is done further applying clamps below the level distal to cervical margin.
- Angles of vaginal vault are fixed with the uterosacral ligaments by many to prevent vault from sagging down and prolapsing.
- Closure of vaginal vault **(Fig. 14)**—lateral vaginal angles are first stitched with transfixing sutures on sides.
- Vaginal vault can be closed by closed method or open method.

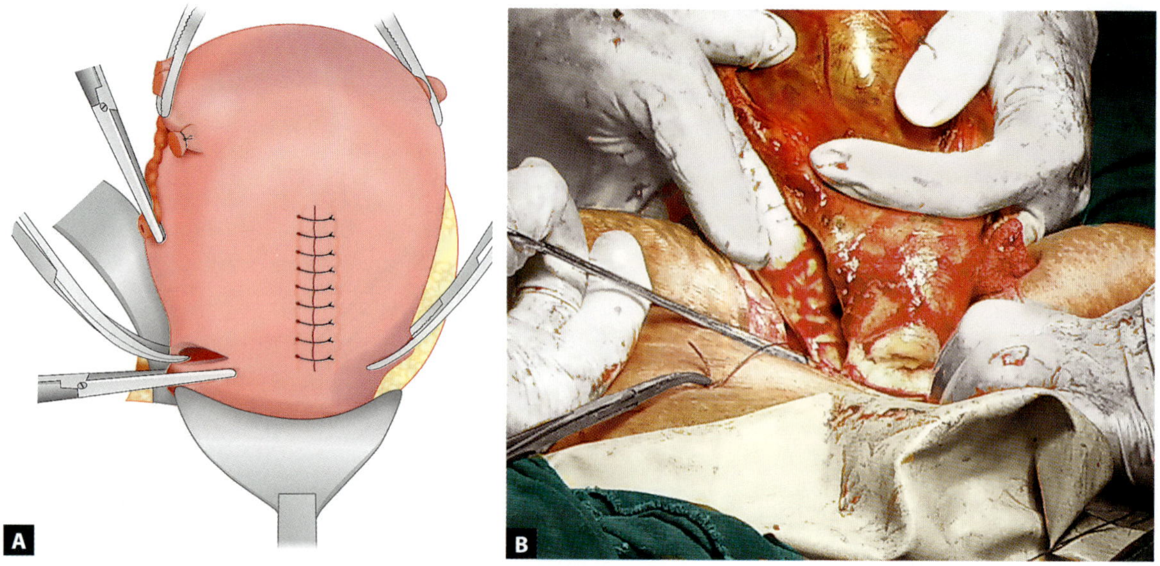

Figs. 13A and B: (A) Just beneath the cervix at the level of cervicovaginal junction two curved hysterectomy clamps are placed one on each side along the lateral fornix over the vaginal vault and proceeded for vault opening; (B) Vaginal vault above the transversely placed clamps is cut from lateral to midline on each side.

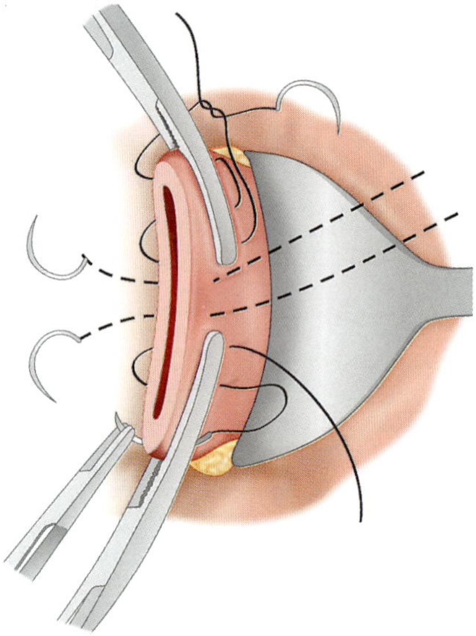

Fig. 14: Vaginal vault is closed with stitches.

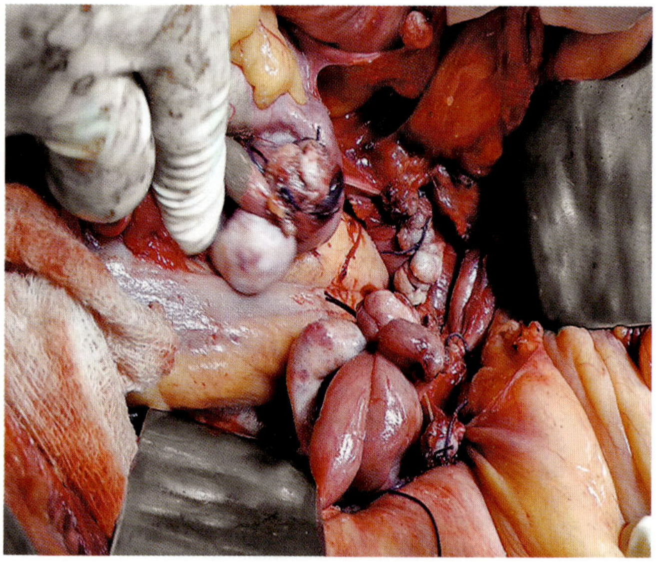

Fig. 15: Vaginal vault after suturing.

- In the close technique, at the angle of vault the wide area of vaginal cuff which is incorporated in the clamp the suture is passed first below the middle of clamp, then passed beyond the tip and then tied securely at the back of clamp with gradual release of clamp and this procedure is done on both sides.
- Now, the middle part of vaginal vault is sutured with figure of eight or interrupted stitches. One must be sure that full thickness anterior and posterior vaginal walls are incorporated during passing of needle. **Figure 15** shows vaginal vault after complete suture.
- The bladder and colon are retracted from the area of suture line.
- In open technique the angles are tied first and the clamps are released and the threads are held by artery forceps and traction given on both sides. The vaginal cut margins are grasped with Allis tissue forceps in the midline one anteriorly and another posteriorly and the cuff is elevated. The vaginal opening is closed either series of figure-of-eight stitches, or by continuous interlocking stitches. After final closure, the vault is inspected for any bleeding, especially on bladder surface. All the pedicles are reexamined whether these are dry without any oozing and any bleeding anywhere is searched for. The whole operative area is irrigated whether complete hemostasis is achieved. The area is pressed with gauze

if there is any oozing. Topical hemostatic agents can also be used. Any injury to bladder or ureter is finally checked for. Before closure of the abdomen instruments, needles, and sponges are counted.

VARIATIONS IN TYPE OF OBSTETRIC HYSTERECTOMY

Variations in the type of obstetric hysterectomy are:

- Total hysterectomy
- *Supracervical (subtotal) hysterectomy instead of total hysterqqectomy:* It is considered in the presence of severe hemorrhage or disseminated intravascular coagulation (DIC) to minimize operative time and to eliminate difficult dissection and blood loss.
- *Modified radical hysterectomy* without lymph node dissection is suggested to dissect the retroperitoneal area and parametrial region so that ureteric and vessels dissection is under direct vision to minimize the chance of injury.
- As obstetric hysterectomy is done in the patients of younger age group the ovaries are not removed except in special rare circumstances as where this is essential to control excessive bleeding or hematoma formation. Recent procedure is to remove the fallopian tubes (salpingectomy) only to reduce the future risk of high-grade epithelial cancer.

VARIATIONS IN TECHNIQUE IN TOTAL HYSTERECTOMY

Variations in the technique in total hysterectomy are:

- Both body and cervix are removed together or fundus is amputated first followed by removal of cervix. The latter will give good exposure to work on lower part.
- Concurrent ligation or delayed ligation of pedicles: In concurrent ligation every pedicle is clamped, cut, and ligated and then proceeded to next. In delayed ligation each pedicle is clamped and cut and laterally displaced. After completion of severing of all six pedicles, i.e., two round ligaments, two tubo-ovarian ligaments, and two for uterine vessels ligation of all the pedicles are done one after another. The later will block the vascular supply of the uterus earlier and bleeding will be less. However, concurrent ligation is preferred by most surgeons.
- *Application of tourniquet:* In this method a tourniquet is used around lower uterine segment through avascular area of broad ligament before proceeding to hysterectomy. But uterine supply from the ovarian arteries is not controlled in this technique during surgery.

POSTOPERATIVE MANAGEMENT

Postoperative care should be given in intensive care with proper clinical and investigation monitoring protocol. Antimicrobials are administered, and thromboprophylaxis is considered.

COMPLICATIONS OF OBSTETRIC HYSTERECTOMY

Peroperative

- Hemorrhage
- Injury to bladder and ureter
- Injury of intestines and rectum
- Anesthetic complications.

Postoperative

- Hemorrhage—reactionary, secondary, intraperitoneal hemorrhage, broad ligament/retroperitoneal hematoma
- Rectus sheath hematoma
- Sequelae of primary morbidity—DIC, renal failure
- Shock
- Urinary retention, urinary tract infection
- Infection—peritonitis, wound sepsis
- Wound dehiscence, burst abdomen
- Paralytic ileus, abdominal distension, intestinal obstruction
- Pneumonia
- Thromboembolism—pulmonary embolism
- Secondary hemorrhage from vault on second week onward
- Urinary fistula—vesicovaginal fistula (VVF), ureteric fistula.

Long-term Complications

- Band adhesion
- Incisional hernia.

PEROPERATIVE COMPLICATIONS

Hemorrhage and injury to bladder and ureter are the two most important complications during surgery.

Peroperative hemorrhage: The two potential areas of bleeding are tubo-ovarian pedicle and uterine vessels pedicle and other site is retrograde bleeding of each clamp. Bleeding from the tubo-ovarian and utero-ovarian anastomosis pedicles may arise due to tear during manipulation, needle prick for transfixing suture, and sometimes, inadequate tightening of the knot due to thickness of the pedicle, retraction of ovarian vessels in postoperative period due to shrinkage. Clamps should not be manipulated or twisted rather only supported otherwise the tissues will be torn due to friability and edema. Pedicles should be double secured, one free tie and, another transfixing, one must be careful not pricking the vessel. Sometimes adnexal bleeding may cause rapid spreading hematoma which should be detected early and managed quickly, even rarely ovary is to sacrifice by adnexectomy to control spread of retroperitoneal hematoma.

URETER AND BLADDER INJURY

It is not very uncommon that bladder and ureter are damaged in obstetric hysterectomy, which occurs more common in emergency obstetric hysterectomy. If it is detected during surgery, the prognosis is excellent. Failure to detection and management during surgery follows a serious consequence.

The bladder is lacerated and damaged commonly during the dissection of uterovesical space particularly in a case with the history of prior cesarean delivery. During clamping of the lower clamp and during the suturing of vaginal cuff bladder may be included that may result future necrosis and sloughing of the bladder with formation of VVF. Abscess at the vault may increase the risk of VVF. Meticulous and careful dissection is done and in suspected cases confirmation of injury is done. For detection of small bladder injury, bladder is filled with opaque (sterile milk) or colored solution (methylene blue in normal saline) into the bladder through the urethra. If detected, it is repaired in two layers followed by continuous bladder drainage for 10–14 days.

Ureter is very vulnerable to be traumatized more than in nonpregnant condition. The crossing of uterine artery during clamping of vessels is one site, another site at the vault when it is entering into the bladder. And the chance of injury increases due to its displacement by hematoma. Lower clamp is always placed medial to the upper clamp and chance of ureteric injury will be less. Ureter may be displaced by hematoma or may be damaged unnoticed. Proper visualization, palpation, and tracing along the course prevent ureteric injury. In suspected injury it should be delineated properly through the broad ligament opening at its base where bifurcation of the common iliac artery is seen above, and the ureter is identified by its location, conduit and peristalsis. It is traced downward from above for inspection. On IV injection of methylene blue or indigo carbamine a blue color fluid is seen coming from ureteral orifice seen through the cystoscopy or intentional cystostomy. If ureteral integrity is suspected retrograde ureteric catheterization is done to check its intactness. If any injury is detected standard management is done preferably with the help of urologist. In PAS, antenatal detection of bladder invasion by ultrasonography (USG) many suggest to use ureteric tent, though it is not universally recommended.

POSTOPERATIVE COMPLICATIONS

Three important complications are bleeding, infections, and wound dehiscence.

Hemorrhage: The potential areas of bleeding in the postoperative period are vaginal cuff, tubo-ovarian, and uterine pedicles as well as parieties in the form of rectus sheath hematoma.

Vaginal bleeding in immediate postoperative period is from vessels of vault and delayed bleeding may be due to secondary hemorrhage or rupture of vaginal cuff hematoma.

Blood may accumulate either in peritoneal cavity or collect in the retroperitoneal space as hematoma. Broad ligament hematoma occurs due to bleeding from uterine vessels which may spread retroperitoneally. Adnexal bleeding accumulates in the peritoneal cavity or may also spread retroperitoneally even up to upper abdomen. Hypotension, pallor, and tachycardia are the important diagnostic signs and oliguria is relatively a late feature. Low/falling hematocrit with or without high-white blood cell (WBC) count is very alarming. Tenderness and fullness of abdomen are the features of hemoperitoneum, but difficult to elicit following laparotomy due to large wound. Sonography and computed tomography (CT) scan are two important diagnostic tools to detect hematoma and hemoperitoneum. Magnetic resonance imaging (MRI) is supplementary in inconclusive cases. Initial management is fluid/blood products transfusion with broad-spectrum antibiotics. Exploratory laparotomy is indicated in large/progressive intraperitoneal bleeding or hematoma. Interventional radiology may be helpful. Small nonprogressive hematoma may not need surgical exploration, however abscess formation is a potential threat. Vaginal cuff bleeding needs proper examination and pressure, if any localized hematoma is drained. Suturing may be attempted, but is not useful as spurting vessel is rarely seen. Vaginal pressure pack is an option. For localized pelvic hematoma drainage through vagina and putting a surgical drain work well. For intraperitoneal bleeding and hematoma exploratory laparotomy is done and all the blood clots are gently removed. Suturing is done in oozing/bleeding sites if possible, or hemostasis done by pressure or topical hemostatic agents. Irrigation done and the abdomen is closed putting a drain. Management of rectus sheath hematoma is discussed elsewhere.

Postoperative Infections

This is one of the important complications after obstetric hysterectomy as the patient is already compromised, anemic, and prolonged exposure time is needed for surgery especially in emergency cases. Sepsis may be evident as cuff abscess, pelvic abscess, peritonitis, and intra-abdominal abscess in the area of hematoma formation. Complete blood count, serum urea, creatinine, electrolytes, and vaginal swab for culture sensitivity and blood culture are done. Broad-spectrum antibiotic is started till the culture sensitivity report comes. Clindamycin and gentamycin are good combination. Others options are combinations are ampicillin, gentamycin, and metronidazole; pipercillin tazobactum or ampicillin sulbactum or third-generation cephalosporine.

In pelvic abscess, drainage can be done through posterior colpotomy approach under general or regional anesthesia with standard lithotomy position using a long Kelly clamp (Pean) passing through the middle of the cuff. In abscess stitches spontaneously fall. A drain (Foley or Malecot catheter) is inserted through the aperture which is removed when the drainage will be minimal. No vaginal wound closure is needed. If abscess is in the peritoneal cavity laparotomy is done, pus is drained, and irrigation done. Laparotomy wound is closed after putting a drain. In abscess drainage in every case pus is sent for culture and sensitivity. Postoperative monitoring of patient both clinical and investigations, fluid electrolyte balance in ICU is very important.

MORTALITY

There is significant mortality following obstetric hysterectomy. Death in nonemergent indication is obviously less. Death is more due to the primary cause of hysterectomy than the surgical procedure itself. Delayed decision of hysterectomy after attempt of conservative treatment and performed by inexperience surgeon is the important factor of death. Preoperative and peroperative care of anesthetic team is very crucial to prevent death.

CHAPTER 23

Laparoscopic Procedures in Obstetrics

Abhinibesh Chatterjee
MBBS DGO DNB (Obst and Gyne) FRCOG (London)
Consultant Gynecologist, Advance Laparoscopic Surgeon and Infertility Specialist, Kolkata, West Bengal, India

Learning Objectives

- History of Laparoscopy in Obstetrics—Past and Present
- Reasons for Difficulties and Challenges of Use of Laparoscopy in Obstetrics
- Advantages of Laparoscopy in Obstetrics
- Indications of Laparoscopy in Obstetrics
- Contraindications of Laparoscopy in Obstetrics

INTRODUCTION

Nonobstetrical surgery in pregnancy is uncommon with an incidence of around 0.2% and when indicated, should be undertaken with proper precautions to minimize fetal risk without compromising the safety of the mother. The mode of surgery, open or laparoscopic, per se does not have a bearing on the outcome, as fetal and maternal outcomes have been similar in both. What matters is timely and accurate diagnosis and a prompt intervention.

Acute appendicitis and cholecystitis are the two most common nonobstetrical surgical emergencies complicating pregnancy. Others are adnexal cysts, masses or torsion, symptomatic cholelithiasis, bowel obstruction, rarely adrenal tumors, splenectomy for refractory severe immune thrombocytopenia (ITP), complicated hernias, inflammatory bowel diseases refractory to medical management or bowel perforation, and other rare conditions.

Pregnancy was considered a contraindication for laparoscopic procedures earlier, due to concerns of uterine and fetal trauma from trocar placement and fetal hypoperfusion due to increased abdominal pressures due to pneumoperitoneum. Down the years, techniques have been developed to avoid these complications and at present laparoscopy is preferred over open surgery, if there are no contraindications, and if the expertise and proper equipment are available.

HISTORY OF LAPAROSCOPY IN OBSTETRICS—PAST AND PRESENT

When laparoscopy was initially used in pregnancy, it was for diagnostic purposes only. The first laparoscopic cholecystectomy was performed in 1980 after one such diagnostic procedure. Schreiber was the first person to perform laparoscopic appendicectomy in 1990. Till late, it was believed that second trimester was the safest time to perform any surgery in pregnancy, but this view has changed and it is accepted that surgery can be safely performed in any trimester (SAGES Guideline 2017).

REASONS FOR DIFFICULTIES AND CHALLENGES OF USE OF LAPAROSCOPY IN OBSTETRICS

Surgical procedures, especially laparoscopic procedures, during pregnancy need special consideration of the following.

Physiological Changes in Pregnancy

Cardiovascular System

Cardiac output is increased. There is reduction of peripheral vascular resistance and plasma oncotic pressure. After 20 weeks, gestation, in supine position, the gravid uterus compresses aorta and inferior vena cava leads to "supine hypotension syndrome".

Gastrointestinal Tract

Stomach is in a more horizontal position and pushed up due to the growing uterus. The bowel is also displaced and so is the appendix, thus altering the localization of pain in appendicitis. The reduced tone of the esophageal sphincter and the increased gastric emptying time leads to gastroesophageal regurgitation and puts the mother at a high risk of aspiration.

Respiratory System

The enlarging uterus causes gradual restriction of the chest movements. Minute ventilation and oxygen consumption are increased. Residual volume and functional residual capacity are decreased. Oxygen content of the mixed venous blood is reduced. Due to the above changes, pregnant women are prone to hypoxemia and hypocapnia. A chronic state of respiratory alkalosis ($PaCO_2$ 28–32 mm Hg) is maintained in pregnancy due to stimulation of the respiratory center by progesterone. Due to edema in the soft tissues in the neck, difficulty might be encountered while inserting an endotracheal tube.

Hematological Changes

Blood volume increases by 30–40% which is due to increase of plasma volume as well as red blood cell (RBC) volume. But the increase in plasma volume is more than that of RBC volume leading to hemodilution and resultant physiological anemia and reduced viscosity in second trimester. Increase in fibrinogen and other clotting factors lead to a hypercoagulable state.

Uterine Size

The uterus grows in size as the gestation advances. The chances of uterine injury during entry and manipulation increase as uterus becomes an abdominal organ after first trimester.

Pneumoperitoneum and its Effects

- Pneumoperitoneum increases the intra-abdominal pressure which decreases inferior vena caval return to the heart, thus reducing cardiac output which diminishes the uterine blood flow leading to impaired placental blood flow and consequently fetal hypoxia and even fetal death.
- Pneumoperitoneum decreases the diaphragmatic movements increasing the peak airway pressure. This decreases functional reserve capacity further, reducing thoracic cavity compliance and increasing ventilation perfusion mismatch.
- Gases used for creating pneumoperitoneum may also contribute: (1) CO_2 absorption and its effects on the fetus is a matter of debate, but there is no data of its detrimental effects in a human fetus is available; (2) Nitrous oxide is safe in that respect but is highly combustible et al.

Patient Positioning

Trendelenburg is the most common position given during pelvic surgeries but for a cholecystectomy a reverse Trendelenburg is needed. Trendelenburg position increases intrathoracic pressure and therefore amplifies the respiratory-related physiologic changes. Reverse Trendelenburg position decreases venous return, hence the cardiac output and subsequently the cardiac index and when this is combined with maternal hypoxia can cause fetal death.

Use of Electrosurgery

Electrosurgery produces smoke which can expose the fetus to carbon monoxide toxicity, if absorbed.

Precautions and Measures to Overcome the Above Challenges and Make Laparoscopy Safer

- Laparoscopic surgery in pregnancy should be performed by advanced laparoscopic surgeons with appropriate training and competencies with trained assistants and where proper equipment is available, in order to reduce complications and operating times.
- Alterations in positioning and the creation of the pneumoperitoneum should be gradual, with monitoring of the woman's hemodynamic status all along.
- The operating pressures should be kept between 10 and 15 mm Hg.
- Maternal blood pressure should be maintained close to baseline.
- CO_2 levels should be monitored with end-tidal carbon dioxide ($ETCO_2$) levels which are maintained between 28 and 32 mm Hg.
- Administering venous thromboembolic (VTE) prophylaxis—use of intermittent pneumatic compression intraoperatively and keeping the operative pressure <15 mm Hg.
- If necessary, uterus may be displaced using methods that do not impact the surgeon's ability to perform the procedure effectively.

ADVANTAGES OF LAPAROSCOPY IN OBSTETRICS

Benefits of laparoscopy during pregnancy appear similar to those benefits in nonpregnant patients.

- Less postoperative pain, hence reduced use of narcotics and less postoperative ileus
- Short hospital stays and faster recovery
- Lower risk of wound complications as the wounds are small.
- Diminished postoperative maternal hypoventilation due to smaller wounds and thus, reduced pulmonary complications such as atelectasis.

- Decreased risk of thromboembolic events as patients are mobilized early.
- Good visualization with a laparoscope, reduces the need to manipulate the uterus and thus lower risk of uterine irritability.

INDICATIONS OF LAPAROSCOPY IN OBSTETRICS

Laparoscopy in pregnancy is indicated in the following conditions:

- Symptomatic gallbladder disease
- Acute appendicitis
- Choledocholithiasis
- Adnexal masses—with symptoms or signs suspicious of malignancy
- Adnexal torsion
- Torsion or incarceration of pedunculated subserous myoma
- Solid organ resection—adrenalectomy, nephrectomy, and splenectomy
- Fetal surgeries
- Cervical cerclage.

CONTRAINDICATIONS OF LAPAROSCOPY IN OBSTETRICS

Patient Independent

- Surgeon with inadequate training and experience
- Poor equipment—operative and monitoring
- Inadequate training of surgical assistants or ancillary staff should be thought of as further contraindications to advanced laparoscopic procedures.
- Unavailability of neonatal intensive care unit (NICU) facilities to care for a preterm viable baby, if the chances of preterm delivery are high.

Patient Dependent

- *Absolute contraindications:*
  - Intestinal obstruction with dilated bowel loops
  - Hemodynamic instability/shock
  - Raised intracranial pressure
- *Relative contraindications:*
  - Cardiac failure
  - Pulmonary failure
  - Soft tissue infection at port sites
  - Extensive adhesions expected
  - Abdominal aortic aneurysm.

Preoperative Assessment and Preparation

Patient Selection

Every patient is assessed carefully for need of surgery and presence of any contraindication to undergoing laparoscopy. Surgery, if indicated, should not be delayed.

Preparation

- The preoperative anesthetic review should be done and relevant features noted, such as the period of gestation, any associated comorbidities, any history of difficult intubation in the past as well as the routine anesthesia history, and examination.
- Aspiration prophylaxis in form of H_2 receptor blocker/proton-pump inhibitors and antiemetics—metoclopramide/ondansetron—should be administered.
- Rh Anti-D immunoglobulin administration is not recommended for laparoscopic surgery.
- *VTE prophylaxis:* Use of intraoperative and postoperative pneumatic compression devices and early postoperative ambulation are recommended.
- A course of antenatal steroids needs to be given, if there are chances of preterm delivery of a viable fetus (>24 weeks and <36 weeks). Magnesium sulfate should be administered for fetal neuroprotection in fetuses <34 weeks [National Institute for Health and Care Excellence (NICE) guideline, 2015]. Urgent surgery should not be delayed for administrating corticosteroids.

Instruments and Gadgets

- CO_2 insufflator
- Suction/irrigation system
- Light source and cable
- Electrosurgery equipment
- Insufflation instruments—Veress needle or Hasson cannula
- Trocar and cannula
- *Laparoscopes:* Both 5- and 10-mm diameter laparoscopes can be used depending upon the surgical requirements and availability of equipment. A 30-degree scope can improve visibility in the pelvis in trained hands.

Sequential Steps and Procedures

Patient positioning: Pregnant patients in their first trimester do not require altered positioning, as the small size of the uterus does not compromise venous return. To avoid the supine hypotension syndrome in patients 18 weeks and above, a partial left lateral decubitus position is given as a complete left lateral decubitus may compromise the ability to operate.

Insufflation pressure: To ensure a safe primary trocar insertion, an insufflation pressure of 20–25 mm Hg can be used since these pressures are only maintained for a short duration and therefore, unlikely to harm the fetus. However, operative pressure should be kept between 10 and 15 mm Hg (SAGES Guideline 2017).

Entry techniques:

- Abdominal access can be gained either by using an open or closed technique.

- Various entry techniques have been studied in pregnant patients. These include, Veress needle, Hasson technique, and direct entry using an optical trocar.
- The use of Hasson's and Veress entry techniques without any entry-related complications have been documented in various studies. The direct entry technique by elevating the umbilicus with a towel forceps and inserting an optical trocar under visual control through it has also been described. The site of entry will be guided by the height of the uterus and history of previous surgeries.

Port placement:

- Primary ports and secondary ports are placed taking into account the size of the uterus and location of the pathology. Primary trocar placement under ultrasound guidance has also been used to avoid uterine injury.
- Secondary port placement should be considered on the same side as the lesion (ipsilateral port placement) as this avoids the need to go across the gravid uterus to reach the pathology, thus avoiding trauma to the uterine surface.

Alternatives to uterine manipulation: In order to improve surgical access without using an intrauterine manipulator, alternative strategies may be used. These include digital vaginal manipulation, planning the placement of surgical ports according to pathology and uterine size, tilting of the surgical table, and use of 30-degree laparoscope. Bearing in mind that uterine surface in pregnancy is more friable and can bleed more easily on contact, even with blunt instruments, it is best to adopt a "no touch" approach.

Energy sources:

- Commonly used energy sources like ultrasound, bipolar, and monopolar can be safely used in pregnant patients.
- General safety rules for monopolar diathermy (e.g., avoiding indirect thermal damage, pedicle effect, coupling, checking for faulty insulation) apply.
- In addition, while using monopolar energy, it is recommended that the uterus should not be in between the electrode and the return plate.
- The smoke produced should be promptly suctioned out to avoid the risk of carbon monoxide exposure.

Specimen retrieval: It might be necessary to avoid spillage of the contents of the pathology in cases of dermoid cysts (to avoid chemical peritonitis) or in suspicious masses (to avoid dissemination of malignant cells inside the peritoneal cavity) and therefore, specimen should be retrieved in a bag. There is no data available on use of power morcellation, which should be discouraged in pregnancy to avoid uterine trauma.

Drains: They are usually placed to drain out blood, pus, or any fluid that may collect inside. The placement of a drain will be decided by the surgeon depending on the case. There is no recommendation for routine placement.

Port closure: As in a nonpregnant patient, ports bigger than 10 mm need a fascial closure to avoid subsequent herniation. The risk of incisional hernia formation is 1–2%. It is greater at the lateral port sites, likely because of the impact of the enlarging uterus stretching the abdominal wall.

Intraoperative fetal heart rate monitoring: In the past, intraoperative fetal heart rate monitoring was considered necessary but as none of the studies have reported any abnormalities during surgery, it is not recommended at present. Instead, only preoperative and postoperative fetal heart rate monitoring is considered sufficient (SAGES Guideline 2017).

Intraoperative CO_2 monitoring: In the past, maternal arterial CO_2 levels were monitored. Recently less invasive $ETCO_2$ monitoring using capnography is considered equally beneficial. $ETCO_2$ measurements to monitor maternal CO_2 levels have been shown to be safe and effective in many studies.

Laparoscopic Procedures

Diagnostic Laparoscopy

Although imaging is preferred for investigating any cause of acute abdominal pain or mass especially in pregnancy, it might not be available promptly or might be inconclusive. In such cases, diagnostic laparoscopy might be helpful (SAGES Guideline 2017). The risks of delaying the diagnosis should be weighed against the risk of negative laparoscopy, which in some studies have shown to increase risks of preterm labor. In case a surgical pathology is detected, the surgeon should be prepared to treat it in the same sitting.

Operative Laparoscopy

Laparoscopic cholecystectomy: Symptomatic cholelithiasis in pregnancy was treated conservatively in the past. At present, early surgical management is the treatment of choice with laparoscopic cholecystectomy and it is shown to be safe in all the three trimesters (SAGES Guideline 2017). In fact, rates of spontaneous abortion and preterm labor have been found to be low with laparoscopic cholecystectomy when compared to laparotomy (Graham G et al., 1998). Uncomplicated cases may be managed conservatively but can present with recurrent symptoms or develop complicated disease requiring repeated hospitalization. Complicated cholelithiasis may result in preterm labor or fetal loss depending on severity.

Laparoscopic appendectomy: Laparoscopic appendectomy is considered the treatment of choice for pregnant women

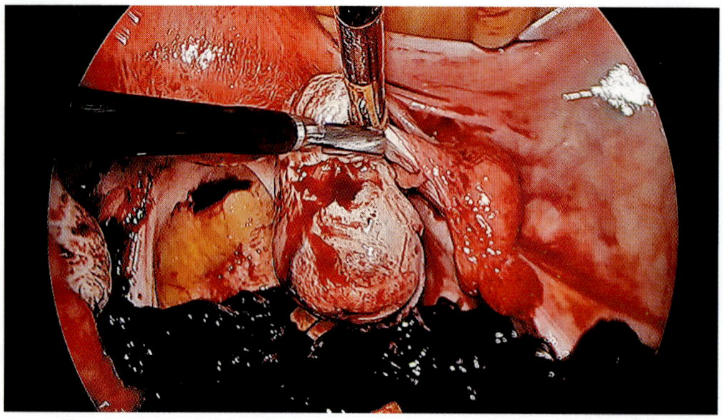

Fig. 1: Rupture of right corpus luteum cyst of pregnancy.

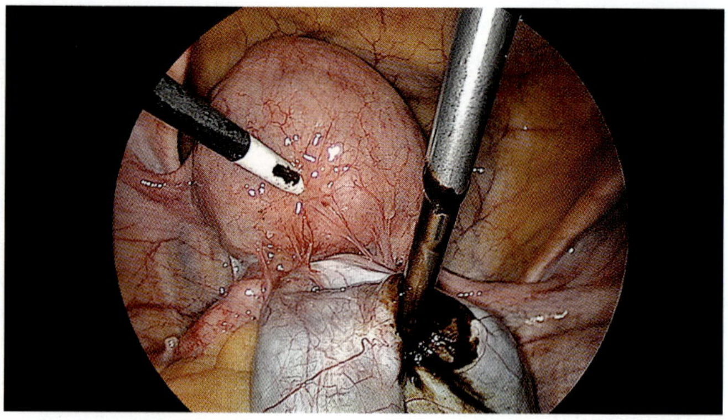

Fig. 2: Ovarian chocolate cyst being drained in early weeks of pregnancy.

with acute appendicitis. Conservative management has no role as it has shown to have higher rates of peritonitis, shock, fetal loss, thromboembolic events as compared to surgical management. Laparoscopic approach is preferred over open surgery (SAGES Guideline 2017). However, there is some level of evidence to show that chances of maternal morbidity, preterm labor, and fetal loss were found to increase after a negative laparoscopy for suspected appendicitis, compared to laparoscopic appendectomy for acute appendicitis. The cause for this observation is not clear and that is why it is important to make an accurate diagnosis before taking the decision to operate. Magnetic resonance imaging (MRI) is useful in these cases and is safer than computed tomography (CT) as it does not use ionizing radiation. It is found to reduce the rate of negative laparoscopy by 50% in a study.

Laparoscopy for adnexal masses: Incidence of adnexal masses in pregnancy is around 2%. These could include ovarian masses or paraovarian cysts. Ovarian cysts detected in first trimester are mostly functional cysts that resolve on their own by the second trimester. Most of the ovarian masses <6 cm and not suspicious of malignancy, not producing symptoms, and with normal tumor markers are observed (ACOG Practice Bulletin, 2007). Due to concern over the need for emergency surgery in event of subsequent complications, rupture **(Fig. 1)**, torsion or of being malignant, an elective removal of masses is generally done for those that persist after 16 weeks and are >6 cm in diameter. Laparoscopy is a safe and effective treatment in such cases (SAGES Guideline 2017). Cyst aspiration, with or without concurrent cystectomy **(Fig. 2)** may also be considered. **Figures 3A to F** show ovarian cystectomy in serous cyst in a patient at 14 weeks of pregnancy who came with pain in abdomen.

Laparoscopy for adnexal torsion and symtomatic subserous fibroid: Torsion of adnexa is uncommon in pregnancy. Laparoscopy is the preferred method of both diagnosis and treatment in the gravid patient with adnexal torsion. If tissue is viable, a simple detorsion is done. However, if it progresses to adnexal infarction, a complete resection is recommended as it may lead to peritonitis, spontaneous abortion, preterm delivery, and death. Progesterone therapy is initiated after removal of the corpus luteum, in pregnancies <12 weeks gestation.

Subserosal pedunculated fibroids can also undergo torsion and present with acute abdomen. These fibroids can be excised laparoscopically. Degeneration of a fibroid, when occurs in a subserosal pedunculated fibroid or a subserosal sessile fibroid with a narrow base, can be managed by myomectomy **(Fig. 4)**.

Laparoscopy for choledocholithiasis: Choledocholithiasis is uncommon in pregnancy. But when it occurs and develops complications such as acute pancreatitis or acute cholangitis, can lead to preterm labor or spontaneous miscarriage. Choledocholithiasis in pregnancy can be managed either by preoperative endoscopic retrograde cholangiopancreatography (ERCP) followed by laparoscopic cholecystectomy or laparoscopic cholecystectomy with common bile duct (CBD) exploration or postoperative ERCP (SAGES Guideline 2017). Both ERCP and laparoscopic CBD exploration are found to be safe in pregnancy hence the choice will depend on the expertise available. Safer alternatives to ERCP are endoscopic ultrasound and choledochoscopy for stone extraction and endoscopic stenting without stone extraction which can be done using minimal radiation.

Laparoscopic cervical cerclage: It can be performed laparoscopically and is as effective as abdominal cerclage for cervical incompetence. Although it is preferably performed as an interval procedure can be safely performed during pregnancy. Marcelene tape or proline suture can be used **(Fig. 5)**.

Laparoscopy for solid organ resection: Laparoscopic resection of organs such as spleen, adrenals, and kidneys might be indicated in a pregnant woman for various conditions. These procedures should be postponed until after delivery,

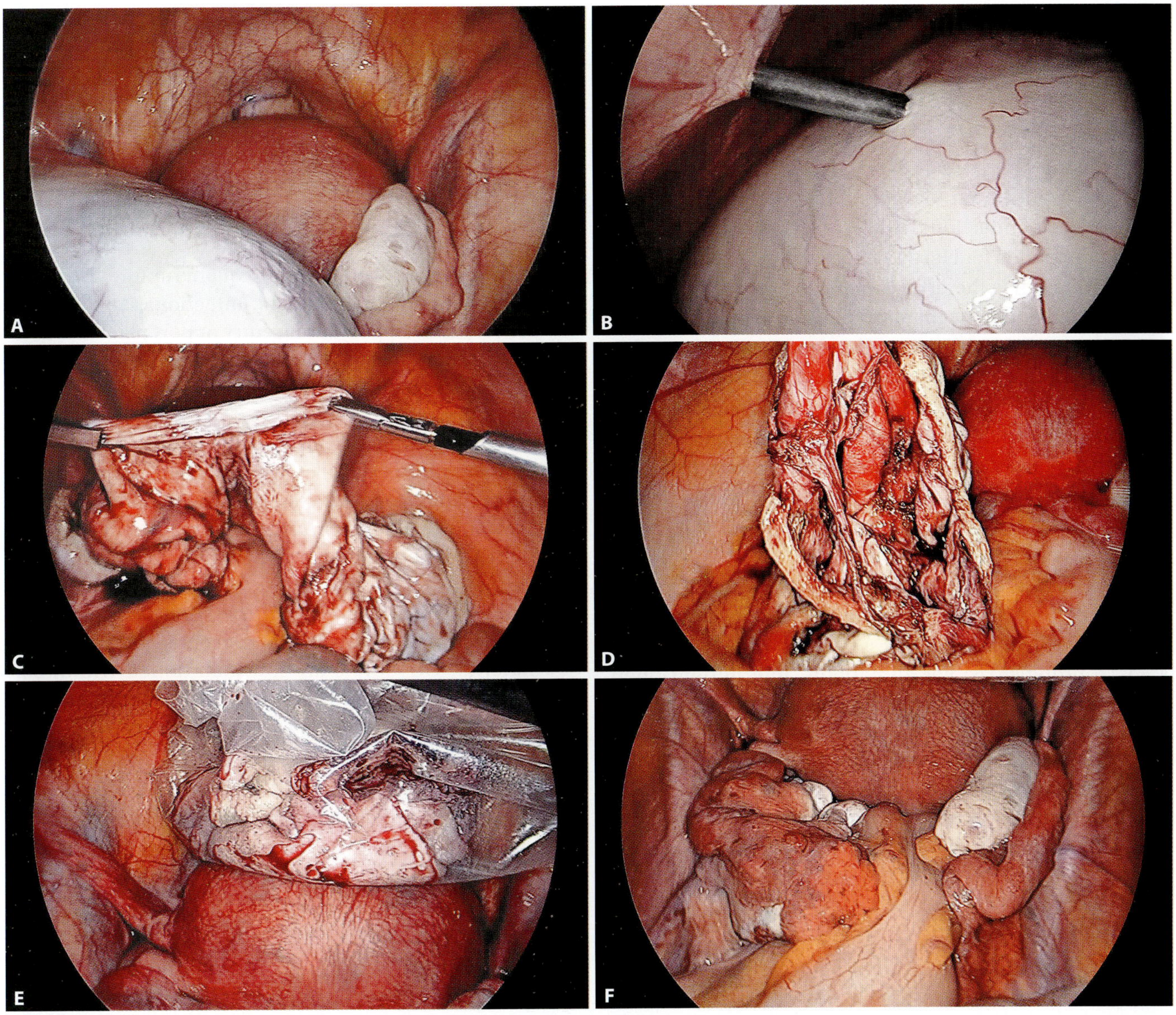

Figs. 3A to F: (A) Ovarian cyst in serous cyst in a patient at 14 weeks of pregnancy who came with pain abdomen. Ovarian cystectomy done; (B) Puncture and aspiration before cystectomy as in patient in Figure 3A; (C) Cystectomy—dissection of cyst wall; (D) Cystectomy; (E) Collection of cyst wall for removal; (F) Final picture after completion of ovarian cystectomy as in patient in Figure 3A.

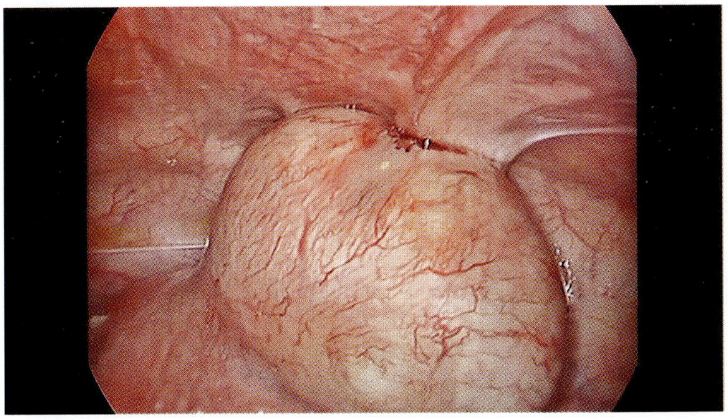

Fig. 4: Degenerated subserous uterine fibroid with pregnancy. Laparoscopy was done for severe pain.

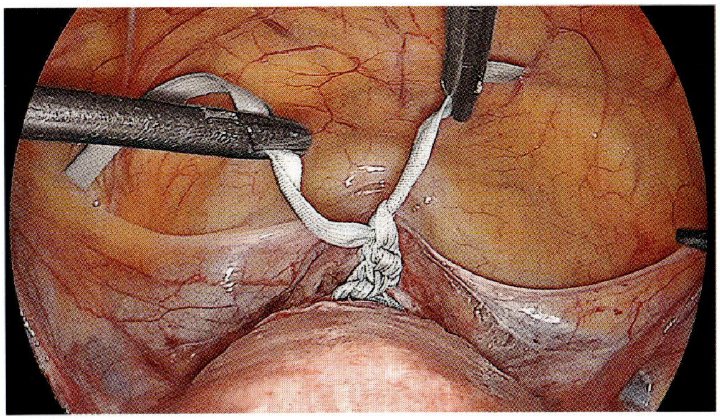

Fig. 5: Laparoscopic method of abdominal cervical cerclage.

if possible but when they threaten the mother's or fetus's life, can be performed safely. The maternal and fetal outcomes have been found to be good.

Postoperative Care

- Antibiotics that are safe in pregnancy and recommended by local antimicrobial guideline should be used in presence of infections. However, they are not routinely recommended for elective surgeries.
- Paracetamol is the drug of choice for postsurgical pain management in pregnant woman and should be used in the lowest possible effective dose and for short periods of time. Opioids—oxycodone, fentanyl, and morphine—are category B and can be used. Tramadol and codeine should be avoided in first trimester as they belong to category C. Nonsteroidal anti-inflammatory drugs (NSAIDs) should be avoided, especially after 32 weeks as they are associated with premature closure of the ductus arteriosus and oligohydramnios.
- Antiemetics are administered to counter any postoperative nausea and vomiting.
- Adequate hydration is necessary to maintain euvolemia.
- *VTE prophylaxis:* For all patients, intermittent pneumatic compression, compression stockings, and early ambulation is advised. Pharmacological thromboprophylaxis is recommended in patients who have intermediate and high risk of VTE.
- Fetal heart monitoring should be carried out in all pregnancies with viable fetuses (SAGES Guideline 2017).
- Tocolytics are recommended in patients only with signs of preterm labor not prophylactically (SAGES Guideline 2017). The choice of the drug will be decided by the obstetrician.

Complications

Even though laparoscopy is considered safe in pregnancy complications can still occur if proper precautions are not taken.

- *Uterine perforation:* With subsequent rupture, laceration of the fetus or the placenta, infections, and preterm delivery can happen during entry or port placement.
- *Bleeding:* As the vascularity of uterus and adnexa is increased in pregnancy, even a minor trauma may result in bleeding.
- *Trauma to adjacent organs and vessels:* Due to the enlarged uterus visualization is limited, increasing the risk of trauma to major vessels and surrounding organs.
- *Cardiorespiratory compromise:* This may occur if creation of pneumoperitoneum and patient positioning are not gradual.
- *Fetal morbidity and mortality:* Fetal health may be compromised if euvolemia, placental perfusion, and maternal CO_2 levels are not maintained within safe ranges. Preterm labor is a risk in the third trimester, and hence there are chances of preterm delivery.

Acknowledgment

The author acknowledges Dr. Smita Jadhav DGO DNB, Consultant Gynecologist for contribution in this chapter.

CHAPTER 24

Anesthesia and Analgesia in Obstetrics

Learning Objectives

- History
- Determining Factors of Perception of Pain During Labor
- Physiology of Labor Pain
- Methods of Pain Relief in Labor
- Local Perineal Infiltration
- General Anesthesia in Pregnancy and Labor

INTRODUCTION

Analgesia and anesthesia are great challenge in obstetric discipline due to the uniqueness of physiological changes during pregnancy. Mortality and morbidity from anesthesia are more in pregnant women in comparison to nonpregnant state. Need of anesthesia in any moment, especially in full stomach and in severe morbid (e.g., preeclamsia, eclampsia, and placental abruption) and compromised women pose very difficult situation. Aspiration of acidic content of stomach in labor is one inheritent problem for maternal adverse outcome. However, improved anesthesia technique, switching to more regional from general anesthesia in pregnancy and labor and wider availability of high dependency unit (HDU) set up have reduced the death of pregnant mother remarkably during last few decades. It is to be remembered that spinal and epidural anesthesia are not always safe and need also good training. Every obstetrician should have a good knowledge of this domain.

HISTORY

In 1591, Eufane MacAyane of Edinburgh, a young mother was dragged from her home just after delivering twin sons and buried alive. Her crime was that she had asked for pain relief during labor. *"Pain of childbirth is a punishment to women as inflicted by God"*—it was the church's teaching of the day. *"Asking relief from pain is against God's wishes—is a sin."* In April 7, 1853 Queen Victoria had asked for pain relief during the birth of her eighth child, Prince Leopold. So, Dr John Snow administered chloroform anesthesia to the queen on request of Sir James Simpson, the queen's obstetrician. Only one decade back (1842), Crawford Long had invented surgical anesthesia in medical history. Alvinst Church of Edinburg, though angry but was compelled to accept the procedure. That is the beginning of introduction of analgesia in obstetric practice. Before that Simpson himself administered labor anesthesia on his niece very confidentially in 1847.

DETERMINING FACTORS OF PERCEPTION OF PAIN DURING LABOR

It depends on mother's emotion, psychological makeup, and preparation during antenatal period. Obstetric factors are parity, more pain in primigravida, much backward pressure in malpresentation and malposition, especially occipitoposterior position, where there is more backward pressure maximum pain occurs in late first stage and second stage of labor.

PHYSIOLOGY OF LABOR PAIN

Visceral (uterine) pain is due to uterine ischemia, stretching of peritoneum, and dilatation of cervix, compression of nerve ganglion, and mainly occurs in first stage of labor with the characteristic of dull ache. Somatic pain (from other structures) is due to stretching and enlargement of pelvic floor structures, vagina, and perineum and occurs in late first stage and second stage of labor.

Pathway of uterine pain in labor: By unmyelinated "c" fibers through sympathetic afferent fibers → uterine, cervical, and hypogastric nerve plexus → main sympathetic trunk → T10 and L1 spinal nerves → posterior nerve roots where pain fibers synapse in dorsal horn of spiral cord. Pain from cervix

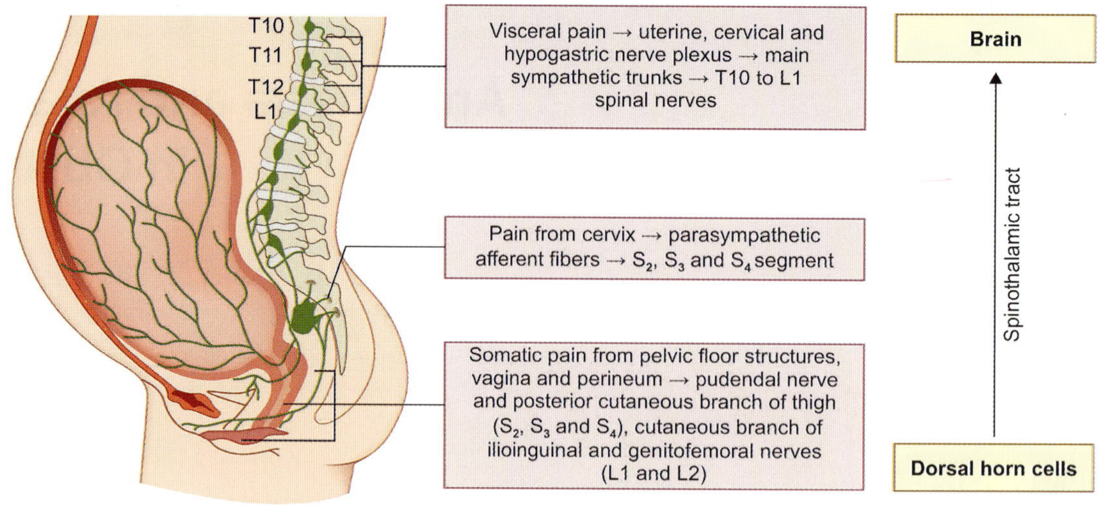

Fig. 1: Pain pathway during labor.

passes through parasympathetic afferent fibers to S2, S3, and S4 segment. **Figure 1** shows the pain pathway in labor.

Pathway of somatic pain in labor: Pain is transmitted by myelinated "A delta fibers" through pudendal nerve and perineal branches of the posterior cutaneous nerve of the thigh to S2, S3, and S4 nerves and cutaneous branches of the ilioinguinal and genitofemoral nerves to L1 and L2. Both visceral and somatic pain is transmitted to dorsal horn cells via spinothalamic tract to brain.

METHODS OF PAIN RELIEF IN LABOR

These are nonpharmacological and pharmacological methods.

Nonpharmacological methods are mother's education and counseling in antenatal period, psychological support, mother's position, relaxation and breathing exercise, acupuncture, hypnosis, and acupressure.

Transcutaneous electrical nerve stimulation (TENS) is less effective analgesia but harmless.

Psychological support is very useful and it minimizes the need of pharmacological analgesia. Midwife or other persons experienced in this process can give support, not necessary husband or doctor.

Mother is allowed to walk and can take any position she desires. Lying back increases the pain. Squatting position and birthing chair reduce the pain. Relaxation in warm water or use of birthing pools are claimed to be effective to reduce pain. However, opioids should not be given to a woman in labor who uses birthing pools.

Pharmacological methods are inhalation analgesia, systemic injection, pudendal block, and paracervical block. Neuraxial analgesia (regional anesthesia) is epidural, spinal and saddle block (low caudal), and combined.

Inhalation Analgesia

Nitrous oxide (Entonox—equal mixture of NO and O_2) is used commonly. Onset of action is rapid, short lasting, and more effective than opiates or TENS. Side effects are nausea, drowsiness, and light headedness. It should not be used for a long period time from the very beginning of first stage of labor because it may cause hypocapnea and fetal hypoxia. It is best used in late labor.

Systemic Analgesics

Narcotic analgesic meperidine combined with tranquilizer antiemetic promethazine is a good analgesia during labor and commonly used. Dose of meperidine (pethidine) is 50–100 mg and that of promethazine is 25 mg administered IM in 3–4 hours interval. Diamorphine is a more effective analgesia, but also more respiratory depressant on the neonate. Meperidine is more sedative than analgesics.

Total dose of meperidine should not exceed 400 mg. A subcutaneous or intravenous (IV) infusion used by the woman as patient-controlled analgesia (PCA) is more effective than intramuscular route. Side effects are nausea and vomiting and for which antiemetic is given with it. It also delays gastric emptying which is not desirable in a mother who may need general anesthesia. Hence, ranitidine should be given as routine. Due to the presence of neonatal depressive action of pethidine, it should not be given when delivery is imminent within 2 hours. The antidote for baby is naloxone hydrochloride 10 μg/kg IV in umbilical vein.

As meperidine crosses the placenta and the half-life of its metabolite normeperidine is 72 hours in new born the other opiates such as butorphanol, fentanyl, and remifentanil are favorably considered as labor analgesia [American College of Obstetricians and Gynecologists (ACOG) 2019]. Fentanyl, a potent synthetic opioid is administered

50–100 µm IV every hourly. Main disadvantage is need of frequent administration. The dose of butorphanol, another opioid receptor agonist-antagonist narcotic is 1–2 mg IV every 4 hourly for which it can be given initially to be followed by fentanyl. Remifentanil, an ultrashort-acting opioid is suitable for PCA.

Pudendal Block

Pudendal nerve (S1, S2, and S3) supplies the vulva and perineum. It passes behind the ischial spine **(Fig. 2)** crossing the sacrospinous ligament along with pudendal artery. Local infiltration of xylocaine at the anatomical landmark of ischial spine blocks the pudendal nerve and provides effective perineal analgesia.

Pudendal block can be done by two routes: (1) transvaginal route **(Fig. 2)** and (2) transperineal route.

Transvaginal Route of Pudendal Block

One 15 cm 18–20-gauge spinal needle fitted with a 20-mL syringe containing 1% xylocaine is introduced under the guidance of left index and middle fingers at the site of ischial spine through the vagina, and the needle reaches above the tip of the ischial spine. After assuring that it has not pierced the blood vessels by aspiration technique; 10 mL is injected at this site. In the similar manner, another 10 mL is injected to block the opposite nerve. Mostly, this method is employed.

Transperineal Route of Pudendal Block

Following local infiltration of 1% lignocaine at a point midway between the anal canal and ischial tuberosity, the needle fitted with syringe-containing lignocaine (as above) is passed transperineally to reach the under surface of ischial spine which is identified by left index finger placed vaginally. Injection lignocaine is injected and the same procedure is applied on other side.

In pudendal block, anesthesia pelvic floor is completely relaxed and the other maneuver like manual removal of placenta can be performed easily. No local infiltration is also needed along with pudendal block.

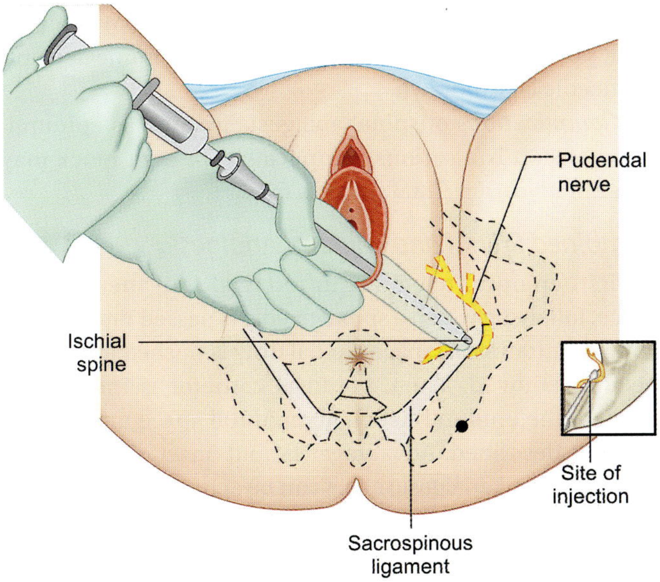

Fig. 2: Pudendal block is administered through transvaginal route.

Neuraxial Regional Block

Regional anesthesia means the administration of analgesic drugs into epidural space or subarachnoid space by which a major part of the body will be anesthetized.

Neuraxial regional block types are: (1) Epidural—drug is injected into extradural or epidural space, (2) Spinal—drug is delivered into the subarachnoid space, and (3) combined spinal epidural.

Epidural analgesic is an effective analgesia in labor making painless labor, whereas spinal anesthesia is not used for routine analgesia in labor, but is administered for cesarean section.

Nerve Blocking Anesthetic Agents

Commonly used agents are bupivacaine, lidocaine, and ropivacaine. Another agent is 2-chloroprocaine. The dose of individual drug depends on particular nerve block and patient profile and the dose varies widely. Inadvertent use of these agents may cause serious toxicity, for which small test dose is administered prior full administration.

Epidural Analgesia (Fig. 3)

Epidural space lies between the dura and periosteum of vertebral canal, which is 4 cm wide. It extends from the foramen magnum above where periosteum and dura fuse to the ligament covering the sacral hiatus below.

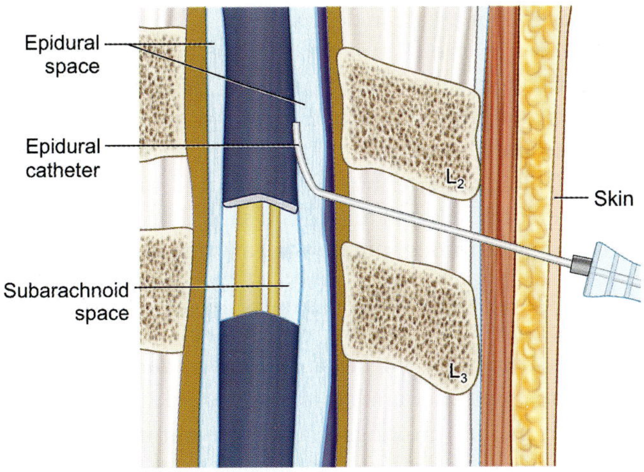

Fig. 3: Epidural space and subarachnoid space. Epidural needle (Tuohy needle) is introduced in epidural space.

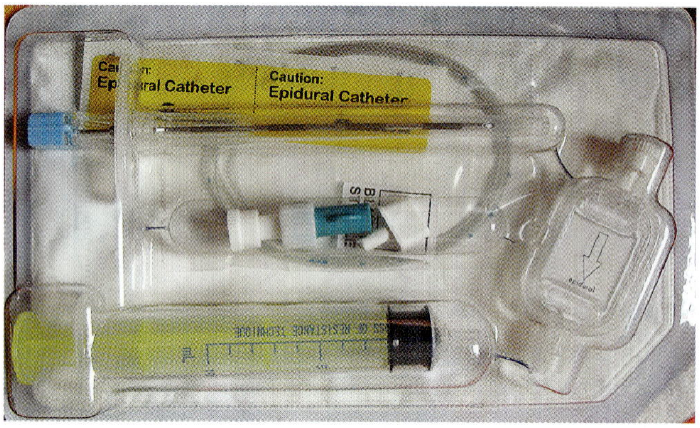

Fig. 4: Kit of epidural set.

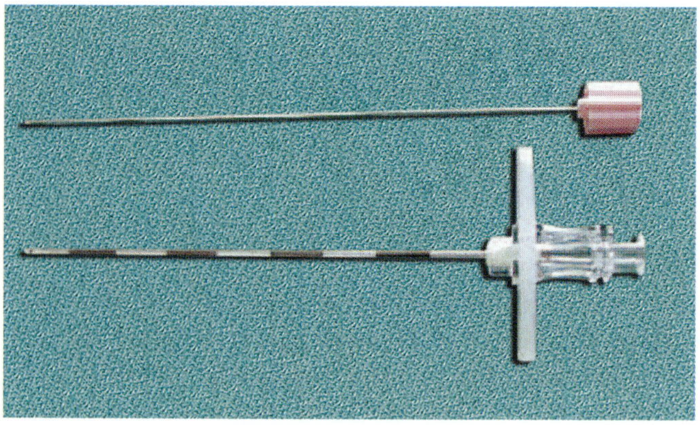

Fig. 5: Epidural needle.

Procedures of continuous epidural analgesia **(Fig. 4)**: Informed consent is taken. Proper hydration is done by IV infusion of crystalloids, ringer lactate, or normal saline before epidural. Purpose is to make a channel so that if hypotension occurs it will be managed promptly and a preload of 500–1,000 mL of ringer lactate is given to avoid hypotension. Woman is kept in left lateral or sitting posture. Epidural needle (Tuohy needle) **(Fig. 5)** is introduced either at L2-L3, L3-L4, or L4-L5 interspace. The epidural space is identified by the loss of resistance technique. Epidural catheter is introduced 3–5 cm into the epidural space. It is aspirated to check the position and if no blood or cerebrospinal fluid (CSF) comes out, a test dose of 3 mL of 1.5% lignocaine with epinephrine or 3 mL of 25% bupivacaine with epinephrine is injected. If no impairment of sensation and motor function of lower limb occurs, catheter is correctly placed. If there is change of sensation or weakness of leg, probably the catheter has gone to the subarachnoid space.

If following the test dose none of the above signs are observed, then a loading dose is given. Woman is placed in right or left lateral position and should not lie in supine position to avoid aortocaval compression. For reduction of pain in labor and vaginal delivery, block is needed T10 to S5 segment and for cesarean delivery T4 to S1 segments.

Blood pressure (BP) is recorded every 5 minutes for the first half an hour. Fetal heart rate (FHR) is monitored continuously. Drug is repeated every 3–4 hours throughout the labor and continued until after third stage for perineal repair. Opioids like fentanyl may be used to supplement epidural block. Epidural anesthesia should be administered and monitored throughout labor by an expert anesthetist.

Advantages of epidural analgesia: It is the most reliable means of effective analgesia in labor and gives complete freedom from pain of labor *(painless labor)*. In some conditions, epidural analgesia has special indications as in hypertension, prolonged labor, premature labor, and multiple pregnancy. Epidural analgesia does not cause prolonged first stage, and as rate of cesarean section does not increase, long-term backache is not increased with it. Operative delivery including cesarean section if needed can be performed by epidural anesthesia.

Contraindications are hypovolemia, coagulation disorder, and presence of local infection.

Complications of epidural analgesia are total spinal (due to large dose in subarachnoid space—accidentally), hypotension, maternal pyrexia, backache, and CNS stimulation—convulsion may occur but rare.

Epidural analgesia prolongs the second stage by abolishing expulsive forces, and lead to higher rate of instrumental delivery but first stage is not affected.

Spinal Analgesia

It is commonly used in cesarean section, instrumental vaginal delivery, and manual removal of placenta. It is not used primarily as labor analgesia. Duration of action persists 2–4 hours. Spinal analgesia is given in single shot.

Procedure: A fine-gauge atraumatic spinal needle **(Figs. 6 and 7)** is introduced into subarachnoid space passing through epidural space and puncturing dura. When CSF comes out, a small volume of local anesthetic is injected and the needle is withdrawn.

Complications of spinal analgesia is same as epidural. Hypotension is a serious complication. A high block may cause bradycardia. Total spinal is rare.

Combined Spinal and Epidural Analgesia

At first, epidural needle is introduced into the epidural space, following which a spinal needle is passed into subarachnoid (intrathecal) space. Spinal drug is pushed and spinal needle removed. Then, epidural catheter is introduced through the epidural needle to epidural space and drug is given as described. Advantage is rapid onset of pain relief, and prolonged analgesic effect can be achieved.

Paracervical Block

Injection lignocaine—1% of 5–10 mL is injected laterally into the cervix at 3 o'clock and 9 o'clock position **(Fig. 8)**. In first stage, pain relief is satisfactory. As it does not block

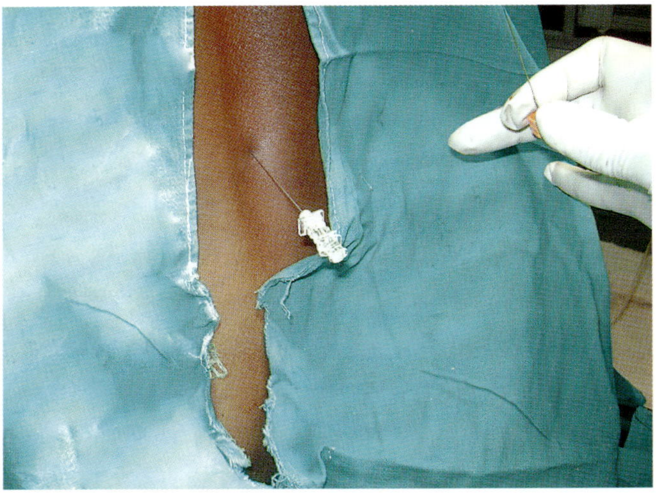

Fig. 6: Insertion of spinal needle.

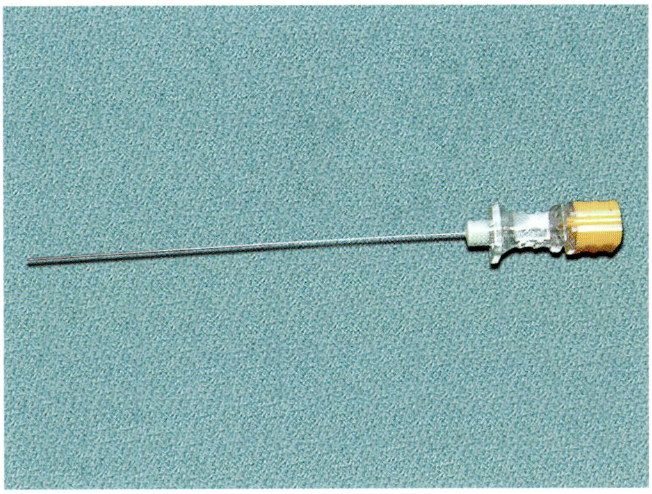

Fig. 7: Spinal needle.

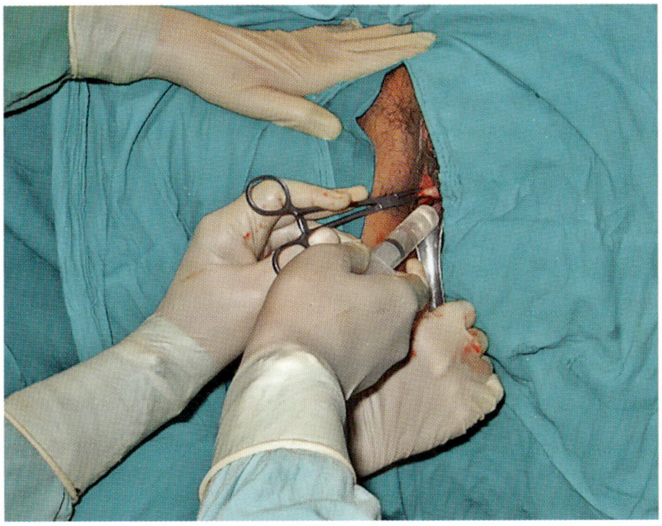

Fig. 8: Procedure of paracervical block.

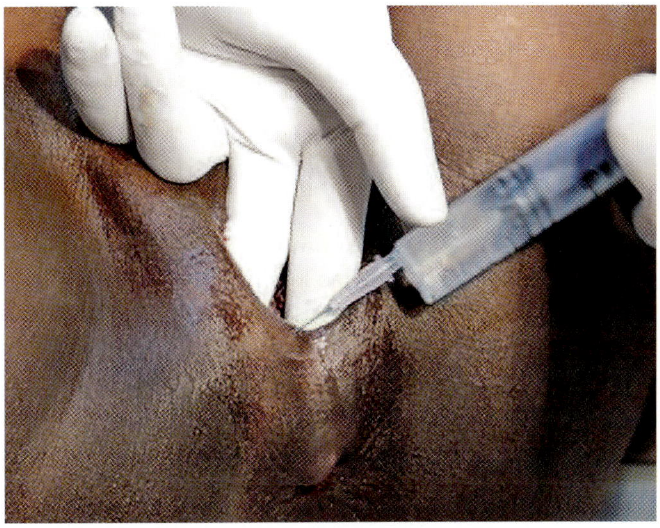

Fig. 9: Perineal infiltration of xylocaine.

the pudendal nerve, additional analgesia is necessary during second stage. Repeated doses are needed during labor as it has short-term effect. Paracervical block may cause fetal bradycardia due to its potential vasospasm action; hence, it should not be used in potential fetal compromise cases. Paracervical block is commonly given in D&E, S&E operation, etc.

Saddle Block

It is a type of regional anesthesia where anesthetic agent is administered in L3-L4 or L4-L5 level. It will produce analgesia on the inner aspects of thigh.

LOCAL PERINEAL INFILTRATION (FIG. 9)

Before episiotomy, injection lignocaine (1%) is locally infiltrated over the perineum to block the cutaneous nerves over the incision line. After pushing the needle, aspiration is done to check whether needle has pricked the blood vessels.

Local Anesthetic Block for Cesarean Delivery

Sometimes, very rarely for cesarean delivery local anesthetic analgesia is needed as a lifesaving measure of fetus when routine anesthesia is not available. There are two techniques. In one method, local agent is infiltrated along the tissue layers of parietes in the incision line. Another technique is the field block. In this second technique, one injection site is midway between the iliac crest and costal margin and another point of blocking is external inguinal ring. Infiltration is done on both sides.

Figure 10 shows nerve distribution and obstetric analgesia.

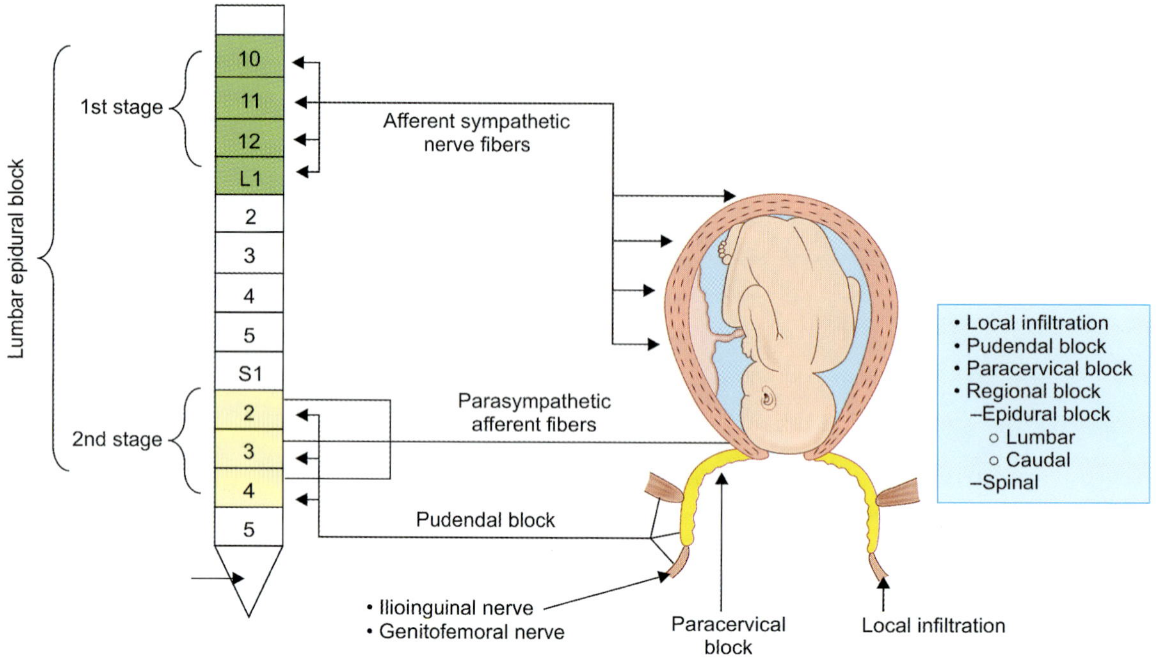

Fig. 10: The schematic diagram shows nerve distribution and various routes of administration of obstetric analgesia.

GENERAL ANESTHESIA IN PREGNANCY AND LABOR

General anesthesia, once commonly employed during cesarean section, has become less popular due to relative increased safety of regional anesthesia. It carries more risk in pregnant state than in nonpregnant state. Thus, regional anesthesia is preferred in pregnant woman.

The risks of general anesthesia in pregnancy are many. These are regurgitation of gastric content, and chance of aspiration are more due to less gastroesophageal tone, increased intra-abdominal volume, and reduced gastric emptying. pH of gastric content is low, and due to increased acidity of gastric content, chance of pneumonitis is more when aspirated. There may be difficult intubation due to pregnancy-related obesity. Failed intubation occurs in about 1 in 250 cases, and is tenfold higher than in nonpregnant state. Case-fatality rate of general anesthesia for cesarean delivery is 32 per million live births whereas that in regional anesthesia is 1.9 per million.

American College of Obstetricians and Gynecologists (ACOG) 2019 suggests neuraxial regional block as the preferred method of pain control in obstetrics due to increased morbidity and mortality of general anesthesia unless contraindicated.

CHAPTER

25

Puerperal Contraception: Postpartum IUCD and Puerperal Sterilization

Learning Objectives

- Types of Contraceptive and Family Planning Methods in Postpartum Period
- Injectable Contraceptives
- Postpartum IUCD
- Postpartum Ligation or Sterilization
- Regret of Permanent Sterilization

INTRODUCTION

India is the second most populous country of the world next to China. It harbors 17.7% of the world's population in only 2.4% of the global land mass. India contributes >20% of births worldwide. At present, World's population is estimated to be almost 7.98 billion (2022). China is the most populous nation. At present (2022), India's population is 1.41 billion contributing 17.7% and that of China is 1.45 billion contributing 18.47% of World's population. Very soon, India will be the most populous country in the World and China will be second.

In India, total fertility rate (TFR) has declined from 2.2 to 2.0 at the national level between the National Family Health Survey 2015–16 (NFHS-4) and the National Family Health Survey 2019–21 (NFHS-5).

According to the NFHS-5, (2019–2021) any modern method used by currently married women age 15–49 years in India is 56.5%. The most popular modern contraceptive in India is female sterilization. Female sterilization accounts for 37.9%, male sterilization 0.3%, IUD/PPIUD 2.1%, pill 5.1%, condom 9.5%, and injectables 0.6%.

Total unmet need for family planning (currently married women age 15–49 years) is 9.4% and unmet need for spacing is 4.0% as per NFHS-5. Significant percentage of women in the first year postpartum have an unmet need for family planning. As institutional delivery has increased remarkably (average 89% according to NFHS-5, in urban 94%), there is abundant scope of postpartum contraception and Government of India has given special stress on postpartum contraception.

TYPES OF CONTRACEPTIVE AND FAMILY PLANNING METHODS IN POSTPARTUM PERIOD

Various methods are as follows:

- Lactational amenorrhea method (LAM)
- Barrier contraceptive
- Postpartum intrauterine contraceptive device (PPIUCD)—CuT 380A, multiload Cu 375, levonorgestrel-releasing intrauterine system (LNG-IUS)
- Progesterone only contraceptive injectable form [injection Depo-Provera or injection norethisterone-enanthate (NET-EN)]
- Subdermal implant—*Implanon* and *Nexplanon* for immediate postpartum placement
- Progesterone only pill (mini pill—Cerazette)
- Puerperal or postpartum sterilization—permanent sterilization in the form of tubectomy.

As combined pill interferes with breastfeeding, it is avoided in first 6 months. Permanent sterilization in the form of tubectomy is done as early as possible after delivery if family is completed. However, first 24 hours are avoided, as this period is very vital so far as neonatal morbidity and mortality is concerned. In LAM, there is 2% chance of conception during first 6 months.

INJECTABLE CONTRACEPTIVES

The two important injectable contraceptives are depot medroxyprogesterone acetate (DMPA) and NET-EN. DMPA is given in a dose of 150 mg every 3 months intramuscularly and NET-EN is given in the dose of 200 mg IM every 2 months.

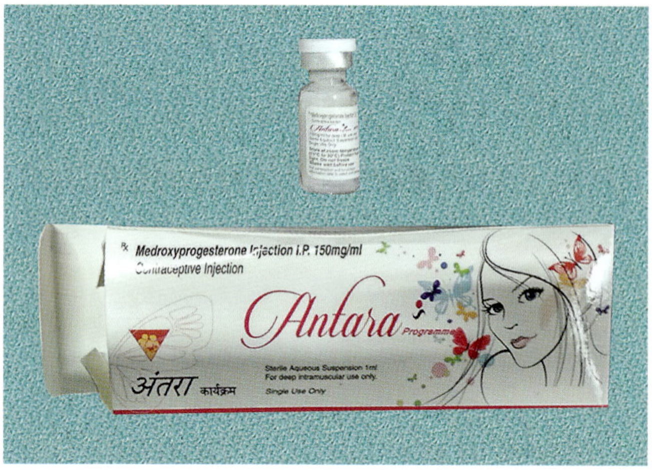

Fig. 1: Antara. Pack of injection depot medroxyprogesterone acetate (DMPA) 150 mg for intramuscular with 1 mL vial (Government of India supply).

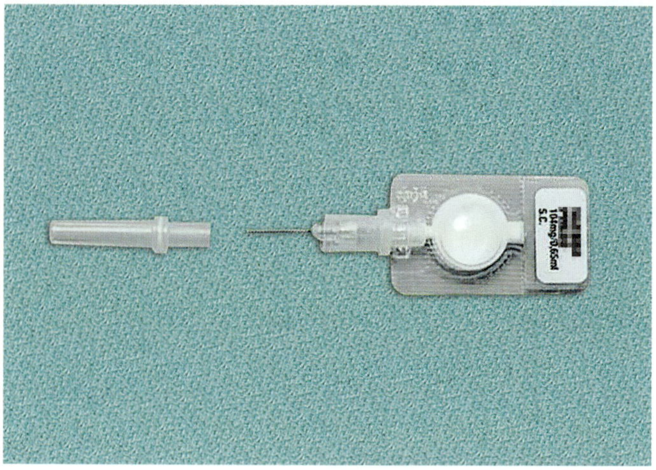

Fig. 2: Sayana-Press.

It is started after 6 weeks of birth in fully or near fully lactating mother and is started immediately or after 3 weeks in nonlactating mother.

The name of injection DMPA (Depo-Provera) supplied by Government of India is "Antara". Injection DMPA containing 150 mg in 1 mL vial for intramuscular injection every 3 months **(Fig. 1)**.

Depo-subQ Provera which is a derivative of DMPA (*Sayana-Press*) containing 104 mg dose (equivalent to 150 mg DMPA intramuscular) for subcutaneous use for every 3 months is available in India **(Fig. 2)** but not supplied by Govt of India in National Family Welfare Programme. Important disadvantages of the injectable contraceptive are amenorrhea and irregular bleeding.

The progesterone only pill Cerazette contains desogestrel 75 μg. It is started from the first day of the cycle and given continuously without any gap. In lactating mother, it is started anytime within 6 months after giving birth if menstruation is not returned and within 4 weeks in nonlactating mother. For details see *Author's "Bedside Clinics in Gynecology" (2nd edition, 2023) published by Jaypee Brothers.*

POSTPARTUM IUCD

Definition

Provision of intrauterine contraceptive device (IUCD) in the immediate postpartum period is called PPIUCD and it offers an effective and safe method for spacing and limiting births. Considering the huge potentiality and abundant scope in India, especially after increase of institutional delivery, Government of India has given special emphasis in PPIUCD and started the training on immediate postpartum insertion of IUCD from 2010 and it is one of the important components of family planning program of India.

PPIUCD is highly justified in India, there is significant percentage of women in the first year postpartum have an unmet need for family planning. Maximum chances of unplanned pregnancy are due to unreliability of LAM, unpredictable ovulation time, and lack of awareness regarding need of contraception.

Advantages

Counseling during antenatal period and in early labor is very successful and woman and family become highly motivated to accept it as a reliable birth spacing method. It is safe to use as it is certain that the woman is not pregnant at the time of insertion. There is minimal risk of uterine perforation because of the thick wall of the uterus. There is reduced perception of initial side effects (bleeding and cramping) and reduced chance of heavy bleeding, especially among LAM users, since they experience amenorrhea. There is no effect on amount or quality of breast milk. It saves time as performed on the same delivery table for postplacental or intracesarean insertions. Additional evaluations and separate clinical procedure are not required. It needs minimal additional instruments, supplies, and equipment. The woman has an effective method for contraception before discharge from hospital. The increased institutional deliveries are the opportunity to provide women easy access to immediate PPIUCD services.

It is an effective long-active reversible contraceptive method.

Effectiveness

Failure rate is low: 0.6–0.8 pregnancies per 100 women in first year of use. The CuT 380A is effective for 10 years for continuous use. Multiload Cu 375 is effective for 5 years.

Disadvantages

Provider needs specific training in postpartum insertion. Expulsion rates appear to be higher. In general, expulsion rates for PPIUCD range between 10 and 14% where in interval, it is 5%. Good technique can reduce expulsion to 4–5%. Nonvisibility of string per vagina may occur in spite of in situ position. The other limitations of the immediate PPIUCD are the same as the interval IUCD.

Timing of Postpartum IUCD Insertion

The PPIUCD can be placed immediately following delivery of the placenta, during cesarean section or within 48 hours following childbirth:

- *Postplacental:* Insertion within 10 minutes after expulsion of the placenta following a vaginal delivery on the same delivery table.
- *Intracesarean:* Insertion that takes place during a cesarean delivery, after removal of the placenta, and before closure of the uterine incision.
- *Immediate postpartum—within 48 hours after delivery:* Insertion within 48 hours of delivery and prior to discharge from the postpartum ward.

Insertion any time after 6 weeks postpartum is called extended postpartum or interval PPIUCD.

The IUCD should not be inserted from 48 hours to 6 weeks following delivery because there is an increased risk of infection and expulsion.

Procedure of IUCD Insertion: Technical Aspects

Both copper containing IUD (CuT 380A, Multiload Cu 375) system and LNG-IUS—Mirena are used **(Figs. 3 to 5)**.

Fundal placement of IUCD is the most important.

Postplacental insertion: Position of the patient is made dorsal lithotomy with or without using labor stirrups. In *postplacental insertion,* long placental forceps (*Kelly's forceps*) **(Fig. 6)** is needed to insert. Negotiation of the "bend" where the uterine body flops over the lower uterine segment is a common challenge during insertion. Insertion

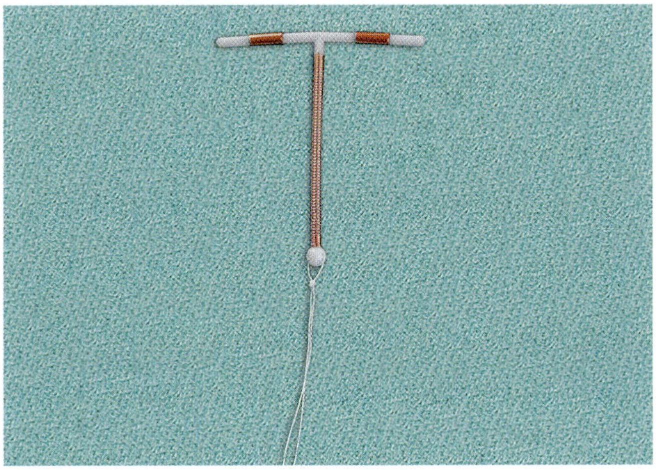

Fig. 3: CuT 380A.

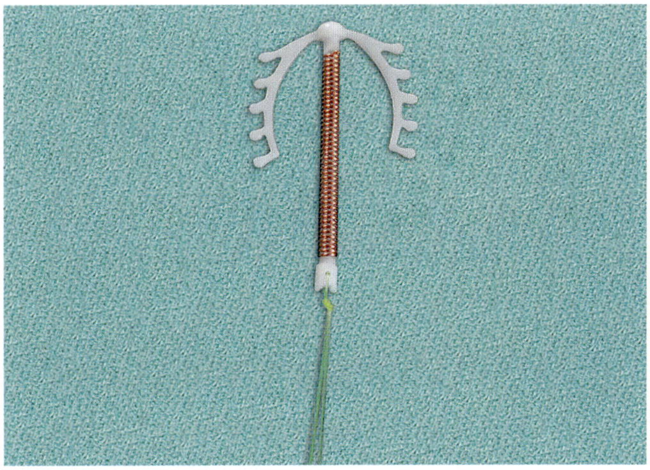

Fig. 4: Multiload Cu 375.

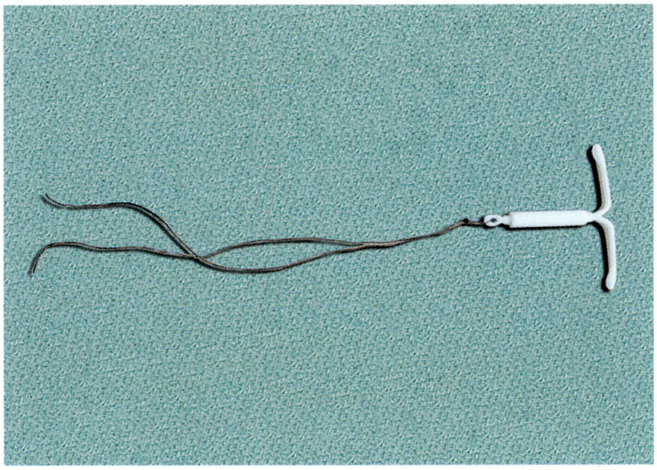

Fig. 5: Mirena [levonorgestrel-releasing intrauterine system (LNG-IUS)].

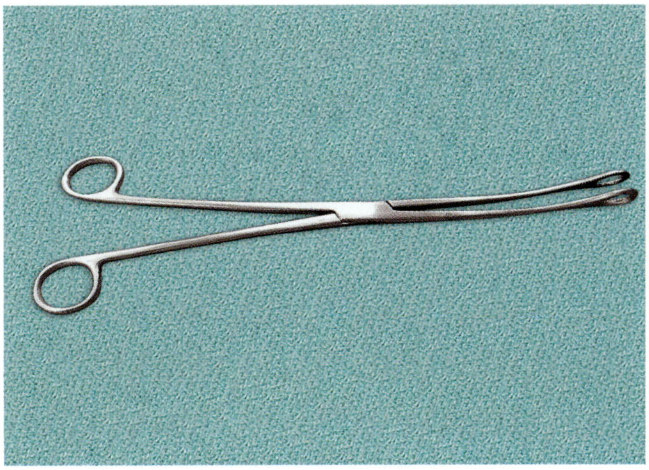

Fig. 6: Kelly's forceps.

technique is shown in the **Figures 7 to 15** with description in legends.

In immediate postpartum (within 48 hours after delivery) insertion, regular ring forceps are sufficient for insertion.

Intracesarean insertion: For intracesarean insertion, it is best done manually with the fingers. Alternatively, regular ring forceps can be used. After the placenta is removed, the provider inserts the IUCD, and then closes the uterine incision. It is important not to attempt to pass the strings of the IUCD through the cervical os before closure of the uterus as this will displace the IUCD and leave it lower down in the uterine cavity. There is no need to fix the IUCD with a ligature.

The provider must insert the IUCD by following all recommended clinical and infection prevention measures for successful insertion.

Selection of Patient

Patient should be selected according to World Health Organization (WHO) medical eligibility criteria.

Contraindications

Medical eligibility criteria—category 3 (relative contraindications): Chorioamnionitis, prolonged rupture of membranes (>18 hours) and 48 hours to 6 weeks within delivery.

Medical eligibility criteria—category 4 (absolute contraindications): Postpartum hemorrhage (unresolved), puerperal sepsis, and extensive genital trauma.

Follow-up

Woman is advised to return to the clinic for postpartum care at 6th week routinely or earlier if she has serious problems.

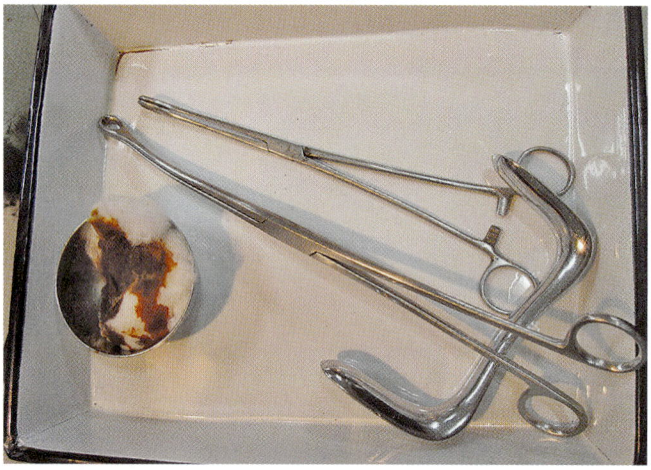

Fig. 7: Instruments necessary for postpartum intrauterine contraceptive device including Kelly's forceps.

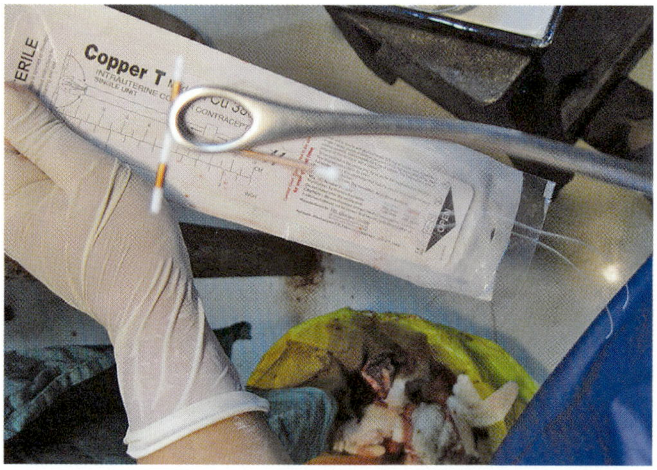

Fig. 8: CuT grasped and taken out with help of Kelly's forceps in non-touch technique.

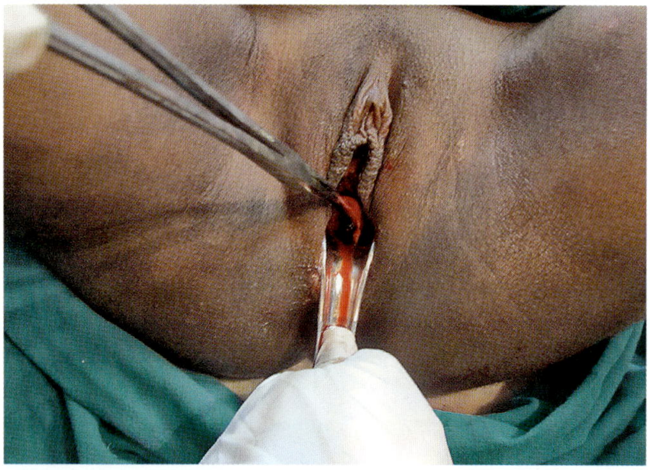

Fig. 9: Following positioning of patient anterior lip of the cervix is held by sponge forceps after retraction of posterior vaginal wall with Sims speculum.

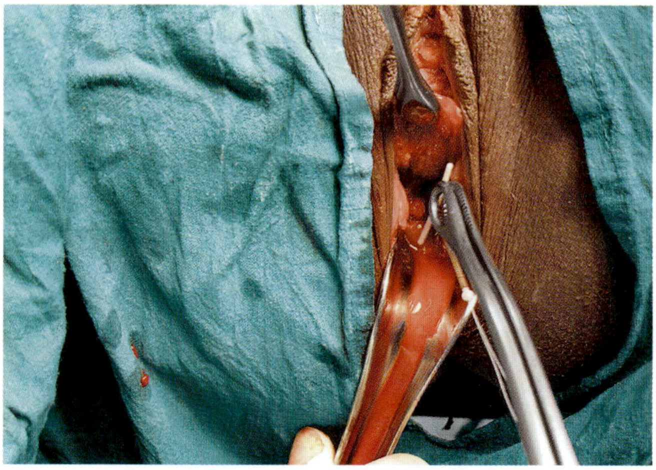

Fig. 10: Intrauterine device is introduced with the help of Kelly's forceps.

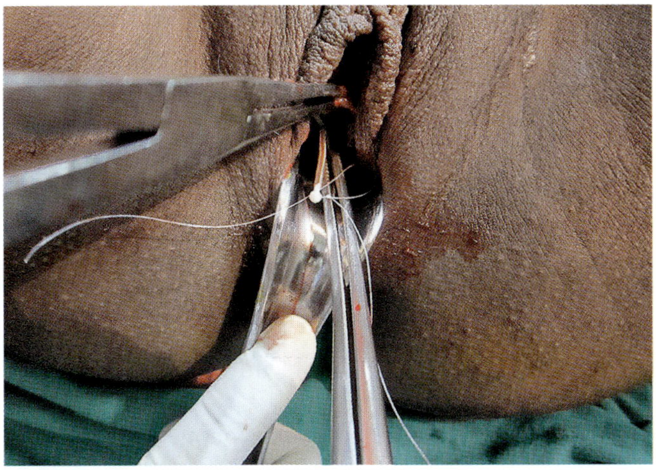

Fig. 11: Now Cu-T is negotiated through the cervical canal.

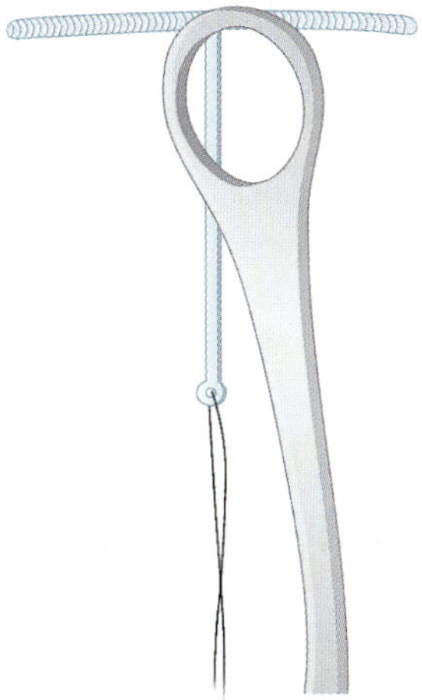

Fig. 12: Method of holding the intrauterine contraceptive device with the Kelly's forceps.

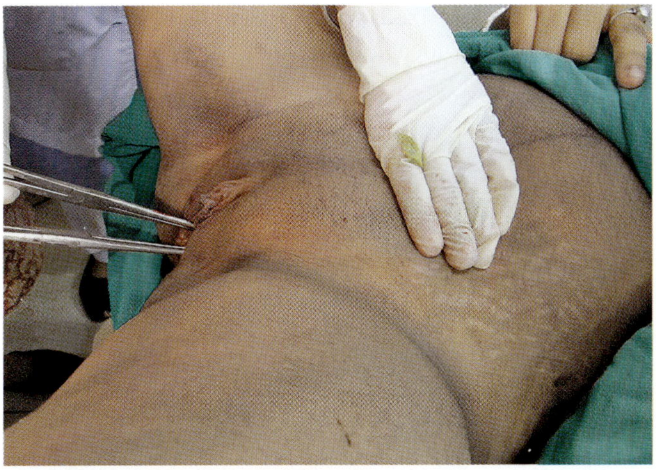

Fig. 13: During insertion, left hand is kept over the uterus to make uterus straighten.

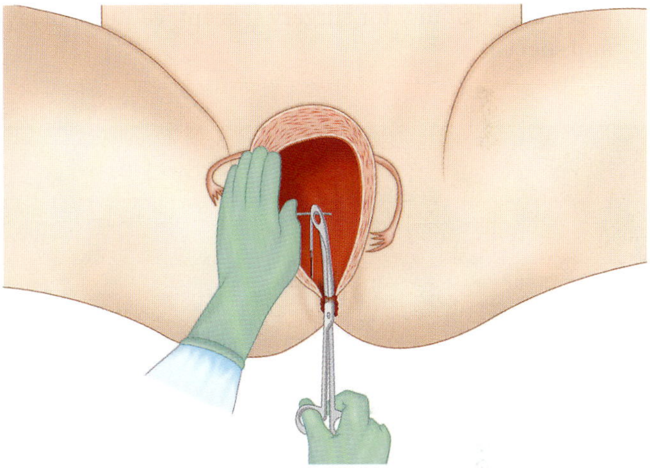

Fig. 14: During insertion, left hand is kept over the uterus to make uterus straighten (diagrammatic).

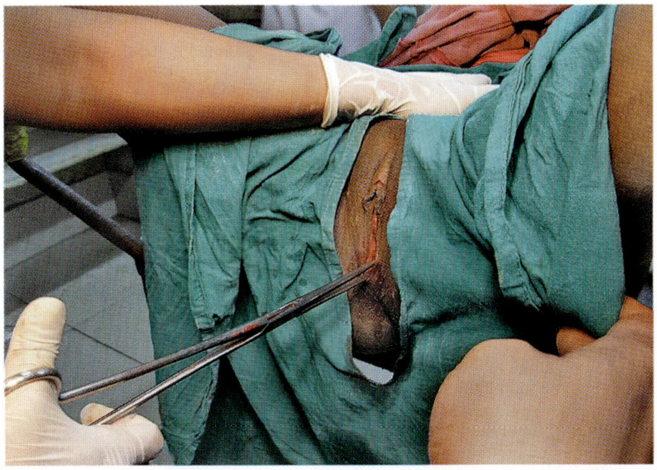

Fig. 15: Before withdrawal of Kelly's forceps, it is opened and shifted to left side away from the device and then withdrawn.

Routine immediate PPIUCD follow-up care should be integrated with standard postpartum services.

A pelvic examination is done to examine the visibility of the strings and to cut them if the woman finds them uncomfortable.

At 6 weeks postpartum, the IUCD strings can be felt by some women and majority within 6 months. It is not necessary for her to check the strings. In suspected expulsion or misplaced IUCD, sonography is advised.

POSTPARTUM LIGATION OR STERILIZATION

Consent for Permanent Tubal Sterilization

Woman herself will give consent. The consent of the partner (spouse) is not required for sterilization. However, the partner should be encouraged to come for counseling.

Eligibility Criteria for Clients Undergoing Female Sterilization

- Self-declaration by the client will be the basis for compiling this information. No eligible client should be denied female sterilization service.

- Clients should be ever married.

> - Female clients should be above the age of 22 years and below the age of 49 years.
> - The couple should have at least one child, whose age is above 1 year, unless the sterilization is medically indicated.
> - Clients or their spouses/partners must not have undergone sterilization in the past (not applicable in cases of failure of previous sterilization).

- Clients must be in a sound state of mind, so as to understand the full implications of sterilization.
- Mentally-ill clients must be certified by a psychiatrist and a statement should be given by the legal guardian or spouse regarding the soundness of the client's state of mind.
- A relevant medical history, physical examination, and laboratory investigations need to be completed to ascertain eligibility for surgery (accept, caution, delay, and special).

Timing of Postpartum Ligation or Sterilization

It should be done as early as possible, within 7 days of delivery. Usually, first 24 hours are avoided as this period is very vital for the neonate. If it cannot be performed early most surgeons prefer to wait for at least 4–6 weeks postpartum for complete involution of uterus and diminished blood flow of fallopian tube.

Various Approaches of Tubal Ligation

Approach may be:

- Abdominal—conventional, minilaparotomy, and laparoscopic
- Vaginal—approach is not suitable for puerperal ligation.

Steps of Abdominal Method (Figs. 16 to 20)

Woman is brought to the table after emptying of bladder herself or catheterized and position is dorsal supine. General, spinal, or local anesthesia is administered. In case

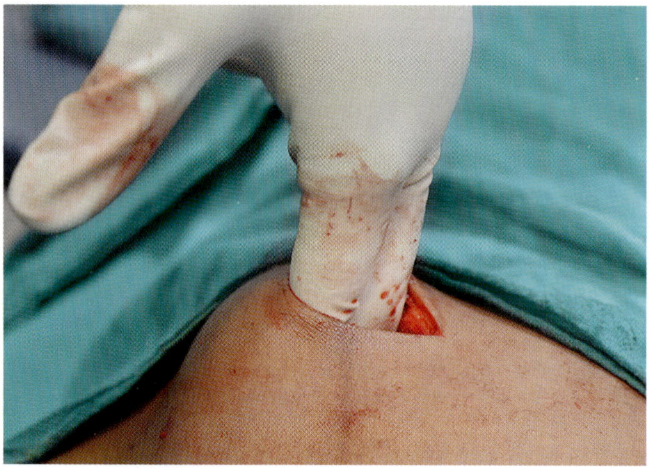

Fig. 16: Tubal ligation—tube is brought out by index and middle finger.

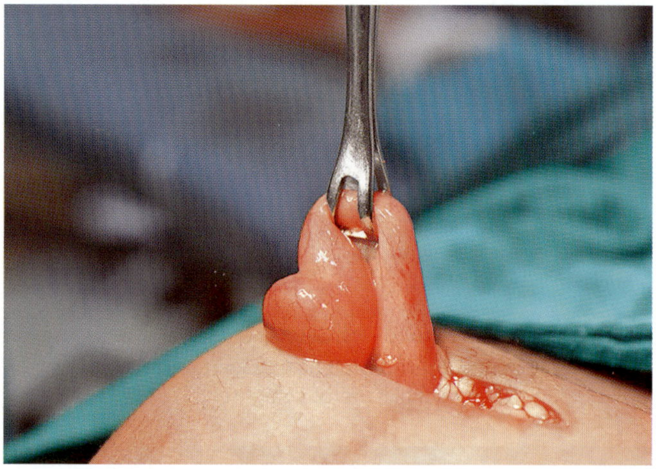

Fig. 17: Tubal ligation—loop of tube is held.

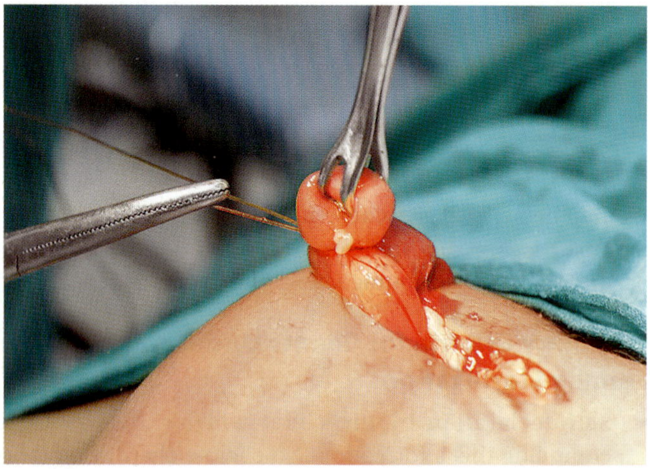

Fig. 18: Ligation by Pomeroy technique.

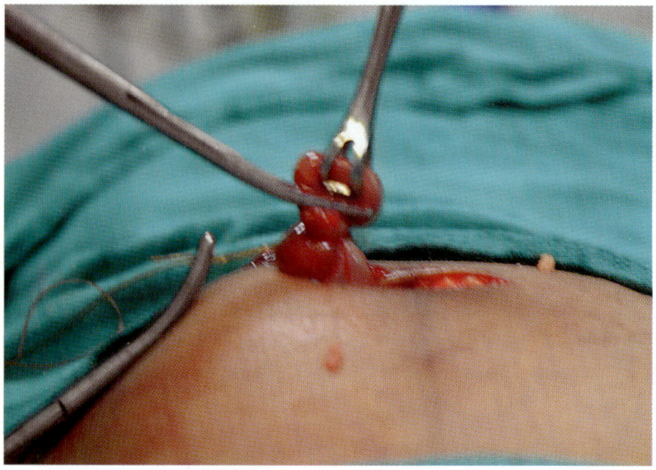

Fig. 19: Pomeroy technique.

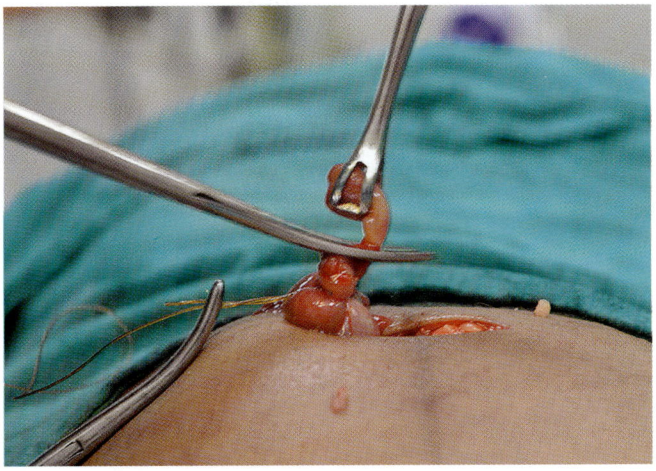

Fig. 20: Pomeroy technique—loop of tube excised.

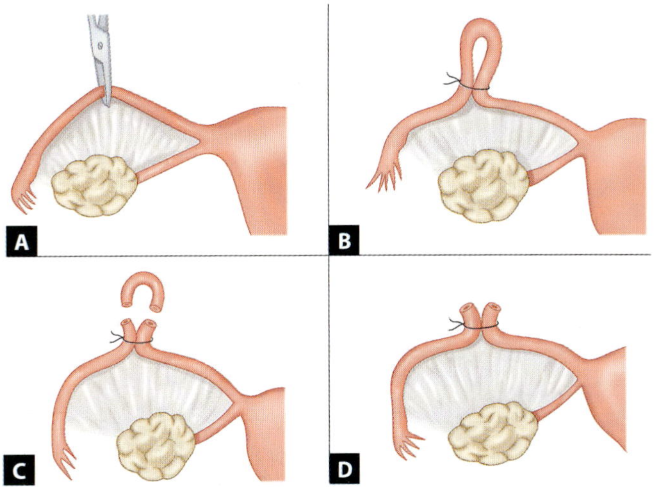

Figs. 21A to D: *Pomeroy method of tubal ligation:* (A) Tube is pulled up by clamp or forceps (Allis or Babcock) to make a loop; (B) The base of the loop is tied with catgut stitches; (C) Loop is excised; (D) Stump after excision.

of local anesthesia, good sedatives are given. After dressing and draping a skin incision of 3–4 cm length is given either transverse, midline vertical, or paramedian. In interval ligation, abdominal incision is given (one finger breadth) 2.5 cm above the symphysis pubis, but in puerperal ligation an incision of 3–4 cm (two finger breadth) is given 2 cm below the highest point of fundus. The index finger is passed behind the uterus then laterally behind broad ligament and the tube is hooked **(Fig. 16)**. Fallopian tube is identified by seeing the fimbria. Pomeroy's procedure should be followed for excision and ligation of tube, using a square knot with 1-0 chromic catgut.

Pomeroy technique (Figs. 17 to 21): After bringing out, the tube through the incision a clamp is placed about 4 cm lateral to the fundus and tube is pulled up so as to form a loop by Allis tissue forceps or Babcock forceps.

Avoiding the blood vessels by observation against light a round bodied needle is passed through the mesosalpinx.

The base of the loop is tied with 1-0 catgut stitches keeping about 2 cm of the loop above. The loop is cut and about 1.5 cm of the loop is removed taking care that the cut margins are not very near to the tie. Care must be taken to avoid damage to the blood vessels, ovaries, and surrounding tissues.

The stumps are inspected carefully to make sure that the tube is cut completely and to ascertain that there is no bleeding from the stump. Tubal mucosa is seen in resected tubal end. The excised segment of the tube is also examined to be sure that tubal segment is removed and sent for histopathological examination. Both sides are done one after other.

The skin incision is to be closed with an absorbable or nonabsorbable suture, and a small dressing, or bandage applied.

Figure 22 shows how the cut ends of the tube are separated away after healing.

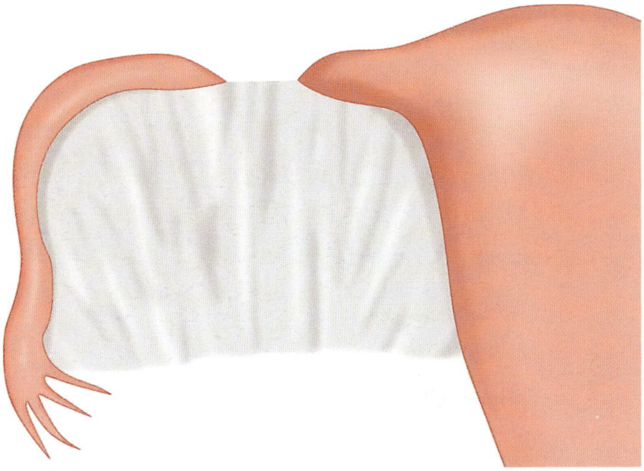

Fig. 22: Cut ends of the tube are found separated away after healing.

Other Techniques of Tubal Sterilization other than Pomeroy

Irving technique ***(Figs. 23 and 24):*** The tube is ligated twice with chromic catgut about 2.5 cm from the uterine cornu and then cut. The medial end is mobilized by dissecting it from mesosalpinx. On the posterior surface of uterus near the cornu, a small tunnel is made in an avascular area. One of the ligatures attached to the medial stump which was kept long is threaded in a needle. The needle is passed through the tunnel to bring about 1.5 cm through the uterine wall. The medial end of tubal is buried and tied in the tunnel. The distal tubal stump is buried in the mesosalpinx which is then closed.

Uchida technique: In the mesosalpinx, saline with epinephrine is infiltrated. The muscle layer of the tube is made

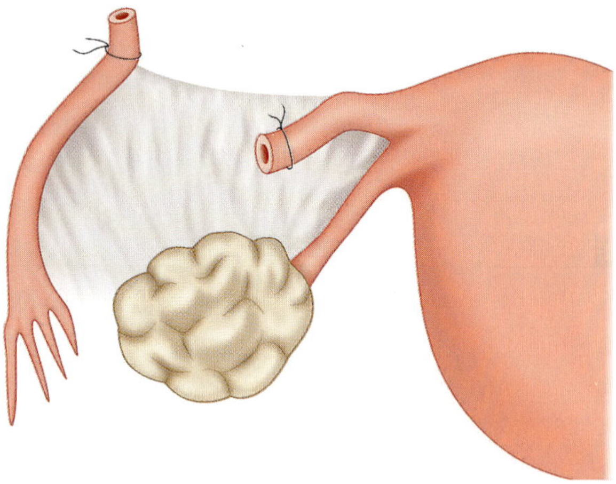

Fig. 23: Irving technique—tube is ligated first.

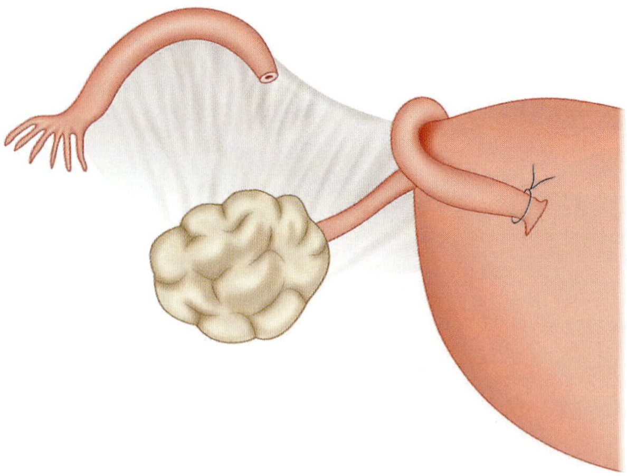

Fig. 24: Irving technique—medial tubal end is buried into a tunnel behind the uterus.

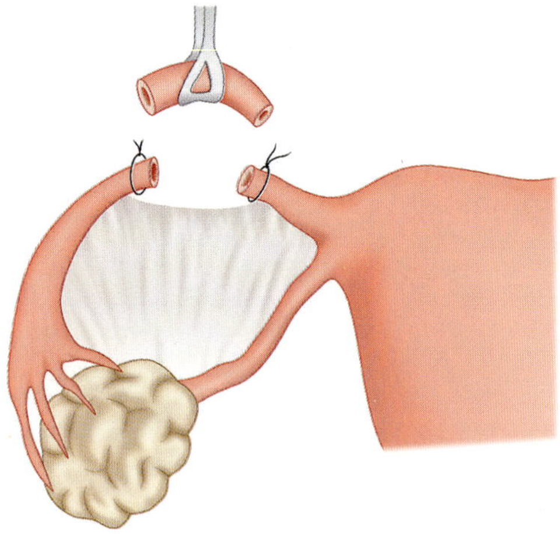

Fig. 25: Parkland technique—intervening segment of tube is excised.

separated from the serosa. The mesosalpinx is incised to open and the denuded tube is pulled out to form a loop. Tube is cut after putting two clamps. The medial end of the tube is made free from the mesosalpinx and 5 cm of the tube is removed. The medial end of the tube is buried inside the mesosalpinx which is then repaired. The lateral stump is kept outside the mesosalpinx after ligation.

*Parkland technique **(Fig. 25)**:* An avascular area in the mesosalpinx is selected adjacent to the tube and perforated with a small artery forceps and the jaws are opened to separate the tube from the mesosalpinx (2.5 cm). The freed tube is ligated proximally and distally and intervening segment of the tube of about 2 cm is excised.

*Kroener fimbriectomy technique **(Figs. 26A and B)**:* The fimbrial end is ligated twice with silk and then excised.

Madlener's technique: In the middle part of the tube, a loop of tube is crushed at the base and ligated with silk suture material.

Risk-reducing salpingectomy is now considered as it reduces the aggressive epithelial cancer. But sterilization reversal is not possible, if needed in future.

However, it is time consuming and somehow difficult in the set-up, it is done. Sterilization at the time of cesarean delivery is easier due to the large operative field and total salpingectomy becomes easy.

Laparoscopic sterilization is not suitable in puerperal ligation. It is described in *Author's Bedside Clinics in Gynecology (2nd edition, 2023) published by Jaypee Brothers Medical Publishers.*

Failure Rate of Tubal Ligation

The overall failure rate in tubal ligation is <1%; lowest in Irving and Uchida and highest in Kroener fimbriectomy (Pomeroy technique 0.3%, Irving technique 0.1%, Kroener fimbriectomy 2–3%, Madlener technique 0.3–2%, and Parkland technique 0.25%).

The reasons for failure are surgical error (30–50%), spontaneous recanalization, or the woman was already pregnant at the time of pregnancy—also called luteal phase pregnancy.

Complications of Tubal Sterilization

Complications of ligation depend on:

- Method of sterilization, method of anesthesia, route of ligation, patient profile, and technical capability of surgeon
- Minor complications may amount to 14% and major complications may reach a maximum of 1–2%. Complications are more in vaginal than abdominal. It is more following cesarean and MTP than in interval ligation.

Operative Complications

- Anesthetic hazards
- Cardiorespiratory arrest
- Respiratory depression

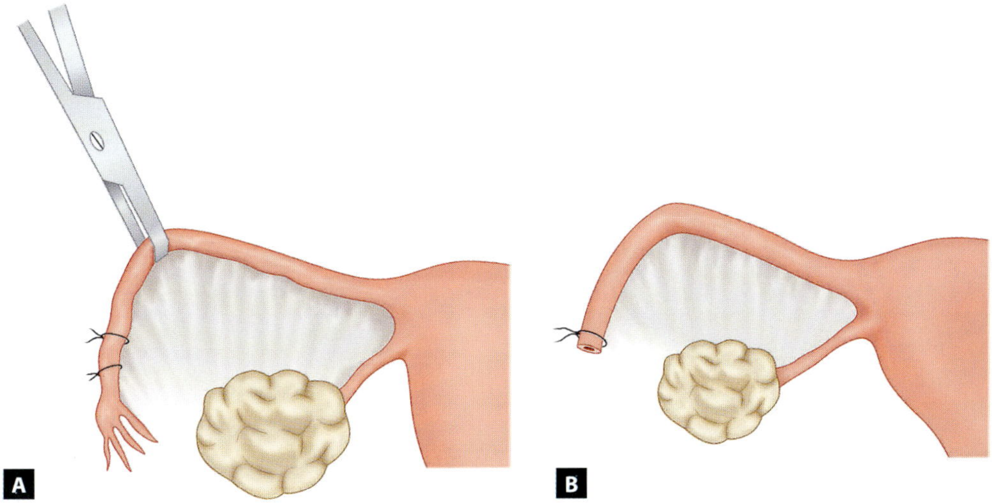

Figs. 26A and B: Kroener fimbriectomy.

- Bowel injury
- Bladder injury
- Injury to tube and ovary
- Broad ligament hematoma
- Bleeding from mesosalpinx
- Convulsion and toxic reaction to anesthetic drugs.

Postoperative Complications

Wound infection, wound hematoma, wound dehiscence, pelvic infection, peritonitis, intestinal obstruction, urinary tract infection (UTI), intraperitoneal hemorrhage, bladder or bowel fistula, and incisional hernia.

Long-term Effects

- *Failure:* 0.4–15%
- *Ectopic pregnancy:* Incidence of ectopic pregnancy is not increased, however following failure ectopic pregnancy may occur and must be excluded. If pregnancy does occur, 15–20% of such pregnancies are likely to be ectopic. Of all ectopic pregnancies poststerilization ectopic contributes 12%. The probable explanation for ectopic gestations after tubal ligation is recanalization or formation of a tuboperitoneal fistula.
- *Post-tubal sterilization syndrome:* Gynecologic and psychologic problems following ligation called "post-tubal sterilization syndrome".
- Psychological problem.

Mortality Following Female Sterilization

1.5/100,000 procedure in USA, in India, it is high 10–70/100,000 procedure. The three major causes of death are anesthetic hazard, sepsis, and hemorrhage.

Efficacy and Failure (WHO) of Female Sterilization

Less than 1 pregnancy per 100 women over the first year after operation (5 per 1,000).

REGRET OF PERMANENT STERILIZATION

Some women regret for sterilization. Women should not undergo tubal sterilization in strong belief that sterilization reversal and assisted reproductive technology (ART) will achieve pregnancy. In both the procedures, success is not guaranteed and both are expensive. Now, various alternative contraceptive procedures including long-acting reversible contraceptive (LARC) are available now.

CHAPTER

26

Destructive Operation

Learning Objectives

- Introduction—Role of Destructive Operation in Present Day Obstetrics
- Types of Destructive Operations in Obstetrics
- Craniotomy
- Decapitation
- Evisceration
- Spondylotomy
- Cleidotomy

INTRODUCTION

Destructive operation is almost an abandoned procedure in most of the places. This chapter is rarely covered by the standard operative obstetrics book today as it is becoming irrelevant in modern day obstetrics. The chapter is incorporated in this book for two reasons. Firstly, destructive operation is still needed in few countries where neglected obstetrics is still prevalent in some areas with low-resource setting. Other reason is that development of obstetrics on safe operative delivery and cesarean delivery is preceded by an era when destructive operative was the only means to save the life of the mother. In fact, many of the renowned obstetricians in 17th and 18th century have passed their career a transitional period from destructive operative surgery to improved obstetric procedure.

TYPES OF DESTRUCTIVE OPERATIONS IN OBSTETRICS

These are: (1) craniotomy—perforation and extraction/cephalocentesis (craniocentesis), (2) decapitation, (3) evisceration, (4) spondylotomy, and (5) cleidotomy.

Craniotomy is a type of destructive operation where the fetal head is perforated and extracted through vagina.

Decapitation refers to the procedure where the fetal neck of the dead fetus is severed by instrument and the fetus is delivered.

Evisceration is destructive operation where the abdominal and thoracic contents of the dead fetus are removed piecemeal through an opening done by embryotomy scissors followed by spondylotomy and delivery of the fetus.

In spondylotomy, the spinal column of the fetus is severed and the trunk is divided in two halves.

Cleidotomy is the division of one or both clavicle with cleidotomy or embryotomy scissors to reduce the bulk of the shoulder (by diminishing the bisacromial diameter of the dead fetus), thus facilitating the delivery of the shoulders.

CRANIOTOMY

Indications of craniotomy are dead fetus with cephalic presentation in case of obstructive labor which may occur due to cephalopelvic disproportion (CPD), impacted occipitoposterior, face and brow, and in arrested aftercoming head of the breech when baby is dead.

Criteria to be fulfilled for destructive operation are fetus must be dead except it may not be in hydrocephalus, the cervix must be fully dilated, there should not be impending rupture or obvious rupture of uterus, and there should not be gross cephalopelvic disproportion.

Instruments required for craniotomy operation are catheter, sponge-holding forceps, perforator, Budin's catheter or sucker, and cranioclast.

Perforator is a nondetachable two-bladed heavy instrument used for perforation of fetal head. In closed condition, the distal end of instrument forms a triangular part with pointed sharp end. The base of the triangle is called shoulder, up to which it is to be introduced during perforation. Lateral edges of the triangular region are sharp which actually cuts the bone. When the handles are closed, the two halves of triangle are opened. There are two types of perforators: (1) Simpson's perforator **(Fig. 1)** with springs and (2) Oldham perforator without any spring.

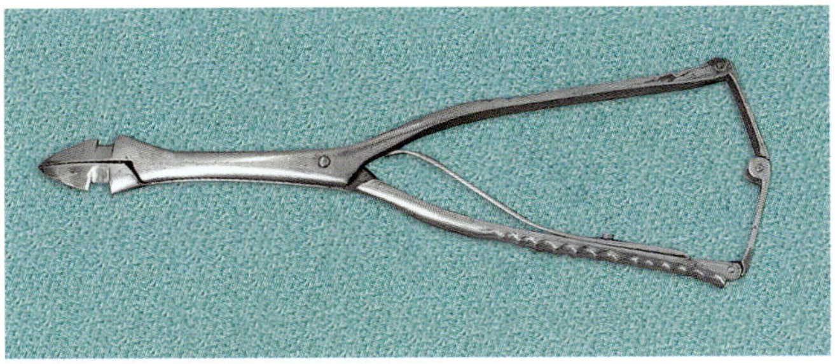

Fig. 1: Simpson's perforator.

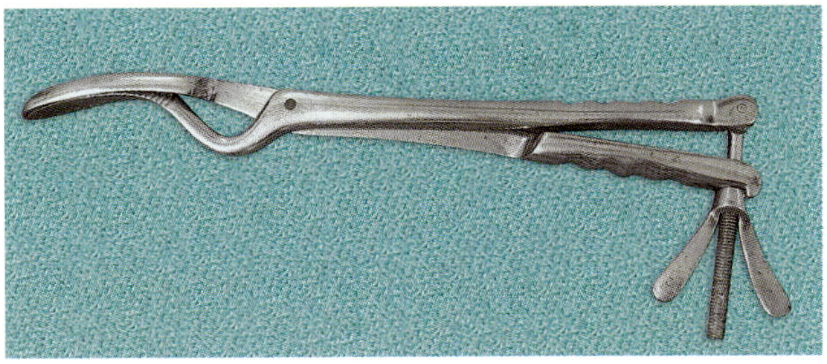

Fig. 2: Cranioclast.

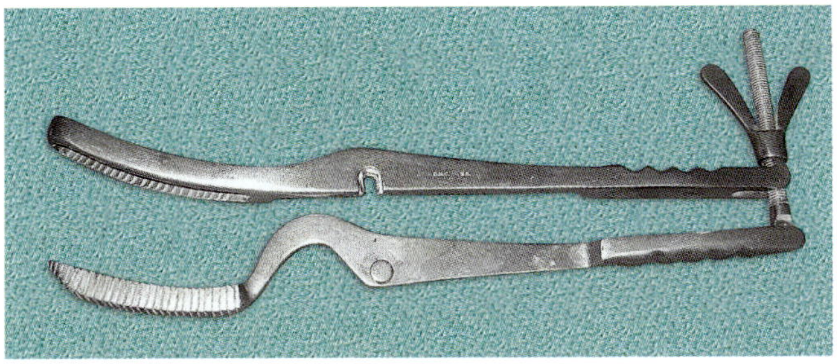

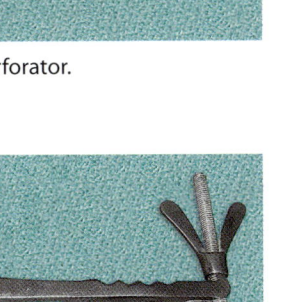

Fig. 3: Blades of cranioclast.

Cranioclast **(Figs. 2 and 3)** is a detachable two-bladed heavy instrument articulated at the lock. The two blades of cranioclast are of different types. One is solid and the other one is fenestrated. Both are curved and fit well to each other when articulated. There is a fixation screw at the proximal part of the solid blade with a corresponding groove on the fenestrated blade. The solid blade is introduced inside the cranial cavity of the fetus keeping the convex edge of blade toward the inner surface of the skull bone. The fenestrated blade is introduced between the skull bone and the sacrum of maternal pelvis, thus fitting the convex edge with the concavity of the sacrum.

Cephalotribe is a three-bladed instrument used in craniotomy (destructive operation) where the perforated head needs diminution in size, when base of the skull is larger than any diameter of pelvis. Such operation is known as *cephalotripsy*. This instrument is rarely used today.

Steps of Craniotomy (Figs. 4A to C)

Basic steps are perforation, drainage of brain matter, and extraction of perforated head.

Detailed history taking, examination, and resuscitation with IV fluid and antibiotics are done. One should be sure that baby is dead and there is no impending rupture or obvious rupture of uterus.

Patient is brought to operation theater and usually general anesthesia is administered. Patient is made lithotomy position. Following antiseptic dressing and draping and catheterization vaginal examination is done to confirm condition of cervix, os, presentation, position, station, and status of membranes (it should be ruptured).

Site of perforation is selected. In vertex, it is on dependent parietal bone, in face—through hard palate or orbit, in brow, it is done through frontal bone and for aftercoming head of breech site of perforation is occipital bone. Fontanel and suture lines are avoided. The assistant will give suprapubic pressure to fix the head.

At the selected site of perforation, two fingers of left hand are placed and the scalp is cut with a pair of scissors. The perforator with closed blades is held in the right hand (in a gun-holding fashion) and introduced through the incised scalp under guidance of the left palm and fingers keeping it at right angle to the surface of the presenting part. The tip of perforator is bored through the skull up to its shoulders. The blades are opened, after pressing on the handles together a linear tear is made. Blades are closed and rotated 90° and again opened thus a crisscross tear is made. After closing the blades again, the perforator is pushed inside the cranial cavity and brain matter is churned. The perforator is then withdrawn under the guidance of left hand.

For drainage of brain matter, a double-channeled Budin's catheter is introduced through the perforation into the cranial cavity and brain matter is washed by running antiseptic solution through the catheter till no more brain matter comes out. Alternatively, sucker tube fitted with electrical sucker may be used to suck the brain matter.

Now, for extraction cranioclast is used. The solid blade is introduced inside the cranial cavity under the guidance of fingers of left hand and is supported by an assistant. The operator's left hand is now placed in sacral hollow and the fenestrated blade (female blade) is introduced from *above* in between the skull and hollow of sacrum over any part of the skull lying posteriorly. Blades are locked and screw is tightened. Left hand is taken out.

Vaginal examination is done to search for any inclusion of maternal soft tissue. A tentative pull is given on the cranioclast to check the proper grip. Now, adequate pull is given to extract the perforated head. The direction of pull is like pull of forceps delivery—first downward and backward, then forward and lastly upward. Instead of cranioclast giant

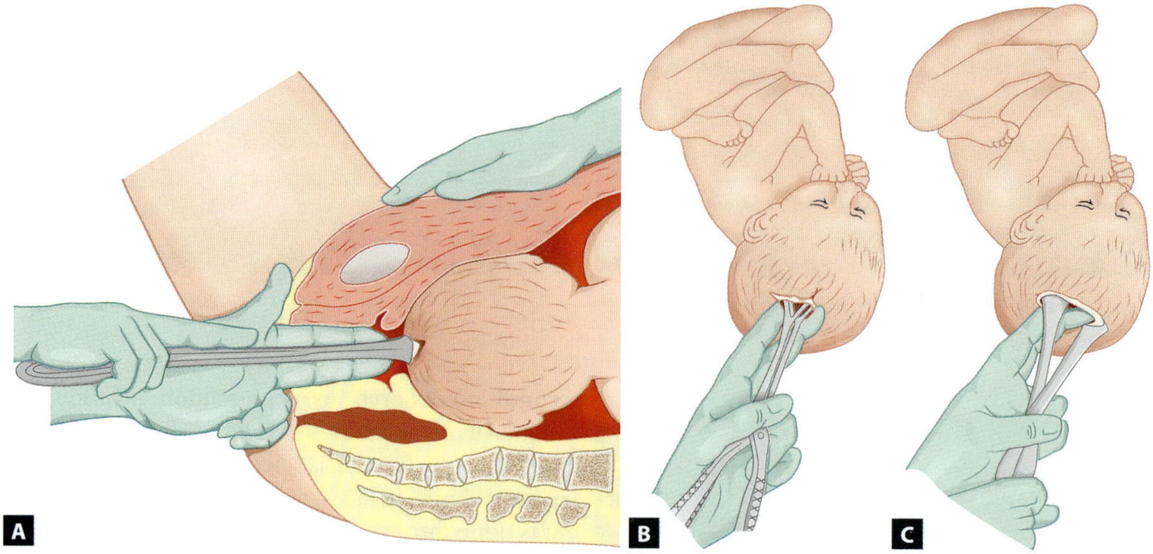

Figs. 4A to C: *Craniotomy:* (A) Perforator is introduced under guidance of left palm and fingers; (B) Tip of the perforator is bored through the skull up to shoulders; (C) Linear tear is made by opening the blades.

vulsellum and Willet's scalp traction forceps can be used to extract fetal head by holding the perforated skull margins.

Placenta is removed manually. Uterine cavity is explored to exclude any perforation and rupture. Cervix and vaginal walls are inspected for any tear or laceration, if any are repaired. Uterine rupture is always excluded before and after any destructive operation.

If this was a case of prolonged obstructed labor, continuous catheterization is done by Foley's catheter and kept for 1 week to prevent vesicovaginal fistula (VVF).

Dealing with Hydrocephalic Head Which is High up Presented by Vertex

A lumbar puncture needle is inserted through a fontanel by fixing the head in pelvis with suprapubic pressure by an assistant, and the head is decompressed with drainage of cerebrospinal fluid (CSF). By this method, baby may be delivered in living condition or dead. However, baby with potential good prognosis is delivered by cesarean method and immediate surgery is performed in neonatal period. Aspiration of CSF with the help of large bore spinal needle to reduce the fetal head size to make birth possible is called *cephalocentesis* or *craniocentesis*. The perforation is made through the posterolateral fontanel behind the ear, if head can be reached per vagina, then traction on the trunk is made to bring the head down as much as possible, and brain matter is washed out and head is delivered by traction. If not approachable through vagina, the trunk is pulled down and a transverse incision is made over the cervical spine as high as possible and the CSF is drained with a metal catheter. In hydrocephalic head (aftercoming head of breech), CSF is drained through abdominal approach by using lumbar puncture needle.

Complications (Dangers) of Craniotomy

Complications are injury to the maternal soft tissues of birth canal, injury to bladder and urethra resulting urinary fistula, commonly vescicovaginal, injury to the uterus—perforation and rupture, and injury to the rectum. Hemorrhage, shock, and sepsis are other complications.

DECAPITATION

Indications of decapitation are impacted shoulder presentation with dead fetus where neck is approachable per vagina. Others are locked twin and double monster.

Criteria to be fulfilled are same as craniotomy operation except a rim of cervix may be present because in shoulder presentation, full dilatation of cervix may not occur.

In impacted shoulder presentation with dead fetus, both decapitation and evisceration can be performed. When neck is approachable decapitation is the choice. When neck is not approachable evisceration is done.

Specific instruments required for decapitation are decapitation hook with knife **(Figs. 5A and B)**, scissors, Blond-Heidler wire and thimble (not used now), and crochet. For extraction of decapitated head obstetric forceps, perforator and cranioclast may be used.

Steps of Decapitation

Preliminary steps are similar to craniotomy. Vaginal examination is done to assess the case whether the conditions are fulfilled, and fetal neck is approachable. If the hand is not prolapsed it is brought down to make it so. Direction of the thumb of outstretched hand will point the side of the head and thus it is determined on which side the head of fetus is. A roller gauze is tied over the wrist of the prolapsed hand and

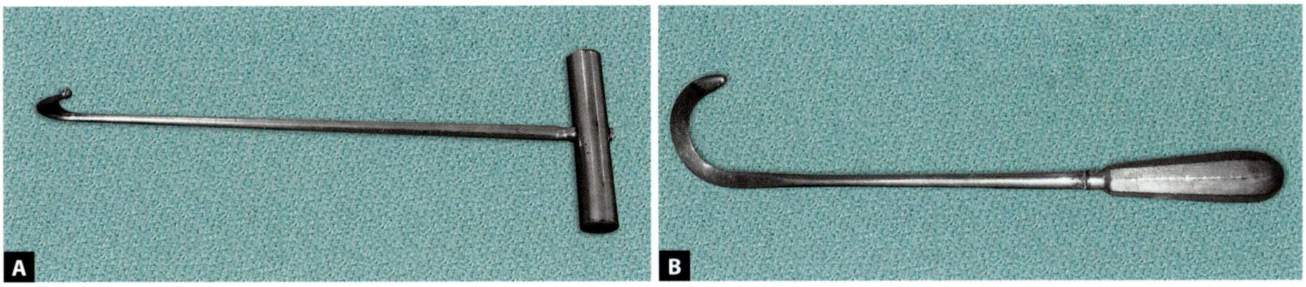

Figs. 5A and B: (A) Jardine's decapitation hook with knife; (B) Ramsbotham decapitation hook with knife.

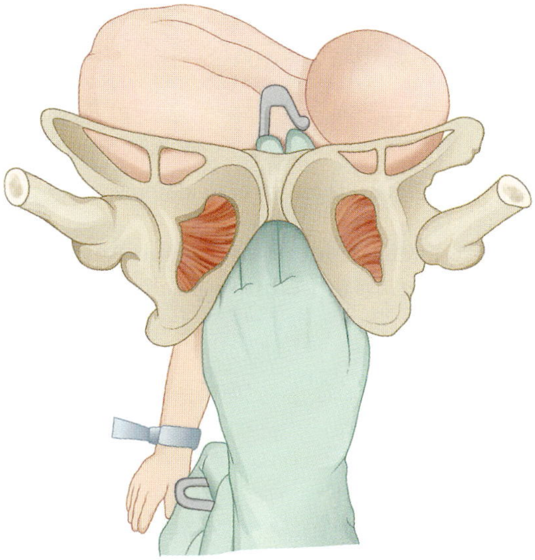

Fig. 6: Decapitation hook with knife is introduced.

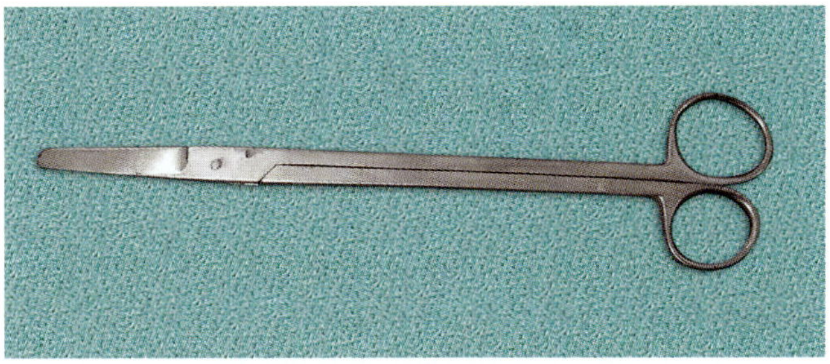

Fig. 7: Embryotomy scissors.

an assistant is asked to pull it in a direction opposite to the head to make the neck steady. The fingers of the left hand are placed over the neck, and the decapitation hook with knife is introduced **(Fig. 6)** per vagina in between the vaginal fingers and the neck, and passed on to a level slightly above the neck. The tip of the hook is kept directing toward the fetal head. The instrument is then rotated at right angle till the curve of the instrument encircles the neck. Then by see-saw movement of the instrument, the neck is severed as far as possible under the guidance of the internal fingers.

The instrument is pushed up, rotated through 90° and is then taken out under the guidance of left thumb and fingers. The last part of the soft tissue of the neck is divided with the help of embryotomy scissors. The head is pushed above to separate it from the trunk. *The trunk is delivered* by pulling the prolapsed arm. Delivery of head is accomplished by any of the methods either by: (i) hooking the finger in the mouth, (ii) using crochet hook, or (iii) forceps. Even craniotomy may be needed in some cases. Rest part and postoperative care is like that of craniotomy.

Complications (dangers) of decapitation are similar to any other destructive operation.

Blond-Heidler wire and thimble is used alternatively in place of decapitation hook with knife where neck is severed by the wire saw tractions after passing the wire loop around the fetal neck. It is difficult to place the wire into position.

EVISCERATION

Indications of evisceration are impacted shoulder presentation with dead fetus and where the fetal *neck is not accessible* per vagina. Fetal malformations such as monsters and fetal ascites can be dealt with evisceration.

Primary steps are same. If there is hand prolapse, it is tied with roller gauze and pulled *toward* the head of fetus (opposite direction of craniotomy). An opening is made at the most accessible site of fetal thorax or abdomen with embryotomy scissors, and viscera are removed piecemeal. The procedure is done under the guidance of internal fingers to protect the maternal tissue from injury. If it is approached through diaphragm, a big opening is done by cutting segments of ribs. A perforator may be needed to perforate the tough diaphragm.

The spine is divided (spondylotomy) by embryotomy scissor **(Fig. 7)** or long Mayo's scissors, and the fetus is delivered by pulling the arm.

SPONDYLOTOMY

The spinal column of the fetus is severed and the trunk is divided in two halves. Evisceration is the preliminary step where the viscera are removed in piecemeal. The spinal column of the lumbar region is hooked by the fingers and cut by embryotomy scissors into two halves. Then soft tissues are cut to divide the fetal body into two halves. The lower half is delivered first followed by the upper part. The procedure is difficult with possibility of uterine rupture and technical skill is needed.

CLEIDOTOMY (FIG. 8)

Indications of cleidotomy are shoulder dystocia in dead fetus (excepting anencephaly where the baby may be living).

Procedures of Cleidotomy

The clavicle is cut by the cleidotomy scissors introduced through the vagina under the guidance of two fingers of left hand. It is better to give a small incision over the skin near clavicle first by any scissor, then introduce the large scissors to cut the clavicle beneath the skin, and this will prevent accidental slipping and injury of adjacent maternal tissues. Cleidotomy scissors is similar to Mayo's or embryotomy scissors, only that there are two knobs—one on each blade at the tip so that the bony clavicle is not slipped during its divisions.

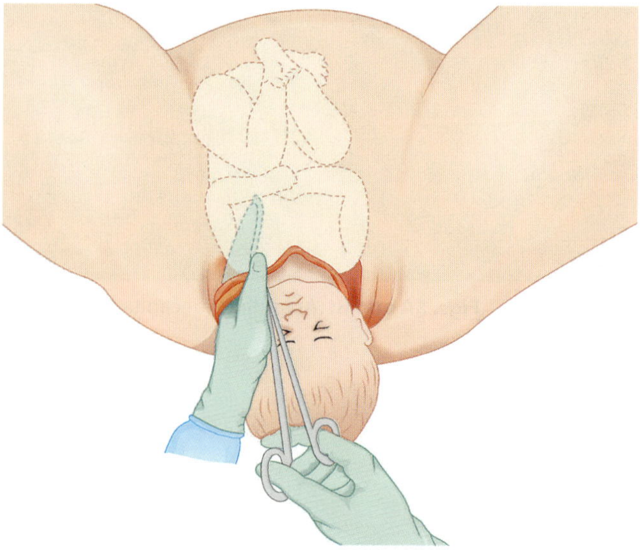

Fig. 8: Procedure of cleidotomy.

For more details reader may consult Author's *Bedside Clinics in Obstetrics,* 5th edition published by Academy Publishers.

CHAPTER 27

Gynecological Diseases in Pregnancy

Learning Objectives

- Pregnancy with Uterine Fibroid (Myoma, Fibromyoma, or Leiomyoma)
- Ovarian Tumor
- Cervical Cancer
- Cervical Polyp
- Pregnancy with Pelvic Organ Prolapse

INTRODUCTION

Gynecological disorder is not uncommonly encountered during pregnancy. Uterine leiomyoma is a common female benign tumor. Most of the cases are asymptomatic. Symptoms of pain appear due to degeneration, rarely due to torsion of subserous variety. Pregnancy outcome depends on size and location. Surgery is rarely indicated. Ovarian masses in pregnancy are common, but most of the cases are small, cystic and benign in nature. Due to its complications such as torsion, rupture, etc. acute emergency may develop. Ovarian malignancy during pregnancy is a real concern, its prognosis is not altered by pregnancy. Cervical cancer screening is similar to nonpregnant state. Sometime conization may be needed. Invasive cancer cervix is treated according to priority of disease stage. Pelvic organ prolapse (POP) during pregnancy is rare event and may have problem during delivery. For appropriate management of the gynecological disorders clear knowledge of individual cases associated with pregnancy is essential to decide the need and to select the proper time of surgery.

PREGNANCY WITH UTERINE FIBROID (MYOMA, FIBROMYOMA, OR LEIOMYOMA)

Incidence

The incidence of fibroid in pregnancy is 2%. It may be much higher (8–18%) depending on racial variation and frequency of routine sonography.

Diagnosis

History

Usually patient is elderly primi and/or has conceived following a period of infertility. Before pregnancy, patient might give history of symptoms of fibroid such as menorrhagia, lump abdomen, and there may be a preconceptional diagnosis of uterine fibroid.

During pregnancy, patient may be asymptomatic. There may be undue enlargement of the abdomen, features of pressure symptoms such as urinary retention [if it is cervical fibroid or fibroid impacted in pouch of Douglas (POD)] or constipation if it gives pressure over the rectum. Pain abdomen is due to degenerative changes or due to torsion of subserous fibroid. Size of the uterus is more than the period of amenorrhea, surface of the uterus becomes nodular, and separate fixed lump or lumps are palpable other than the fetal parts, frequently confused with diagnosis of ovarian tumor. Definite diagnosis is done by sonography.

Effects of Pregnancy over Fibroid

Fibroid may become enlarged or regressed in size, softened, and flattened. Majority do not become enlarged. They are frequently displaced upward. Red generation is common during pregnancy. There may be pain even acute in nature, tenderness, nausea, vomiting, and mild fever with high WBC counts. It is very difficult to differentiate from appendicitis, abruption, kidney stone, or pyelonephritis. Sonography is useful. Bed rest and analgesics are usually sufficient. Sometimes, pain becomes severe. With conservative treatment symptoms usually disappear within 1–2 weeks, however with chance of recurrence. Subserous vein over the fibroid becomes prominent and engorged, even may be ruptured causing intraperitoneal hemorrhage. There may be torsion of pedunculated subserous fibroid which needs laparotomy and myomectomy. Torsion commonly occurs following delivery; infection of fibroid is uncommon during antenatal period and may occur during puerperium.

Effects of Fibroid over Pregnancy

In most of the cases, fibroid during pregnancy do not cause unfavorable outcome. It depends on the size of the tumor, site of the tumor, and the type of tumor whether it is submucous, intramural, or subserous.

Complications are mostly in submucous variety, least in subserous variety except the torsion. More low down the fibroid higher chance of malpresentation and obstructed labor. There is more chance of miscarriage and preterm labor and increase placental abruption. Malpresentation and nonengagement may occur due to low down fibroid. Obstructed labor may occur due to cervical fibroid or low corporeal fibroid. There is chance of uterine inertia during labor. Cesarean delivery rate in fibroid is higher. Third stage complications like postpartum hemorrhage (PPH) are common and during puerperium subinvolution and sepsis may occur.

Diagnosis of Fibroid in Pregnancy

Most of the leiomyomas are asymptomatic. Height of the uterus is more than the period of amenorrhea. Additional swelling other than fetal parts is palpable over the uterus. There may be malpresentation. Sonography is mandatory for diagnosis, size determination, and to determine location **(Fig. 1)**. Magnetic resonance imaging (MRI) may be required and performed after first trimester if sonography becomes inconclusive. Sonographic monitoring of fibroid during pregnancy is not recommended in otherwise uncomplicated fibroid.

Management of a Case of Pregnancy with Fibroid

During antenatal period—usually pregnancy becomes uneventful except pain abdomen. If there is pain abdomen, it is necessary to rule out whether due to red degeneration or due to torsion of subserous fibroid. Effect of progesterone on growth of myoma is unpredictable. Red degeneration is managed conservatively and torsion needs laparotomy. Myomectomy is not advocated during antenatal period except in torsion of subserous fibroid. Myomectomy in antenatal period in selected cases with good outcome has been reported.

Mode of Delivery in Pregnancy Associated with Myoma

In most of the cases, vaginal delivery is possible as fibroids are usually displaced upward except in cervical fibroid. Active management of third stage is mandatory to prevent PPH. Fibroid itself is not an indication for cesarean delivery except in few cases as written here.

Myomectomy Scar Rupture during Labor

Risk of rupture in trial of labor in previously myomectomized woman is not much. It is 0.47%, almost similar to that of trial of labor (0.2–0.9%) in prior lower uterine cesarean delivery.

Indication of Cesarean Delivery in Fibroid in Pregnancy

Elective cesarean section (CS) is done in cases of cervical fibroid. In prolonged labor, in pregnancy with bad obstetric history or in elderly primi with long period of infertility CS is also contemplated.

Difficulty during Cesarean Delivery

If there are multiple fibroids occupying the whole uterus cesarean delivery also becomes difficult to deliver the baby by lower uterine segment cesarean section (LUCS) **(Fig. 2)**. Sometimes, classical cesarean delivery (upper uterine) is needed if fibroid occupies the whole lower uterine segment.

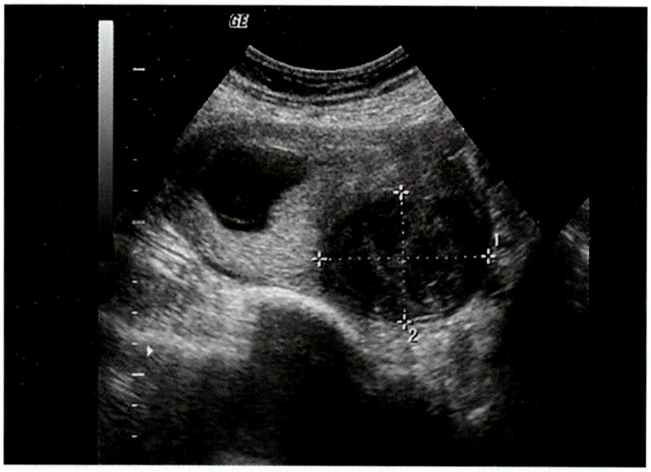

Fig. 1: Ultrasound (USG) showing early pregnancy with fibroid. *Courtesy:* Professor Kamal Oswal, Head, Department of Radiodiagnosis, Vivekananda Institute of Medical Sciences, Kolkata, West Bengal, India.

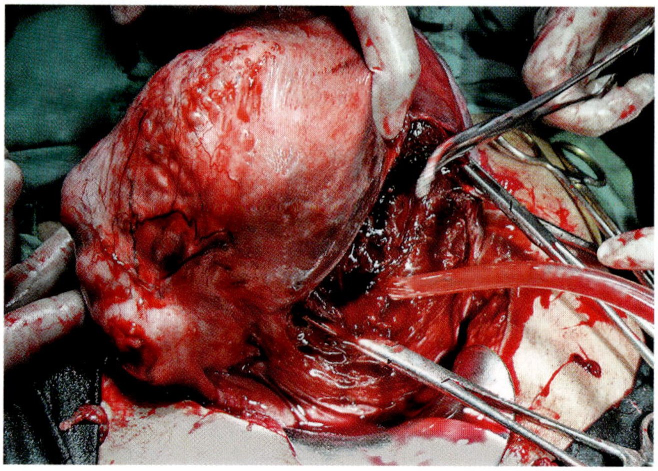

Fig. 2: Cesarean section (CS) in a case of multiple leiomyoma before CS wound repair after baby and placenta delivered.

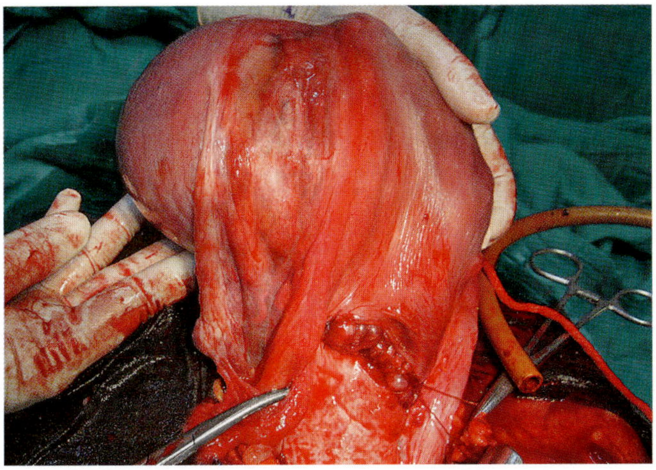

Fig. 3: A large myoma in right fundo-posterior region following lower uterine segment cesarean delivery.

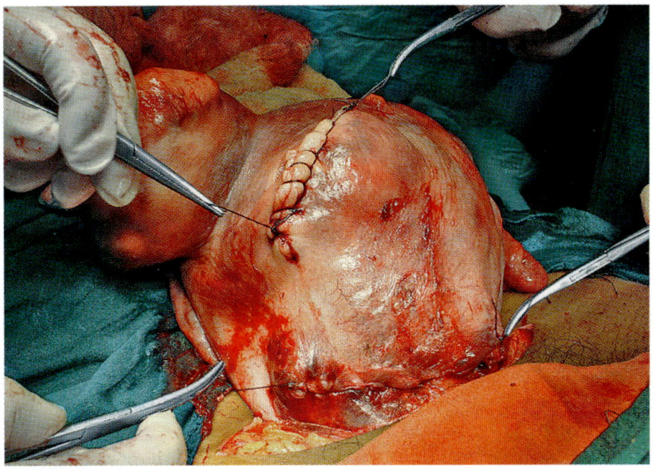

Fig. 4: After repair of cesarean wound, cesarean myomectomy done removing one large myoma and other myoma right part of fundal region remained intact.

Figure 3 shows repair of cesarean wound in a pregnancy with fibroid.

Role of Myomectomy during Cesarean Delivery

Myomectomy is usually not recommended during cesarean delivery for fear of torrential hemorrhage. Myomectomy during cesarean delivery is indicated only in pedunculated subserous fibroid or if a small fibroid lies over or near the incision line. In recent days, there is increase tendency of myomectomy during cesarean delivery **(Fig. 4)** due to availability of blood and good vasopressor agents. Routine myomectomy during cesarean delivery is not recommended.

OVARIAN TUMOR

Clinically detectable ovarian masses are thought to affect about 1 in 1,500 pregnancies. Ultrasound scanning probably detects prevalence of adnexal masses in early pregnancy of about 1 in 200. These are mostly cysts of the corpus luteum and do not persist beyond second trimester. Ovarian malignancy is very rare at approximately 1 case per 20,000–50,000 pregnancies.

Types of Adnexal Mass Found in Pregnancy

It is mostly benign and very rarely malignant. *Benign cystic teratoma* (dermoid cyst) is relatively common during pregnancy. The different ovarian masses seen during pregnancy are endometrioma, corpus luteum cysts, benign cystadenomas **(Fig. 5)**, and benign cystic teratoma. Pregnancy-related ovarian swellings are pregnancy luteoma, hyperreactio luteinalis, and ovarian hyperstimulation syndrome due to the effects of pregnancy hormones. Hyperreactio luteinalis is the development of multiple and large theca-lutein cysts after the first trimester due to the exceptionally high hCG level. They are commonly found in multiple pregnancy, gestational trophoblastic disease (GTD), and fetal hydrops.

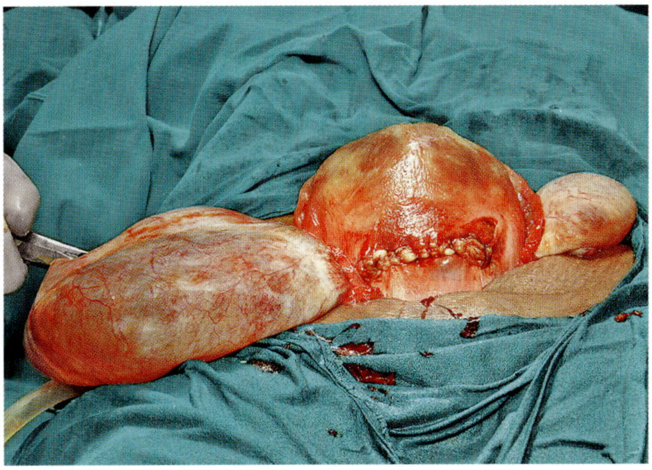

Fig. 5: Bilateral septate mucinous cystadenoma. Right side 18 × 20 cm, left side 8 × 6 cm—bilateral cystectomy done during lower uterine segment cesarean section (LUCS) at 36 weeks.

Diagnosis

Clinical Presentation

Many are asymptomatic. Most adnexal masses are detected coincidentally during routine antenatal ultrasound. A small proportion of cases may be large enough to be detected clinically during bimanual palpation. There may be undue enlargement, increase breathlessness, pain, bladder, and rectal symptoms. The mass may also present with complications. Woman may present with acute abdomen in complications such as rupture and torsion **(Fig. 6)**. Per abdominally height of the fundus becomes more than period of amenorrhea. Two separate masses may be palpable. Small ovarian tumor may be hidden lateral and behind the large gravid uterus.

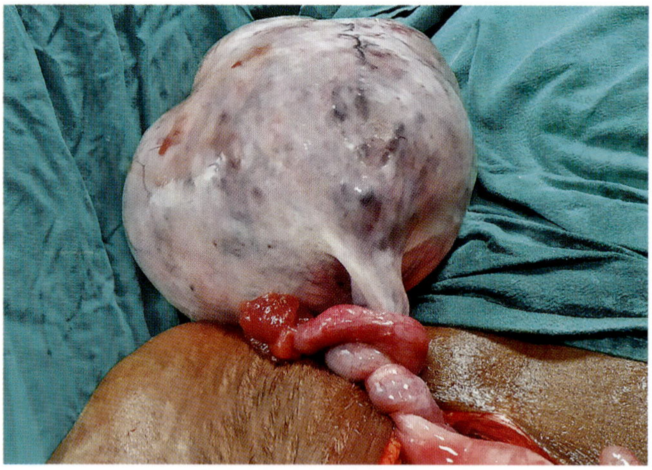

Fig. 6: Torsion of ovarian tumor.

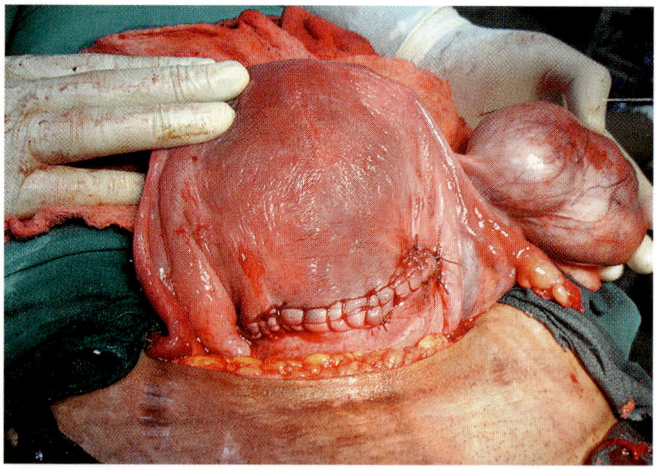

Fig. 7: Ovarian dermoid cyst (benign cystic teratome) in pregnancy. Lower uterine segment cesarean section (LUCS) done followed by cystectomy.

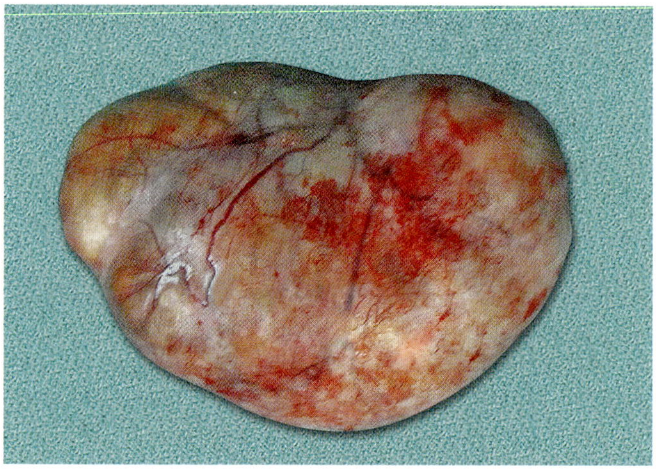

Fig. 8: Following cystectomy in the dermoid cyst as in the patient shown in Figure 7.

Investigations

Ultrasound (USG) scanning including Doppler is done to detect the size, location, appearance, and to assist decisions on management. Morphological criteria can differentiate benign ovarian cyst from malignant one. Ovarian tumor markers are used mainly to monitor disease status during treatment. Several markers can be elevated due to pregnancy itself, e.g., CA-125, β-human chorionic gonadotropin (β-hCG). In confirmed malignancy, investigations to stage the tumor (such as MRI scanning of the pelvis) may be used, as the risk to the mother is considered to outweigh that to the fetus. Computed tomography (CT) is less commonly used during pregnancy due to adverse fetal exposure.

What are the effects of ovarian tumor over pregnancy and labor?

Increase chances of abortion, premature labor—iatrogenic or spontaneous are there. Any complication of ovarian tumor may adversely affect the pregnancy outcome. There may be undue enlargement of abdomen and its consequences such as there will be more respiratory distress and increase abdominal pain. Malpresentation and nonengagement of presenting part and obstructed labor. There is difficulty in clinical examination.

Effects of Pregnancy over Ovarian Tumor

Many of the complications of ovarian tumor increase during pregnancy. There is increase chance of (1) torsion—at least double than that of nonpregnant state; torsion commonly occurs *early second trimester and after delivery,* (2) intracystic hemorrhage, (3) rupture due to impaction and hemorrhage, and (4) infection.

Management of a Case of Ovarian Tumor during Pregnancy

If the mass is thought to be benign and unlikely to cause complications, expectant management and follow-up scans are recommended. There is little evidence to support the routine laparoscopic excision of presumed benign ovarian tumors. Surgery is indicated for large (>5–10 cm in diameter) and/or symptomatic tumors and those that appear highly suspicious for malignancy (solid or mixed solid and cystic) on ultrasound. The optimal surgical window being around 16–20 weeks of gestation. Risk of abortion increases after surgery. In second half of pregnancy asymptomatic tumor can be observed till delivery after which surgery is done.

Surgery: The extent of surgery is decided by the intraoperative findings showing whether the tumor is benign or malignant. Conservative surgery, preferably cystectomy or salpingo-oophorectomy is indicated for benign ovarian cyst **(Figs. 7 to 9)**. If surgery is not done in pregnancy, diagnosed ovarian tumor should be removed as early as possible after delivery. More extensive surgery (including staging biopsies) for confirmed higher-grade malignancies may be needed.

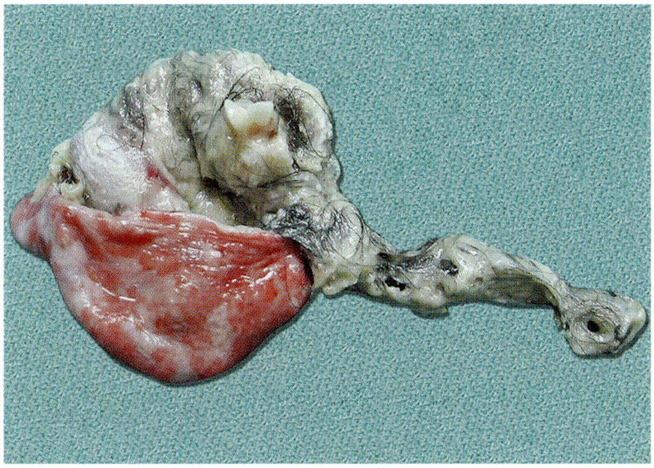

Fig. 9: To cut open to show teeth, hair, and sebaceous material in enucleated dermoid cyst (cut section of same specimen as Figures 7 and 8).

Rarely, chemotherapy may be given after delivery or at least after 20 weeks in order to minimize the potential fetal toxicity. The short- to medium-term fetal outcome appears to be relatively good.

Labor and Delivery

If the tumor lies above pelvic brim, there is no problem for vaginal delivery. If it lies in the pelvis, cesarean delivery is done followed by salpingo-oophorectomy (ovariotomy) or cystectomy. Following delivery, chance of torsion increases as already stated.

Prognosis

It is excellent in benign cases. Prognosis in cases of ovarian malignancy is related to tumor grade and stage, but one series shows 70% maternal survival and relatively good fetal outcomes. Earlier diagnosis gives a better prognosis.

CERVICAL CANCER

The incidence of cancer cervix during pregnancy is very low estimated to be 1.2 in 10,000 pregnancy.

Diagnosis of Cancer Cervix during Pregnancy

In pregnancy, routine Pap test screening has advantage of diagnosing preinvasive lesions. Screening of cancer cervix is similar to nonpregnant state. Invasive lesions may have symptoms.

Management of Cases with Abnormal Cytology

Most of them should undergo prompt colposcopy and the aim is to exclude invasive cancer. In lesions of high-grade disease and invasive cancer, biopsy is done. Cervical intraepithelial neoplasia (CIN) during pregnancy is allowed to deliver vaginally with re-evaluation postpartum provided that invasive disease is excluded.

If invasive lesion is suspected *conization* with loop electrosurgical excision procedure (LEEP) or by cold knife conization is indicated. Extensive excision is limited for fear of membrane rupture. Conization is avoided in pregnancy as far as possible as there is increased risk of membrane rupture, hemorrhage, abortion, and preterm delivery.

Clinical Manifestations

It may present with bleeding per vagina or excessive white discharge. There may not be any period of amenorrhea. Per speculum examination shows an unhealthy cervix with growth which bleeds on touch. Per rectal examination is done to determine the extent of lesion.

Investigations

Pap test, in suspected early lesion—colposcopic-directed biopsy is performed. In unavailability of colposcope Schiller's iodine test is done. In obvious lesion, punch biopsy is performed. Cone biopsy is avoided during pregnancy for fear of membrane rupture, hemorrhage, infection, and abortion (33%).

Differential Diagnosis

Normal cervical changes during pregnancy (hyperemia), cervical erosion, and cervical polyp may mimic cancer cervix. Careful examination, cytology, and biopsy findings differentiate from normal cervix.

What are the effects of pregnancy over cancer cervix?
Course of the disease is usually unaffected. Increase vascularity and inflicted trauma over cervix during vaginal delivery as causes of dissemination of tumor cell are not well documented, but a possibility.

Effects of Cancer Cervix over the Pregnancy

There may be increase chance of miscarriage, preterm labor, fetal growth restriction, anemia, difficulty of vaginal delivery due to nondilation of cervix, hemorrhage during delivery, PPH, infection, and cesarean delivery rate.

Staging of Cervical Cancer in Pregnancy

Cancer cervix is staged clinically. Staging incorporates pelvic examination, renal USG, chest X-ray, cystoscopy, proctoscopy, and cone biopsy. Cancer cervix in pregnancy is diagnosed in stage I in 75% of cases. Extent of cancer is often underestimated due to pregnancy-induced softening of cervical, paracervical, and parametrial tissue.

Management

It depends on period of gestation when detected and stage of the disease and desire of continuation of pregnancy.

In microinvasive disease continuation of pregnancy and vaginal delivery is safe followed by definitive therapy. In early stage of the disease (stage I and early stage IIA) surgery in the form of radical hysterectomy and pelvic lymphadenectomy is the preferred treatment.

In first half of pregnancy immediate treatment is advised.

In later half, pregnancy can be continued until fetal lung maturity develops. In first half of pregnancy, radical hysterectomy is performed with fetus in situ or following medical termination of pregnancy (MTP)/hysterotomy in the mid trimester after proper counseling. In later half of pregnancy hysterotomy (cesarean delivery) is performed first followed by radical hysterectomy in the same sitting. In advanced stages, radiotherapy is given. External beam therapy (EBR) induces spontaneous abortion in early pregnancy. If product of conception is not expelled curettage is done. Hysterotomy may be needed in second trimester before radiotherapy as dilatation and evacuation may cause severe hemorrhage.

Except very near to term in no case definitive treatment is not deferred for long time (longer than 4 weeks) in expectation of a viable baby.

Mode of Delivery

Vaginal delivery can be allowed in early cases. There may be uterine dystocia and bleeding during delivery and PPH. In large growth, where dilatation of cervix is a problem, cesarean delivery is performed. Growth in the episiotomy scar has been reported following vaginal delivery which apparently seems to be "seeding" of tumor cells in episiotomy scar. Hence, classical cesarean delivery followed by radical hysterectomy with pelvic lymphadenectomy is the preferred treatment.

Prognosis

There is no difference in-between pregnant and nonpregnant situation. Majority (75%) have stage I disease and thus, have slightly better prognosis.

CERVICAL POLYP

Polyp is grasped with sponge holding forceps and twisted to strangulate feeding vessels. If pedicle is thick surgical ligation and excision is needed.

PREGNANCY WITH PELVIC ORGAN PROLAPSE

Pregnancy may occur in a woman with POP (**Fig. 10**). There may be cystocele, uterine descent, rectocele, and even enterocele depending upon the presence of which complication may occur in pregnancy and labor.

Prevalence

Pelvic organ prolapse is mostly found in developing countries in multiparous women and incidence varies from 1 in 200–500 labors.

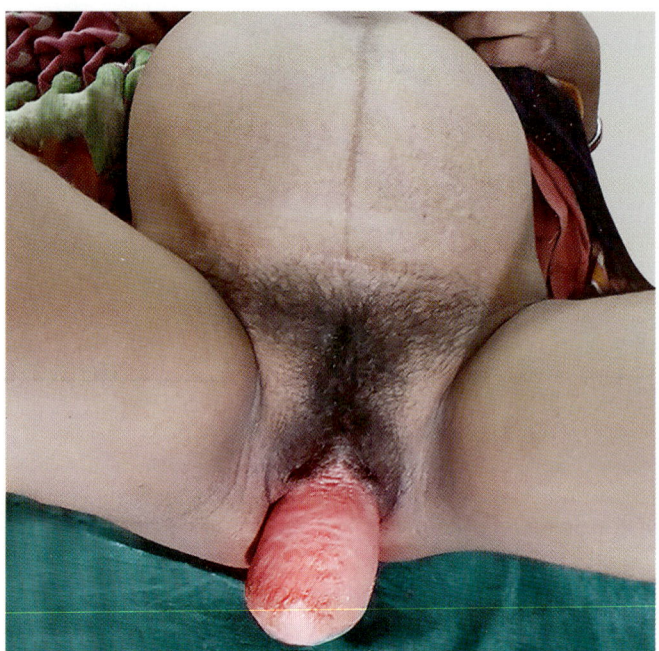

Fig. 10: Pelvic organ prolapse in term pregnancy.

Effect of Pregnancy over POP

The protruded cervix with prolapsed uterus usually ascends as the uterus becomes abdominal organ after 12 weeks of pregnancy and patient may relieve of symptoms. If uterus persists in prolapsed position incarceration may occur at 12–14 weeks of pregnancy for which the uterus needs to be replaced sometimes in early pregnancy and suitable pessary is needed to keep the uterus in correct position as a preventive measure.

Effects of POP over the Course of Pregnancy and Labor

In early pregnancy, POP causes distressing symptoms such as something coming down sensation, white discharge, backache and bladder symptoms of frequency, incomplete evacuation, and stress incontinence. Presence of cystocele may increase urinary stasis which predispose to urinary tract infection. Urinary stress incontinence becomes worsened as urethral closure pressure is not increased sufficient enough to compensate increased bladder pressure. Presence of large rectocele may cause constipation. There may be premature onset of labor.

During labor—delayed dilatation, slow effacement and edema of cervix may cause cervical dystocia, and prolonged first stage. There is increase chance of early rupture of membranes. As the cervix descends in pelvic floor, there is early bearing down effort by mother and mother becomes exhausted. Presence of cystocele, rectocele, and large enterocele may hinder the fetal descend and second stage becomes prolonged if they are not pushed out of the way.

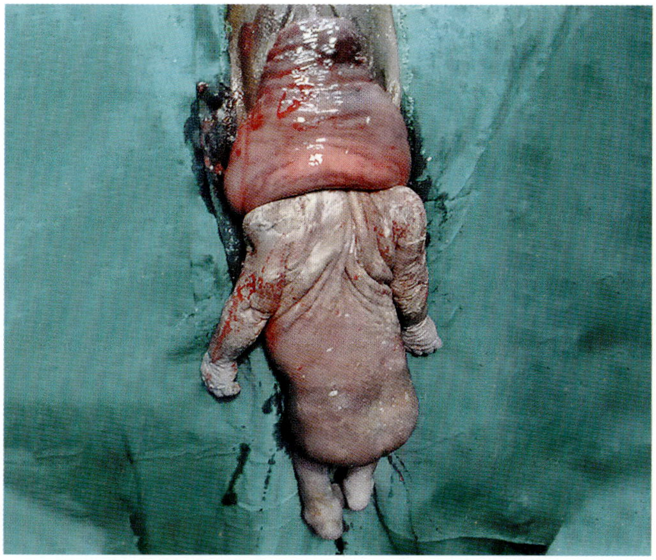

Fig. 11: Arrest of aftercoming head of breech in undilated cervix in a case of genital prolapse.
Courtesy: Dr Anirban Mondal, Associate Professor, Bankura Sammilani Medical College and Hospital, Bankura, West Bengal, India.

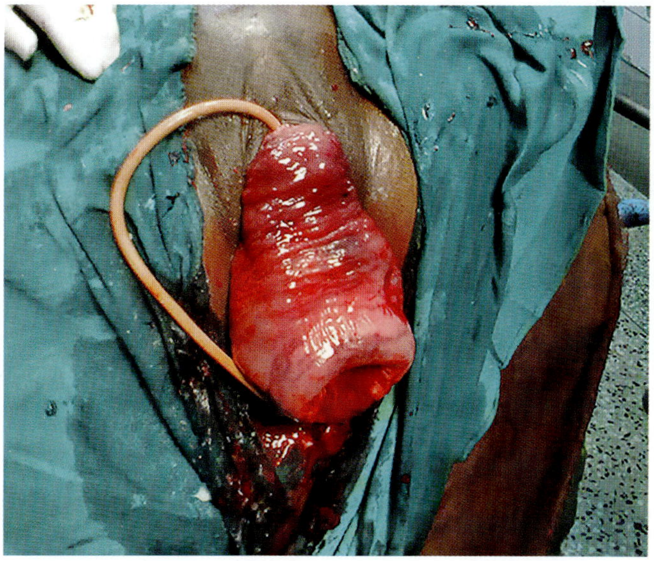

Fig. 12: Appearance of thick and edematous cervix in POP after delivery of aftercoming head of breech as shown in Figure 11.

Figure 11 shows arrest of aftercoming head of fetus in breech presentation in undilated cervix in case of genital prolapse. **Figure 12** shows the appearance of cervix in POP after delivery of aftercoming head of cervix.

Management of POP

Rest is advised in early pregnancy. In large prolapse, patient may be admitted in first trimester till uterus becomes abdominal organ. Ring pessary is needed sometimes (see earlier). During early labor, if cervix looks edematous glycerin-acriflavine pack is given. In late first stage, if cervix is not dilated fully Duhrssen's incision (rarely) on cervical lip is given and delivery is accomplished by ventouse or forceps application. Sometimes cesarean delivery is needed when the head is high up with edematous nondilating cervix.

CHAPTER 28

Surgical Illness in Pregnancy

Learning Objectives

- Introduction—Importance of Surgical Illness in Pregnancy
- Appendicitis
- Peptic Ulcer
- Cholecystitis and Gallstone
- Pancreatitis
- Renal Stone

INTRODUCTION

With the alteration of physiology, anatomy, and functions of the reproductive tract during pregnancy, various aspects of other systems also change to cope up with the burden of pregnancy and also to support it. The anatomy, physiology, and functions of the gastrointestinal (GI) system alter remarkably during pregnancy. Clinical manifestations of the disease of different systems alter and many new symptoms arise due to pregnancy that mimic the features of other systems. Clinical findings including pain, tenderness, etc., are obscured due to a hugely enlarged uterus and displacement of the organs. Besides, few investigations such as X-ray and computed tomography (CT) scan are generally contraindicated in pregnancy. Laparoscopy is safe in pregnancy only in expert hands. Pregnant women also suffer from surgical diseases that are common in general population. Every obstetrician must be acquainted with the character of these diseases with change of clinical manifestations and modification of management including operative techniques during pregnancy.

APPENDICITIS

The incidence of appendicitis during pregnancy is 0.02–0.1%.

Diagnosis

Pain in the right iliac fossa, nausea, vomiting, and tenderness on McBurney's point are the usual manifestations.

Difficulties in diagnosis of appendicitis in pregnancy are due to the following:

- There is lack of a typical presentation of appendicitis. Site of pain and tenderness migrate with upward displacement of appendix by growing uterus.
- Nausea and vomiting which are the common symptoms of appendicitis are also common in the first half of pregnancy.
- Leukocytosis is common in normal pregnancy. Sonography is helpful. Typical finding of graded compression sonography is not obvious. Appendiceal CT scan is accurate to diagnose but modified to reduce radiation; MRI is best if available. Diagnostic accuracy is inversely proportional to the gestational age.

Differential diagnoses are cholecystitis, pyelonephritis, labor pain, and abruption.

Effect of Appendicitis on Pregnancy

There are more chances of abortion and preterm labor if peritonitis occurs. Infertility is unlikely later due to appendicitis.

Effect of Pregnancy on Appendicitis

As the appendix ascends, entrapment of infection by omentum becomes less. The incidence of perforation increases with advancement of gestation.

Management

Surgery is the treatment as soon as diagnosed as peritonitis makes the pregnancy worse. The laparoscopic approach is preferred by many in the first and second trimesters. Intravenous (IV) antibiotic with second-generation cephalosporin or third-generation penicillin is preferred. Tocolytic is not recommended as it may increase pulmonary-permeability edema by sepsis syndrome.

PEPTIC ULCER

Peptic ulcer is less common in pregnancy. Pregnancy improves the peptic ulcer probably due to gastroprotective effects caused by decreased gastric secretion, reduced motility, and increased mucus secretion. In active ulcers, *Helicobacter pylori* is searched by urea breath test, serological test, and endoscopy.

Management

Nonsteroidal anti-inflammatory drug (NSAID) is avoided. The first line of treatment is H2 receptor or proton-pump inhibitors (omeprazole). Sucralfate provides a protective coat. All of these are safe in pregnancy. Endoscopic evaluation is not contraindicated in pregnancy. In *H. pylori* positive cases, a combination of antimicrobials and proton-pump inhibitors is prescribed.

Perforation and hemorrhage are rare in pregnancy.

CHOLECYSTITIS AND GALLSTONE

Acute cholecystitis during pregnancy or in puerperium is common and usually associated with gallstones or sludge. The incidence of gallstone in pregnancy is about 2% and that of biliary sludge (forerunner of gallstones) is 30%. Acute cholecystitis results from obstruction of cystic duct and is mostly bacterial in origin. Half of the patients have history of pain in the right upper hypochondrium due to gallstones.

Diagnosis

In acute cholecystitis, there is pain, low-grade fever, nausea, vomiting, anorexia, and tenderness in the right hypochondrium. Complete blood count (CBC) shows leukocytosis. Ultrasound (USG) can visualize gallstones. A patient with gallstone may be asymptomatic in up to 10% cases.

Management of Acute Cholecystitis

Initial management is medical therapy which consists of IV fluid, nasogastric suction, analgesic, and antibiotics.

In contrast to the previous approach, earlier surgery is commonly done in pregnancy and operative and endoscopic intervention is preferred to the conservative approach. Laparoscopic cholecystectomy is the treatment of choice. The rationale of early surgery is that the recurrence rate is high and recurrent cholecystitis in late gestation is associated with preterm labor, unplanned labor induction, and more cesarean delivery; moreover, surgery becomes technically difficult. Cholecystectomy is safe during pregnancy and does not increase preterm labor and maternal and fetal mortality.

PANCREATITIS

Acute pancreatitis in pregnancy is rare and usually occurs in the third trimester. Up to one-tenth becomes necrotizing pancreatitis. It is characterized by cell membrane breakage, proteolysis, edema, hemorrhage, and necrosis. The most common cause of acute pancreatitis in pregnancy is gallstone. Other predisposing factors may be trauma, acute fatty liver of pregnancy (AFLP), hypertriglyceridemia, and alcohol abuse.

Effect of Pancreatitis on Pregnancy

Pancreatitis during pregnancy leads to increased chance of preterm delivery, intrauterine fetal demise (IUFD) and also maternal death. The outcome depends on the severity of pancreatitis. There is an increased risk of preeclampsia. Necrotizing pancreatitis has a high mortality rate of 15%.

Diagnosis

Clinical: There is mild-to-severe epigastric pain, nausea, vomiting, low-grade fever, tachycardia, hypotension, and abdominal distension. Tenderness over abdomen is present. Few patients may develop acute respiratory distress syndrome (ARDS).

Laboratory findings: Serum amylase (n = 28–100 IU/mL) and lipase (n = 7–59 IU/L) become very high. Amylase becomes three times than normal. CBC shows leukocytosis. Raised bilirubin and raised aspartate transaminase (AST) are suggestive of cholelithiasis. Sonography is helpful to diagnosis. Various prognostic scoring systems are designed to classify pancreatitis.

Management of Acute Pancreatitis

Treatment is supportive. IV fluid, stoppage of oral fluid, analgesics, and broad-spectrum antibiotics are started. Endoscopic retrograde cholangiopancreatography (ERCP) is suggested in common bile duct stone. Cholecystectomy is done after the acute stage is over to prevent recurrent pancreatitis. A small number of patients need intensive care treatment due to complications such as peritonitis involving cardiac, renal, and gastrointestinal (GI) systems.

RENAL STONE

The incidence of renal stone varies from 0.02% to 0.2%. In pregnancy, stones are either calcium phosphate or hydroxyapatite though in a nonpregnant state they are mostly calcium oxalate.

Effect of Urinary Tract Stone on Pregnancy

There is an increased chance of a low-birth-weight baby and preterm labor.

Effect of Pregnancy on Course of Urinary Stone

Pregnant women are less symptomatic due to urinary tract dilatation. Up to 80% women may respond to conservative therapy and spontaneous expulsion of stone may occur.

Diagnosis

Urinary stone mostly presents with loin to groin pain and hematuria. Sonography is useful to diagnosis. CT scan is very useful but due to the issue of radiation exposure, it is avoided in pregnancy and MRI is suggested.

Management

Medical management includes hydration, analgesic, and antimicrobial in presence of infection. 60–80% women respond to conservative therapy.

Definitive treatment: Various options are ureteric stenting, percutaneous nephrostomy, laser lithotripsy (transurethral), flexible basket extraction via cystoscopy, and ureteroscopy.

CHAPTER 29

Gastrointestinal Tract Injury and Urinary Tract Injury

Learning Objectives

- Risk Factors
- Gastrointestinal Tract Injury
- Rectovaginal Fistula
- Urinary Tract Injuries during Child Birth

INTRODUCTION

Injuries of urinary tract and that of gastrointestinal (GI) tract are important potential complications in obstetric patients. During vaginal delivery injury of urinary tract is restricted to urethra and rarely bladder lacerations and lower part of ureter are involved in instrumental delivery or when repair of high up vaginal laceration is attempted. Vesicovaginal fistula (VVF) is an important sequel of prolonged labor and prevalent in many undeveloped countries. Urinary bladder and urinary tract injury are potential serious complications in extreme laceration during cesarean delivery, management of broad ligament hematoma, and more especially in peripartum hysterectomy.

In vaginal delivery, injury of GI tract is restricted to lower rectum and anal canal sphincter complex (OASIS) which is discussed in Chapter 15. Gut injury in obstetrics is uncommon but may happen during laparotomy for cesarean delivery and relaparotomy cases where there is extensive adhesion. Altered anatomy during pregnancy, and performing surgery in emergency, and stressful situations are important contributory factors for intraoperative accident.

Sometimes undetected cases of both bowel and urinary tract injury present in very morbid conditions either urinary tract fistula or renal damage. In undetected gut injury, patient comes with severe abdominal distention and features of septic and fecal peritonitis.

All obstetricians should have ability to recognize those injuries in spot and in case of simple injury management can be done by generalist with good outcome. In extensive injuries, assistance of respective specialized consultant is sought for. Failure to detect immediately may have severe morbidity and serious consequences.

RISK FACTORS

Identification of risk factors: Prior detection of risk factors not only helps to take precautionary measures but also where injury is a possibility preparation with expert team will make the outcome better.

The important risk factors are previous cesarean delivery, previous pelvic or abdominal surgery, pelvic adhesions, emergency delivery with surgical haste, cesarean delivery following prolonged labor, placenta previa, morbid adherent placenta, cesarean hysterectomy, internal iliac ligation, and endometriosis.

GASTROINTESTINAL TRACT INJURY

As mentioned gut injury during cesarean delivery though uncommon, may occur in some situations such as abdominal and pelvic adhesions during opening of abdomen. Majority of the injuries are lower rectum and anal canal following child birth. The incidence of Bowel injury cesarean delivery is about 0.05% during.

Small Gut Injury

Diagnosis is done by examination of the suspected area of gut and finding the spilling of bowel content.

Management depends on time of injury, size, depth, site, and blood supply of the injured area. In case of injury incurred before delivery of the baby, the part is covered with mop (laparotomy sponge) to keep aside which will be repaired after delivery of baby and cesarean wound closure.

The procedure of repair for type of injury is as follows:

Serosal injuries: Serosal injuries which are small usually need no repair. Large serosal injuries are repaired with 2-0 or 3-0 absorbable or permanent oversewing suture followed by reinforcing the serosa and muscularis with interrupted stitches. Sutures are placed parallel to the lumen of bowel to prevent narrowing of lumen.

Full Thickness Opening of Small Gut

If the size is less than or equal to circumference of gut, local primary repair is adequate if blood supply is not jeopardized. 3-0 Vicryl or silk suture with taper needle is used. Both angles are included. Suture line should be perpendicular to direction of gut lumen to prevent future stricture. If the rent is longitudinal, it will be repaired transversely to make it transverse wound to prevent constriction. Wound is closed with the same suture in imbricating fashion with 3–4 mm spacing including muscularis and lamina propria of the intestine. Final diameter should be at least 1–2 cm after repair. Any leaking is tested by giving slight pressure. If size is more the half circumference and/or their multiple injuries and blood supply is jeopardized and the part of gut is devitalized resection anastomosis **(Figs. 1 to 3)** is done. General surgeon or gynecologic oncologist is consulted. Resection is done either manually or with intestinal stapler, the latter is preferred due to less leakage and better blood supply. Gut is inspected thoroughly for any other injury. Peritoneal cavity is washed with normal saline. A drain is given if there was significant spillage.

Large Gut Injuries (Colon)

Small serosal laceration: It is repaired like that of small intestine. Where there is extensive injuries and compromised blood supply resection should be done and general surgeon or gynecologic oncologist is consulted. Most of the penetrating colon injuries can be treated with primary repair, resection, and anastomosis. In case of definite evidence of or suspicious of ischemia, inflammation **(Fig. 4)** compromised gut, need of repair with tension or delayed diagnosis with fecal peritonitis and infection diverting colostomy is done. It is to be remembered that colonic vasculature is very prone to be jeopardized due to its pattern of blood supply and before deciding local repair blood supply to be assured to prevent postoperative leakage. The author encountered a pregnant moth who was referred during antenatal period with colostomy wound which was done distal colon obstruction. Cesarean delivery was done with the colostomy wound **(Figs. 5 and 6)**.

Prevention of Gut Injury

If there is previous surgery or chance of adhesion due to previous history of any septic or Koch's peritonitis, peritoneum should be opened very cautiously. Opening site is selected or extension of the incision is done away from the previous incisional area. The gut should be separated from the adhesions with sharp dissection keeping the scissor away from the gut not by blunt pressure or traction. The internal structure is dealt with very gentle traction, meticulous tissue handling, and with good exposure under vision. Use of diathermy should be limited and is used away from the hollow structure. In adhesions and suspected gut injury gut should be thoroughly and systematically examined along its whole length.

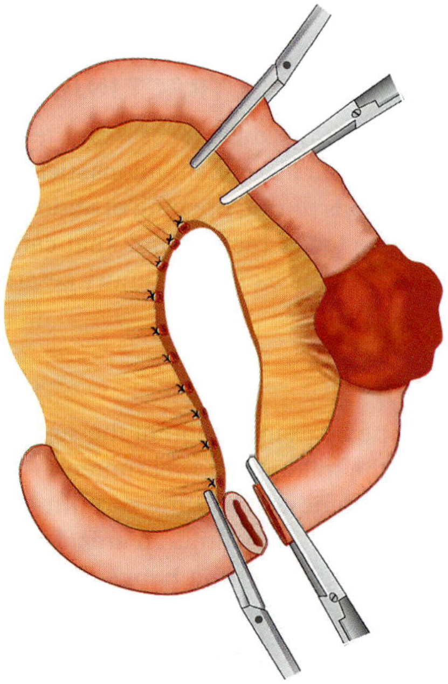

Fig. 1: Diagrammatical representation of resection of small intestine.

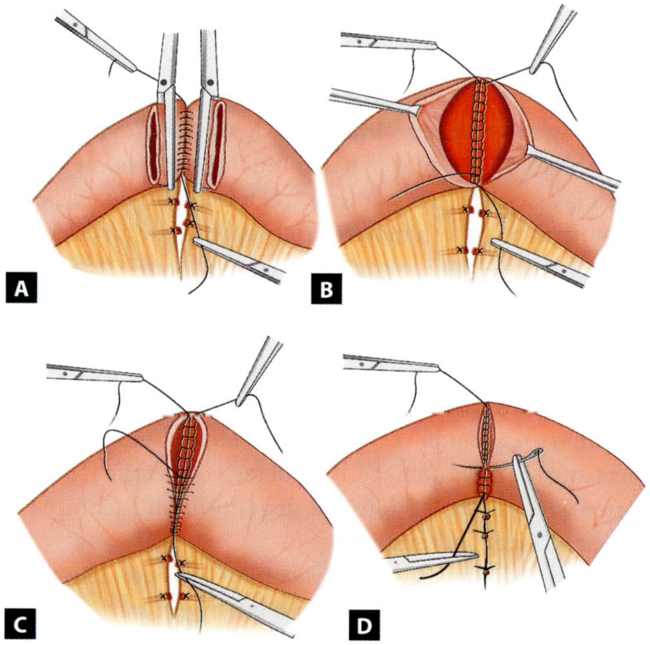

Figs. 2A to D: End-to-end anastomosis: (A) Repair of seromuscular layer on posterior surface; (B) Suture of bowel margins—posterior; (C) Apposition of bowel margins—anterior; and (D) Seromuscular layer repair on anterior surface along with repair of mesentery.

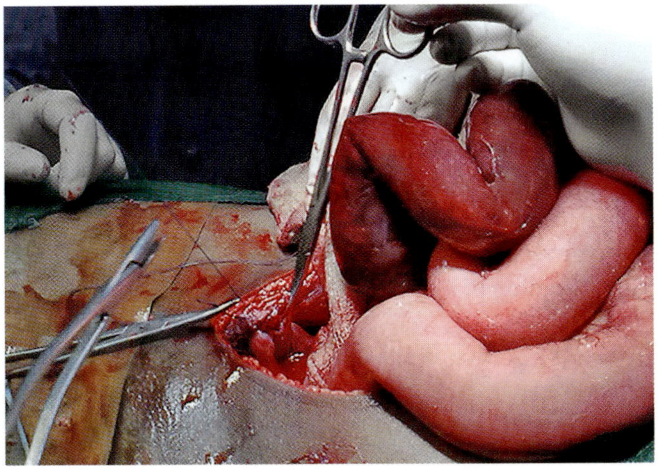

Fig. 3: Anastomosis after resection of devitalized part of small intestine.

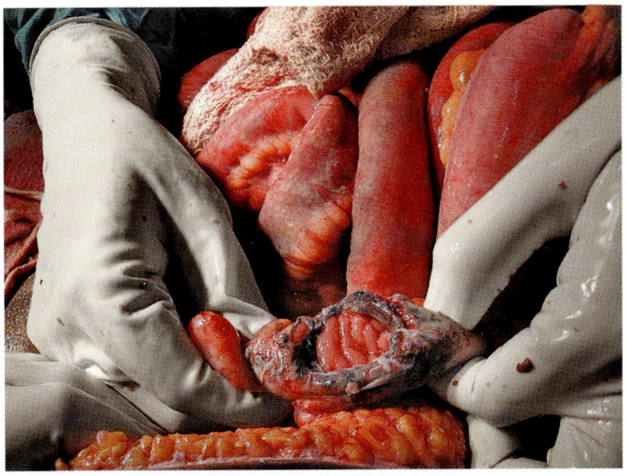

Fig. 4: Injury of sigmoid colon after perforation of uterus on attempt of mid-trimester abortion (D&E).

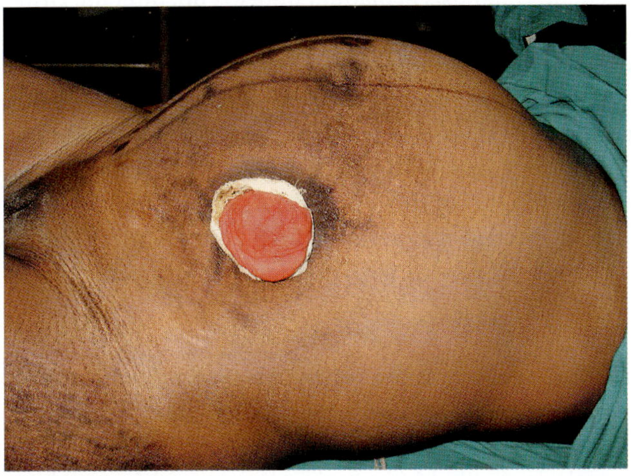

Fig. 5: Colostomy wound in a 19-year primigravida near term. Emergency colostomy was done due to an annular stenotic growth (benign stricture) in rectum about 5 cm from anal verge for intractable intestinal obstruction. At that time, period of gestation was 8 weeks and pregnancy was not disturbed.

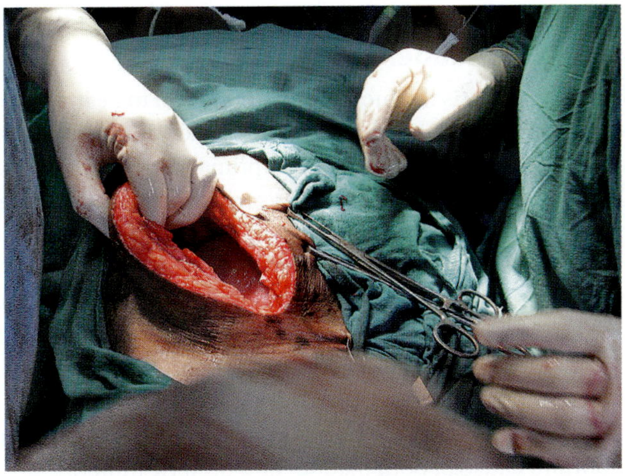

Fig. 6: Cesarean delivery was done at 38 weeks by midline incision of skin in the patient as shown in Figure 5. Colostomy wound is covered seen on left side.

RECTOVAGINAL FISTULA

This is due to abnormal communication between rectum and vagina with epithelial lined tracts. This results because of involuntary escape of flatus and feces into the vagina.

Obstetric causes are: (A) Obstetric trauma—(1) faulty repair of obstetric CPT or nonhealing of repaired CPT, (2) obstructed labor, (3) instrumental delivery, and (4) inclusion of rectal mucosa during episiotomy repair [Discussed in the chapter of Episiotomy and Obstetric Anal Sphincter Injuries (OASIS)].

Management of Rectovaginal Fistula

Surgical repair is done after 8–12 weeks if not done immediately. Sometime small fistula heals spontaneously.

For low or middle fistula, vaginal approach is sufficient. In upper fistula, abdominal method is needed.

Fistula situated in lower third of vagina: It is converted into complete perineal tear and repaired as CPT.

Fistula situated at middle or upper part: Repair is done by flap splitting method. Fistula situated near vault is difficult to repair from below and abdominal approach may be needed. Details are described in Author's *Bedside Clinics in Gynecology*, 2nd edition, 2023 by Jaypee Brothers Medical Publishers.

URINARY TRACT INJURIES DURING CHILD BIRTH

Urinary tract injuries during child birth occur mostly in difficult cesarean delivery, especially in previous cesarean delivery, morbid adherent placenta, cesarean in second stage, extensive laceration of wound, internal iliac ligation, etc. as have been mentioned.

Urethral injury ranges from 0.025 to 0.09% and bladder injury ranges from 0.08 to 0.095%

Injuries of Urethra

Minor injury to distal urethral meatus and laceration on paraurethral region is common during vaginal birth. Due to restrictive use of episiotomy, the preferred forces are more directed to anterior wall and mild anterior inner laceration occurs. Periurethral area is highly vascular and in presence of brisk hemorrhage repair may be needed with fine stitches. Few interrupted stitches with 3-0chromic catgut are given to restore anatomy of urethral meatal ring. Urinary retention is common. Foley catheter is given routinely or given when there is retention and kept for few days. Perineal care in the form of warm sitz bath or alternatively cool pack may be applied. Local anesthetic spray gives pain relief as the region is highly painful.

Injuries of Bladder

Urinary bladder is the most vulnerable organ to be injured in pelvic surgery. In obstetrics, cesarean delivery is the important cause. Recently, with rise of rate of primary cesarean delivery number of women with prior cesarean delivery has been increased. Bladder injury has been increased fourfold due to repeat cesarean delivery than primary cesarean. Injury is more common in cesarean after attempt of trial of labor after cesarean (TOLAC) than direct cesarean delivery without trial. The incidence of bladder injury is ninefold increased in obstetric hysterectomy in comparison to gynecological hysterectomy. Emergency obstetric hysterectomy is another important cause of both bladder and ureteric injury.

Timing of bladder damage: Bladder injury commonly occurs in two times (1) during opening the peritoneal cavity at the time of laparotomy and (2) dissecting the vesicouterine space to retract the bladder downward **(Fig. 7)** both during hysterotomy (cesarean) and obstetric hysterectomy. More than 90% cases dome of the bladder is injured. The bladder is lacerated and damaged commonly during the dissection of uterovesical space particularly in a case with history of prior cesarean delivery. During clamping of the lower stump and during the suturing of vaginal cuff bladder may be included that may result future necrosis and sloughing of the bladder with formation of VVF. Abscess at the vault may increase the risk of VVF.

Intraoperative diagnosis is the most essential part, otherwise later there will be formation of fistula in the form of vesicovaginal, vesicouterine, and ureterovaginal.

Diagnosis of Bladder Injury

If bladder injury is detected during surgery, the prognosis is excellent. Diagnosis of bladder injury is not difficult. Urine is seen in the operative field, sometimes small amount of urine is obtained, bulb of the Foley catheter is visible, lacerated bladder wall becomes visible, and hematuria in the urinary catheter pipe is seen. For detection of small injury of bladder, bladder is filled with opaque (sterile milk) or colored solution (methylene blue in normal saline or indigo) into the bladder through the urethra. Total 200–300 mL is needed. In all suspected cases, confirmation of injury is done.

Management of Bladder Injury

Size and location of the injury are ascertained. In case of involvement of trigon, distance of ureteric orifice from the injury site is evaluated. Injury closure to orifice needs ureteric tent. Bladder opening is repaired in two layers, first layer simple continuous with 3-0 absorbable or delayed absorbable suture and second layer in imbricating technique including muscularis and submucosa **(Fig. 8)**.

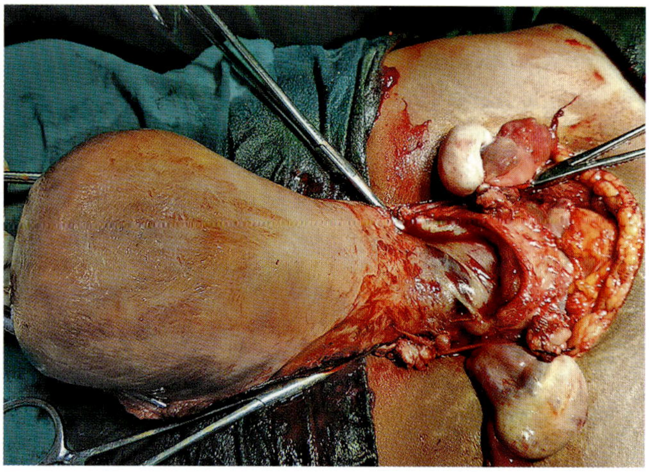

Fig. 7: Meticulous dissection with great care of the vesicouterine space to retract the bladder downward.

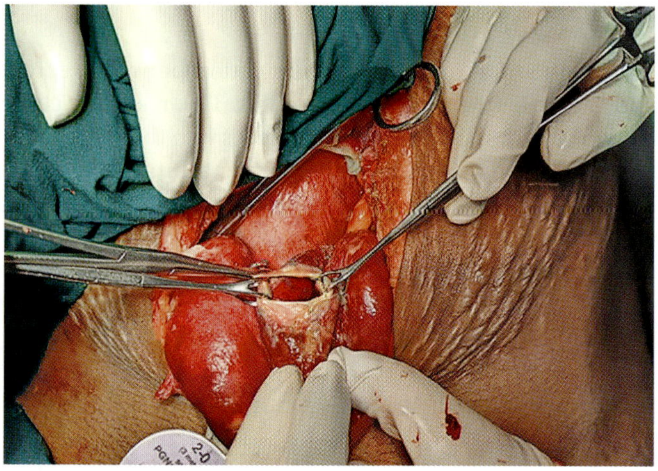

Fig. 8: *Bladder injury:* Patient referred from outside after vaginal delivery following prolonged labor.
Courtesy: Dr Madhurima Kar and Dr Bharat Mandi, RG Kar Medical College, Kolkata, West Bengal, India.

Chromic catgut or Vicryl (polyglactin 910) is used. Following repair leaking test is done with methylene blue or sterile milk. In case of leaking, few interrupted stitches are given. An additional continuous suture can be given to make the inner stitches tension free. Continuous bladder drainage with Foley catheter is given for 10–14 days. Suprapubic catheterization is usually not required.

In undetected cases, hematuria, pain abdomen, ascites, peritonitis, urinoma sepsis, and abnormal renal function test result. Computed tomography (CT) with cystography and retrograde cystography and cystoscope are helpful to diagnose.

Prevention of Bladder Injury

Risk factors for bladder injury are kept in mind. Preoperative continuous bladder drainage is given. Adhesion prevention protocol is maintained in primary cesarean delivery. Meticulous and careful dissection of bladder, maintenance of moistening of tissue, and complete hemostasis are some important steps. Closure of the cesarean wound by two layers prevents adhesion formation than in second layer claimed by a group of workers. Chance of inadvertent bladder injury is more in midline skin incision than Pfannenstiel incisions.

Injuries of Ureter

Injury of ureter is rare in simple cesarean delivery. In cesarean hysterectomy, chance of injury rises remarkably.

Ureter is very vulnerable, to be traumatized in pregnancy than in nonpregnant condition during hysterectomy (seven times more). Extension of cesarean wound during clamping of bleeding vessels (uterine), ureter may be injured.

Danger Points of Injury of Ureter (Fig. 9)

(1) At the infundibulopelvic ligament at pelvic brim during infundibulum ligament clamping; (2) Crossing of uterine artery and ureter at the base of broad ligament during ligation of uterine artery; (3) Clamping of Mackenrodt's ligament where ureter enters ureteric tunnel at internal os level; and (4) Lateral angle of vault of vagina where ureter enters the bladder during clamping or suturing of vaginal vault.

In obstetric hysterectomy, the crossing of uterine artery during clamping of vessels and another site at the vault when it is entering into the bladder is most frequent site of injury. And the chance of injury increases due to its displacement by hematoma.

Diagnosis of Ureteric Injury

Intraoperative diagnosis of ureteric injury is difficult in contrast to bladder injury where it is possible during surgery in majority of cases. Injury of ureter may be (a) division by through and through cutting, (b) partial occlusion by kinking or by crushing due to accidental clamping, (c) ligature or clamping, and (d) devascularization resulting ischemic necrosis. Injury is not always division by through and through to diagnose ureteric damage, high index of suspicion is needed.

Diagnosis during surgery can be done by giving intravenous dye (intravenous methylene blue or indigo carmine). Urine in jets can be seen from urethral orifices by transurethral cystoscopy, suprapubic telescopy, or direct visualization by through intentional cystotomy. Retrograde passage of ureteral catheters by cystoscopy either per urethra

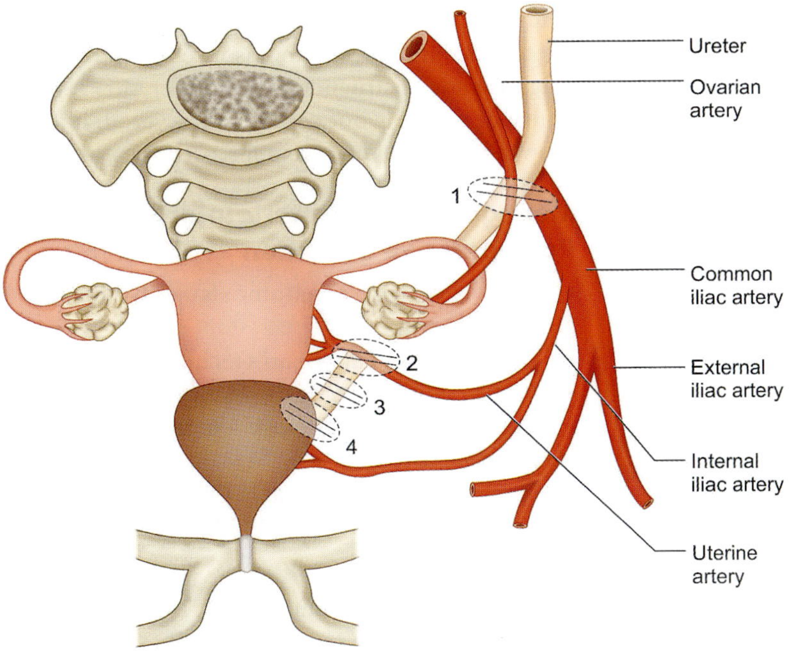

Sites of injury of ureter
1. At the infundibulopelvic ligament at pelvic brim
2. Crossing of uterine artery and ureter at base of broad ligament
3. Clamping of Mackenrodt's ligament where ureter enters ureteric tunnel at internal os level
4. Lateral angle of vault of vagina where ureter enters in bladder

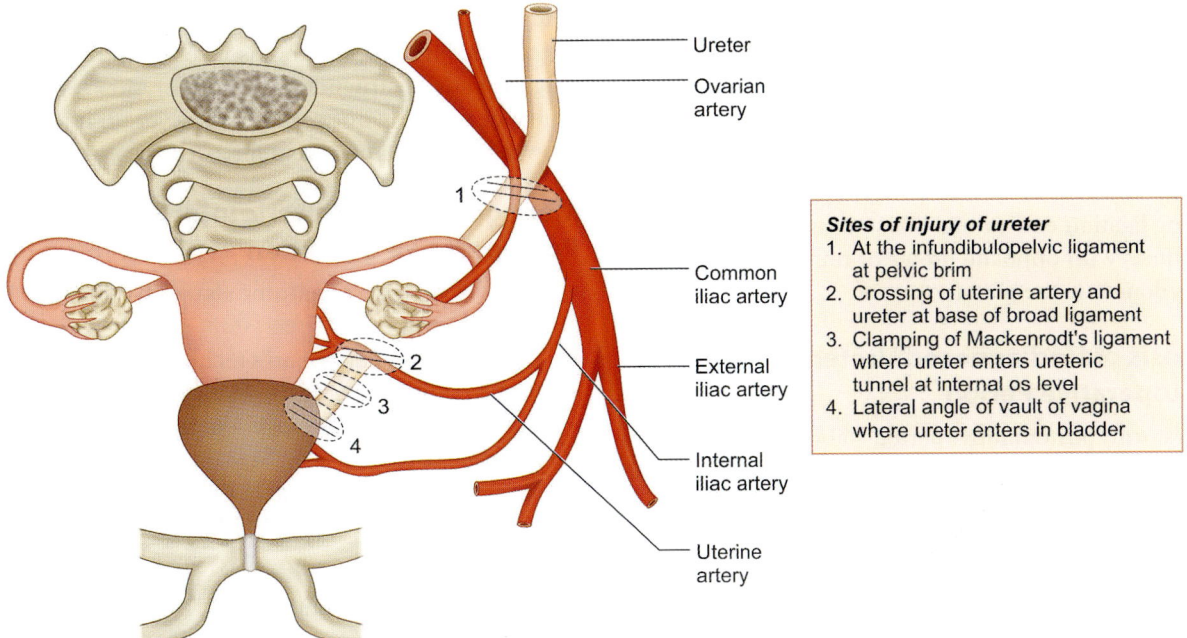

Fig. 9: *Course of ureter:* Four danger points where injury of ureter may occur during hysterectomy.

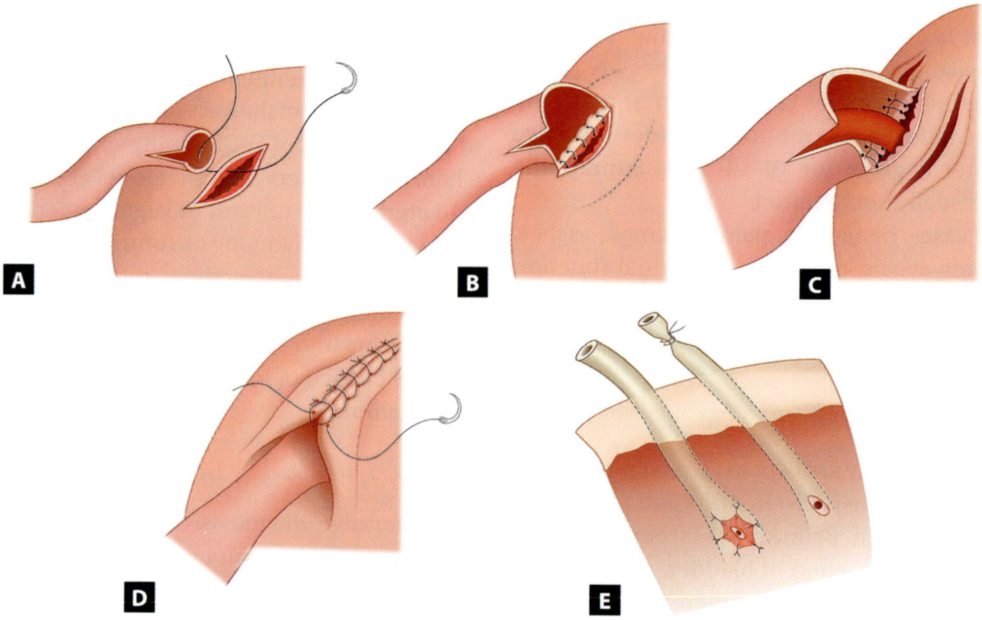

Figs. 10A to E: Ureterovesical anastomosis with ureteric catheter.

or cystostomy wound is the most definitive diagnostic technique. In suspected injury, it should be delineated properly through the broad ligament opening at its base where, bifurcation of the common iliac artery is seen above, and the ureter is identified by its location, conduit, and peristalsis. It is traced downward from above for inspection.

In placenta accreta spectrum (PAS), antenatal detection of bladder invasion by ultrasonography (USG) may suggest to use ureteric tent, though it is not universally recommended. The outcome is definitely good if it is diagnosed and managed intraoperatively. If any injury is detected, standard management is done preferably with the help of urologist.

Management of Ureteric Injury Detected Intraoperatively

In case of crush injury by ligature or clamp, the ligature or clamp is released and a ureteric tent is introduced. Following ligation end-to-end anastomosis, ureteroureteric anastomosis with opposite ureter or reimplantation of the ureter is done into the bladder.

Diagnosis of Undiagnosed Ureteric Injury in Postoperative Period

There is stormy postoperative period—abdominal distension and pain, rigor, persistent fever due to urinoma formation, tenderness at costovertebral angle and oliguria. In unilateral injury, there may not be severe symptoms and kidney on that side becomes atrophic and nonfunctioning. There will be escape of urine per vagina few days following a history of surgery, from drain or from surgical incision indicating fistula formation. Patient can pass urine per urethra as bilateral involvement is unlikely. Combined three swab test and combined pyridium tests are done to differentiate ureterovaginal or VVF. Intravenous pyelography, USG, CT may detect hydronephrosis, urinoma, or abscess. In cystoscopy, no urine is seen to come from damaged ureteric side. If injury is confirmed retrograde or antegrade stent is tried, if unsuccessful define management is done by re-exploration.

Role of Ureteral Stents

(a) It is inserted at the beginning of surgery in high-risk cases of ureteric injury, many prefers in PAS. At the end of surgery, the tent is removed; (b) Tent is inserted intra-operatively to diagnose any obstruction also; and (c) After repair, in crush injury or ureter is not completely severed, it is inserted to keep the patency and is kept for 2–8 weeks.

Management of Ureteric Injury Following Postoperative Detection

- Ureterovesical anastomosis with/without bladder mobilization.
- Using bladder flap (Boari's technique).
- End-to-end anastomosis—done over a ureteric catheter.
- Transureteric anastomosis—ureter is anastomosed with opposite ureter.
- Nephrostomy immediately followed by definite surgery in later date.
- Nephrectomy.

Ureterovesical anastomosis (Figs. 10A to E): Ureterovesical anastomosis is done in injury at the base of broad ligament or near the bladder so that it can be implanted in bladder.

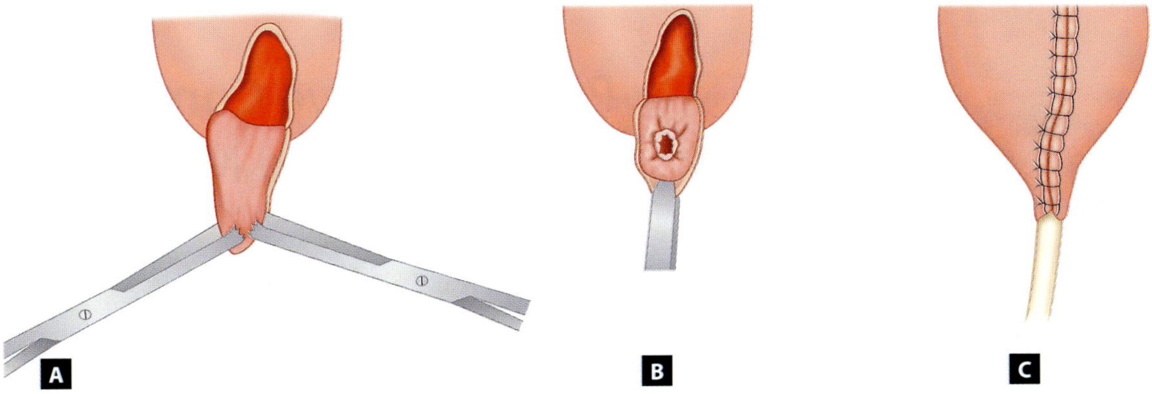

Figs. 11A to C: Ureterovesical anastomosis with bladder flap (Boari's flap method).

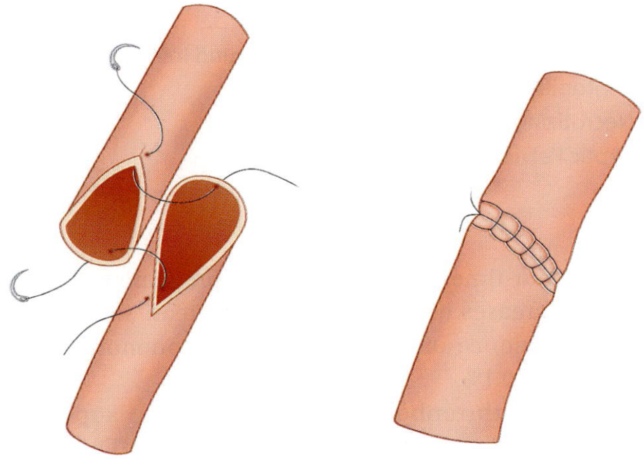

Figs. 12A and B: Ureteroureteric anastomosis.

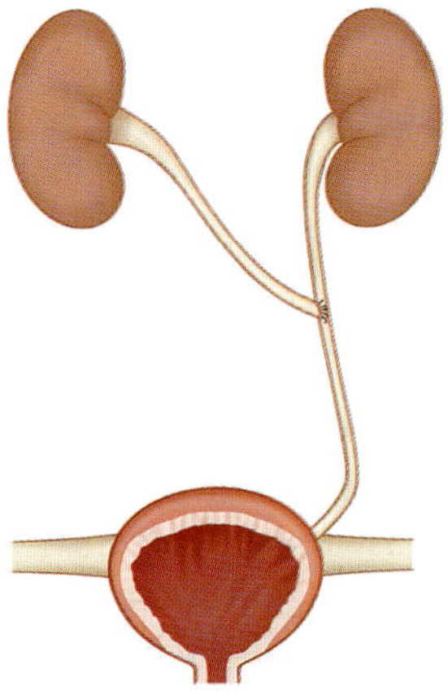

Fig. 13: Transureteric ureteroureteric anastomosis.

Procedure of ureterovesical anastomosis: The distal end of the proximal part of cut end of ureter is split longitudinally for 0.5 cm and fine suture is passed through the flaps. A ureteric catheter is passed through the ureter and fixed.

The end of distal part of the ureter is tied. Cavity of the bladder is opened by 4 cm incision at the fundus. An artificial ureteric tunnel is made by putting an artery forceps inside the cavity near original orifice and pierced through the wall with small incision. The ureteric catheter and the threads are drawn inside the bladder by the forceps and ureteric wall is fixed to the bladder wall. The end of catheter is passed through the urethra to bring it through external urinary meatus (EUM). Bladder is closed in layers. To prevent the stenosis, tunnel is made in such a way that the ureter traverses through the wall obliquely to some extent not directly through and through.

Ureterovesical anastomosis with bladder flap (Boari's flap method) ***(Figs. 11A to C):*** In case, fistula is high-up, a tongue of bladder wall is separated from the bladder wall and made ureteric like tube and anastomosis is done without tension.

End-to-end anastomosis: Following accidental ligation of ureter end-to-end anastomosis over a ureteric catheter **(Figs. 12A and B)**, ureteroureteric anastomosis with opposite ureter **(Fig. 13)** or reimplantation of the ureter is done into the bladder.

Prevention of Ureteric Injury

Preoperative risk assessment is done to consider in which case chance of ureteric injury may occur. Extension of cesarean wound is a potential condition. Surgeon must be ureteric conscious during pelvic surgery. Four danger points must be remembered and surgeon will be very careful during dealing with those areas. If there is extension of the uterine wound and laceration extends to broad ligament precaution to be taken. Ureter may be displaced by hematoma or may be damaged unnoticed. After suturing ureter must be identified and suspicious cases patency is evaluated. During peripartum, hysterectomy of vesicouterine space is separated adequately before clamping the uterine stump. Lower clamp is always placed medial to the upper clamp and chance of ureteric injury will be less. The dictum is to cut nothing until ureter is identified and isolated in its entire extent. Visualization of the peristalsis, the ureter is best way to identify it. If in doubt always trace the ureter from pelvic brim by opening medial leaf of peritoneum. Too much skeletonization of ureter is prohibited. Preoperative stenting in anticipated cases is preferred in many settings.

CHAPTER 30

Postoperative Complications and Management

Learning Objectives

- Venous Thrombosis
- Pulmonary Embolism
- Anticoagulants Used in Thromboembolic Phenomenon
- Infections
- Wound Problems and Surgical Site Wound Infection
- Peritonitis
- Necrotizing Fasciitis
- Septic Pelvic Thrombophlebitis

INTRODUCTION

Cesarean delivery is the most common major surgery in obstetrics. In the last few decades, the rate of cesarean delivery has increased significantly throughout the world. The reasons have been discussed in the chapter on cesarean delivery (Chapter 16). At present, the cesarean delivery rate in India is 21.5% (urban 32.3%, rural17.6%) as per National Family Health Survey 5 (NFHS-5) (2019–2021) data. Cesarean delivery has significant morbidity and mortality. The average maternal mortality in a developed country is 2–4/100,000 which is 10 times more than vaginal birth; in a developing country, the maternal mortality rate of cesarean delivery is 10–20/100,000. Causes of maternal death in cesarean delivery are hemorrhage, infection, anesthetic complications, and pulmonary embolism. Various immediate postoperative morbidities are shock, hypotension, postpartum hemorrhage (PPH), rectus sheath hematoma, broad ligament hematoma, abdominal distention, intestinal obstruction, thromboembolic phenomena—pulmonary embolism and problems related to skin wound—dehiscence, collection of blood, serous fluid and pus, and burst abdomen. Many of those are discussed in respective chapters; some need elaborate discussions and management strategy as these complications are not uncommon in day-to-day practice in the era of a higher rate of cesarean delivery.

VENOUS THROMBOSIS

Pregnancy and puerperium are at risk of venous thromboembolism (VTE) and pregnancy is associated with a 6–10-fold increase of thromboembolic manifestations in comparison to a nonpregnant state. In puerperium, the risk is about four times than that of term pregnancy. The risk further increases after emergency cesarean section. The overall incidence of a thromboembolic phenomenon in pregnancy is 0.1%.

Different thromboembolism events are superficial venous thrombosis, deep vein thrombosis (DVT), and pulmonary embolism.

The reason of increased risk of VTE is a hypercoagulable state in pregnancy and puerperium due to the rise in concentration of the coagulation factors I, II, VII, VIII, IX, X, XII, etc. Venous stasis due to compression of enlarged uterus and immobilization of lower limbs after delivery is also an important etiological factor. Other factors are trauma to the vessel wall, dehydration, anemia, infection, multiparity, and advanced age. The thromboembolic phenomenon is more common in Western countries in comparison to Asian and African countries. Death from a thromboembolic event has decreased due to early ambulation in the postpartum period.

Risk Assessment of Postnatal Thromboprophylaxis (Royal College of Obstetricians and Gynaecologists 2015)

High risk: Any previous thromboembolism and anyone requiring antenatal low molecular weight heparin (LMWH).

Intermediate risk: Cesarean section in labor, asymptomatic thrombophilia (inherited or acquired), body mass index (BMI) >40 kg/m^2, prolonged hospital admission, and medical comorbidities such as heart or lung diseases, systemic lupus erythematosus (SLE), cancer, inflammatory conditions, nephrotic syndrome, sickle cell disease, intravenous drugs, etc.

Lower risk: Age >35 years, obesity (BMI >30 kg/m^2), parity ≥3, smoker, elective cesarean section, any surgical procedure in the puerperium, gross varicose veins, current systemic infection, immobility, e.g., paraplegia, long distance travel, SPD, preeclampsia, midcavity rotational operative forceps, prolonged labor (>24 hours), and PPH >1 L or blood transfusion

Indications of Prophylactic Anticoagulant in Puerperium with Duration of Therapy

Risk assessment is done first and then the following guideline is followed:

- In high-risk cases—at least 6 weeks postnatal prophylaxis with LMWH.
- In intermediate risk group—at least 7 days postnatal prophylaxis is given. Extended prophylaxis is given if persisting or there are more than three risk factors.
- In lower risk group—if there are two or more factors.
- In case of less than two lower risk factors, mobilization and avoidance of dehydration are advised.

Superficial Venous Thrombosis

Superficial venous thrombosis during pregnancy or puerperium is usually found with superficial varicosities or following intravenous catheterization. This type is confined to the superficial veins of the saphenous venous system. The treatment consists of rest, analgesics, and elastic support. Anticoagulation therapy is not needed.

Deep Vein Thrombosis

Diagnosis of DVT is based on clinical findings and imaging:

Symptoms

Pain over the calf with redness and swelling is the usual symptom. However, in more than two-third cases in pregnancy, it is limited to the iliac and femoral veins whereas in nonpregnant cases it starts from the calf veins. There is tenderness over calf muscle on squeezing when the lower extremity is involved. Homan's sign and Moses' sign become positive. In calf muscle involvement, *Homan's sign* **(Fig. 1)** is the elicitation of pain in calf muscles on sudden dorsiflexion of the foot. Presence of this sign signifies DVT. Tenderness on squeezing the calf muscles with the examiner's finger is called *Moses' sign* which also becomes positive in DVT.

Investigations

Compression ultrasound of the proximal vein is the initial test as recommended by American College of Obstetricians and Gynecologists (ACOG 2014). In case of doubtful findings in ultrasound, MRI is suggested. Invasive test—venography with contrast media gives a good view of veins. The other test is estimation of D-dimer.

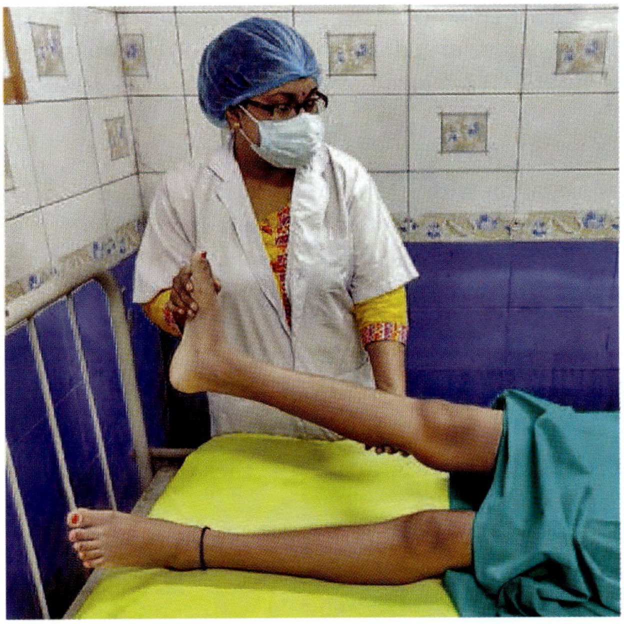

Fig. 1: Demonstration of Homan's sign.

Management includes bed rest, raising of foot end, good analgesia, anticoagulants, graduated elastic stocking, and streptokinase and antibiotics.

PULMONARY EMBOLISM

Pulmonary embolism is one of the most common causes of maternal mortality in a developed country. The incidence is 1 in 7,000 deliveries. It is more common in puerperium, but may occur in the antenatal period at any time. Diagnosis is the same in two groups. More than 75% cases are preceded by DVT. As high as 50% cases of DVT may be complicated with pulmonary embolism for which diagnosis and appropriate management are very important. If not diagnosed in time, it may be fatal. A high index of suspicion is the key to diagnosis.

The most common symptoms are mild respiratory distress or inspiratory chest pain, cough, syncope, slight tachycardia (>90/bpm) and low-grade temperature.

In massive pulmonary embolism, there may be cardiorespiratory collapse, severe chest pain, air hunger, and death.

Investigations

Sonography of the lower limb is done to diagnose DVT. ECG, X-ray of chest, and arterial blood gas (ABG) are done to exclude other causes. A ventilation-perfusion (V/Q) scan or CT pulmonary angiogram is done in suspected pulmonary embolism. D-dimer test is done as a screening test for thromboembolism; its value is less in pregnancy. MRI is used to diagnose pulmonary embolism but is not useful for detection of subsegmental thrombus. Pulmonary angiography is said to be the gold standard to diagnose pulmonary embolism. Dye-induced allergy, renal failure and longer time to perform limit the use of pulmonary angiography and CT angiography has become preferred imaging.

Management

Resuscitation with intravenous (IV) fluid, O_2 inhalation, cardiac massage, dopamine/ adrenaline, anticoagulant (IV bolus dose followed by infusion), and streptokinase for thrombolysis are the line of treatment. To prevent recurrence, a vena cava filter is used.

ANTICOAGULANTS USED IN THROMBOEMBOLIC PHENOMENON

The anticoagulants used in the thromboembolic phenomenon are:

- Unfractionated heparin—conventional heparin
- LMWH—enoxaparin, dalteparin
- Oral anticoagulants—warfarin.

Low molecular weight heparin is preferred and the treatment of choice can be oral warfarin in prolonged therapy. The advantages of LMWH are that it is safe, effective, easy to administer, with lower hemorrhagic complications, and does not cross placenta. The patient can self-administer it. LMWH and warfarin are safe in breast-feeding women.

Dose for Thromboprophylaxis

Unfractionated heparin—10,000 units twice daily SC.

LMWH—now the treatment of choice: Enoxaparin—40 mg SC once daily up to 6–11 days and dalteparin—5,000 units SC daily.

Dose for Treatment of Deep Vein Thrombosis and Pulmonary Embolism

Unfractionated heparin—IV bolus dose (80 units/kg body weight) followed by IV infusion (18 units/kg/3 hourly), maximum 40,000 units in 24 hours, changed to SC after 5–7 days. Monitored by activated partial thromboplastin time (APTT) and platelet count.

LMWH—Enoxaparin 1 mg/kg SC twice daily or dalteparin 100 units/kg SC twice daily. Anti-Xa levels are monitored.

Oral anticoagulants—can be given simultaneously with parenteral therapy or to start after few days of parenteral therapy and monitored by prothrombin time and international normalized ratio (INR) (2–3).

INFECTIONS

The common manifestation of puerperal infection is puerperal pyrexia. Puerperal pyrexia or fever is defined as a maternal temperature of 100.4°F (38°C) or higher during the first 10 days of puerperium occurring on two occasions with more than 6 hours apart, exclusive of the first 24 hours. About 15% of puerperal mothers suffer mild fever due to breast engorgement, called milk fever, which is a rise of temperature by 1–2°F due to engorged breasts, which usually lie below 38°C, rarely above 39°C, and passes usually within 24 hours. The earliest reference of puerperal fever is found in the works of Hippocrates from the 5th century.

Causes of puerperal pyrexia are urinary tract infections (UTIs) (cystitis and pyelonephritis), breasts infection (mastitis, breast abscess), puerperal sepsis (most common), respiratory complications, septic pelvic thrombophlebitis, and intercurrent infections, e.g., respiratory tract infection, enteric fever, influenza, and pulmonary tuberculosis.

Urinary Tract Infections

Cystitis and pyelonephritis are common in puerperium. The reasons are bladder catheterization, operative delivery, and trauma during labor. Physiological changes during pregnancy facilitate the occurrence of UTI. Hydroureter, decreased ureteric muscle tone, and peristalsis favor pyelonephritis. Spiking temperature, dysuria, and tenderness at the costovertebral angle are the usual features. Routine urine examination shows pyuria and bacteriuria, and confirmation is done with culture. As there is possible contamination with lochia during collection of urine, it should be sent after collection through the catheter. Treatment is antipyretic, antibiotic, and proper hydration. Ampicillin and gentamycin combination or cefazoline/ ceftriaxone is started before availability of the culture report. A total of 7–14 days' course of antibiotic is adequate to control infection.

Breast Infections

In mastitis, the patient complains of breast pain which is usually unilateral. There are tenderness and warmth over the affected breast. The common organism is *Staphylococcus aureus*. Treatment comprises support to the breast, analgesics, and antibiotics. Antistaphylococcal penicillin or erythromycin in penicillin-sensitive cases is given for 10–14 days.

Breast abscess is diagnosed by the physical finding of suppuration and confirmed by sonography which shows a cystic cavity with surrounding inflammation. Incision and drainage under general anesthesia is the usual treatment.

Breastfeeding is allowed in the unaffected breast.

Lung Complications during Puerperium

Respiratory complications are aspiration pneumonitis (Mendelson syndrome), atelectasis of lungs, and common respiratory infections.

Mendelson syndrome (aspiration pneumonitis) is common in labor and in induction of general anesthesia due to increased aspiration of stomach content (which has very low pH <2.5) as there is delayed gastric emptying and relaxation of lower esophageal sphincter and increased intra-abdominal volume. Gastric emptying time is further prolonged due to labor. In the past general anesthesia and aspiration of stomach content into lungs resulting in severe chemical pneumonitis (Mendelson syndrome) was an important cause of maternal death in obstetrics. Switching to regional and precautions taken during pre- and intraoperative steps have reduced this complication. Acid neutralizing agents, such as sodium citrate, are now given liberally before induction of anesthesia. ACOG (2015) recommends a diet of moderate amount of clear liquid during uncomplicated labor. But avoidance of solid food for 6–8 hours before elective cesarean delivery is recommended.

Following aspiration of gastric contents, severe hypoxemia develops. There is fall of oxygen saturation, tachypnea, tachycardia, cyanosis, bronchospasm, atelectasis, and hypotension. Changes develop in X-ray. Treatment is supportive with oxygenation and ventilation. Corticosteroid and antibiotics are given empirically, but there is no convincing evidence of benefit. The patient is closely watched for infection and development of acute respiratory distress syndrome (ARDS).

Pulmonary atelectasis is the most common lung complication in the postoperative period. It develops within 24 hours of cesarean delivery or following an obstetric procedure under general anesthesia. X-ray of chest shows linear densities in the base of the lungs. Use of spirometry and encouragement of cough and deep breathing prevent atelectasis. Atelectasis is self-limiting.

Any other concurrent respiratory infection in the postoperative ward is not uncommon and that should be cared for.

Genital Infection and Puerperal Sepsis

Puerperal infection, either following vaginal delivery or by cesarean delivery, is a common complication in puerperium.

Organisms Responsible for Puerperal Sepsis

- Most of the genital tract infections are polymicrobial.
- Aerobes are gram positive: Group A streptococcus, Group B streptococcus, *Staphylococcus* and gram negative: *Escherichia coli*, *Klebsiella*, and *Pseudomonas*.
- Anaerobes are anaerobic *Streptococcus*, *Bacteroides* and *Clostridia*
- Miscellaneous are *Chlamydia trachomatis*, *Mycoplasma hominis*, *Neisseria gonorrhoeae*, and *Ureaplasma urealyticum*.

Risk factors are as follows:

- Patient profile—obesity, immune-compromised, and diabetes
- Antenatal—PROM and chorioamnionitis
- Intranatal—repeated vaginal examinations, prolonged labor, instrumental delivery, cesarean delivery, retained bits, manual removal of placenta, and genital lacerations.

Ascending of Infection and Spread of Infection through Vagina

Infection from the lower genital tract ascends to cause endometritis, metritis, parametritis, salpingoophoritis (abscess), pelvic abscess, peritonitis and by the lymphatic and blood vessels to distal sites, e.g., septic thrombophlebitis, pulmonary infection, septicemia, and endotoxic shock.

Prevention by the aseptic approach and good safe surgical techniques and routine use of prophylactic antibiotic before cesarean delivery have reduced the infection remarkably.

Mild-to-moderate puerperal infection is treated with broad-spectrum antibiotics, e.g., co-amoxiclav or cephalosporin with metronidazole combination orally or intravenously as the case may be. In severe infection, more intensive treatment is needed with the multidisciplinary team. There may be septicemia and endotoxic shock which are described (Chapter 2).

Infection Following Cesarean Delivery

Cesarean delivery is one of the high risk factors for postpartum infection involving uterus and the surrounding organs. Prolonged labor, rupture of membranes, and multiple vaginal examinations increase the risk of infection. Infection following cesarean delivery may manifest as endometritis, metritis, parametritis, adnexal abscess, and peritonitis. Those may cause hysterotomy (cesarean) and wound disruption and also extend to parieties including skin wound.

Etiology are polymicrobial, and the organisms involved are already described.

The most vulnerable site of harboring of bacteria is hysterotomy incision site following which infection from endometritis and metritis later spread to parametrial tissue and the surrounding regions. Fever and lower abdominal pain are the usual features of metritis. On vaginal examination, there will be parametrial tenderness and foul-smelling lochia. Exceptionally, in β-hemolytic streptococci infection, there may be scanty and odorless lochia. The blood picture shows leukocytosis (18,000–30,000). It should be interpreted properly as leukocytosis is common in puerperium. Routine vaginal swab culture is not mandatory.

Treatment

A broad-spectrum antimicrobial agent is administered in the intravenous or oral route depending on severity. Combination of clindamycin and gentamicin is a standard and effective regimen. Ampicillin may be added from the beginning or if there is no clinical response with the two. As gentamycin is nephrotoxic, a combination of clindamycin and second-generation cephalosporine or a combination of clindamycin and aztreonam are given in a renal compromised patient. Metronidazole is a good substitute of clindamycin. Metronidazole, ampicillin, and gentamicin are age-old treatment and a very effective combination. Imipenem, a carbapenem, has good broad-spectrum coverage against the metritis. Cilastatin is added with it to inhibit renal metabolism of imipenem.

Perioperative prophylactic antibiotic during cesarean delivery has reduced the infection morbidity significantly and is more effective when given before skin incision rather than after cord clamping. ACOG (2016) recommends prophylactic administration of antibiotic to all women undergoing cesarean delivery. A first-generation cephalosporine single agent is recommended by ACOG except in patients who are allergic to the drug or have already received proper antibiotic.

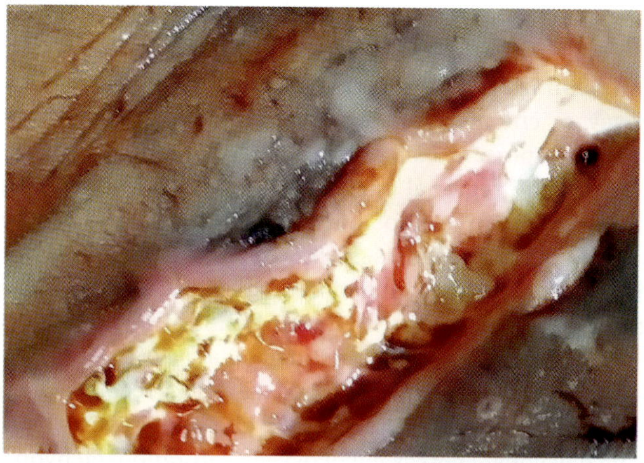

Fig. 2: Infected skin wound with pus and infected debris following cesarean delivery.
Courtesy: Dr Anirban Mondol, Associate Professor, Bankura Sammilani Medical College, Bankura, West Bengal, India.

WOUND PROBLEMS AND SURGICAL SITE WOUND INFECTION

Wound Hematoma

Small collection of blood or serous fluid is common in cesarean wound and vulvovaginal wound. Those of the vulvovaginal site are discussed in respective chapter. Diagnosis is done by clinical features, and sonography or CT scan is needed in equivocal cases or more larger swelling. Small abdominal hematoma following CD absorbs spontaneously in most of the cases. Larger or progressive swelling needs surgical evacuation. If an obvious bleeding source is found, diathermy coagulation or suture is given.

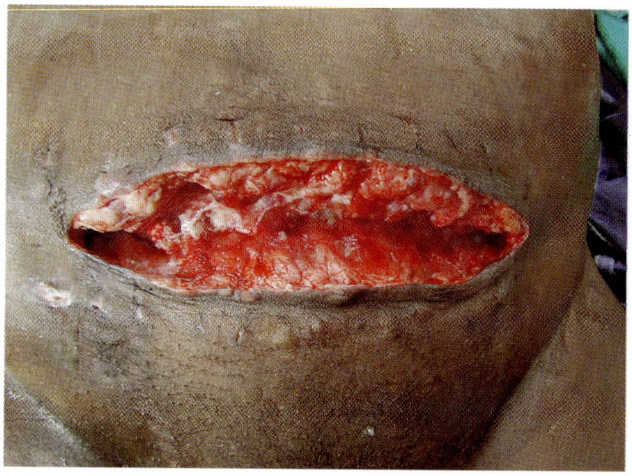

Fig. 3: Superficial wound gaping following cesarean delivery.

Surgical Site Infection

The incidence of surgical site infection (SSI) varies and following prophylactic antibiotics the incidence is reduced; still, the average incidence is 5%.

Types of SSI are categorized into superficial incisional, deep incisional, and the involvement of organ and other sites. The criteria of SSI are clearly defined by Centres for Disease Control and Prevention (CDCP) (2014).

Superficial Surgical Site Infection

Patient usually has history of metritis and not responding to treatment. There is erythema, induration, swelling, and/or purulent discharge from the wound site usually appearing usually from 5th or 6th day onward **(Fig. 2)**.

Treatment

Mild infection responds well with oral antibiotic without abscess formation.

If there is abscess formation, quick drainage is needed. All the purulent materials are removed and breakage of loculations is done **(Fig. 3)**. Pus is sent for culture sensitivity.

During drainage, the integrity of fascia is checked. If it is intact, debridement and dressing are sufficient and expected to improve. Dressing is done daily at least once or twice. The use of any antiseptic agent such as iodine, savlon, or hydrogen peroxide is controversial. One group suggests to use only normal saline. The wound heals by secondary intention or by delayed primary closure using nonabsorbable suture nylon or polypropylene **(Fig. 4)**. Delayed primary closure is preferable by many for quick healing and good scar. The ideal time of primary closure is determined by the formation of healthy granulation tissue which usually takes 5–6 days after the first debridement. Many prefer retention suture and others use short segment of rubber catheter through which suture is passed before tying and the latter is inexpensive and ideal for low-resource settings **(Fig. 5)**. An alternate method is use of a vacuum-assisted negative pressure wound therapy system **(Figs. 6 to 9)**.

Wound Dehiscence

Wound dehiscence means separation of wound with disruption of fascial layer and it usually occurs after

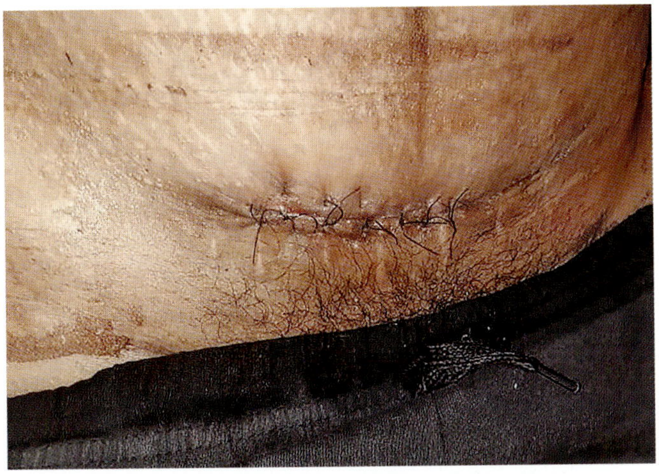

Fig. 4: Delayed primary closure using nonabsorbable suture.
Courtesy: Dr Anirban Mandol, Associate Professor, Bankura Sammilani Medical College, Bankura, West Bengal, India.

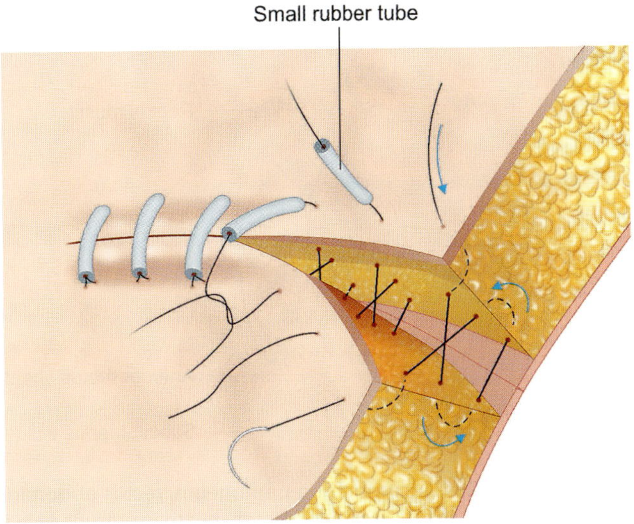

Fig. 5: Wound closure using small rubber tubing (diagrammatic).

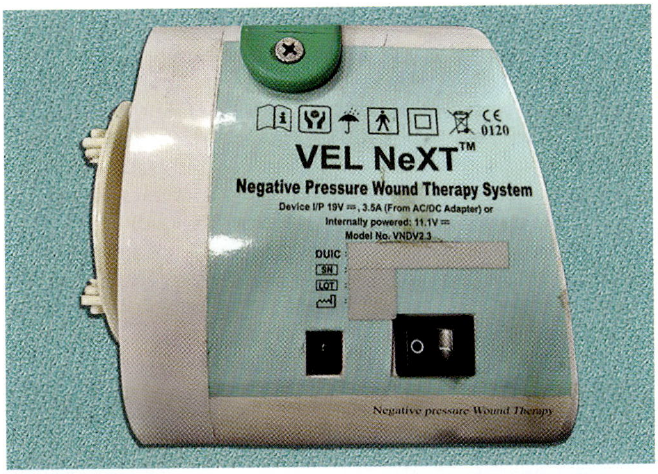

Fig. 6: Vaccum-assisted negative pressure wound therapy system.
Courtesy: RG Kar Medical College, Kolkata, West Bengal, India.

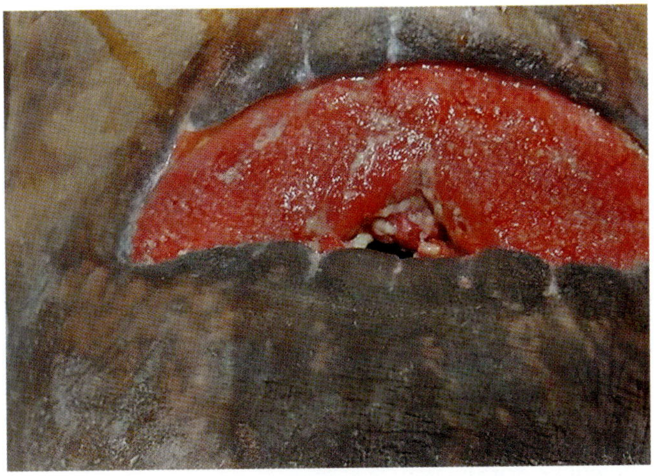

Fig. 7: Wound before application of vacuum-assisted negative pressure wound therapy system.

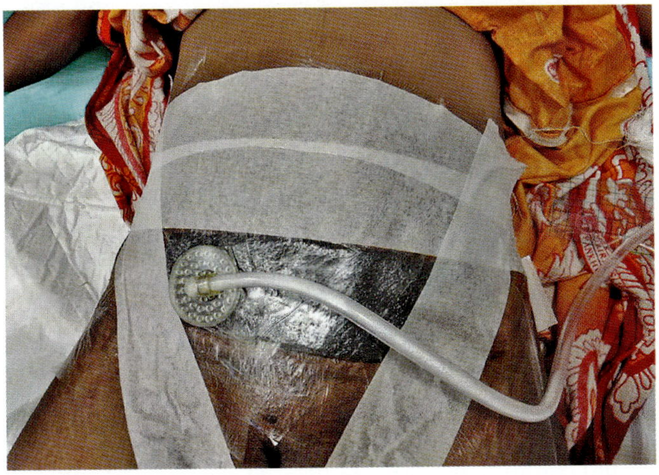

Fig. 8: Patient fitted with vacuum-assisted negative pressure wound therapy system as in Figure 7.

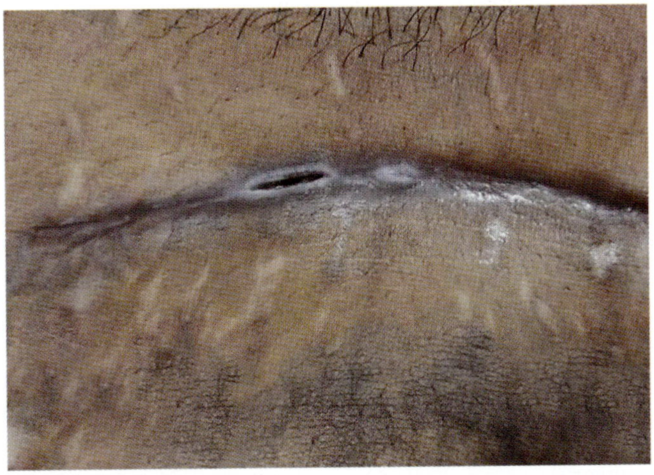

Fig. 9: Wound healed by secondary intention using vacuum-assisted negative pressure wound therapy system as in Figure 7.
Courtesy: Dr Poulomi Sarkar, RG Kar Medical College, Kolkata, West Bengal, India.

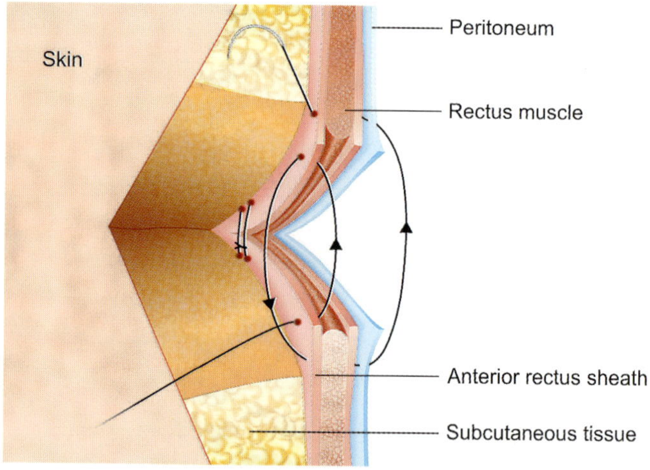

Fig. 10: Mass closure incorporating peritoneum, rectus abdominis muscle, and rectus sheath. Posterior rectus sheath is present only in the supraumbilical region (diagrammatic).

5 days of surgery preceded by discharge of serosanguinous fluid. Sometimes, parieties open in full depth with the intestines and omentum protruding through the wound. Classically, it is also called "burst abdomen." The patient is immediately taken to the operation theater after covering bowel and abdominal contents with sterile packing soaked with normal saline. Broad-spectrum antibiotic is started. Under general anesthesia, the abdomen and pelvis are explored. If there is abscess formation, all are cleared and the peritoneal cavity is irrigated. Fascial margins are debrided to reach heathy tissue. This type of wound opening needs secondary closure. If the rectus fascia looks healthy, Smead–Jones or mass closure is done **(Fig. 10)**. After packing the subcutaneous area, delayed closure of superficial structure is performed.

PERITONITIS

Peritonitis is very uncommon following cesarean delivery. It occurs in metritis or following gut injury or following forgotten foreign body **(Figs. 11 to 13)**. Generalized peritonitis is a grave complication of cesarean delivery. Nausea, vomiting, pain in the abdomen, and abdominal distention are the features. Broad-spectrum antibiotic and supportive management are given. If not improved, the decision of laparotomy is taken to know the cause and drainage of pus.

Ogilvie syndrome, a rare cause of postoperative abdominal distension, is due to adynamic colonic ileus as described in chapter (Cesarean Delivery). Causes of postoperative distension following cesarean delivery and stepwise approach are discussed in chapter 16 (Cesarean Delivery).

Tubo-ovarian abscess in puerperium is a rare complication. Usually, it occurs on one side and is evident after 1–2 weeks. The patient may present with rupture

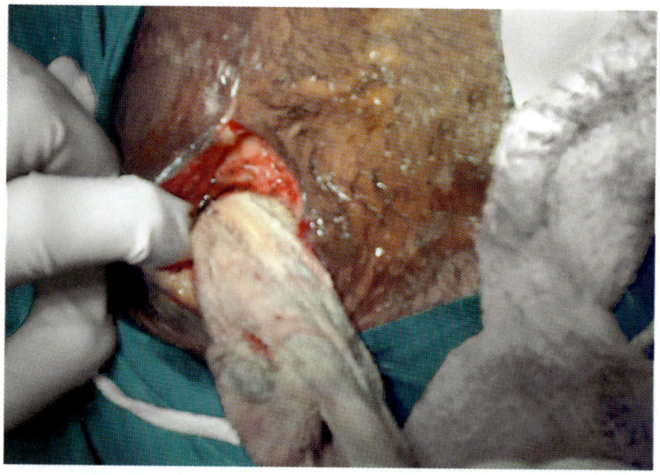

Fig. 11: Forgotten mop (gauze) coming out through the skin wound. Patient underwent laparotomy, and hysterectomy was performed in a remote place. She developed abdominal distension in postoperative days following which her condition improved. She used to visit the hospital infrequently for abdominal discomfort and constipation. After 3 months of laparotomy, she attended the emergency because of a white cloth like structure that came out through one angle of skin wound. On examination and traction, it was found to be abdominal gauze (mop). Surprisingly, the patient's vitals were stable. The decision of laparotomy was taken and performed with difficulty. The average-sized gauze was found to be densely adhered to the surrounding abdominal structures, intestines, and omentum and it was removed with difficulty. There were injuries in jejunum and necrosis over significant areas of jejunal and ileum. Resection anastomosis was performed. The patient recovered and was discharged in a healthy condition 4 weeks after surgery (see Figs. 12 and 13).

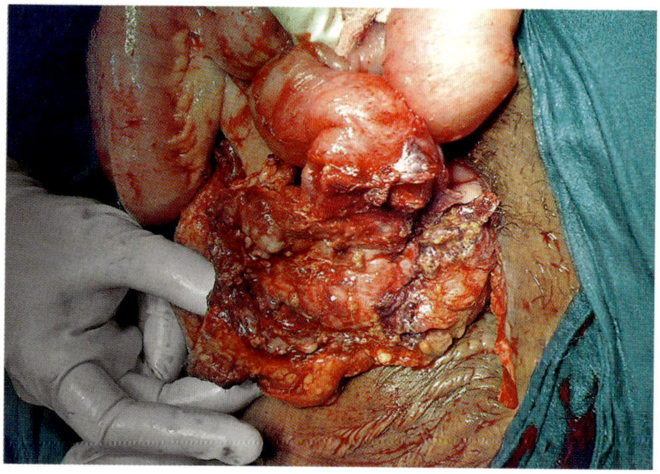

Fig. 12: Laparotomy findings following removal of abdominal gauze of the patient as shown in Figure 11.

of abscess when laparotomy is mandatory. In localized case, a conservative approach with antibiotic and image-guided drainage is adequate.

Phlegmon is the intense form of parametrial cellulitis and formation of an area of induration following cesarean delivery. The patient usually improves with prolonged therapy with antibiotics.

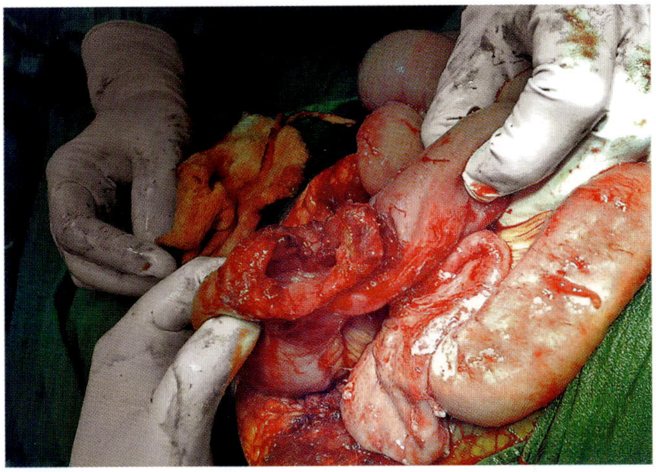

Fig. 13: There were injuries in jejunum and necrosis over significant areas of jejunum and ileum. Resection anastomosis was performed (in patient shown in Figure 11).

Very uncommonly, the cesarean wound is disputed in severe peritonitis and intra-abdominal abscess formation. Surgical exploration is done and hysterectomy may be needed. In case of difficulty in total hysterectomy, supracervical hysterectomy is considered, with removal of infected tissues as much as possible.

NECROTIZING FASCIITIS

Necrotizing fasciitis is a very rare but potentially fatal wound infection involving the skin, fascia, and muscle. In obstetrics, it may occur following cesarean delivery and also in episiotomy and perineal lacerations. It may occur following MiniLap, diagnostic laparoscopy, and even after suprapubic catheterization. Necrotizing fasciitis may follow vulvar infection in a diabetic and immunocompromised patient

Necrotizing fasciitis is caused by various organisms; anaerobes are common and *C. perfringens* is identified along with aerobes *Bacteroides fragilis* and *E. coli*.

Initially, skin changes are erythema, edema, and tenderness. A woman complains of fever, malaise, and looks toxic. Skin remains intact initially; later, there is extensive gangrene, crepitus, and inflammation. Buttocks, thigh, and lower abdominal walls are rapidly involved in perineal tears. In cesarean delivery, the initial symptoms appear after 3–5 days. The patient may ultimately go into septic shock. Extensive wound debridement under general anesthesia and intensive management of septic shock with proper antimicrobial therapy in an intensive care unit with multidisciplinary team management are absolutely needed to save the mother. Mortality is inevitable without surgery and half of the patients die even after surgery. Skin grafting and use of synthetic mesh are needed in the later period after recovery of the patient.

SEPTIC PELVIC THROMBOPHLEBITIS

Pelvic thrombophlebitis is an infective complication following both vaginal and cesarean delivery. The overall incidence is 1 in 2,000–3,000 deliveries. From the reported study, the incidence of pelvic thrombophlebitis is found to be more following vaginal delivery than cesarean birth.

Risk factors and etiology including premature rupture of membranes (PROM) and chorioamnionitis are described above under the heading of puerperal sepsis. The infection of septic phlebitis extends along the venous drainage of uterus and other pelvic organs including ovarian venous plexus with inflammation inside the vessels leading to formation of thrombosis.

Clinical diagnosis is based on suspicion when fever persists in spite of proper antibiotic therapy for endometritis. Despite the relief of pain, fever persists. The concept of surgical excision of involved veins once considered for diagnosis and treatment is discarded now. CT and MRI confirm the diagnosis. An appropriate antimicrobial agent in the intravenous route is the key treatment. Intravenous heparin on an empirical basis is advocated by most authorities.

Phlegmasia Alba Dolens (White leg)

Phlegmasia alba dolens or white leg is a condition where there is development of indurated painful swollen white leg which occurs due to *thrombosis of the femoral veins*. This is due to extrapelvic spread of infection from pelvic thrombophlebitis.

It develops usually in the second week of puerperium. Symptoms are severe pain and swelling in the lower limbs and high fever with rigor. Pain is due to arterial spasm following irritation from the thrombosed veins.

There will be high temperature and tachycardia. Tender-indurated parametrium, subinvolution of uterus, and foul-smelling lochia are the per vaginal findings.

The legs become swollen, pale, glistening, and pit on pressure.

Leukocytosis is found on blood investigations. USG, CT scan, and MRI are done for confirmation of diagnosis.

Management includes rest to the foot in elevated position and administration of analgesic, antibiotics, and anticoagulants. LMWH is the treatment of choice.

Index

Page numbers followed by *f* refer to figure, *fc* refer to flowchart, and *t* refer to table.

C

D

E

H

I

N

O

P

T